INTRODUCTION TO COMMUNICATION DISORDERS

A Lifespan Evidence-Based Perspective

Fourth Edition

ROBERT E. OWENS, JR.
State University of New York at Geneseo

DALE EVAN METZ
State University of New York at Geneseo

KIMBERLY A. FARINELLA
University of Arizona

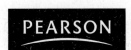

Boston   Columbus   Indianapolis   New York   San Francisco   Upper Saddle River
Amsterdam   Cape Town   Dubai   London   Madrid   Milan   Munich   Paris   Montreal   Toronto
Delhi   Mexico City   Sao Paulo   Sydney   Hong Kong   Seoul   Singapore   Taipei   Tokyo

Vice President and Editor in Chief:
Jeffery W. Johnston
Executive Editor and Publisher: Stephen D. Dragin
Editorial Assistant: Anne Whittaker
Vice President, Director of Marketing:
Quinn Perkson
Senior Marketing Manager: Christopher D. Barry
Senior Managing Editor: Pamela D. Bennett
Senior Project Manager: Linda Hillis Bayma
Senior Operations Supervisor:
Matthew Ottenweller

Senior Art Director: Diane Lorenzo
Cover Designer: Candace Rowley
Photo Coordinator: Monica Merkel
Cover Art: SuperStock
Media Project Manager: Rebecca Norsic
Full-Service Project Management: Thistle Hill
Publishing Services, LLC
Composition: Integra Software Services
Printer/Binder: Edwards Brothers
Cover Printer: Lehigh-Phoenix Color/Hagerstown
Text Font: ITC Mendoza Roman Book

Credits and acknowledgments borrowed from other sources and reproduced, with permission, in this textbook appear on appropriate page within text.

Every effort has been made to provide accurate and current Internet information in this book. However, the Internet and information posted on it are constantly changing, so it is inevitable that some of the Internet addresses listed in this textbook will change.

Photo Credits: Jupiter Unlimited, pp. 2, 154, 164, 234; Spencer Grant/PhotoEdit Inc., p. 10; Michal Heron/Michal Heron Photography, p. 15; iStockphoto.com, pp. 24, 48, 89, 190, 214, 314, 356, 441; Kim Farinella, pp. 59, 265, 386; Patrick White/Merrill, pp. 78, 480; Pearson Learning Photo Studio, p. 82; Katelyn Metzger/Merrill, p. 102; Peter M. Fisher/Corbis–NY, p. 113; Photos to Go, p. 145; David Mager/Pearson Learning Photo Studio, p. 173; Photo Researchers, Inc., pp. 227, 369; Corbis RF, p. 258; Christina Kennedy/PhotoEdit Inc., p. 280; Barbara Schwartz/Merrill, p. 342; PH College, p. 376; © Owen Franken/Corbis, All Rights Reserved, p. 400; Phanie/Photo Researchers, Inc., p. 404; Eliseo Fernandez/Landov Media, p. 462; Scott Cunningham/Merrill, p. 466; Krista Greco/Merrill, p. 488.

Library of Congress Cataloging-in-Publication Data

Owens, Robert E.
  Introduction to communication disorders : a lifespan evidence-based perspective/Robert E. Owens, Jr., Dale Evan Metz, Kimberly A. Farinella.—4th ed.
    p. cm.
  Includes bibliographical references and index.
  ISBN-13: 978-0-13-700008-1 (pbk.)
  ISBN-10: 0-13-700008-1 (pbk.)
  1. Communicative disorders. I. Metz, Dale Evan. II. Farinella, Kimberly A. III. Title.
RC423.O95 2010
616.85'5—dc22

2009053064

10 9 8 7 6 5 4 3 2

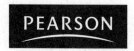

www.pearsonhighered.com

ISBN-13: 978-0-13-700008-1
ISBN-10: 0-13-700008-1

Preface

Introducing a new edition is always an exciting endeavor. The thrill of a new book is tempered with the anxiety of "getting it right." As an author you want readers and professors to appreciate all the work you've put into the project. So it is with the fourth edition. We hope that those of you who are familiar with the previous editions will agree with us that this one is a worthy contribution to the education of young speech-language pathologists and audiologists.

It is with mixed emotions that we bid farewell to our colleague Adelaide ("Addie") Haas, PhD, and a warm welcome to Kimberly Farinella, PhD, from the University of Arizona. Dr. Haas is enjoying a well-deserved retirement, jetting all around the globe, sampling cultures and living life to the fullest. Addie has always had a thirst for new knowledge and experiences, and we wish her all that life has to offer. Dr. Farinella is a young PhD with intellect and curiosity who is already making a name for herself as a researcher.

Within each chapter, we have attempted to describe a specific disorder and related assessment and intervention methods. In addition, we have included lifespan issues and evidence-based practice to provide the reader with added insights. Each disorder is also illustrated by personal stories of individuals with that disorder. Reader interest and reflection are stimulated by thought questions at the end of each chapter and by margin notes. Further knowledge can be gained by the suggested readings and the Internet locations provided at the conclusion of each chapter.

Students will find the accompanying CD-ROM helpful as a learning device and study tool. Many disorders are presented in sound and video format on this disk. In addition, self-study questions follow the outline of each chapter and highlight important information.

NEW TO THIS EDITION

The fourth edition of *Introduction to Communication Disorders* has many new features that strengthen the existing material in the previous edition. These include the following:

- The addition of evidence-based practice (EBP) throughout the text. As in many health-related fields, the American Speech-Language-Hearing Association (ASHA) has undertaken to have audiologists and speech-language pathologists provide the most effective and efficient assessment and intervention practices possible, which is reflected in our text. In recognition of this, the subtitle of the text has been altered to *A Lifespan Evidence-Based Perspective.* Beginning in the first chapter, we introduce students to the concepts of EBP.

- Each chapter has been updated. We have added over 400 new and relevant research studies. Professors will appreciate the effort involved in staying current in our ever-changing fields of study.

- We have worked to improve readability throughout the book and to provide the right mix of information for those getting their first taste of this field. Although some chapters have been altered, several have been rewritten with this goal in mind.

- In each chapter, in addition to the discussion of EBP, we have added new boxes that include the best practices in assessment and intervention for the disorders discussed. These boxes give students a quick reference.

- In recognition of the growing importance of the Internet in our lives, we have included references to Web sites in each chapter to further students' knowledge and to explore the topics discussed.

- Based on feedback from several instructors, we have added new diagrams and figures to demonstrate for students the locations of various disorders, especially those with a neurological basis.

- Additional disorders have been added. For example, on the advice of several instructors who requested that we discuss childhood motor-speech disorders and mention other types of language disorders, we added these to the disorders section.

- New examples of disorders have been added to the accompanying CD-ROM to offer students more examples of the disorders discussed.

- The text's Companion Website has been redesigned to be more user friendly and to help students learn the material included in the text. This includes links to other sites of interest.

We hope that you'll agree with us when we claim that this is a more user-friendly and informative text than the previous editions. Please feel free to contact us with suggestions for further strengthening our work.

ACKNOWLEDGMENTS

Robert Owens

I would like to thank the faculty of the Department of Communicative Disorders and Sciences at State University of New York at Geneseo for their forbearance and assistance with this book. Ms. Wendy Metz, who has taught our introductory course, was especially helpful in her review of the manuscript and insistence that the text adhere to high standards of inclusiveness and content coverage. A clinical perspective was provided by Ms. Linda Deats, Ms. Irene Belyakov, and Dr. Linda Spencer. Dr. "Hugo" Ling-Yu Guo helped with his critique. Finally, my and Dr. Metz's chair, Dr. Linda House, has been extremely helpful both with her expertise and her understanding of the magnitude of our writing task. We are especially indebted to Ms. Jordan Nieto for her gathering of new material for the accompanying CD-ROM.

My most personal thanks goes to my partner, who supported and encouraged me and truly makes my life fulfilling and happy. I'm looking forward to our life together.

Dale Evan Metz

I gratefully acknowledge Dr. Donald Warren, University of North Carolina, Chapel Hill, for the photographs of children with cleft lip and palate, and Dr. Robert Orlikoff, West Virginia University, for the photographs of laryngeal pathology and for the audio samples of voice disorders. I also greatly appreciate Dr. Bright Russell for contributing the CD-ROM video segments of vocal fold behavior.

Ms. Janice Masterson kindly contributed video fluoroscopic samples of swallowing, which can be seen on the book's CD-ROM. Kelly Julian and Julie Klejdys were invaluable to the development of the book's CD-ROM and they also, along with Shanna Wiech, were significant contributors to selected tracks of the CD-ROM. We are especially appreciative of the video-tape segments supplied for the CD-ROM by the Prentke-Romich Company of Wooster, Ohio, a developer of augmentative and alternative communication equipment.

Kay PENTAX, Lincoln Park, New Jersey, kindly provided pictures of some of their clinical instruments, and we thank them for their cooperation. I deeply appreciate the efforts of my wife, Wendy, for her tireless reading of this book during various stages of development and for her love and boundless forbearance with me.

Kimberly Farinella

I would like to thank Bob Owens, Dale Metz, and Steve Dragin for including me on this edition of the textbook. It has been an amazing experience and I'm truly honored to be a coauthor with people I greatly respect and admire. A very sincere thanks to Sarah A. Orjada-Dachtyl, PhD, for developing the Instructor's Manual, Test Bank, and PowerPoint information. We so appreciate your time and creative efforts. Thank you to Alice E. Smith, PhD, for her help and expertise in cleft palate. Thank you to Tony DeFeo, PhD, for sharing all of his books, articles, notes, expertise, and wisdom whenever I needed it.

I wish to thank my late mentor, Dr. Thomas J. Hixon, for teaching me everything I know about speech science and for inspiring me to become who I am today. I also want to sincerely thank my dearest friend and mentor, Jenny Hoit, for her help and support in all of my professional endeavors. I am truly grateful for her wisdom and genuineness. Thank you to my great friend, Cynthia M. Fox, PhD, for the LSVT audio samples provided on the CD-ROM, as well as for all of the glee and laughter throughout the years. Thank you for keeping my life fun. Finally, I am forever grateful to Todd Hixon for always encouraging me to follow through with my career goals and for reminding me not to take everything so seriously.

The following reviewers offered many fine suggestions for improving the manuscript: Latha Bhushan, Lock Haven University; Roberta Chapey, CUNY Brooklyn College; James Panico, Southern Illinois University; and Deborah Weiss, Southern Connecticut State University. Their efforts are sincerely acknowledged.

Brief Contents

Contents

INTRODUCTION TO COMMUNICATION DISORDERS

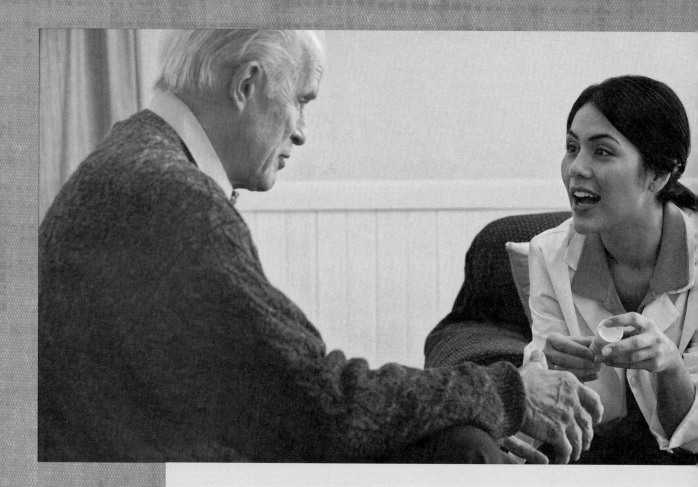

CHAPTER LEARNING GOALS

When you have finished this chapter, you should be able to:

- Describe the roles of audiologists, speech-language pathologists, and speech, language, and hearing scientists

- Explain the process of going from student to professional in the field of communication disorders

- Identify the functions of the American Speech-Language-Hearing Association

- Outline the history of changing attitudes toward individuals with disabilities over the centuries and especially legislation over the past several decades

A Journey: From Student to Professional

Can you imagine life without communication? No talking, no listening, no interacting with others? Communication is part of what makes us human. Even minor or temporary problems with communication, such as laryngitis, are often frustrating. Many individuals, including those who choose to study communication disorders, have experienced a problem in speaking or listening at some time in their lives, or someone close to them is in this situation.

We hope throughout this text to offer some insights into the nature of **communication disorders**. In this first chapter, we take you on a journey from student to professional, outlining the steps for becoming an audiologist, speech-language pathologist, or speech scientist. We'll also explore other professional team members, where speech-language pathologists and audiologists work, and what they do, plus explain the nature of evidence-based practice (EBP).

You will learn about the various types of credentials that are needed in different employment settings and about the organizations through which professionals can address issues, learn, and advocate for the people they serve. This first chapter also provides a historical perspective and outlines the laws that mandate appropriate care for those in need. Along the way, we'll find out why people choose these careers.

HELPING OTHERS TO HELP THEMSELVES

Why do people decide to become speech-language pathologists or audiologists? It is mostly because of the satisfaction that they receive from helping others to live a fuller life. Box 1.1 contains excerpts from student applications to communication disorders programs. Many students cite a personal or family encounter with a communication disorder. Almost all write about a desire to be useful to society.

BOX 1.1
Reasons for Selecting a Major in Communication Disorders

Students who applied to major in communication disorders were asked to write a brief essay explaining their motivation. Some excerpts from these essays follow:

Erika B.: When I was a little girl, I can painfully remember being picked on by the other children about the way I spoke. My once cute lisp was no longer cute at 8. I was told that "I talked like a baby" or sometimes the kids would mimic what I said in an exaggerated way. At age 10, my family moved to a new school district. A speech-language pathologist there worked with me on my lisp and other articulation problems. People who meet me today can hardly believe that I ever had a problem! I want to help people who are in similar situations. I know the hurt that accompanies the humiliation of being teased because you can't communicate properly.

Dana C.: One of my best friends was born with a complete bilateral cleft lip and palate. After 13 operations and over 9 years of speech therapy, a stranger would never know that my friend ever had a communication problem. I want to have the opportunity to help to make a similar difference in someone's life.

Victoria F.: All of her life, my cousin Jackie's family had been told that she had a common disfluency problem and that she would outgrow it. However, Jackie was a teenager and continued to be dysfluent. Finally Jackie's parents took her to a speech-language pathologist in private practice. The speech therapy resulted in transforming Jackie from a shy child with a reluctance to speak to a gregarious adolescent. At her Sweet 16 party, Jackie took the microphone and read her own speech of thanks and recognition and everyone cried. That's when I realized that I wanted to be a speech pathologist.

Tara F.: My interest in speech science began soon after I graduated from our local community college with a business degree. I knew this would result in a monotonous desk job, and I wanted my career path to take a different direction but I did not yet know what. That August my grandmother had quadruple heart bypass surgery and a stroke followed. I entered the world of speech science 3 days after she slipped into a semi-coma. When she awoke, she couldn't speak at all. I went to my library and checked out a book about strokes and read it cover to cover that night. I learned that even though she couldn't express herself through spoken word, she might be able to do so in writing, and she did. Each day was frustrating, but my grandmother improved and was soon able to grunt. From grunting, she moved to words like "No!" and she laughed aloud. Often words would come out, but they did not make sense. It was as though she was speaking a foreign language. She eventually recovered, but not fully. Although she regained her ability to speak, she speaks more slowly and more thought is required than before the stroke. My grandmother is the motivation behind my anticipated speech pathology career choice.

Denise F.: I had always considered attending college after completing my high school education, but due to unfortunate financial circumstances at that time, I was unable to do so. I took a job with an insurance agency and through 18 years of employment developed a satisfying career. About 12 years ago, at the age of 2, my oldest son was classified as Speech Impaired and Learning Disabled. He is now in the ninth grade and has made tremendous progress. He is mainstreamed for all subjects with only minimal Resource Room time. He is no longer classified as Speech Impaired. Although I tried to help him at home, I know my son would never have made the progress that he has without the professional services of special educators. I want the opportunity to provide these services and benefits to other families and their children.

Devon T.: My mother is hard-of-hearing. She has less than 50% hearing in each ear. Growing up was a little bit different because of this. I had to repeat myself most of the time while talking to her. I had to speak clearly, and most of all, I could not cover my mouth. My mother reads lips. Whenever the phone rings in my house, a lamp in my mother's room lights up. My mother bought her first hearing aid several years ago and cried all night. The only thing I could think of was how amazing that this little machine could help her hear better. I loved looking at it, and I admired my mother for overcoming her hardships and handicap.

John T.: I am a 40-year-old successful pastry chef. Since I have a family, a career change took lots of planning

BOX 1.1
(Continued)

and the beginning of a dream being fulfilled. When my son was 3 years old, he still was only babbling. His doctor was wonderful, but from Korea and did not see any problems with Jimmy's speech. Since my wife and I were worried, we had Jimmy evaluated by a speech-language pathologist. He was diagnosed with language and articulation difficulties. We took him to the clinic at St. John's University. The therapy made a difference in my son's life. It also crystallized my desire to work with children in a helpful and meaningful way.

THE PROFESSIONALS

Today, professionals who serve individuals with communication disorders come from several disciplines. They often refer clients to one another or work together to provide optimal care. Specialists in communication disorders are employed by preschools, schools, colleges and universities, hospitals, independent clinics, nursing care facilities, research laboratories, and home-based programs. Many are in private practice. Speech-language pathologists and audiologists receive similar basic training but in their advanced study concentrate on one profession or the other.

> Opportunities for speech-language pathologists and audiologists include serving individuals of all ages from infancy through the aged with varied disorders, from mild to profound, in a wide assortment of settings.

Audiologists

Audiologists are specialists who measure hearing ability and identify, assess, manage, and prevent disorders of hearing and balance. They use a variety of technologies to measure and appraise hearing in people from infancy through old age. Although they work within educational settings to improve communication and programming for people with hearing disabilities, audiologists also contribute to the prevention of hearing loss by recommending and fitting protective devices and by consulting to government and industry on the effects and management of environmental noise. In addition, audiologists evaluate and assist individuals with **auditory processing disorders [(C)APD]** and select, fit, and dispense hearing aids and other amplification devices and provide guidance in their care and use (DeBonis & Moncrieff, 2008). Licensed audiologists are independent professionals who practice without a prescription from any other health care provider (ASHA, 2001b). Box 1.2 contains an audiologist's comments on some of the challenges and rewards of the profession. As you will note, being a good detective, or problem solver, is one of the skills that is needed. Web sites of interest are found at the end of the chapter.

CREDENTIALS FOR AUDIOLOGISTS

At the present time, the entry-level requirement for audiologists is a master's degree. Prospective audiologists study hearing science, the assessment and

BOX 1.2
An Audiologist Reflects

Stella T.: I love the detective work of diagnostic procedures and the closure of rehab. I am given the clues from case history and my test findings. My job is to quickly and efficiently come up with an accurate diagnosis, recommendations, and rehabilitative plan. I have to be able to explain these in terms my patients can understand. I have to have completed all of this in less than one hour before moving on to save the rest of the world. I get closure by being able to measure the success of my rehabilitative plan within a relatively short span of time (a few weeks) and make adjustments in my plan as needed. I love making another person's life a little easier.

Beginning in the year 2012, a doctoral degree will be required for professional employment as an audiologist.

remediation of hearing loss, anatomy and physiology, and related subjects and obtain supervised clinical experience. See Appendix A: "Requirements for Becoming an Audiologist." Beginning in the year 2012, individuals wishing to work as audiologists will need 3 to 5 years of education beyond the bachelor's degree. Their studies will culminate in a doctoral degree that may be an audiology doctorate (AuD), doctor of philosophy degree (PhD), or doctor of education degree (EdD).

After a person has earned either a master's degree (prior to 2012) or a doctorate (after 2012), obtained the required preprofessional as well as paid clinical experience, and passed a national examination, she or he is eligible for the Certificate of Clinical Competence in Audiology (CCC-A) awarded by the American Speech-Language-Hearing Association (ASHA). ASHA CCC-A (sometimes referred to as ASHA "Cs") is the generally accepted standard for most employment opportunities for audiologists in the United States. In addition, states require audiologists to obtain a state license. The requirements tend to be the same or very similar to the ASHA standards (ASHA, 2001b, 2001c).

Speech-Language Pathologists

Speech-language pathologists (SLPs) are professionals who provide an assortment of services that relate to communicative disorders. The distinguishing role of the SLP is to identify, assess, treat, and prevent communication disorders in all modalities (including spoken, written, pictorial, and manual) both receptively and expressively. This includes attention to physiological, cognitive, and social aspects of communication. Speech-language pathologists also provide services for disorders of swallowing and may work with individuals who choose to modify a regional or foreign dialect. Like audiologists, licensed speech-language pathologists are independent professionals who practice without a prescription from any other health care provider (ASHA, 2000a, 2000b, 2000c). Box 1.3 contains reflections by two speech-language pathologists; the first one has been in private practice as a

BOX 1.3
Two Speech-Language Pathologists Reflect

Phillip S.:   Gladys was 12 when I met her. She had NO voice, no laugh, no cry, no moan, no words, and no song. The administrators of the school for multiply handicapped children said not to work with her because she could not be helped—after all, she had no voice. Why? Why no voice? Why no way to help? Why such pessimism? Against the will of the institution, we began to explore, and she sang in the school show 5 months later. It was not until the following fall that she began to speak normally, as though she had been doing it all her life. It was experiencing the birth of Gladys's voice that sent me back to school for my doctoral studies. Was this a miracle? I guess a miracle is when something is possible, and does happen, but it was beyond your imagination. In our work we must first see something that is not yet there and believe in it long enough to become a partner in making it come about.

Robert O.:   For me, the exciting part of my job is the problem solving and the satisfaction of helping others.

Similar to a fictional detective who collects all the clues, synthesizes the information, and deduces the guilty party, I evaluate each client and determine the best course of intervention. The more severe the impairment, the greater the challenge, and I love a challenge. How can I help a young man who attempted suicide and is now brain injured to access the language within him? How can a young child with autism begin the road through communication to language? How can I help parents communicate with their infant who has deafness, blindness, and cerebral palsy? When is the best time to introduce signing with a nonspeaking client? These are all challenges for me and the children and adults I serve. We work together as I try to solve each communication puzzle and propose and implement possible intervention strategies. Sometimes I'm very successful and sometimes I have to reevaluate my methods, but as I said, I love a challenge.

clinician for about 25 years. Although sometimes frustrated by the lack of support within his work setting, he believes in setting his imagination free and not giving up in the challenge to help others. The other SLP notes the detective-like work and satisfaction of helping others.

CREDENTIALS FOR SPEECH-LANGUAGE PATHOLOGISTS

With technology, the task of the SLP is changing. The technology for digital speech recording and analysis are now readily available, as are new and exciting assistive technologies for those with great difficulty communicating via speech (Ingram et al., 2004). Speech-language pathologists have a master's or doctoral degree and have studied typical communication and swallowing development; anatomy and physiology of the speech, swallowing, and hearing mechanisms; phonetics; speech and hearing science; and disorders of speech, language, and swallowing.

Three types of credentials are available for speech-language pathologists:

1. Public school certification normally stipulates basic and advanced coursework, clinical practice within a school setting, and a satisfactory score on a state or national examination. At the least, prospective

school SLPs need a bachelor's degree, although in most states, a master's degree either is the entry-level requirement or is mandated after a certain number of years of employment. The exact requirements to become a school SLP vary from state to state. The American Speech-Language-Hearing Association encourages the same standards for SLPs in all employment settings, as described in the following paragraph.

2. The American Speech-Language-Hearing Association issues a Certificate of Clinical Competence in Speech-Language Pathology (CCC-SLP) to individuals who have obtained a master's degree or doctorate in the field. Ongoing professional development must be demonstrated through any of a variety of continuing education options. As of 2004, the United States, United Kingdom, Australia, and Canada allow mutual recognition of certification in speech-language pathology (Boswell, 2004). See Appendix B, "Requirements for Becoming a Speech-Language Pathologist."

3. Individual states have licensure laws for speech-language pathologists that are usually independent of the state's department of education school certification requirements. A license is needed if you plan to engage in private practice or work in a hospital, clinic, or other setting apart from a public school. Most states accept a person with ASHA CCC-SLP as having met licensure requirements, although you will need to check with your state licensing board on the specifics.

> The professions of speech-language pathology and audiology require lifelong learning. Clinicians need to be able to intelligently use relevant research findings in their practice.

Table 1.1 shows the credentials that are needed in the professions of audiology and speech-language pathology. These are also found on the ASHA Web site.

Speech, Language, and Hearing Scientists

Individuals who are employed as speech, language, or hearing scientists typically have earned a doctorate degree, either a PhD or an EdD. They are employed by universities, government agencies, industry, and research centers

TABLE 1.1

Credentials for speech-language pathologists and audiologists

Credentialing Organization	Speech-Language Pathologist	Audiologist
American Speech-Language-Hearing Association	Certificate of Clinical Competence in Speech-Language Pathology (CCC-SLP)	Certificate of Clinical Competence in Audiology (CCC-A)
State department of education	Certification as Teacher of Students with Speech and Language Disabilities*	—
State professional licensing board	License as Speech-Language Pathologist	License as Audiologist

*The title for the school-based speech-language pathologist varies from state to state.

to extend our knowledge of human communication processes and disorders. Some may also serve as clinical speech-language pathologists or audiologists.

WHAT SPEECH, LANGUAGE, AND HEARING SCIENTISTS DO

Speech scientists may be involved in basic research exploring the anatomy, physiology, and physics of speech-sound production. Using various technologies, these researchers strive to learn more about typical and pathological communication. Their findings help clinicians to improve service to clients with speech disorders. Recent advances in knowledge of human genetics provide fertile soil for continuing investigation into the causes, prevention, and treatment of various speech impairments. Some speech scientists are involved in the development of computer-generated speech that may be used in telephone answering systems, substitute voices for individuals who are unable to speak, and many new purposes. Box 1.4 contains some observations by a speech-language scientist who enjoys the interdisciplinary nature of his work. His current research involves the study of tongue placement in the production of speech sounds.

Language scientists may investigate the ways in which children learn their native tongue. They may study the differences and similarities of different languages. Over the past half a century or so, the United States has become increasingly linguistically and culturally diverse; this provides an excellent opportunity for cross-cultural study of language and communication. Some language scientists explore the variations of modern-day English (dialects) and how the language is changing. Others are concerned with language disabilities and study the nature of language disorders in children and adults. An in-depth knowledge of typical language is critical to understanding language problems.

BOX 1.4
A Speech-Language Scientist Reflects

James D.: What I like best about speech-language science is the way it combines disciplines. When I was in high school, my favorite subjects were English and biology. Studying speech-language science is like studying English and biology at the same time. To be a good speech-language scientist, or a good speech-language pathologist, or a good neurolinguist, you have to know about BOTH language and physiology. It is not enough to be just a linguist or just a physiologist. And you have to know how these two things, one primarily a product of the "mind" (however one chooses to define that) and the other a function of the body, interact. Furthermore, the physiology of speech and language encompasses a broad range of bodily systems, including the neurologic, respiratory, laryngologic (or phonatory), and upper vocal tract articulatory. As if that wasn't enough in itself, you must know something about the physics of sound to really understand speech and its production. If you choose to explore speech modeling or have a clinical interest in augmentative communication systems, you could even touch on areas that we normally think of as associated with engineering. Thus, the study of speech-language science is a truly interdisciplinary study, in any number of ways. In that respect, it is a continual challenge, intellectually, and provides an opportunity to interact with a tremendously broad range of other professionals.

Hearing scientists investigate the nature of sound, noise, and hearing. They may work with other scientists in the development of equipment to be used in the assessment of hearing. They are also involved in the development of techniques for testing the hard-to-test, such as infants or those with severe physical or psychological impairments. Hearing scientists develop and improve assistive listening devices such as hearing aids and telephone amplifiers to help people who have limited hearing. In addition, hearing scientists are concerned with conservation of hearing and are engaged in research to measure and limit the impact of environmental noise.

PROFESSIONAL AIDES

Paraprofessionals usually have an associate's or bachelor's degree; they work closely with and are supervised by professionals with more training and experience.

Professional aides, sometimes referred to as paraprofessionals or speech-language pathology or audiology assistants, are individuals who work closely with SLPs or audiologists. In those states in which professional aides are permitted, the title, educational requirements, and responsibilities of these individuals vary.

Speech-language pathology assistants (SLPAs) typically participate in communication screenings. They often engage in routine therapy tasks under the direction of an SLP. They may engage in clerical tasks and assist the SLP in the preparation of assessment and treatment materials. SLPAs may work in any of the settings in which a fully credentialed SLP is found. Audiology assistants may conduct screenings, participate in calibration of audiological instrumentation, and engage in a variety of clerical tasks.

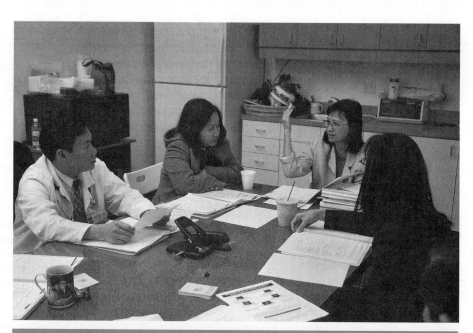

Speech-language pathologists often work as part of a professional team.

Support personnel may work only with supervision and are not permitted to perform such tasks as interpretation of test results, service plan development, family/client counseling, or determination of when to discharge a client from treatment (ASHA, 1995; Paul-Brown & Goldberg, 2001).

Related Professions: A Team Approach

Specialists in communication disorders do not operate in a vacuum. They work closely with family members, regular and special educators, psychologists, social workers, doctors and other medical personnel, occupational, physical, and music therapists. They may collaborate with physicists and engineers. Box 1.5 contains a speech-language pathologist's schedule, showing a tremendous amount of teamwork.

BOX 1.5
A Team Approach

Alicia is the senior speech-language pathologist in a community-based rehabilitation center in New York state. During the mornings, Alicia works with infants, preschoolers, and school-age children at the center. In the afternoons, she directs the Augmentative/Alternative Communication Program and assists severely impaired individuals of all ages to improve their communication abilities. The schedule outlined below has a bit more collaboration than is normally found in any one day, but it suggests the kinds of activities that are typical within a workweek.

8:30 A.M.	Education staff meeting for preschool children: classroom teacher, psychologist, social worker, occupational therapist, physical therapist.
9:00	Preschool class activity: eight children ages 3–4, one classroom teacher, two aides.
10:00	Individual half-hour therapy sessions with children in the preschool and school programs.
11:30	Combined physical and speech therapy for Jeramy, age 4, diagnosed with spastic cerebral palsy; work with physical therapist.
noon	Lunch
12:30 P.M.	Prepare for the afternoon.
1:00	Consult with engineer on wheelchair switch for Lucretia, age 7, who is multiply handicapped.
1:30	Outpatient, David, aged 24, had been in a motorcycle accident and experiences some speech and language difficulties.
3:00	Conference with Sally Brown, Bettina's foster mother, and Barbara Sloane, the social worker for the family.
3:30	Communication Disorders Department Meeting. Malcolm, an audiologist, reports on three-hour course he took on Saturday on cochlear implants.
4:30	The workday is officially over, but Alicia stays until 5:00 to read the professional journal *Language, Speech, and Hearing Services in the Schools*, which arrived today. Alicia is especially interested in the article about using children's books in working with preschoolers and photocopies it to share with other staff members.

SERVICE THROUGH THE LIFESPAN

Individuals with communication disorders may be of any age, and professionals address their needs from birth through old age. According to U.S. Census Bureau reports, 1 in 5 people has a disability. In general, the likelihood of having a disability increases as we age. Unfortunately, according to ASHA (2008), "it is difficult to assess the aggregate number of individuals in the U.S. who have speech, voice, and/or language disorders."

Infants may be screened for hearing loss and a host of other disabilities soon after birth. The U.S. Census Bureau reports that about 2% of all children born in the United States have some disabling condition, and hearing loss occurs more often than any other physical problem (Brault, 2005). Babies and toddlers may exhibit developmental delay and mental retardation. They may have physical problems including those involving movement, hearing, and vision. These disabilities may be due to a wide range of causes, discussed later in this text, and may impact the youngster's communication and feeding abilities. An interdisciplinary approach is necessary in the assessment and treatment of young children, and an Individualized Family Service Plan (IFSP), developed for each child treated, must be directed at the entire family with sensitivity to its language and culture. Early intervention has been demonstrated to be highly valuable in facilitating optimum results and potentially preventing later difficulties.

Preschoolers with communication difficulties must also be identified and helped. For some, services begun earlier may now be handled by different agencies. The youngster may be placed in a special preschool; professionals may continue to assist the family in addressing the child's needs.

Almost half of all speech-language pathologists are employed by school systems. They work with youngsters in all grades, addressing a full range of communication and swallowing problems. These are described in the chapters that follow. School-age children with communication difficulties often also suffer academically and socially, thereby adding additional urgency to the work of communication experts.

Some young adults such as those who were identified earlier as being developmentally delayed or with physical disabilities may continue to receive certain services until they are 21 years old. At this point some of these women and men may enter day-treatment programs, and/or find employment in workshops where speech-language pathologists and audiologists may be available to serve their needs.

Other individuals may find themselves in need of communication services for the first time later in life. For example, between 1.5 and 2 million Americans sustain traumatic brain injury each year in the United States (see Chapters 5 and 7) stemming from bicycle, motorcycle, or car accidents or from falls. As a result, they may have cognitive and/or motor problems that interfere with their ability to communicate and/or eat normally. The speech-language pathologist may play an important role in rehabilitative efforts.

Among those over age 65, stroke, neurological disorders, and dementia may interfere with effective communication and swallowing. Hearing loss may affect at least 1 in 4, creating a need for assessment and treatment.

Speech-language pathologists and audiologists work directly with such individuals. They often also work with spouses and children, as well as staff members of nursing homes and other adult facilities in providing counseling and guidance directed at improving quality of life in these later years (Lubinski & Masters, 2001).

Evidence-Based Practice

Throughout this text, we've tried to report the best information we can based on the research evidence available. As an SLP or audiologist, if that is your career choice, it will be your responsibility to provide the best, most well-grounded intervention that is humanly possible. In other words, you should do what works and is most effective.

Deciding on the most efficacious intervention is a portion of something called evidence-based practice (EBP). EBP is an essential part of effective and ethical intervention. The primary benefit is the delivery of optimally effective care to each client (Brackenbury et al., 2008). Using EBP, clinical decision making becomes a combination of scientific evidence, clinical experience, and client needs. In other words, research, specifically the small portion of research directly relevant to decisions about practice, is combined with reason when making decisions about treatment approaches (Dollaghan, 2004).

EBP is based on two assumptions (Bernstein Ratner, 2006):

- Clinical skills grows not just from experience but from the current available data, and
- The expert SLP or audiologist continually seeks new therapeutic information to improve efficacy.

Professional journals, called peer-reviewed journals, in which each manuscript is critiqued by other experts in the field and accepted or rejected on the basis of the quality of the research, are the best source of clinical evidence.

The philosophy and methods of EBP originated in medicine but have now been adopted in many other health care professions and related services. In the fields of audiology and speech-language pathology, EBP is a work in progress. Although ASHA has established the National Center for Evidence-Based Practice in Communication Disorders, it will take years to establish comprehensive assessment and intervention guidelines. Evidence on some key issues may still be weak or unavailable. In addition, new information may come to light through research that changes previous assumptions about that evidence. None of this relieves SLPs and audiologists of the responsibility to provide the best, most efficacious assessment and intervention possible. See the ASHA online resource at the end of the chapter.

In this discussion, we've used two terms: *efficacy* and *effectiveness*. These are sometimes difficult to discern given the heterogeneous nature of the existing research studies, so it's important that you understand the generally accepted meanings of these terms from a clinical and research perspective. Technically, **efficacy** as it relates to clinical outcomes is "The probability of benefit to individuals in a defined population from a medical technology applied for a given medical problem under ideal conditions of use." (Office of Technology Assessment, 1978). There are three key elements to this definition:

- It refers to an identified population, such as adults with global aphasia, not individuals,
- The treatment protocol should be focused and the population should be clearly identified, and
- The research should be conducted under optimal intervention conditions (Robey & Schultz, 1998). Actual results in real-life clinical situations may be less than under the more ideal situation mentioned.

Of interest is the therapeutic effect or the positive benefits resulting from treatment. The ideal treatment, then, would seem to be the one that results in largest changes to meaningful client outcomes with only limited variability across clients (Johnson, 2006).

Unfortunately, in the fields of speech-language pathology and audiology, only a small percentage of the articles concern intervention efficacy. Making clinical decisions, therefore, is not particularly easy, especially given potentially competing claims, varying clinical expertise, and client values. Still, SLPs especially are tasked to determine which treatment approach is best for each client. It is also important for SLPs to recognize that efficacy is never an all-or-nothing proposition (Law et al., 2004; Rescorla, 2005). We cannot, for example, promise a "cure," so we are left to ponder the relative effectiveness of various therapeutic approaches.

Effectiveness is "The probability of benefit to individuals in a defined population from a medical technology applied to a given medical problem under average conditions of use." (Office of Technology Assessment, 1978). Thus the effectiveness of treatment is the outcome of the real-world application of the treatment for individual clients or subgroups. In short, effectiveness is "what works." Valid clinical studies must be realistically evaluated for the feasibility of applying them to intervention with specific populations and individuals (Guyatt & Rennie, 2002).

One way of determining potential effectiveness, but not the only one, may be a clinical approach's reported **efficiency** (Kamhi, 2006a). Efficiency results from application of the quickest method involving the least effort and the greatest positive benefit, including unintended effects. For example, an unintended benefit of working to correct difficult speech sounds is that it improves the production of untreated easier sounds, although the reverse is not true (Miccio & Ingrisano, 2000). Targeting more difficult sounds would seem to be more efficient.

Other factors in decision making include the clinician's expertise and experience, client values, and service delivery variables. In addition to clinical experience and expertise, individual SLP factors such as attitude and motivation are important. Clients vary widely and respond differently to intervention based on each client's unique characteristics, such as family history and support, age, hearing ability, speech and language reception and

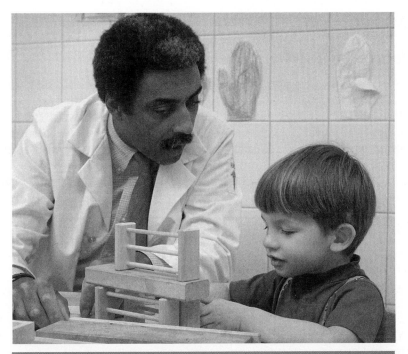

As in other professions, SLPs and audiologists use evidence-based practice to provide the best services possible.

production, cognitive abilities, and psychosocial traits, such as motivation. Finally, service delivery factors include the targets and methods selected, the treatment setting, participants, and the schedule of intervention.

The SLP or audiologist must carefully discuss possible intervention options with the client and/or family, including an explanation of the research evidence. The goal is to provide sufficient information to enable the client and/or family to make an informed choice or to collaboratively plan and refine the options to suit the client and/or family preferences.

Making good clinical decisions is never easy. High-quality evidence-based research must be evaluated critically by each SLP and applied to specific clients with specific communication disorders. Evidence-based practice requires the judicious integration of scientific evidence into clinical decision making (Johnson, 2006). Although EBP can improve and validate clinical services, we must acknowledge that it can be difficult to incorporate into everyday clinical settings because of the time required for SLPs to comb through relevant research. In addition, evidence may be limited, contradictory, or nonexistent (Brackenbury et al., 2008). In the last analysis, however, the necessity of providing the best intervention services possible must be the foremost professional concern.

PROFESSIONAL ORGANIZATIONS

American Speech-Language-Hearing Association

ASHA is a nonprofit organization of speech-language pathologists, audiologists, and speech and hearing scientists that was founded in 1925. In 2009, it had 135,000 members and affiliates from throughout the United States and the world. It is the largest association for those concerned with communication disorders. ASHA's mission, found on its Web site referenced at the end of the chapter, is to empower and support speech-language pathologists, audiologists, and speech, language, and hearing scientists by:

- Advocating on behalf of persons with communication and related disorders,
- Advancing communication science, and
- Promoting effective human communication (ASHA, 2009c).

SCIENTIFIC STUDY OF THE PROCESSES AND DISORDERS OF HUMAN COMMUNICATION

ASHA encourages study of typical and disordered communication by mandating a curriculum of study for prospective speech-language pathologists and audiologists. In addition, ASHA provides financial grants to individuals who are engaged in research that furthers our knowledge of communication and assessment, treatment, and prevention of pathologies. ASHA works closely with governmental agencies that may sponsor relevant scientific investigation.

Students who join the National Student Speech-Language-Hearing Association (NSSLH) receive professional journals, attend conferences at reduced rates, and pay less for their initial ASHA certification and membership.

To dispense knowledge among professionals, ASHA publishes several scholarly periodicals: *Journal of Speech, Language, and Hearing Research; Language, Speech, and Hearing Services in Schools; American Journal of Speech-Language Pathology: A Journal of Clinical Practice*; and *American Journal of Audiology: A Journal of Clinical Practice*. ASHA also holds an annual convention at which members and others share information and learn through scientific sessions, exhibits, seminars, and short courses. Additional institutes, workshops, conferences, and teleseminars are held throughout the year. Continuing education for professionals is fostered through these activities.

CLINICAL SERVICE IN SPEECH-LANGUAGE PATHOLOGY AND AUDIOLOGY

Programs that provide clinical services to people with communicative disorders may be accredited by ASHA. This means that representatives of ASHA will review the procedures that are used in diagnosis and treatment. A site visit will ensure that equipment, materials, and record keeping adhere to the highest professional standards. Clinical service will be the responsibility of individuals who meet ASHA standards for the CCC-SLP or CCC-A (see Appendixes A and B).

MAINTENANCE OF ETHICAL STANDARDS

To ensure that the highest moral and ethical principles are followed within the professions of speech-language pathology and audiology, ASHA provides a code of ethics, which is found on the ASHA Web site referenced at the end of the chapter. The basic principles are as follows:

1. The welfare of the persons served by communication disorders specialists is paramount.

2. Each professional must achieve and maintain the highest level of professional competence. The ASHA Certificates of Clinical Competence (CCC) are considered the minimal achievement for independent professional practice. Clinicians should provide service only within their own areas of competence. Professional development and continuing education should be ongoing. New technology requires that speech-language pathologists and audiologists continually update their skills so as to safely and accurately address patient needs.

3. Professionals must promote understanding and provide accurate information in statements to the public.

4. Professionals are responsible for assuring that ethical standards are maintained by themselves, colleagues, students, and members of allied professions. All members of ASHA are responsible for the monitoring and maintaining of ethical standards throughout the profession (ASHA, 2001a).

> Ethical questions pervade our lives as individuals and professionals. At all times, it is up to each individual to know the code of ethics and to seek consultation in assuring adherence to the highest possible standards.

ADVOCACY FOR INDIVIDUALS WITH COMMUNICATIVE DISABILITIES

The American Speech-Language-Hearing Association is active in encouraging members of Congress and state legislatures to pass legislation that provides for appropriate services for communication-impaired individuals. Bills such as the Individuals with Disabilities Education Act and the Americans with Disabilities Act became law in part because of the extensive promotional activities of organizations such as ASHA.

The needs and characteristics of people with speech, language, and hearing disabilities are clarified and publicized by ASHA on radio, on television, and through print media. In May, which is "Better Speech and Hearing Month," you are especially likely to hear public service announcements that advocate for understanding, prevention, and treatment of communication disorders.

Related Professional Associations

Although ASHA is the largest organization for communication disorder professionals, other groups are also active and worthwhile. Some speech-language

FIGURE 1.1
....

Selected professional associations relevant to communication disorders.

Academy of Dispensing Audiologists	American Auditory Society	National Hearing Conservation Association
Academy of Rehabilitative Audiology	American Speech-Language-Hearing Association	National Student Speech-Language-Hearing Association
American Academy of Audiology	Audiology Foundation of America	Orton Dyslexia Society
American Academy of Otolaryngology–Head and Neck Surgery	Canadian Association of Speech-Language Pathologists	Stuttering Foundation of America
	Council on Education of the Deaf	

pathologists and audiologists belong to several associations. Figure 1.1 lists some of those most closely affiliated. Prospective speech-language pathologists and audiologists are advised to take courses in biology, psychology, and sociology to better understand their clients and to work more effectively with professionals from other disciplines.

COMMUNICATION DISORDERS IN HISTORICAL PERSPECTIVE

It is believed that in many early human groups less able individuals were shunned. Children who were malformed or who had obvious physical disabilities were sometimes abandoned. The aged who could no longer contribute might also be abandoned, deprived of food, or even killed.

Over the centuries attitudes changed somewhat and by the late 1700s in some parts of the world, societal efforts were being made to help those who were unable to care for themselves. Individuals began to be classified and grouped according to their disorder. Special residences for individuals with deafness, blindness, mental illness, and intellectual limitations were established, although most were little more than warehouses providing no services other than what was necessary to keep the residents alive (Karagiannis et al., 1996).

The first U.S. "speech correctionists" were educators and others in the helping or medical professions who took an interest in speech problems (Duchan, 2002). These were accompanied by a few "quacks" who promised curing therapies or drugs. The more legitimate therapists came from already established professions. Among them were Alexander Melville Bell and his father, Alexander Graham Bell, of telephone fame. Other Americans trained with famous "speech doctors" in Germany and

Austria or became interested in speech correction because of their own difficulties, often with stuttering. The first professional journal, *The Voice*, appeared in 1879 and focused primarily on stuttering research and intervention.

Early interest groups were formed primarily among teachers within the National Education Association and among physicians and academics belonged to the National Association of Teachers of Speech. The latter group formed the American Academy of Speech Correction in 1925, a precursor to the ASHA, and attempted to promote scientific inquiry and to set standards for training and practice. ASHA has had varying names over the years, finally settling on the American Speech-Language-Hearing Association in 1978.

The profession of audiology originated in the 1920s when *audiometers* were first designed for measuring hearing. Interest surged in the 1940s when returning World War II veterans exhibited noise-induced hearing loss due to gunfire or to prolonged and unprotected exposure to noise. Others had psychogenic hearing loss as a result of trauma. The Veterans Administration provided hearing testing and rehabilitation.

Gradually, ASHA was able to establish professional and educational standards and to advocate for the rights of individuals with disabilities. During the 1960s in the United States and elsewhere, intense energy was directed toward the advancement of civil rights for all people. Just as the rights of women, ethnic minorities, gays, and lesbians have been and are being recast, the status of individuals with disabilities has been reevaluated, and bold reforms initiated. The American Coalition of Citizens with Disabilities was created in 1974; legislative action on behalf of all Americans with handicapping conditions began in earnest around the same time. In many cases, people with disabilities occupied leadership roles in the push for change. As a result of this work, providing opportunities for individuals with disabilities to develop to their full potential was no longer simply an ethical position. It became federally mandated through a series of laws.

Congress enacted the Education for All Handicapped Children Act (EAHCA) as Public Law Number 94–142 in 1975. It mandated that a free and appropriate public education must be provided for all handicapped children between the ages of 5 and 21. Several years later, Public Law 99–457 extended the age of those served to cover youngsters between the ages of birth and 5. In 1990, Congress reauthorized the original law and renamed it the Individuals with Disabilities Education Act (IDEA). IDEA addressed the multicultural nature of U.S. society. The needs of individuals with limited English proficiency and those from racial and ethnic minorities were targeted for special consideration. Reauthorized in 2004, IDEA established birth-to-six programs and established new early intervention services. ASHA has been a vital advocacy agency throughout this long legislative process. Figure 1.2 summarizes major federal legislation that has implications for individuals with communication disorders.

A series of laws passed by the U.S. Congress over the past 50 years mandate appropriate treatment for individuals with disabilities.

1965: *Elementary and Secondary Education Act (Public Law 89-10)*
- States were provided federal funds so that students with special needs, including the gifted, would be evaluated and educated.

1966: *Handicapped Children's Early Education Act (Public Law 90-247)*
- Model programs for educating children with disabilities were federally funded.

1973: *Section 504 of the Vocational Rehabilitation Act (Public Law 93-112)*
- Forbids discrimination of services or employment to people with disabling conditions.

1975: *Education of All Handicapped Children Act (EAHCA) (Public Law 94-142)*
- All school-age children with disabilities must be provided a free, appropriate public education in the least restrictive environment.
- All related services (including speech-language therapy, physical therapy, and occupational therapy) that are needed for the child to benefit from the education must be provided.
- To benefit from this law, children must be evaluated and found to have a disabling condition as defined in the law.
- An Individual Education Plan (IEP) must be written for each child and must stipulate:
    Present level of performance
    Annual long-term goals and short-term objectives
    Designated instruction, services, and placement
    Date services are to be initiated and anticipated duration of services
- A Committee on Special Education (CSE) composed of the child's parents (or person designated by them), school administrator, and relevant educators and teachers must meet to review and endorse the IEP.
- Parents must agree to the initial evaluation in writing and approve and sign the IEP.
- The IEP must be reviewed each year.

1986: *Education of the Handicapped Amendments (Public Law 99-457)*
- Federal funds were provided to states that wanted to develop programs for disabled infants and toddlers from birth through age 2.
- The provisions of P.L. 94-142 were extended to disabled children between the ages of 3 and 5 years.
- Services must be provided by qualified personnel who meet the criteria for licensure stipulated by the state. (The intent was to end the double standard with one set of requirements needed to provide services in a school setting and another set needed to work in hospitals or private agencies.)
- An Individualized Family Service Plan (IFSP) must be written for each child with special needs that may include home-based instruction and therapy and parent education.

1988: *Technology-Related Assistance for Individuals with Disabilities (Public Law 100-407)*
- Included funding for centers to serve children and adults who may benefit from augmentative and alternative communication (AAC).
- Additional technological support became available.

1990: *Individuals with Disabilities Education Act (IDEA)*
- Recognized and made provisions for increasing diversity of U.S. population.
- Required free, appropriate public education (FAPE) for children with disabilities.
- Part B outlined programs for preschool children as described in each child's Individualized Education Program (IEP).
- Part C specified programs for infants and toddlers as provided by an Individualized Family Service Plan (IFSP).

1990: *Americans with Disabilities Act (ADA) (Public Law 101-336)*
- Mandated improved access to buildings and facilities that provide goods or services to the public through provision of ramps, parking facilities.

FIGURE 1.2
············

It's the law: Major provisions of important federal legislation affecting people with communicative disabilities.

- Mandated accessible rest rooms.
- Provided for effective communication with people with disabilities, including use of interpreters, appropriate signage; and telecommunication devices for the deaf (TDDs).

1997: *Reauthorization of the Individuals with Disabilities Education Act (Public Law 105-17)*
- Specified what is to be included in an IEP.
- Specified that FAPE is only terminated upon graduation.
- Added attention deficit disorder and attention deficit hyperactive disorder under some circumstances.
- Part C strengthened the requirement that services for birth–3 be provided within the context of family. Family members are part of the interdisciplinary team and primary decision makers in the collaborative effort.

2000: *Developmental Disabilities Assistance Act and Bill of Rights Act (Public Law 106-402)*
- Stated educational rights for individuals with disabilities.
- Defined developmental disability as a severe, chronic disability of an individual 5 years of age or older that
    - is attributable to mental or physical impairment or a combination of impairments;
    - is manifested before the age 22 years;
    - is likely to continue indefinitely;
    - results in substantial functional limitations in three or more areas of life activity, such as

self-care, receptive and expressive language, learning, mobility, self-direction, capacity for independent learning, and economic self-sufficiency; and
- reflects the individual's need for a combination and sequence of special, interdisciplinary, or generic services, individualized supports, or other forms of assistance that are of lifelong or of extended duration and are individually planned and coordinated.

2004: *Individuals with Disabilities Education Improvement Act* (IDEIA)
- Required that individualized programs in IFSPs or IEPs be offered in the natural environment or the least restrictive environment (LRE).
- Guaranteed the rights of parents in determining their child's education
- Outlined that early intervention services (birth–3 years) should be
    - Transdisciplinary in nature, optimizing the participation of children and their families,
    - Family centered and responsive to families' priorities as well as the culture and values of the family,
    - Individualized for the child and family,
    - Developmentally appropriate,
    - Provided in the least restrictive and most natural environment for the child and family, and
    - Based on empirical evidence on intervention effectiveness.

FIGURE 1.2
....
(Continued)

SUMMARY

Speech-language pathologists, audiologists, and other specialists work together to assist those with communicative impairments. They work in a variety of settings and with people of all ages. They are rewarded by contributing to the well-being of others. Professionals who are engaged in clinical service for those with communication disorders have a minimum of a master's degree and supervised clinical experience. They generally have earned the American Speech-Language-Hearing Association Certificate of Clinical Competence (ASHA-CCC) in their area of specialization.

Services are provided to individuals from birth through advanced age. The American Speech-Language-Hearing Association (ASHA) is the largest organization of professionals working with communication disorders. ASHA's missions include the scientific study of human communication, provision of clinical service in speech-language pathology and audiology, maintenance of ethical standards, and advocacy for individuals with communication disabilities. As a result, federal legislation currently mandates services for people with disabilities.

THOUGHT QUESTIONS

- What do speech-language pathologists and audiologists do?
- What do speech, language, and hearing scientists do?
- What are the requirements for becoming a professional in the fields of communicative disorders?
- What services might be needed for individuals at different ages?
- What are the missions of the American Speech-Language-Hearing Association?
- How have attitudes toward people with disabilities changed through the centuries?

SUGGESTED READINGS

Nicolosi, L., Harryman, E., & Kresheck, J. (2003). *Terminology of communication disorders: Speech, language, hearing* (5th ed.). Baltimore: Williams & Wilkins.

Nolan, C. (1987). *Under the eye of the clock: The life story of Christopher Nolan.* New York: St. Martin's Press.

Peterson's Guides. (Ed.). (2009). *Peterson's graduate & Professional Programs: An overview 2009.* Princeton, NJ: Peterson's (published annually).

Singh, S. (Ed.). (2000). *Singular's illustrated dictionary of speech-language pathology.* San Diego: Singular.

ONLINE RESOURCES

Acoustical Society of America
http://asa.aip.org/
Of special interest to hearing scientists and audiologists.

American Academy of Audiology
www.audiology.org/
Consumer and professional information regarding hearing and balance disorders as well as audiological services.

American Speech-Language-Hearing Association
www.asha.org/default.htm
Information for professionals, students, and others who are interested in careers in speech-language pathology, audiology, or speech, language, or hearing science.

www.asha.org/docs/html/TR2004-00001.html
ASHA site describes evidence-based practice.

National Institute on Deafness and Other Communication Disorders (NIDCD)
http://nidcd.nih.gov/
The U.S. governmental agency site containing relevant health and research information.

Peterson's
www.petersons.com/
Offers helpful advice for graduate school and a student planner.

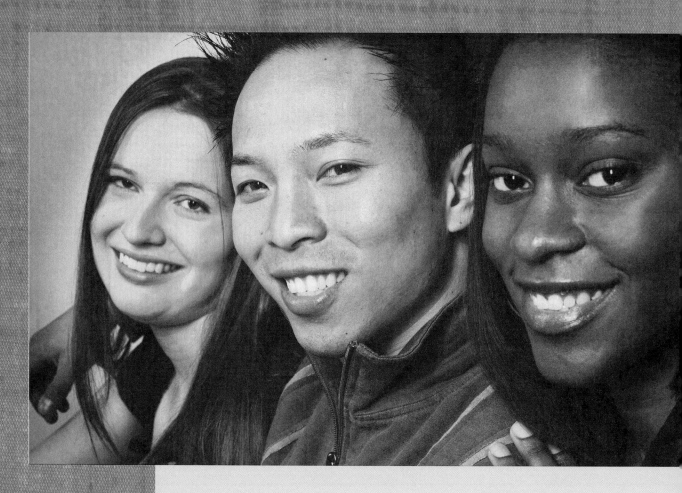

CHAPTER LEARNING GOALS

When you have finished this chapter, you should be able to:

- Explain the role of culture and environment in communication
- Describe what is involved in human communication
- Demonstrate how communication disorders may be classified
- Name some types of communication disorders
- Discuss and estimate the frequency of occurrence of communication disorders

2

Typical and Disordered Communication

HUMAN COMMUNICATION

· ·

The Social Animal

Possibly the worst punishment that can be given to a prisoner is to be sentenced to isolation. Discipline for a teenager might include limitations on telephone or e-mail use. These restrictions are punitive because we humans are social beings. We have powerful drives to be with and to communicate with others.

What is **communication?** In general, we can say that communication is an exchange of ideas between sender(s) and receiver(s). It involves message transmission and response or feedback. "Someone does or says something, and others think or do something in response to the action or the words as they understand them" (Beebe et al., 1996, p. 6). We communicate to make contact, to reach out to others. We communicate to satisfy our needs, to reveal feelings, to share information, and to accomplish a host of purposes. If your mother ever said, "Talking to you is like talking to the wall," you recognized that she was unhappy because you did not respond. Communication is interactive; it is a give-and-take. The importance of effective communication is highlighted in Box 2.1.

Several variables affect communication and its success or failure. These include cultural identity, setting, and participants. The study of these influences on communication is called **sociolinguistics.**

CULTURAL IDENTITY

Each of us is a member of a language community. The more you understand about your own culture and that of the people with whom you communicate, the more effective your interaction will be. If this text were written in perfectly good Mandarin Chinese and you could not read that language, it would

BOX 2.1
Mundo Pax

Mundo Pax means "world peace" in Latin. A school superintendent we know uses this as his e-mail address. As an educator, he deeply believes that peace on earth comes through education. As communication specialists, we suggest that the key element of education that may lead to peace is effective communication. Visualize a 2-year-old child, whom we'll call Donna. Unable to use language well enough to express her needs, she will push, hit, cry, grab, and engage in temper tantrums. If Donna were older and had words to ask for what she craved, all that fussing might have been avoided. This might be especially true if she had the words "please" and "thank you" to open opportunities for her. If what Donna wants was possessed by another child who was not easily swayed by polite requests, Donna, if able to use sophisticated language, could trade, negotiate, or bargain. She could offer a toy that she had in exchange for the one she wanted, or she might suggest taking turns or playing together. Now picture nations that are greedy for wealth, building up military might to enable them to attack to obtain what they desire. Could improved communication skills spare us warfare? Can effective communication lead to mundo pax?

It is axiomatic to say, "We cannot *not* communicate" (Watzlawick et al., 1967, p. 48). Even a lack of response to someone sends a message to "leave me alone."

communicate nothing meaningful to you. Speakers and listeners must share competence in a common language if they are to communicate fully.

Perhaps you have traveled to a country in which a language that you did not know was spoken. You might have been able to communicate by gesture and pantomime; however, you would have to agree that while you could exchange some meaning, it fell far short of optimal communication. Even when two people come from the same language background, "perfect" communication is rare. This is because successful communication depends on related factors such as age, socioeconomic status, geographical background, ethnicity, and gender.

Jennifer and John were college sweethearts; however, they recognized significant differences in ways of relating. When Jennifer was growing up, her family openly discussed issues and disagreements, often to the point of forceful argumentation and yelling. These heated discussions sometimes led to tears, but eventually they typically terminated in hugs. John's family was more reserved. When two people did not agree, it was considered polite to keep your thoughts to yourself. In her relationship with John, Jennifer soon learned that she could not criticize him without his becoming sullen and hurt. However, she often wished that he would comment more frankly on decisions she was making. They both recognized that each would have to make major adjustments if their future marriage was to succeed.

SETTING AND PARTICIPANTS

The location of communication influences its nature. Where you interact affects how and what you'll say. You communicate differently at home, in school, in a noisy restaurant, and at a ballgame. Similarly, you might speak quite differently to your best friend, your mother, your father, your boss, your grandmother, and large audiences.

Means of Communication

Communication takes many forms and can involve any or a combination of our senses, including sight, hearing, smell, and touch. It can include both verbal and nonverbal means, such as the spoken word, naturalistic gesture, or sign. The primary vehicle of human communication is language, and speech is the primary means of language expression for most individuals.

LANGUAGE

Language may be defined as "a socially shared code or conventional system for representing concepts through the use of arbitrary symbols and rule-governed combinations of those symbols" (Owens, 2008, p. 460). Some characteristics of language follow:

- Socially shared tool
- Rule-governed system
- Arbitrary code
- Generative process
- Dynamic scheme

Language is a tool for relating to others and for accomplishing a variety of objectives. As we pointed out earlier, others must share the code if communication is to occur. When an infant utters, "ga da da ka," we cannot call this language, because this "code" is not shared.

Many people are so accustomed to their own language that they fail to recognize its arbitrary nature. Is there anything in the sound combination or the written letters of the word "water" that resembles the wet stuff? Is the French word "l'eau" or the Italian "l'acqua" any more or less moist? A comparison of different languages rapidly confirms this very arbitrary nature. The equivalent of the English word "butterfly" is "farfalla" in Italian, "mariposa" in Spanish, and "Schmetterling" in German—four very different renditions of that graceful creature. Some words have no equivalent in other languages.

Each language, in addition to being composed of arbitrary but agreed upon words, consists of rules that dictate how these words are arranged in sentences. In English, an adjective precedes a noun; for example, we say, "brown cow." In French, as in many other languages, this sequence is reversed, and they say, "le vache brun" ("the cow brown"). The rules of a language make up its **grammar.** Interestingly, you do not have to be able to explain the rules to recognize when they have been broken. Take, for example the sentence, "The leaves of the maple green tree in the breeze swayed." Most American students will simply know that the sentence is wrong and say, "It doesn't sound right." This recognition of "wrong" and "right" grammar is called **linguistic intuition** and is possessed by native speakers of a language.

Parents often assume that their infant's earliest "ma ma" or "da da" are uttered in reference to themselves. These sound combinations are not considered true words unless there is evidence that they are used meaningfully.

Language is **generative;** this means that each utterance is freshly created. We do not just quote or repeat what has been heard. We paraphrase and modify and present our own ideas in an individual way. Imagine a conversation if all we could do was imitate one another.

Languages are also **dynamic;** they change over time. The famous Academie Française has tried to keep French "pure" and true to its origins. The Academie still attempts to keep "foreign" words from infiltrating French. For example, it has tried to ban the English words "jet" and "drugstore." But "le jet" is apparently easier to use than the French "l'avion à réaction," and so it stays. No academy, no school, no law, and no army can keep languages from being modified. In American English, we add five or six new words each day. Pronunciation, grammar, and ways of communicating also change.

All human languages consist of similar basic ingredients. The primary components have been labeled form, content, and use (ASHA, 1993; Bloom, 1970). See Figure 2.1.

Form   Form consists of phonology, morphology, and syntax. The sound system, or **phonology,** of English consists of about 43 phonemes (unique speech sounds). Although different languages use many of the same phonemes, variations exist. Spanish and German, to name only two, do not use the English "th." As a consequence, because this sound is not learned as a child, it is difficult for some nonnative English speakers to produce.

Phonotactic rules specify how sounds may be arranged in words. Like rules of grammar, phonotactic rules are not universal. For example "k" and "n" cannot be blended in spoken English, although this combination is acceptable in German. For this reason the "k" in "knife" and "Knoxville" is silent for native English speakers but might be pronounced by Germans speaking English as a second language.

Morphology involves the structure of words. A **morpheme** is the smallest grammatical unit within a language. Words contain both **free morphemes** and **bound morphemes.** A free morpheme may stand alone as a word. For example, "cat," "go," "spite," "like," and "magnificent" are all free morphemes. If you attempt to break them into smaller units, you lose the meaning of the word. In contrast, "cats," "going," "spiteful," "dislike,"

FIGURE 2.1
....

Components of language.

Source: From *Language Development: An Introduction* (5th ed.) (p. 19) by R. Owens, Needham Heights, MA: Allyn & Bacon. Copyright 2001 by Robert E. Owens. Reprinted with permission.

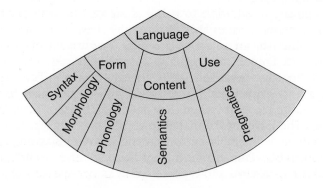

and "magnificently" each contain one free and one bound morpheme. The bound morphemes (-s), (-ing), (-ful), (dis-), and (-ly) change the meanings of the original words by adding their own meanings but can be used only as attachments to free morphemes.

Syntax pertains to how words are arranged in a sentence. In an English declarative sentence, the subject comes before the verb: "John is going to the opera." When we reverse the order of the subject and the auxiliary or helping verb, we change the meaning of the sentence and end up with a question: "Is John going to the opera?" In the sentence "Mary was kissed by John," who is doing the kissing? Even though "John" comes after the verb, he is the actor because this sentence is in the passive voice. Although you probably don't consciously know and can't recite the rules for active and passive sentences, your linguistic intuition makes it easy for you to comprehend their meaning (Chomsky, 1965).

Content   Because language is used to communicate, it must be about something, and that is its content, meaning, or **semantics. Semantic features** are the pieces of meaning that come together to define a particular word. For example, "girl" and "woman" share the semantic features of *feminine* and *human*, but *child* is generally considered a feature in "girl" and not in "woman." You'll notice that we said "generally" because, although most of us think of a "girl" as being young, it is common among some groups of people to refer to any woman as a "girl." Each word has multiple meanings, as you can quickly verify by looking in the dictionary. It is the other aspects of language, such as use and form, that determine the appropriate definition in context.

If you are beginning to think that this is complicated, you are right. As we said earlier, social and cultural factors influence the way language is used. The more two people know about one another, the more effectively they will be able to communicate.

Use   Use, or **pragmatics,** is the driving force behind all aspects of language. We speak for a reason. It is the purpose of our utterance that primarily determines its form and content. For example, if you are with a friend and are hungry, you might say, "Let's get something to eat." If function was a simple biological drive, then "eat" grunted out might suffice. But who and where you are, whom you are with, and the time of day also influence what you say. If you are at your home and you have invited the friend to dinner, you might say, "Dinner is ready." If you are working with someone as noon approaches, you might suggest, "Let's break for lunch."

Pragmatic rules of communication have been identified (Grice, 1975), some of which vary with culture (Gumperz & Hymes, 1972). For example, in the United States, business meetings tend to be very task oriented. Very little time is spent on social exchanges; the work to be done has center stage. In Saudi Arabia, however, when two people meet for the first time for business purposes, they might spend the entire session talking about family and friends and not get to the meat of the business until the second meeting. The rules for business conversations in each of these societies are different. A few general rules for speakers of American English are presented in Figure 2.2

> While all are important, it is the use or purpose of communication that dictates form and content.

1. Only one person speaks at a time. Each person should contribute to the conversation.
2. Speakers should not be interrupted.
3. Each utterance should be relevant.
4. Each speech act should provide new information.
5. Politeness forms reflect the relationship of the speakers.
6. Topics of conversation must be established, maintained, and terminated.
7. The speaker should be sensitive to successfully communicating the message, avoiding vagueness and ambiguity.
8. The listener should provide feedback that reflects comprehension of the message.

SPEECH

Speech is the acoustic representation of language. Features such as articulation, fluency, and voice interact to influence the speech production signal. The final product reflects the rapid coordination of movements associated with each of these features.

Articulation Articulation refers to the way in which speech sounds are formed. How do we move our tongue, teeth, and lips to produce the specific phonemes of a language? How do we combine these individual sounds to form words? After all, we don't speak in a series of isolated sounds such as "h-e-ll-o" or we'd sound like robots. Chapter 10 explains the nature of speech sound production and describes the problems that may occur.

Fluency **Fluency** is the smooth, forward flow of communication. It is influenced by the rhythm and rate of speech. Every language has its own rhythmic pattern; we often think of rhythm as timing. Do we pause after each word that we speak? Do we pause after each sentence? If we do, how long do the pauses last? What is our phrasing? You'll note that timing is not an isolated feature of speech. A word or syllable that is held tends to be emphasized and said more loudly. A skilled storyteller uses pauses and rhythmic variations for dramatic effect.

The speed at which we talk is our **rate.** Overall rate can reveal things about us. It may provide clues as to where we come from. For example, people from New York usually speak more rapidly than those from Georgia. However, if you habitually speak very quickly, it may suggest that you are in a hurry, are impatient, or have a great deal to say. By contrast, slow speech may connote a relaxed or casual personality.

The component of speech that includes rate and rhythm is referred to as *prosody*. Prosodic features are also known as suprasegmentals. *Supra-* means "above" or "beyond," so suprasegmental features go beyond individual speech sounds (or segmental units) and are applied to whole phrases or sentences. Stress and intonation are also suprasegmental features of speech production that are discussed later in this chapter.

Although most of the time we attempt to use a clear, sufficiently loud voice, sometimes our meaning may be more effectively communicated by a whisper, a whine, or a throaty rasp. When you are upset, your voice might sound angry to the point where someone says, "Don't use that tone of voice with me." Clearly, tone communicates information.

VOICE

Voice can reveal things about the speaker as well as about the message. A woman with a hoarse voice might (correctly or not) communicate to others that she smokes. A person with a soft, high-pitched voice might be communicating youth or immaturity. A deep, throaty voice might connote masculinity or authority.

Both the overall level of loudness and the loudness pattern within sentences and words are important. A generally loud voice may communicate strength; a soft one may suggest timidity. By stressing different words within a sentence, you are also conveying different meanings. Say the following sentence in each of the ways listed here, with the emphasis or increased loudness on the underlined word. Notice how the meaning changes.

I got an "A" on my Physics final.

I got an "A" on my Physics final.

I got an "A" on my Physics final.

I got an "A" on my Physics final.

Placing the stress on different syllables within certain words also changes the meaning. Contrast the following:

record/record

recess/recess

present/present

You might have noticed that as you vary the stress, the pitch, duration, and pronunciation of different speech sounds may also change. The pitch tends to go up as the loudness is increased. Similarly, you are likely to prolong the syllable that receives stress. The first vowel in the noun "record," meaning a log or old-fashioned musical platter, is usually pronounced /ɛ/, as in "bed," whereas in the verb "record," as in the act of jotting something down or making a tape or CD, that "e" is more likely a schwa, /ə/, the first sound in "above," or an /ɪ/, as in "bid."

Pitch is a listener's perception of how high or low a sound is; it can be physically measured as frequency or cycles per second, called hertz. **Habitual pitch** is the basic tone that an individual uses most of the time. Women usually have higher pitched voices than men, and children have higher voices than adults of both sexes. So our habitual pitch tells something about who we are.

> The symbols /ɛ/, /ə/, and /ɪ/ represent phonemes or speech sounds to be described in more detail in Chapter 10, "Disorders of Articulation and Phonology."

Punctuation and font type and size may contribute to the meaning of an email. A century ago, perfumed letter paper modified the written word.

Pitch movement within an utterance is called **intonation.** A rising intonation turns a statement into a question. First say the following sentence by bringing your pitch down for the last word, then say it by raising your pitch at the end:

I want to do the dishes.

You'll notice that intonation influences meaning. You should also observe that as you alter intonation, your rhythm and loudness patterns also change.

NONVERBAL COMMUNICATION

Although most humans rely heavily on spoken communication, some researchers report that about two thirds of human exchanges of meaning take place nonverbally (Zeuschner, 1997). The term *nonverbal* encompasses both the suprasegmental aspects of speech that we described in the previous section and the **nonvocal** (without voice) message exchange that we present in the following paragraphs.

Artifacts The way you look and the way you have decorated your personal environment communicate something about you. Even the car that you drive can deliver a message. One young man we know impressed a woman on their first date by correctly selecting her car out of 30 in a parking lot. He did this by evaluating the make and year as well as the items on the seat and dashboard. If you walk into the best hotel in your area dressed in a business suit and ask for the rest room, you will be treated better than if you were wearing shabby jeans and looking unkempt. Assumptions are made about our personalities and trustworthiness on the basis of our possessions, clothing, and general appearance.

Music, art, architecture, and furniture are also artifacts that communicate. They communicate messages from the artists who designed and produced them and also from the people who purchase, patronize, or in some way support them.

Kinesics **Kinesics** refers to the way we move our bodies, or *body language*. This includes overall body movement and position as well as gestures and facial expression. Although there is some overlap with signing, gesturing typically lacks **explicit** (clearly defined) movements. In signing, the meanings of particular movements are well specified. For example, in American Sign Language (ASL), a thumb stroke down the cheek means "girl." Kinesics tend to be more general, subtle, or **implicit.** Gestures such as a "brush-off" have explicit meanings, and they support and contribute to the larger speech system. By contrast, signing is a primary means of communication that is used by many people who are deaf. ASL is described in greater detail in Chapter 14, "Audiology and Hearing Loss," and Chapter 15, "Augmentative and Alternative Communication."

Space and Time The study of the physical distance between people as it affects communication is called **proxemics.** Proxemics not only reflects the relationship between people but is also influenced by age and culture. Infants, children, people from Middle Eastern and Latin cultures, and those with strong emotional attachments, such as lovers, tend to interact in intimate or close proximity, very near one another. One young U.S. student we know reported feeling "backed into a corner" by an exchange student from Spain whom she had just met at a social gathering. It is likely that the Spanish woman felt that the American was "too distant."

Tactiles are touching behaviors. Who touches whom and how and where on the body the touch occurs can reveal a great deal. For example, some friends hug and kiss, others shake hands, and still others simply greet with a smile and a nod. Children in our society learn that touching others is usually not appropriate and are told early on to "keep your hands to yourselves." In contrast, infants' earliest interactions normally include considerable parental and caretaker touch.

Chronemics is the effect of time on communication. Again, cultural and age factors influence this nonvocal aspect of communication. People from German and Scandinavian backgrounds tend to be exactingly prompt, while those from Latin and African cultures may permit greater time flexibility. When two individuals come from cultures with different time rules, conflicts can easily arise. Status and context also affect chronemics (Poyatos, 1983). You might be kept waiting at the doctor's office, but your doctor does not expect to have to wait for you. Promptness is part of the U.S. work ethic. If you are routinely late to class or to a job, you've violated a chronemic norm and might have to pay a price in terms of a lowered grade or lost employment.

Young children operate in the here and now. When infants cry to be fed, they do not accept "Dinner will be ready in half an hour." Most toddlers do not normally patiently wait to have their needs and desires fulfilled. During these years, their communication is also only about the present. With increasing maturity, youngsters learn to tell time, to wait, and to talk about past, future, and nonpresent events, people, and things.

Age, sex, education, and cultural background influence every aspect of communication. These variations in communication are not impairments. Differences reflect regional, social, cultural, or ethnic identity and are not a disorder of speech or language (ASHA, 1993). Table 2.1 offers a sampling of typical communication features at different life stages. We describe communication impairments in the next section.

> Speech-language pathologists recognize the heterogeneous nature of the U.S. population and strive to be sensitive to both verbal and nonverbal variations.

COMMUNICATION THROUGH THE LIFESPAN

The most complex and challenging task newborns face is learning the abstract code called language that those around them use to communicate. To do this, infants must first learn the rudiments of communication and begin to master the primary means of language transmission, called speech. The early establishment of communication between children and their caregivers fosters the development of speech and language, which in

TABLE 2.1

A lifespan view of typical communication

Age Range	Receptive Communication	Expressive Communication								
		Language			Speech			Nonverbal Communication		
		Form	Content	Use	Articulation	Fluency	Voice	Artifacts	Kinesics	Space/Time
Infancy	Quiets/turns to human voice; Distinguishes speech sounds	Prelinguistic sound-making	No "true" speech; vocalizations, body movement focus on here and now	Obtain assistance; imitate; respond to others	Gurgles, coos, babbles	Rhythm and rate begin to resemble that of surrounding language toward end of year	Varies volume, rate, pitch	Toys, materials given to child, may "give" objects to others	Gestures precede meaningful spoken language	Close proximity/immediacy
Toddler	Responds to some verbal commands	Vocabulary growth from 4 to 300 words; moves from single word to short utterances	Familiar names, actions	Imitate, greet, protest, question	Simplified phonology		High (childish) pitch, more variability than adults	Toys, begins to construct things, start of imaginary play	Gestures slowly take second place to spoken language	Proximity decreases, begins to comprehend "now" and "later"
Preschool	Comprehension far exceeds expression; enjoys stories, books; follows increasingly complex commands; comprehends simple humor	Vocabulary grows from 1,000 to more than 2,000 words; uses complete sentences	Immediate to imaginary, includes past, present, and future	Greet, request, protest, inform, pretend, entertain	Almost all speech sounds correctly produced by the end of this period	Part-word, whole word, and phrase repetition not uncommon	Adjusts to listener; often used effectively to enhance verbal communication	Tremendous variability, reflects social/cultural background	Gestures used to enhance verbal communication	Begins to understand personal space

TABLE 2.1
....
(Continued)

School-Age	Reading skills improve; receptive language grows to 50,000 words by sixth grade, 80,000 words end of high school; comprehension becomes adult-like	Vocabulary grows to 25,000 to 30,000 words; slang important; written language more complex than spoken language	Very broad, includes distant as well as near and abstract concepts	Many enjoy talking, sharing thoughts, raising and answering personal as well as abstract questions; narrative skills expand	Speech sounds correctly produced	Rate may be rapid, fluency is good	Pitch drops to adult levels with puberty, voice used to supplement verbal message	Clear indication of what is wanted, reflect peer group, gender	Gestures used in wide array of means to supplement speech	Becomes territorial, mature understanding of space and time
Early and Middle Adulthood	Comprehension increases	Education and occupation may be reflected in vocabulary	Full range of topics; written language continues in importance and sophistication	Instructing, directing others may be added if not there earlier	Mature articulation	Use of rhythm and rate to enhance message	Mature pitch, full-bodied vocal quality	Tremendous variety dependent on sociocultural and individual variables	Body movement and gesture continue to supplement verbal communication	Space may reflect relative "importance" in environment as well as cultural factors
Advanced Age	Comprehension may decrease	Vocabulary may reflect "older" generation	May focus more on past than future	May have limited communication partners, speech may be major way to achieve companionship	Normally not impaired	Rate may slow	Pitch may increase, vocal quality become "thinner"	Old/familiar items may become increasingly treasured	Body movement may be less forceful	May crave touch, as significant others become less available

Sources: Information from Owens, (2010), Shadden & Toner (1997).

Note: This is a sampling of communication behaviors. Variability within each age group is the norm.

Communication is established very early between the child and caregiver.

turn influences the quality of communication. This intricate pattern is further complicated by physical, cognitive, and social development as children mature. We can go even further to suggest studies in several languages that reveal that language proficiency is critical to development of higher cognitive skills, even nonverbal ones (Oller et al., 2001).

Every person's speech and language continue to change until the end of life. Communication reflects the changes occurring in us and around us. Even the means of communication can change. Your great-grandparents might have begun life without a telephone and had to learn this new means of communication. Your grandparents probably began life without television. We, the authors, had to learn to use computers to communicate when we were well into our adult lives. You, in contrast, grew up with the Internet.

Languages change too. New words and phrases have entered American English within your lifetime, such as *Internet, Blu-ray disc, iPod, rollerblade, text message, hip hop,* and *hybrid vehicle.* Other cultures and languages have contributed *mullah, sushi, Reggaeton, salsa,* and *tsunami.* The competent communicator continues to adapt to changes in the language and in the commnication process.

Children become communicators because we treat them as if they already are.

The key to becoming a communicator is being treated as one. Although both speech and language depend on physical and cognitive maturation, neither is sufficient to account for the rapid developments in children's communication. Most linguists would also agree that language has strong biological underpinnings, although this too is an insufficient explanation in itself of the language learning process.

The process of learning speech and language is a social one that occurs through interactions of children and the people in their environment. Speech and language are learned within routines and familiar activities that shape children's days and within conversations about food, toys, and pets and later about school, social life, and the like. As listeners, we use a variety of lexical, syntactic, and stress-pattern cues flexibly to break continuous speech into more readily interpretable chunks (Sanders & Neville, 2000).

In different cultures, the type of child-caregiver interaction, the model of language presented to the child, and the expectations for the child differ, but each is sufficient for the learning of language. Learning to become an effective communicator is a dynamic and active process in which children in our culture become involved in the give-and-take of conversations. Even the more formal educational processes of learning to read and write are initially social and occur within book-reading activities in the home involving children and caregivers.

COMMUNICATION IMPAIRMENTS

Now that we have an idea of the complexity and varied nature of communication, it should be easy to see that much can go wrong. The American Speech-Language-Hearing Association (ASHA) defines communication and related disorders as "disorders of speech (articulation, voice, resonance, fluency), orofacial, myofunctional patterns, language, swallowing, cognitive communication, hearing, and balance" (ASHA, 1997, p. I-64iii). Notice that this definition does not confine itself to speech and hearing; also included are reading and writing, as well as manual and other communication systems, in addition to processes such as swallowing and balance that share anatomy and physiology with parts of the communication mechanism. Communication disorders may be categorized on the basis of whether reception, processing, and/or expression is affected. Is the problem primarily one of hearing, comprehending and manipulating language, or speaking? In fact, the three dimensions may be intertwined, reflecting the "interaction and interdependence among the processes of speech, language, and hearing" (ASHA, 2001b, Standard 3.4). Figure 2.3 presents various systems for categorizing communication disorders.

Etiology, the cause or origin of the problem, may be used to classify a communication problem. Disorders may be due to faulty learning, neurological impairments, anatomical or physiological abnormalities, cognitive deficits, hearing impairment, or damage to any part of the speech system.

Sometimes a dichotomy is made between **congenital** and **acquired** problems. Congenital disorders are present at birth; acquired ones are the result of illness, accident, or environmental circumstances anytime later in life. Finally, disorders may range from borderline or mild to profoundly severe.

Variations in communication are not impairments. Communication **dialects** are differences that reflect a particular regional, social, cultural, or ethnic identity and are not disorders of speech or language (ASHA, 1993).

In this text, we provide a **holistic** approach to diagnosis and treatment of people with communicative impairments. We have separate chapters

Reception	Expression	Etiology	Time of Onset	Severity
Hearing Acuity:	*Speech:*	Neuromotor	Congenital	Borderline
Conductive	Articulation	1abnormalities	Acquired	Mild
Sensorineural	Fluency	Hearing impairment		Moderate
Mixed	Voice	Environmental/		Severe
Auditory Processing:	*Language:*	learning factors		Profound
Decoding	Form	Cognitive deficits		
Integration	Phonology	Anatomical or		
Organization	Morphology	physiological		
Understanding speech	Syntax	impairments		
under adverse	Content			
conditions	Vocabulary			
Short-term memory	Use			
Multiple categories	Pragmatics			

FIGURE 2.3

Possible classification of speech communication disorders.

Speech-language pathologists are concerned with both verbal and non-verbal disorders of communication.

that discuss speech characteristics such as voice, fluency, and phonology, but we also provide chapters that are organized on the basis of etiology such as neurogenic and craniofacial disorders. Within each chapter, we examine the interconnectedness of age, time of onset, social and cultural factors, cause of the presenting disorder, and describe evidence-based assessment and treatment practices. We observe that it is common for an individual who demonstrates difficulties with one aspect of communication to be affected in other areas as well. We demonstrate that differences and dialects do not constitute disorders, and we examine the sometimes perplexing contrast between "typical" and "impaired."

Language Disorders

DISORDERS OF FORM

As explained earlier, language form includes phonology, morphology, and syntax. We speak in sounds (phonemes) that are combined into words (morphemes), which in turn are combined into phrases and sentences (based on syntactical rules). Errors in sound use, such as not producing the ends of words ("hi shi i too sma" for "his shirt is too small), constitutes a disorder of phonology. Incorrect use of past tense or plural markers ("the girl wented home" for "the girls went home") is an example of a disorder of morphology. Note that these patterns are sometimes a reflection of a particular speech dialect. The SLP must distinguish between dialectal variations, which do not signify impairment, and disorders (see Chapter 4, "Assessment and Intervention"). Syntactical errors include incorrect word order and run-on sentences (for example, "I want to go mall and go skate and buy peanuts and you come with me 'cause I want you to but not Jimmy 'cause he's not big enough to go skate"). These errors in school-age children may affect academic achievement and social well-being.

Disorders of form may be due to many factors, including sensory limitations such as hearing problems or perceptual difficulties such as learning disabilities. Limited exposure to correct models may also hinder a child's language development. For many children who are delayed in their production of mature language forms, the cause is not apparent.

DISORDERS OF CONTENT

Children and adults with limited vocabularies, those who misuse words, and those with word-finding difficulties may have disorders of content or semantics. Similarly limited ability to understand and use abstract language as in metaphors, proverbs, sarcasm, and some humor suggests semantic difficulties. A persistent pattern of avoiding naming objects and referring instead to "the thing" is another indication of a disorder of content. Limited experience or a concrete learning style may contribute to this problem in youngsters. Among older people, cerebrovascular accidents (strokes), head trauma due to accidents, and certain illnesses may result in word-retrieval problems and other content-related difficulties.

Disorders of Use

Pragmatic language problems may stem from limited or unacceptable conversational, social, and narrative skills; deficits in spoken vocabulary; and/or immature or disordered phonology, morphology, and syntax. Examples of impaired pragmatic language skills might include difficulty staying on topic, providing inappropriate or incongruent responses to questions, and constantly interrupting the conversational partner. Culture, group affiliations, setting, and participants described earlier in this chapter play a major role in judgments regarding pragmatic competence.

> It is not uncommon for an individual to have an impairment in more than one aspect of communication.

Speech Disorders

Disorders of speech may involve articulation (the production of speech sounds), fluency (rhythm and rate), or **voice** (pitch, loudness, and quality). They may affect people of all ages, be congenital or acquired, be due to numerous causes, and reflect any degree of severity.

Disorders of Articulation

Production of speech requires perception and conceptualization of the speech sounds in a language as well as motor movements to form these sounds in isolation and in context. You must have both a mental/auditory image of the sound you are going to say and the neuromuscular skills to produce the sound. The cognitive and theoretical concepts of the nature, production, and rules for producing and combining speech sounds in language is known as phonology. The actual production of these sounds is called **articulation.**

It is not always possible to determine whether an individual's speech-sound errors indicate an impairment of phonology or articulation. To sort this out, speech-language pathologists (SLPs) identify the phonemes that are incorrectly produced and look for error patterns that may point to phonological disturbances. The sound system of a language is usually fully in place by age 7 or 8. Children with multiple speech-sound errors past age 4 may have *phonological* difficulties. The causes are often not known but may be the result of faulty learning due to illness, such as ear infections, hearing or perceptual impairments, or other problems in the early years.

The SLP also assesses the client's ability to move the structures needed in speech, such as the jaw, lips, and tongue. The causes of articulation disorders include neuromotor problems such as cerebral palsy, physical anomalies such as cleft palate, and faulty learning. When paralysis, weakness, or poor coordination of the muscles for speech result in poor speech articulation, the disorder is called **dysarthria.** Apraxia of speech also results in poor articulation due to neuromotor difficulties; however, the difficulty appears to be in programming the speech mechanism while muscle strength is normal. Dysarthria and apraxia can affect children as well as adults. Assessment and treatment of phonological and articulatory disorders are described in Chapter 10, "Disorders of Articulation and Phonology."

DISORDERS OF FLUENCY

As we described earlier, fluency is the smooth, uninterrupted flow of communication. Certain types of fluency disruptions are fairly common at different ages. For example, many 2-year-olds repeat words: "I want-want-want a cookie." Around age 3, youngsters often make false starts and revise their utterances: "Ben took . . . he broked my crayon." Because these speech patterns are so common, they are sometimes referred to as **developmental disfluency.** Typically fluent adults occasionally use **fillers** ("er," "um," "ya know," and so on), **hesitations** (unexpected pauses), **repetitions** ("g-go-go"), and **prolongations** ("wwwwell"). However, when these speech behaviors exceed or are qualitatively different from the norm or are accompanied by excessive tension or struggle behavior, they may be identified as **stuttering.** Appropriate diagnosis and intervention when warranted are the task of the SLP (Yairi et al., 2001).

Fluency disorders are generally first noticed before 6 years of age. If remediation efforts are not made or are unsuccessful, this condition might continue and even worsen by adulthood. Adult onset of disfluency also occurs. Advancing age, accidents, and disease can all disrupt the normal ease, speed, and rhythm of speech. The causes of nonfluent speech are typically unclear; this is explored further in Chapter 8, "Fluency Disorders."

> Speech language pathologists use several indices to differentiate developmental disfluency from early stuttering.

VOICE DISORDERS

As in other areas of speech, voice matures as the child gets older. From uncontrolled cries to carefully modulated whispers, shouts, and variations in pitch, the development of voice follows a predictable pattern. Although occasionally children are born with physiological problems that interfere with normal voice (such as a congenital laryngeal web; to be described in Chapter 9, "The Voice and Voice Disorders"), more common is the pattern of **vocal abuse.** It is characterized by excessive yelling, screaming, or even occasional loud singing that results in **hoarseness** or another voice disorder.

Habits such as physical tension, yelling, coughing, throat clearing, smoking, and alcohol consumption can disrupt normal voice production. These behaviors may result in pathology to the vocal folds such as polyps, nodules, or ulcers. Disease, trauma, allergies, and neuromuscular and endocrine disorders may also affect voice quality. For example, individuals with Parkinson disease, a progressive neurological disorder, may have a soft voice with limited pitch and loudness variation.

Hearing Disorders

According to ASHA, a hearing disorder "is the result of impaired auditory sensitivity of the physiological auditory system" (ASHA, 1993, p. 40). It may affect the ability to detect sound, to recognize voices or other auditory stimuli, to discriminate between different sounds, such as mistaking the phoneme /s/ for /f/, and to understand speech.

DEAFNESS

When a person's ability to perceive sound is limited to such an extent that "the primary sensory input for communication [is] other than the auditory channel," the individual would be considered deaf (ASHA, 1993, p. 41). Deafness may be congenital or acquired.

Total communication, including sign, speech, and speechreading, is often considered the most effective intervention. **Assistive listening devices (ALD), cochlear implants,** and **auditory training** may be helpful. These are explained in Chapter 14.

> Universal neonatal hearing screening is mandated by law in many states. In this way, congenital deafness can be identified and addressed very early.

HARD OF HEARING

A person who is hard of hearing, in contrast to one who is deaf, depends primarily on audition for communication. Hearing loss may be temporary due to an illness, such as an ear infection, or permanent, caused by disease, injury, or advancing age. Hearing loss is usually categorized in terms of severity, laterality, and type. The severity of a hearing loss may range from mild to severe. It may be **bilateral,** involving both ears, or **unilateral,** affecting primarily one ear. Finally, the loss may be **conductive, sensorineural,** or **mixed.** A conductive loss is caused by damage to the outer or middle ear; people with this type of loss usually report that sounds are generally too soft. A sensorineural loss involves problems with the inner ear and/or auditory nerve; this type of damage is likely to affect a person's ability to discriminate and consequently understand speech sounds, although they may "hear" them. A typical pattern is that of older people who report that they hear just fine but wish others would not mumble. Mixed hearing loss, as the name implies, is a combination of both conductive and sensorineural loss (see Chapter 14 for further discussion).

Auditory Processing Disorders

An individual with an auditory processing disorder (APD) may have normal hearing but still have difficulty understanding speech. Individuals with APDs struggle keeping up with conversation, understanding speech in less than optimal listening conditions (i.e., degraded speech signal, presence of background noise), discriminating and identifying speech sounds, and with integrating what they hear with nonverbal aspects of communication (DeBonis & Moncrieff, 2008; Stecker, 1998). These difficulties are sometimes traced to tumors, disease, or brain injury, but often the cause is unknown. APD can occur in both children and adults. A special battery of auditory diagnostic tests is used to determine or rule out APD; however, there is currently no "gold standard" to ensure correct identification of the disorder (McFarland & Cacase, 2006). APD may coexist with other disorders including attention deficit hyperactivity disorder (ADHD) and speech-language and learning disabilities (ASHA, 2005).

How Common Are Communication Disorders?

Before we attempt to estimate the numbers of people who have disorders of communication, we examine the concepts of normalcy and patterns of disability.

WHAT IS "NORMAL"?

A recent cartoon showed an empty room and a sign reading "Meeting of Members of Functional Families." The implication was that there are no functional or "normal" families. Likewise, we could ask, "Is anybody normal?" If anything, variability is the norm. We humans are remarkable in our diversity. Just as no two snowflakes are identical, no two individuals, even twins, are exactly alike. Our faces, fingerprints, and manner of communication are unique.

The bell-shaped normal curve graphs measurements that are used to distinguish those who are average from those who perform above and below others of the same population (see Figure 2.4). Many language tests use a

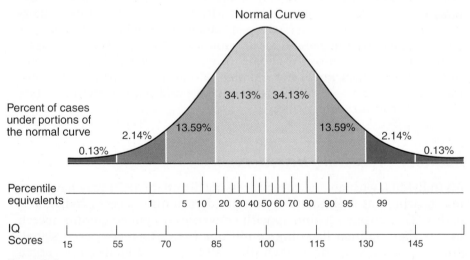

FIGURE 2.4

The normal curve, percentile equivalents, and IQ scores.

Source: Based on information from *Assessing and Screening Preschoolers*, by E. V. Nuttall, I. Romero, and J. Kalesnik, 1992, Boston: Allyn and Bacon: and *Measurement and Assessment*, by E. H. Wiig and W. A. Secord, 1992, Chicago: Riverside Publishing Co.

scoring system comparable to IQ scores. Most people (a little over 68%) of those tested will have IQ scores between 85 and 115. Higher or lower scores are above or below average. An individual who performed in the lowest 5 to 10% achieved a score that is significantly below average (Haynes & Pindzola, 1998).

Because the word *normal* suggests "without problems," we prefer to use the term *typical* when we mean "like most others of the same age and group." Classifying people on the basis of a bell curve, using a statistical percentage cutoff, may be little more than disability "by decree" (Lubker, 1997, p. 4). A more valid approach requires clear definitions of speech and language disorders. We discuss this further in Chapter 4, "Assessment and Intervention."

COMMUNICATION DISORDERS AS SECONDARY TO OTHER DISABILITIES

Most communication disorders are secondary to other disabilities. For example, children with a cleft palate have physical health problems as well as voice and articulation disorders. People with cerebral palsy have motor deficits beyond speech. Children with learning disabilities are especially likely to have language difficulties but may also have articulation, voice, fluency, and/or hearing deficits (Gibbs & Cooper, 1989). In addition, they experience academic and social difficulties.

ESTIMATES OF PREVALENCE

Prevalence refers to the number or percentage of people within a specified population who have a particular disorder or condition at a given point in time. If you determined the prevalence of stuttering in the entire U.S. population, among first-grade children, among college seniors, among U.S. males, or among U.S. females, you would get different prevalence figures in each case. For this reason, prevalence statistics must specify the population on which they are based.

Current estimates suggest that about 17% of the total U.S. population have some communicative disorder. About 11% have a hearing loss, and approximately 6% have a speech, voice, or language disorder. Many of those with hearing losses also have speech, voice, or language disorders. Six to 10 million Americans (about 3% of the population) have a disorder of swallowing (Castrogiovanni, 1999b, 1999c), and many of these individuals also have a communicative impairment. Although these figures are relatively low, it is likely that more, generally mild, cases are not reported (Tierney et al., 2000).

The percentage of people with hearing loss increases with age. Between 1% and 2% of people under 18 years of age have a chronic hearing loss, compared with approximately 32% of those over age 75. Exposure to noise has contributed to the hearing loss in about a third of those affected (Castrogiovanni, 1999a).

Impairments of speech-sound production and fluency are more common in children than adults and more common among males than females.

The terms *incidence* and *prevalence* are often confused. Incidence refers to the number of *new* cases of a disease of disorder in a particular time period. Prevalence is the number of *new and old* cases in a particular time period.

Communication disorders also vary with gender. For example, certain disorders, such as autism spectrum disorder, are four times as prevalent in males.

Speech disorders due to neurological disorders or brain and spinal cord injury occur more often among adults. It has been estimated that anywhere between 3% and 10% of Americans have voice disorders; this percentage is greater among school-age children and people over age 65 (Castrogiovanni, 1999b).

Language disorders occur in 8% to 12% of the preschool population; the prevalence decreases through the school years. Language deficits in older adults may be associated with stroke or dementia. It is likely that 5% to 10% of people over age 65 experience language disabilities related to these disorders (Bello, 1994; Castrogiovanni, 1999b). Table 2.2 highlights some communication disorders that may appear through the lifespan.

TABLE 2.2
....
Communication disorders that may manifest themselves through the lifespan

Age Range	Disorders	Receptive Communication	Expressive Communication	Swallowing
Infancy	Hearing impairment Fetal alcohol or drug-exposure syndrome Parental neglect/abuse Cerebral palsy	Limited response to sound/speech Limited response to others Atypical physical postures and movement	Atypical birth and other early cries Deaf infants vocalize normally for first 6 mos. Others may have little vocalization Passivity	May have difficulties with breast or bottle; later problems with solid foods
Toddler	Autism/Pervasive developmental disorder may be identified (hypersensitive to stimuli) Mental retardation not suspected earlier may now become apparent Brain injury due to falls	Comprehension of spoken language limited	Delay in first spoken word Utterances limited May use objects ritualistically	Rigid food preferences/dislikes Caution needs to be taken to prevent putting small objects in mouth that may be swallowed/ choked on
Preschool	Delays that were suspected earlier may become more pronounced Fluency difficulties may emerge Specific language disabilities Middle ear problems common	Interactions with peers and others may be difficult	Inappropriate use of toys/objects Vocabulary may be limited, utterances short Alternative/ augmentative communication may be recommended Excessive dysfluency; delayed phonology and grammatical development	Food preferences may be more entrenched

TABLE 2.2
....
(Continued)

Age Range	Disorders	Receptive Communication	Expressive Communication	Swallowing
School-Age	Language learning problems Hyperactivity/ Attention deficit disorder Brain injury due to falls and other accidents	Difficulties attending, following directions, speech and reading comprehension	Narrative and other pragmatic skills may be affected	Inappropriate eating habits may become established
Young Adulthood	Brain injury due to bike, motorcycle, car, and other accidents most prevalent in these years	Comprehension affected, generalized confusion, abstract thinking impaired	Pragmatic skills affected Life plans altered Dysarthria and apraxia may affect speech intelligibility	Neuromotor injury may impact on swallowing
Middle Adulthood	Hearing often starts to decline Life-threatening illnesses such as cancer may be diagnosed Neurogenic problems may appear; multiple sclerosis, ALS, Parkinson's, and Alzheimer's diseases; stroke (aphasia)	Speech in noise may be difficult to comprehend Aphasia and Alzheimer's may result in comprehension difficulties	Illness-related depression may affect expressive communication Dysarthria and apraxia may impair speech intelligibility Alzheimer's and aphasia cause language difficulties	Eating/swallowing may be impaired initially following stroke; swallowing difficulties often present in degenerative neuromotor diseases (e.g., multiple sclerosis, ALS)
Advanced Age	Hearing deficits common Neurogenic problems become progressively worse	Difficulty understanding speech may cause "tuning out"	Voice may be weak Word-finding problems Inappropriate speech Perseveration	Disinterest in food, swallowing impairments may lead to aspiration pneumonia

Sources: Information from Owens (2010); Shadden & Toner (1997).

Note: This is a sampling of problems that may be seen. Variability within each age group is the norm.

SUMMARY

Communication is an exchange of ideas; it involves message transmission and response. Human communication is remarkable and may take many forms. It is strongly influenced by culture and environment. Not only do people speak different languages, but within language groups, age, gender, socioeconomic status, geographical background, ethnicity, and other factors influence our communication.

The primary vehicle of human communication is language. It may be spoken, written, or signed and has been described in terms of form, content, and use. Form refers to the sound system, or phonology; word structure, or morphology; and syntax, or how the words are arranged in sentences. Content is semantics or meaning, and use is the purpose or pragmatics of the communication. Communication is also transmitted by nonverbal behaviors and characteristics.

A breakdown can occur in any aspect of communication. When communication is unimpaired, we tend to take it for granted, but when it fails us, we may feel frustrated and isolated. About 17% of the U.S. population currently experience some limitation of hearing, speech, and/or language. See the American Speech-Language Hearing Association Web site at the end of the chapter to learn more about various disorders.

THOUGHT QUESTIONS

- How do social and cultural aspects of human beings influence communication?
- In what ways can disorders of communication be described and classified?
- What communication disorders are likely to be diagnosed in different age groups?
- How do the sociolinguistic factors that describe you influence your communication? What variations in communication might be due to age, gender, and ethnicity?

SUGGESTED READINGS

Axtell, R. (1998). Gestures: *The do's and taboos of body language around the world.* Rev. ed. New York: Wiley.

Hirsh-Pasek, K., & Golinkoff, R. (1999). *The origins of grammar: Evidence from early language.* Cambridge, MA: MIT Press.

Ruben, B., & Stewart, L. (2006). *Communication and human behavior* (5th ed.). Boston: Pearson Education.

ONLINE RESOURCES

American Speech-Language-Hearing Association
www.asha.org
ASHA Web site discusses various disorders that affect children and adults who may benefit from the help of the speech-language pathologist.

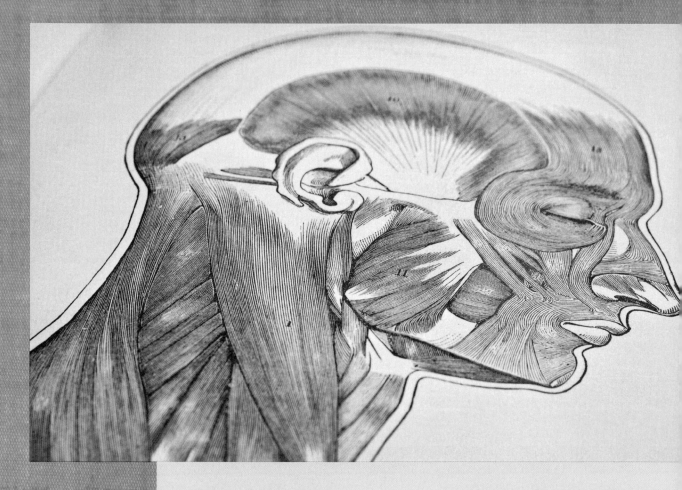

CHAPTER LEARNING GOALS

When you finish this chapter, you should be able to:

- List and describe the structures of the respiratory, laryngeal, and articulatory/resonating systems

- Explain the respiratory processes for quiet breathing and for speech breathing

- Explain the phonation process

- Explain the articulatory and resonating processes for human speech

- Explain the motor speech production process

3

Anatomy and Physiology Related to Speech, Hearing, and Language

Speech production is generally taken for granted as a biological function that takes care of itself; your thoughts and ideas are expressed with little or no apparent effort. But for all its apparent simplicity, the production of speech requires an incredibly complex coordination of biophysical events involving hundreds of muscles and millions of nerves. It is paradoxical that such complex physiological behavior appears to be so effortless. This natural paradox, however, is probably necessary. If we had full conscious comprehension of what we are doing when we speak, we would probably be unable to utter a single word. Monitoring all the nerves and muscles, the tone of the voice, facial expression, and word order would be an impossible intellectual feat (Thomas, 1979).

For many individuals, however, speech production is anything but effortless. Sometimes abnormalities of anatomical structures and physiological systems that support speech interfere with the speech production process. Thus knowledge of the anatomy and physiology of the speech mechanism is fundamental to understanding many different communication disorders that are evaluated and treated by speech-language pathologists. Successful treatment of voice and swallowing disorders, laryngectomy (the surgical removal of the larynx), and cleft palate requires a thorough understanding of the anatomy and physiology of the speech mechanism.

THE PHYSIOLOGICAL SUBSYSTEMS SUPPORTING SPEECH

Anatomy is the study of the structures of the body and the relationship of these structures to one another. **Physiology** is a branch of biology and is defined as a science concerned with the functions of organisms and bodily structures.

Harvard neuroscientist Steven Pinker says, "One easy way to understand speech sounds is to track a glob of air through the vocal tract into the world, starting in the lungs." (Pinker, 1995, p. 163). Obviously, the production of speech is more complicated than Pinker's musing, but speech production does require control of air pressure and air flow from your lungs through your vocal tract into the atmosphere. Three physiological subsystems are involved in speech production: (1) the **respiratory system** provides the driving force for speech by generating positive air pressure values beneath the vocal folds; (2) the vocal folds, anatomical structures in the **laryngeal system** or *larynx*, vibrate at high rates of speed, setting air molecules in the vocal tract into multiple frequencies of vibration; and finally, (3) the **articulatory/resonating system** acts as an acoustic filter allowing certain frequencies to pass into the atmosphere while simultaneously blocking other frequencies. In this chapter, we discuss the structures, muscles, and physiology of the subsystems of speech production, and address the changes in each across the lifespan.

The Respiratory System

The primary biological functions of your respiratory system are to supply oxygen to the blood and to remove excess carbon dioxide from the body. This process is automatic and controlled by the respiratory centers located within the brainstem of the central nervous system. Although the primary function of respiration is to sustain life, it also serves as the generating source for speech production. Air is inhaled into your lungs to become the potential energy source for sound production. The air is then expelled in a controlled manner, to be modified by your vocal folds and articulators to generate speech sounds.

STRUCTURES OF THE RESPIRATORY SYSTEM

Figure 3.1 illustrates the primary components of the adult respiratory system, including (1) the pulmonary apparatus, which is further subdivided into the lungs, the trachea (windpipe), and the pulmonary airways, and (2) the chest wall (thorax), comprising the rib cage wall, the abdominal wall, the abdominal content, and the diaphragm (Hixon & Hoit, 2005). The structures of the chest wall surround and encase the pulmonary apparatus, and together they form a single functional unit (Hixon et al., 2008).

The **lungs** are a pair of air-filled elastic sacs that change in size and shape and allow us to breathe. They are cone shaped and have a porous, spongy

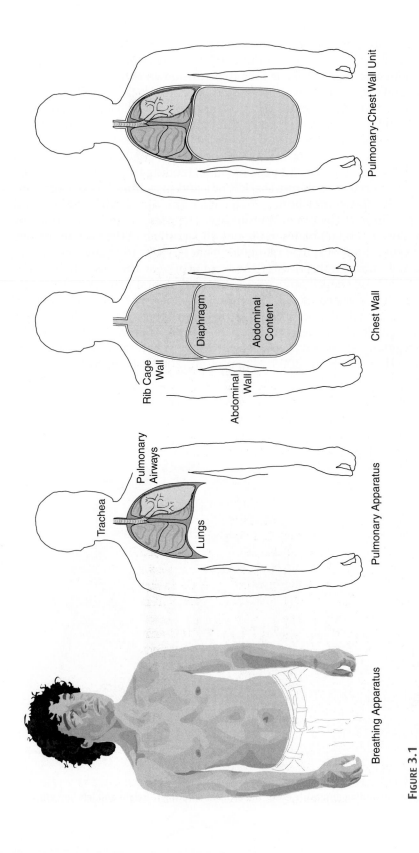

FIGURE 3.1
....
Breathing apparatus and its subdivisions.

Source: From *Evaluation and Management of Speech Breathing Disorders: Principles and Methods* (p. 13), by T. Hixon and J. Hoit, 2005, Tucson, AZ: Redington Brown. Copyright 2005 by Thomas J. Hixon and Jeannette D. Hoit. Reprinted with permission.

texture. The left lung is smaller than the right to allow room for the heart. Air moves to and from the lungs via the **trachea,** or windpipe. The trachea is a cartilaginous and membraneous tube that runs down through the neck into the torso and divides into two smaller tubes, one into each lung. These are the mainstem *bronchi*. As these two tubes continue on, they divide over and over, extending and traveling further down through the lungs, creating an intricate network of *pulmonary airways*. Refer to Figure 3.2.

The rib cage wall is a framework of bone and cartilage that surrounds the lungs. It consists of the 12 pairs of ribs extending from the thoracic segment of the vertebral column (backbone) and attaching to cartilage connected to the flat center bone, or the sternum, along with the pectoral (shoulder) girdle at the top of the rib cage. The pectoral girdle is formed by the two clavicle (collar) bones in the front that attach at the back to the two flat, triangular bony scapulae (shoulder blades). Refer to Figure 3.3a.

The abdominal wall provides the framework for the lower half of the torso. It is oblong shaped and consists of the vertebral column at the back, with 15 of the 32 vertebrae (i.e., 5 lumbar, 5 sacral, 5 coccygeal) that extend from approximately the bottom of the rib cage to the coccyx (tailbone) and the pelvic girdle (bony pelvis). The pelvic girdle is comprised of the two large, irregularly shaped hip bones together with the sacral and coccygeal vertebrae (Hixon & Hoit, 2005; Hixon et al., 2008). Refer to Figures 3.3a and 3.3b.

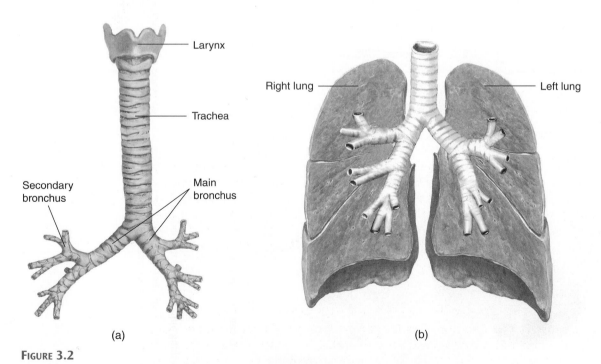

(a)   (b)

FIGURE 3.2

Anterior view of the trachea and bronchi (a) and an anterior view of the bronchi entering the right and left lungs (b).

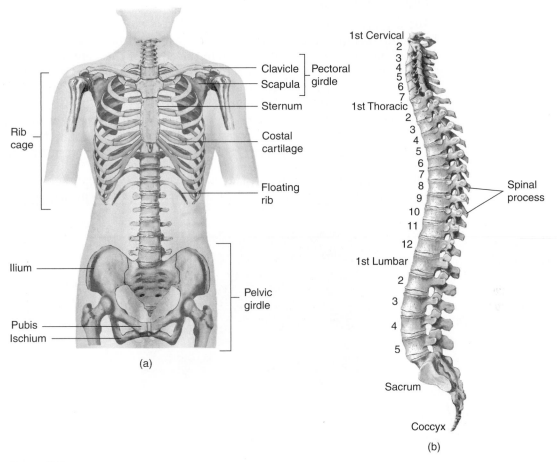

FIGURE 3.3
....
Anterior view of the thorax and pelvis (a) and a lateral view of the vertebral column (b).

The abdominal wall is covered by two broad sheets of connective tissue; the one in the front is called the **abdominal aponeurosis,** and the one in the back is the lumbodorsal fascia. The abdominal aponeurosis, along with the abdominal muscles (discussed later in this section), enclose and help support the abdominal content, which include all of the structures in the abdominal cavity such as the stomach and intestines (Hixon & Hoit, 2005).

MUSCLES OF THE RESPIRATORY SYSTEM

The respiratory muscles are divided functionally into muscles of inspiration and muscles of expiration. Inspiratory muscles are generally found above the diaphragm; expiratory muscles are located below the diaphragm. With the exception of the diaphragm, all respiratory muscles are paired (i.e., located on both the right and left sides of the body).

INSPIRATORY MUSCLES

The diaphragm is the principal muscle of inspiration. It is a dome-shaped structure composed of a thin, flat, nonelastic central tendon and a broad rim of muscle fibers that radiate up to the edges of this central tendon. The central tendon is in direct contact with each lung as shown in Figure 3.4a. The diaphragm separates the thorax (chest) from the abdomen. At rest, it looks like an inverted bowl (Hixon & Hoit, 2005). Figure 3.4b shows the relative position of the diaphragm at rest. When the diaphragm contracts during inspiration, it pulls downward and forward, thus enlarging the thorax. The lungs in turn are pulled in a downward direction, resulting in an increase in lung volume.

In addition to the diaphragm, numerous thoracic and neck muscles contribute to inspiration. For example, *external intercostals*, which include

FIGURE 3.4
....

Anterior view of the relationship of the diaphragm to the lungs (a) and an anterior view of the diaphragm at rest (b).

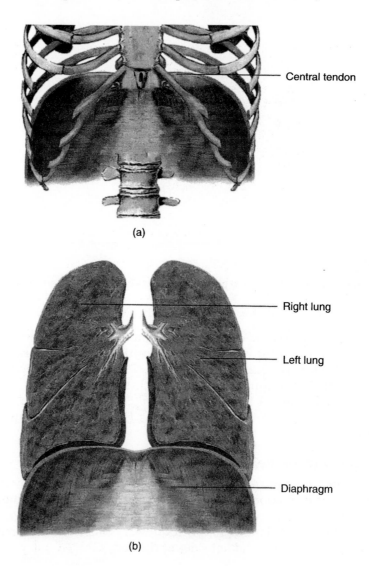

Central tendon

(a)

Right lung

Left lung

Diaphragm

(b)

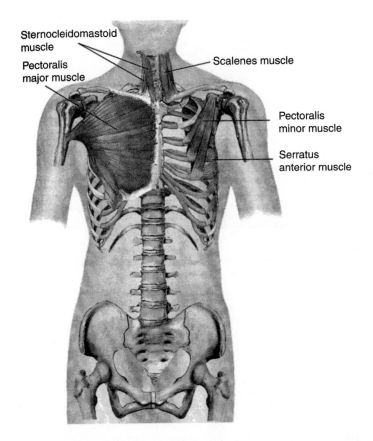

FIGURE 3.5

Anterior view of thoracic muscles.

Sternocleidomastoid muscle

Pectoralis major muscle

Scalenes muscle

Pectoralis minor muscle

Serratus anterior muscle

11 (paired) muscles located in the spaces between the outer portions of the ribs, elevate the rib cage when they contract. The external intercostals thereby assist in increasing the size of the thoracic cavity during inspiration. Other muscles that serve to elevate the ribs and expand the thorax during inspiration include the *pectoralis major muscle, pectoralis minor muscle, serratus anterior muscle*, and *levatores costarum*. These muscles, with the exception of the *levatores costarum* muscles located on the posterior rib cage wall, are illustrated in Figure 3.5.

The *sternocleidomastoid* is a major muscle of the neck that also assists in elevating the rib cage. When it contracts, it pulls up on the sternum and the first two ribs during inspiration. A similar action is performed by the scalene muscles, which are also muscles of the neck shown in Figure 3.5.

MUSCLES OF EXPIRATION

Expiration allows carbon dioxide to be expelled from the body via the lungs and for speech to be produced. The *internal intercostal muscles*, which lie underneath the external intercostals, are important for speech production because they help control the descent of the rib cage during expiration. Recall that the external intercostal muscles are important during inspiration. Figure 3.6 illustrates the internal and external intercostal muscles.

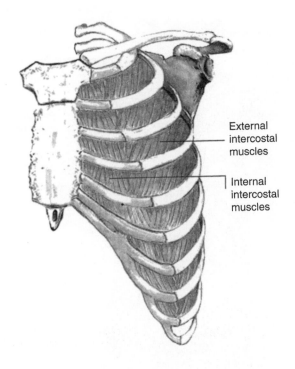

External
intercostal
muscles

Internal
intercostal
muscles

The most important muscles of expiration are located in the front and on the sides of the abdomen. The *external oblique, internal oblique, transverse abdominis,* and the *rectus abdominis* are four paired muscles that encase a portion of the abdominal wall. Contraction of the abdominal muscles pulls the lower ribs and sternum downward and forces the abdominal wall inward. During expiration, these muscles, depicted in Figure 3.7, assist the diaphragm's movement back to its relaxed dome-shaped configuration. Abdominal muscles are attached to the skeleton by means of the *abdominal aponeurosis,* the broad sheet of connective tissue that covers the front of the abdominal wall.

Numerous other muscles located on the front and back of the thorax may also contribute to respiration. The use of other muscles during inspiration and expiration may be related to body position, certain pathological states, and environmental conditions.

THE PHYSIOLOGY OF TIDAL BREATHING AND SPEECH BREATHING

Quiet breathing, or **resting tidal breathing,** is breathing to sustain life. As you are reading this chapter, you are using tidal breathing. The rate and depth of breaths taken during tidal breathing are determined by your body's oxygen needs and the amount of carbon dioxide in the blood. Resting tidal breathing involves contraction of the diaphragm, moving it downward and slightly forward, which in turn expands the rib cage wall and moves the abdominal wall outward (Hixon & Hoit, 2005). Expansion of the rib cage wall also causes expansion of the lungs. This results in an increase in lung volume and a decrease in **alveolar pressure** (i.e., pressure within the lungs) below that of atmospheric pressure. Air then rushes into the lungs,

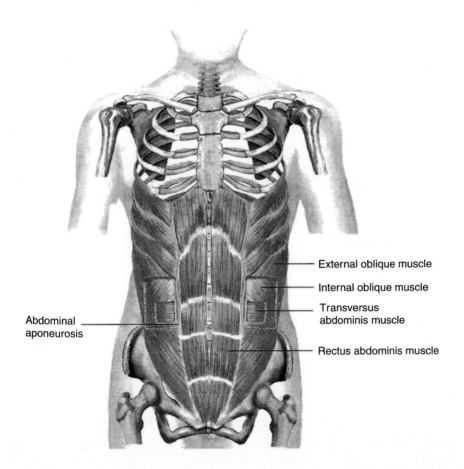

FIGURE 3.7

Anterior view of abdominal musculature. Muscles are cut to illustrate the different layers of muscle.

External oblique muscle

Internal oblique muscle

Transversus abdominis muscle

Rectus abdominis muscle

Abdominal aponeurosis

equalizing alveolar pressure with atmospheric pressure. Approximately 0.5 L of air are inhaled during quiet breathing.

When the resting tidal inspiratory cycle ends, expiration (or exhalation) begins. Expiration results from the decrease in the size of the rib cage wall, and thus compression of the lungs, which in turn increases the pressure within the lungs (Hixon & Hoit, 2005). Air then rushes out of the lungs until equilibrium with atmospheric pressure is reached. Expiration during quiet breathing does not require active muscle contraction. Rather, it is achieved by gravity and the natural tendency (i.e., passive recoil) of the pulmonary-chest wall unit to return to its relaxed state. A respiratory cycle is defined as one inhalation followed by one exhalation. During resting tidal breathing, the duration of inspiration and expiration are relatively equal.

Breathing for purposes of speech production differs from resting tidal breathing in a number of ways. First, contraction of the diaphragm produces rapid, forceful inspirations. Furthermore, the time spent inhaling is short relative to the time spent exhaling which is much longer. You may inhale as much as 2 L of air during speech breathing depending on the specific demands of the utterance. Most people begin speaking at lung volumes that are higher than those achieved during resting tidal breathing. This allows for the generation of more passive recoil pressures that can be

Speech breathing differs from quiet breathing in many ways, but the oxygen and carbon dioxide ratio in the blood is the same for both types of breathing.

FIGURE 3.8

Volume, pressure, and shape events for an extended steady utterance produced in the upright body position.

Source: From *Evaluation and Management of Speech Breathing Disorders: Principles and Methods* (p. 57), by T. Hixon and J. Hoit, 2005, Tucson, AZ: Redington Brown. Copyright 2005 by Thomas J. Hixon and Jeannette D. Hoit. Reprinted with permission.

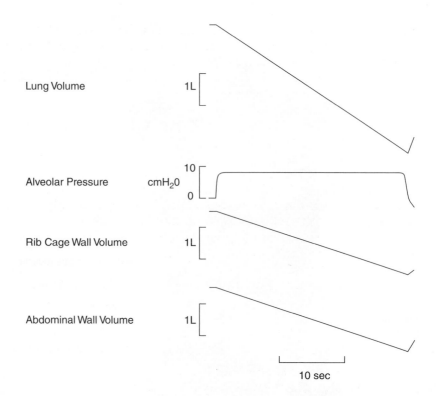

used during expiration to produce running speech. Unlike expiration during quiet breathing, active muscle contraction of both inspiratory and expiratory muscles is needed during speech to prevent all of the air from rushing out of the lungs too quickly. At the beginning of an utterance, muscles of inspiration may be active (i.e., diaphragm and external intercostals), along with active contraction of expiratory muscles of the rib cage and abdominal wall, which is especially important in sustaining alveolar pressure for longer utterances. Of note, expiratory muscle activation is maintained during inspiration, which allows these muscles to be in a state of readiness for speech production, thereby increasing efficiency. Refer to Figure 3.8.

LIFESPAN ISSUES OF THE RESPIRATORY SYSTEM

At birth, you had a rest breathing rate between 30 and 80 breaths per minute. By age 3, your tidal breathing rate decreased to values between 20 and 30 breaths per minute. This change in rate is due to the fact that newborns have very few alveoli, the areas where gas exchange occur in the lungs. Alveoli increase in number with age such that by adulthood, there are several hundred thousand (Kent, 1997; Zemlin, 1998). Watch preschool children and make note of their more frequent and deeper inhalations relative to adults. By age 7, the number of alveoli approaches adult values; however, children this age tend to use larger lung volumes, larger abdominal wall volumes, and generate greater lung pressures during speech compared to adults, even though loudness levels are similar. By 10 years of age, the respiratory system functions in a more adultlike fashion. Tidal breathing rates are between 17 and 22 breaths per minute, and lung and abdominal wall volumes and lung pressures during speech production more closely approximate those used by adults (Hixon & Hoit, 2005).

As children grow, the structures of the respiratory system increase in size, and, in turn, lung capacity increases. Maximum lung capacities are reached in early adulthood and remain fairly constant until middle age. Respiratory function is affected by age beginning in the seventh or eighth decade of life. Hoit and Hixon (1987) found that 75 year-old adults use larger lung volumes and larger lung volume excursions during speech production when compared to 25-year-old adults. This is presumably to compensate for potential air loss at the level of the larynx (due to age-related changes of the vocal folds discussed later in this chapter) and air wastage occurring during pauses (Sperry & Klich, 1992).

Respiratory function is also affected by exercise, health, and smoking. It is estimated that smoking in older people could result in a 500 mL (approximately 1 pint) cumulative loss in pulmonary function every 10 years (Kent, 1997).

The Laryngeal System

The **larynx** is an air valve composed of cartilages, muscles, and other tissue. It is the principal sound generator for speech production, colloquially known as the "voice box," and sits on top of the trachea opening up into the pharynx (throat). The larynx's primary biological function is to prevent foreign objects from entering the trachea and lungs. Additionally, the larynx can impound air for forceful expulsion of foreign objects that threaten the lower airways.

The structural support of the larynx, its musculature, and how it is used for speech production are discussed in this section. Figure 3.9 illustrates the skeletal framework of the larynx and its principal components.

STRUCTURES OF THE LARYNGEAL SYSTEM

The hyoid bone is a horseshoe-shaped structure that serves as the point of attachment for both laryngeal and tongue musculature. It lies horizontally in the neck and is positioned at the top of the larynx. It is considered free floating because it is not connected to any other bones in the body. The larynx appears to be suspended from the hyoid bone by various attachments. You can locate the two posterior ends

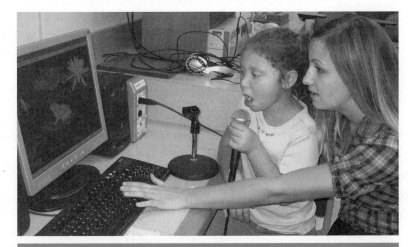

This client is using biofeedback to monitor speech production.

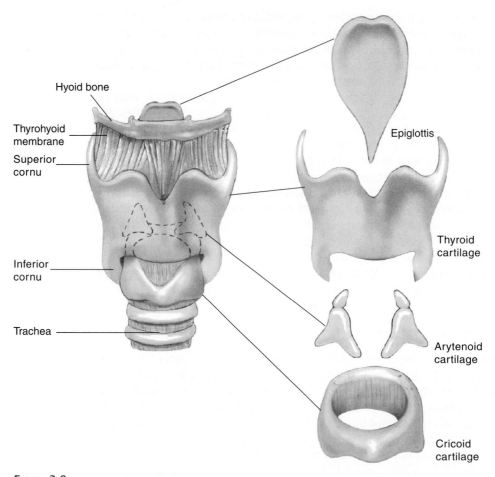

Figure 3.9
....

Anterior view of the skeletal framework of the larynx.

of the major horns of your hyoid bone. Place your thumb and middle finger on the lower angle of your jaw. Slide your fingers down about 1 inch and push in. You will feel two prominences that you can move from side to side. These prominences are the posterior projections of your hyoid bone.

The larynx consists of several cartilages connected to one another by ligaments and membranes. The *thyroid cartilage* is the largest laryngeal cartilage. It forms most of the front and sides of the laryngeal skeleton. The upper part has a V-shaped depression called the thyroid notch. It can be felt by palpating the front of the neck. Just below this notch is a jutting protrusion called the *thyroid prominence,* or Adam's apple (Hixon et al., 2008), which can be very prominent in some adult men.

The back edges of the thyroid cartilage have two long upper horns, called the *superior cornua,* and two short lower horns, called the *inferior cornua.* The upper horns connect the thyroid cartilage with the hyoid bone, and the lower horns connect the thyroid and cricoid cartilages.

The *cricoid cartilage* is a ring-shaped structure that sits immediately above the first tracheal ring and directly below the thyroid cartilage. It forms the lower aspect of the laryngeal skeleton. On the upper, sloping rim of the posterior border of each cricoid cartilage are the *arytenoid cartilages*. These paired cartilages are pyramidal shaped and have an apex (top), a base, and three sides. The base of each arytenoid cartilage has a forward pointed projection called the *vocal process*, and a rounded broad projection extending toward the back called the *muscular process* (Hixon et al., 2008).

The epiglottis is a large leaf-shaped cartilage attached at its lower end to the thyroid cartilage just below the thyroid notch. Its midportion is attached to the body of the hyoid bone and its upper part is free, extending to the root of the tongue. The epiglottis has no role in speech production. Rather it assists in preventing food from entering the larynx and lower airways during swallowing.

The Vocal Folds

The vocal folds are attached at the front near the midline of the thyroid cartilage and at the back to the vocal processes of the arytenoid cartilages via the vocal ligament. When viewed from above, the paired vocal folds appear to be ivory-colored bands of tissue. They abduct (move apart) during respiration and adduct (move together) during phonation.

The vocal folds are made up of five different layers. The outermost layer is a thin, stiff epithelial tissue, followed by three layers of lamina propria, and finally, an innermost layer of muscle fibers, with the *thyroarytenoid muscle* forming the bulk of each vocal fold. These five layers are subgrouped into the *body*, which includes the muscle fibers and the deepest layer of lamina propria, and the *cover*, consisting of the intermediate and superficial layers of lamina propria and the epithelium (Hixon et al., 2008).

Figure 3.10 depicts the human vocal folds during a single vibratory cycle. Sustained vocal fold vibration is shown on the book's CD-ROM.

Muscles of the Larynx

The laryngeal muscles are divided into three groups: intrinsic, extrinsic, and supplementary muscles (Zemlin, 1998). The intrinsic muscles, illustrated in Figure 3.11, are critical for phonation and for modifying the pitch and loudness of the voice. Intrinsic muscles have both points of attachment on the larynx itself. They are the posterior cricoarytenoid, lateral cricoarytenoid, interarytenoid, thyroarytenoid, and cricothyroid muscles.

The *posterior cricoarytenoid muscle* is the sole muscle of abduction. Contraction of this muscle rotates the vocal processes of the arytenoid cartilages away from the midline, separating the vocal folds and opening the *glottis*, or area between the vocal folds. Muscles of adduction include the *lateral cricoarytenoid* and the *interarytenoid*. The lateral cricoarytenoid is a small fan-shaped muscle that rotates the arytenoids toward midline when it contracts, drawing the vocal folds together and closing the glottis. Contraction of the interarytenoid muscle pulls the arytenoids together, thereby assisting in vocal fold adduction.

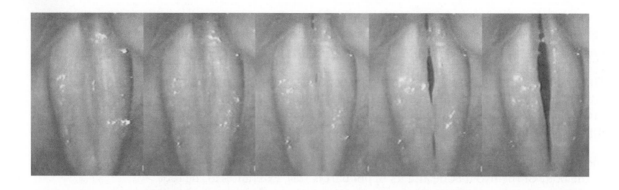

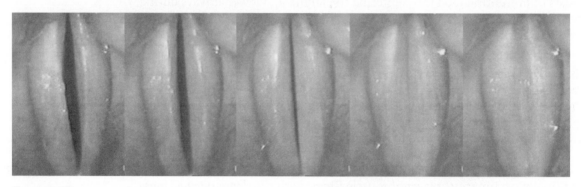

FIGURE 3.10

Stroboscopic film images of the vocal folds during one complete vibratory cycle. (Photograph courtesy of Robert Orlikoff, Ph.D., West Virginia University).

Muscles that tense the vocal folds include the *thyroarytenoid muscle* and the *cricothyroid muscle.* The thyroarytenoid muscle is attached to the inside surface of the thyroid cartilage and arytenoid cartilage on the same side (see Figure 3.11). It is often described as having two distinct bundles: the external thyroarytenoid muscle (thyromuscularis) and the internal thyroarytenoid (thyrovocalis). The thyrovocalis makes up the main vibrating mass of the vocal folds. Contraction of the thyroarytenoid muscle draws the arytenoid cartilages forward, reducing the distance between the thyroid and arytenoid cartilages, thus tensing the vocal folds. The thyroarytenoid muscle is important for adjusting (raising or lowering) pitch, and with increased activation, is also associated with higher loudness levels, particularly in the low pitch range (Hirano et al., 1970; Isshiki, 1964).

The *cricothyroid* is a fan-shaped muscle with its fibers extending outward as they course from the cricoid cartilage to the thyroid cartilage. Contraction of this muscle pulls the thyroid away from the arytenoid cartilages, altering the length and tension of the folds. The cricothyroid muscle is therefore important for increasing pitch.

Extrinsic laryngeal muscles support and stabilize the larynx. They are the *sternothyroid, thyrohyoid,* and *inferior constrictor muscles.* Two extrinsic laryngeal muscles are shown in Figure 3.12.

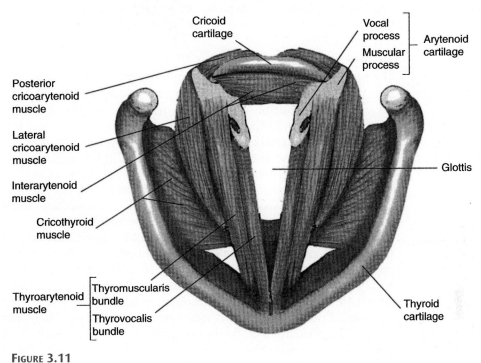

Cricoid cartilage

Vocal process

Muscular process

Arytenoid cartilage

Posterior cricoarytenoid muscle

Lateral cricoarytenoid muscle

Interarytenoid muscle

Cricothyroid muscle

Glottis

Thyroarytenoid muscle

Thyromuscularis bundle

Thyrovocalis bundle

Thyroid cartilage

FIGURE 3.11

Superior view of intrinsic laryngeal muscles.

Supplemental muscles generally have one point of attachment on the hyoid bone and are subdivided into the suprahyoid and infrahyoid groups. Muscles in the suprahyoid group are generally located above the hyoid bone and assist in laryngeal elevation. Those in the infrahyoid group are generally located below the hyoid bone and assist in laryngeal depression. Place your

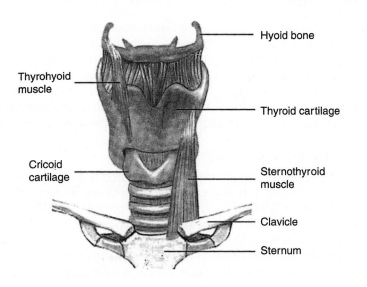

Hyoid bone

Thyrohyoid muscle

Thyroid cartilage

Cricoid cartilage

Sternothyroid muscle

Clavicle

Sternum

FIGURE 3.12

Anterior view of two extrinsic muscles of the larynx.

hand on your larynx and swallow. Note that your larynx is pulled upward and then lowered. This motion is a result of supplemental muscle contraction.

LIFESPAN ISSUES OF THE LARYNGEAL SYSTEM

The laryngeal system also goes through significant changes as a function of age. In the newborn, the larynx is small and positioned very high in the neck. The high position of the larynx near the hyoid bone allows the newborn to breathe and nurse simultaneously while protection of the airway is maintained. The larynx begins to move downward in the neck during the first year of life and reaches its final position in the region of the seventh cervical vertebra between 10 and 20 years of age (Hixon et al., 2008).

The laryngeal cartilages also increase in size and become less pliable with age. The hyoid bone ossifies (turns to bone) by 2 years of age. The vocal folds are approximately 4 to 6 mm long in the newborn. By age 6, they increase to about 8 or 9 mm in length. The increase in length of the vocal folds is equal in boys and girls until puberty. During puberty, the vocal folds increase to approximately 12 to 17 mm in girls, and 15 to 25 mm in boys. By adulthood, females' vocal folds are about 21 mm in length; males' are about 29 mm in length (Kent, 1997). The sex difference in adult vocal fold length accounts for the fact that men normally have lower pitched voices than women.

With advancing age, laryngeal cartilages begin to ossify, although the female larynx, unlike the male's, never completely ossifies. The vocal folds begin to lose muscle tissue (atrophy) while the more superficial layers of vocal fold tissue thicken and lose their elasticity. As a result, the vocal folds become stiffer and less flexible with age. Age effects are realized in men as an increase in pitch, likely due to muscle atrophy and loss of mass of the folds. Women, in contrast, experience a decrease in pitch with age, likely due to hormone-related changes associated with menopause (Stoicheff, 1981).

The Articulatory/Resonating System

The articulatory/resonating system extends from the opening of the mouth to the vocal folds, and comprises the oral cavity, the nasal cavity, and the pharyngeal cavity as shown in Figure 3.13. Together these three cavities form your vocal tract, which is a resonant acoustic tube that shapes the sound energy produced by the respiratory and laryngeal systems into all of the English speech sounds (Kent, 1997). Structures important for speech production such as the teeth, tongue, and velum (soft palate) are housed within these three cavities.

STRUCTURES OF THE ARTICULATORY/RESONATING SYSTEM

The articulatory/resonating system consists largely of the 22 bones that make up the facial skeleton and cranium (braincase). Some of these bones are shown in Figure 3.14. With the exception of the *mandible* (lower jaw), the bones of the face and cranium are fused tightly together by sutures. The mandible articulates with the temporal bone by means of a complex joint known as the *temporomandibular joint (TMJ)*. This joint allows the mandible to move up and down and side to side, which is necessary for chewing.

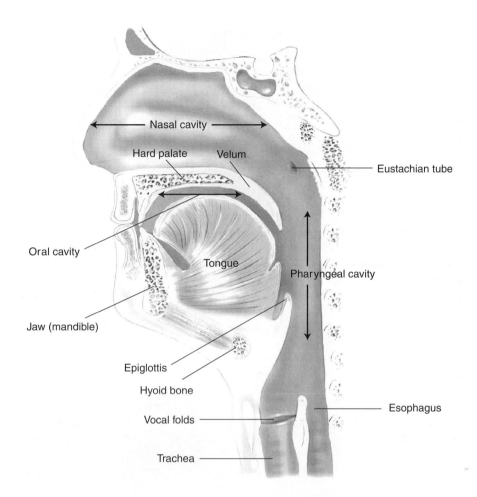

FIGURE 3.13
················
Schematic of the human
vocal tract.

TEETH

Adults have a total of 32 teeth that are held within the *alveolar processes* (thick spongy projections) of the mandible and *maxilla* (upper jaw) inside the oral cavity. The obvious biological function of teeth is chewing food, but the teeth are also important for production of some English speech sounds.

Horizontal bones of the maxilla form the bony hard palate, which comprises the front two thirds of the roof of the mouth. Figure 3.15 shows the structures of the bony hard palate and the relationship of the maxillary teeth.

TONGUE

The principal structure within the oral cavity important for speech production is the tongue. The tongue is a muscular hydrostat, meaning it has no bone or cartilage, much like an elephant's trunk. It provides its own structural support through contraction of its muscles but also has a "soft skeleton" of connective tissue that surrounds and separates its different components (Hixon et al., 2008; Kent, 1997). It can be functionally divided into five parts: the *body*, or central mass, the *root*, which forms the front wall

FIGURE 3.14

Anterior (a) and lateral (b) views of skull bones.

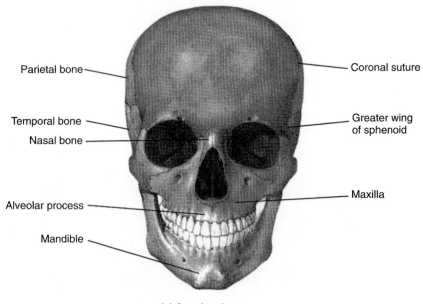

Parietal bone

Coronal suture

Temporal bone

Nasal bone

Greater wing of sphenoid

Alveolar process

Maxilla

Mandible

(a) Anterior view

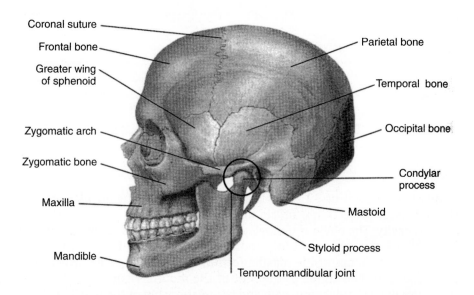

Coronal suture

Frontal bone

Greater wing of sphenoid

Zygomatic arch

Zygomatic bone

Maxilla

Mandible

Parietal bone

Temporal bone

Occipital bone

Condylar process

Mastoid

Styloid process

Temporomandibular joint

(b) Lateral view

of the pharyngeal cavity, the broad surface called the *dorsum;* the *blade* that makes up its front surface and lies just behind the *tongue tip* (Kent, 1997).

The tongue is made up of four intrinsic muscles and four extrinsic muscles. Intrinsic tongue muscles are confined to the tongue itself and include the *superior longitudinal, inferior longitudinal, vertical,* and *transverse* muscles.

The *superior longitudinal muscle* pulls the lateral margins of the tongue up, forming a trough-like shape. Contraction of the *inferior longitudinal*

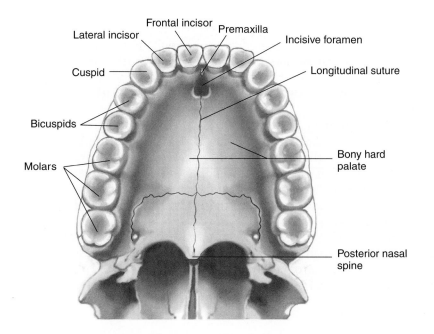

FIGURE 3.15

Inferior view of an adult bony hard palate and teeth.

muscle shortens the tongue and pulls the tongue tip downward. The tongue can be narrowed and elongated or broadened and flattened by contraction of the *transverse* and *vertical* muscles, respectively.

The extrinsic tongue muscles originate from structures outside the tongue and insert on various locations within the tongue, blending with intrinsic muscle fibers. They are the *styloglossus, palatoglossus, hyoglossus,* and *genioglossus* muscles. The extrinsic muscles are responsible for changing the position of the tongue in the oral cavity. Figure 3.16 shows the locations of some of the intrinsic and extrinsic tongue muscles.

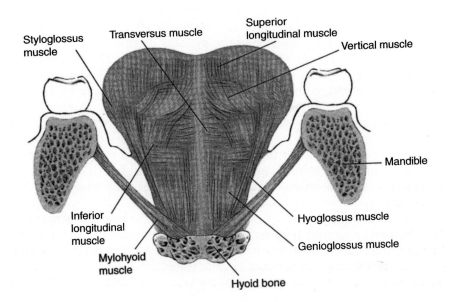

FIGURE 3.16

Coronal section of the tongue.

VELUM

The velum, or soft palate, located in the pharynx, is an important structure for both speech and swallowing. You can see a portion of your velum by looking into a well-illuminated bathroom mirror. You will see a structure projecting downward called the **uvula;** the uvula is the termination of your velum.

When you breathe through your nose, the velum hangs like a curtain from the posterior aspect of the bony hard palate. During swallowing and speech production, the velum elevates and decouples (separates) the nasal cavity from the pharyngeal cavity, leading to **velopharyngeal closure,** or contact of the velum with the lateral and posterior pharyngeal walls (Kuehn & Henne, 2003). Failure to separate these cavities during swallowing would result in food passing through the nasal cavity.

During speech production, velar elevation is necessary to prevent air from escaping through the nose and allow sufficient air pressure to build up in the oral cavity for production of pressure sounds (e.g., /p/, /b/). Any air that escapes through the nose during speech can result in a nasal-sounding resonance (quality).

LIFESPAN ISSUES OF THE ARTICULATORY/RESONATING SYSTEM

The bones of the skull grow rapidly during the first years of life and reach adult size by about 8 years of age. At birth, the newborn has 45 separate skull bones that ultimately fuse into 22 bones by adulthood. Once they fuse together, the cranium appears to be one solid bone.

The bones of the lower portion of the face grow at a much slower rate than bones of the skull. These lower facial bones do not reach maximum adult size until about 18 years of age. Because of these different growth patterns of the skull bones and the facial bones, the face is able to grow downward and forward relative to the cranium (Kent, 1997).

Dentition in the infant begins to emerge at about 6 months of age. This first set of teeth is temporary and is usually referred to as primary or deciduous dentition. Emergence of the primary dentition is usually complete by 3 years of age. At approximately 5 years of age, the primary teeth begin to fall out and the permanent or secondary teeth begin to appear. The emergence of the secondary teeth is usually complete by 18 years of age.

The tongue of the newborn occupies most of the oral cavity (Kent, 1997). During the first several years of life, the posterior portion of the tongue descends into the pharyngeal cavity. The tongue reaches its mature size at about 16 years of age. In general, the growth of the tongue is similar to the growth of the mandible (lower jaw) and to the lips (Kent, 1997).

Finally, as one ages, the length and volume of the oral cavity increases. This anatomical change influences the overall resonant characteristics of the vocal tract in males and females by lowering the frequencies at which the vocal tract naturally resonates (Xue & Hao, 2003).

THE SPEECH PRODUCTION PROCESS

The production of speech begins with the sound produced by vocal fold vibration, or **phonation.** Phonation is initiated by approximating or adducting the vocal folds and closing the glottis or opening. Once the vocal folds are closed, air pressure generated by the respiratory system increases beneath the vocal folds. Recall that the air pressure generated by the respiratory system that builds beneath the vocal folds is called alveolar pressure. Figure 3.17 is a simple illustration of the vocal folds during one cycle of vibration.

The air pressure from below displaces the lower edges of each vocal fold laterally (apart). This is followed by lateral displacement of the upper edges of each vocal fold, until the vocal folds are fully separated, opening the airway (frames 1, 2, 3, and 4 of Figure 3.17). Following maximum opening of the folds, the vocal folds' natural elastic restoring forces causes the lower edges of the folds to begin to move inward toward midline, followed by the upper edges until the vocal folds collide with each other, closing off the airway (frames 5, 6, and 7 of Figure 3.17). The entire process is repeated in a cyclical fashion at the **fundamental frequency** of vibration, or the number of cycles (i.e., opening and closing of the vocal folds) per second (Story, 2002).

Because lateral displacement of the lower portion of the vocal folds precedes lateral displacement of the upper portion, the upper and lower portions of the vocal folds are said to be out of phase. It is this *vertical phase difference* that contributes to self-sustained vibration of the vocal folds and not the *Bernoulli effect* (i.e., high air velocity through a narrow tube creates a partial vacuum that serves to "suck" the vocal folds back together), as historically described.

For each vibratory cycle, the air in the vocal tract is set into vibration and sound is produced. The sound that results from vocal fold vibration is complex, consisting of a fundamental frequency, or the lowest frequency component that corresponds to the rate of vocal fold vibration mentioned earlier, and approximately 40 additional higher frequencies called **harmonics.** The harmonic frequencies are whole-number multiples of the fundamental frequency. For example, when the fundamental frequency is 100 Hz, the second harmonic is 200 Hz, the third is 300 Hz, and so on. Figure 3.18 is a stylized spectrum of the complex sound produced by vocal fold vibration. A spectrum

1	2	3	4	5	6	7

     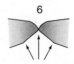

FIGURE 3.17

Anterior view of the vocal folds during one cycle of vibration. Air from the lungs creates a pressure beneath the vocal folds (1, 2, and 3). This pressure causes the vocal folds to separate (4). The natural elastic restoring forces of the vocal folds and the time delay with respect to the upper and lower portions of the vocal folds causes the vocal folds to begin to close (5 and 6). The vocal folds close the glottis to end the cycle, and the next cycle begins (7).

FIGURE 3.18

Spectrum illustrating a
fundamental frequency
of 200 Hz and related
harmonics (a) and a
spectrum of a fundamen-
tal frequency of 100 Hz
and related harmonics (b).

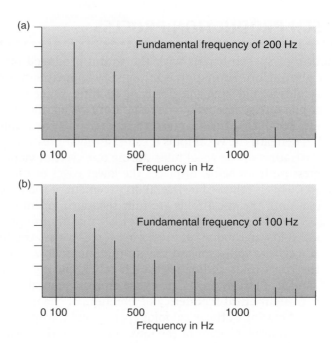

represents the frequencies of a complex sound along the horizontal (x) axis,
and their relative intensity is represented on the vertical (y) axis. Note that
the relative intensity decreases systematically with increases in harmonic frequency. See the Web site listed at the end of the chapter to perform your own
spectral analysis.

The vocal tract is an acoustic resonator that will modify the quality of
the sound produced by your larynx. In any acoustic resonator, some frequencies are reduced or attenuated and other frequencies are enhanced
dependent on certain physical aspects of the resonator.

Movement of the tongue, lips, and larynx will change the shape of the
vocal tract and in turn modify the sound emanating from the larynx. Produce
the vowels /i/ (as in the word "bee") and /u/ (as in the word "boot"). Try to
sense how your tongue and lips change position for the production of these
two vowels. Changes in the position of your lips and tongue in turn change
certain physical characteristics of the vocal tract that directly affect the
quality of the sound that emanates from your mouth.

Air-filled cavities are
acoustic resonators.
The frequency or
frequencies at which
a filled cavity will res-
onate are determined
by the volume of the
cavity, the area of the
opening of the cavity,
and the length of the
opening of the cavity.

Figure 3.19 represents how changes of vocal tract shape influence which
frequencies are enhanced and which are attenuated. A complex sound is
produced by vocal fold vibration (a), and the vocal tract acts as a filter
attenuating some frequencies and enhancing others (b). The sound that
emanates from the mouth during vowel production (c) is related directly to
the general shape of the vocal tract determined largely by tongue position.
Note that for the /u/ vowel, low frequencies are enhanced, whereas high
frequencies are somewhat attenuated. For the /i/ vowel, low frequencies are
somewhat attenuated, whereas high frequencies are enhanced.

During consonant production, your tongue is sometimes used to
momentarily occlude your vocal tract for the production of stop sounds

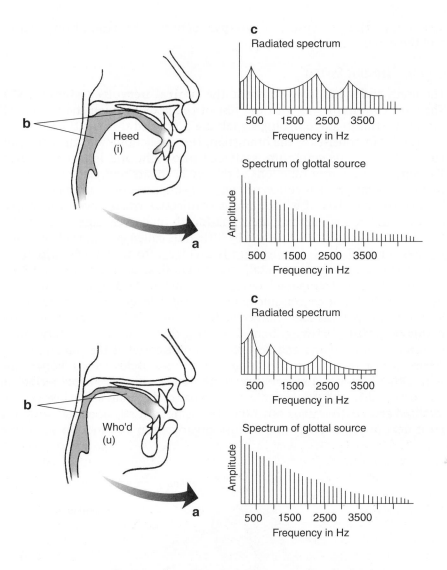

FIGURE 3.19
··················

Spectra of glottal sound source (a) that sets the air in the vocal tract (b) into vibration. The vocal tract filters the glottal sound source differently for the vowels /i/ and /u/ as seen in the radiated spectra (c).

such as /t/, /d/, /k/, and /g/. Production of sounds such as /s/ and /sh/ require your tongue to form a constriction in the vocal tract that will produce frication noise when air is passed through the constriction.

The Nervous System

The nervous system consists of the brain, spinal cord, and all associated nerves and sense organs. The **neuron** is the basic unit of the nervous system. Each neuron has three parts: the *cell body,* a single long *axon* that transmits impulses away from the cell body to the next neuron, and several branching *dendrites* that receive impulses from other cells and transmit them toward the cell body. A nerve is a collection of neurons. Neurons do not actually touch but are close enough such that electrochemical impulses can "jump" the tiny space, or **synapse**, between the axon of one neuron and the dendrites of the next.

CENTRAL NERVOUS SYSTEM

The brain and spinal cord comprise the **central nervous system (CNS).** The CNS communicates with the rest of the body through the nerves. All incoming stimuli and outgoing signals are processed through the CNS.

The brain consists of the brainstem, the cerebellum, and the cerebrum (upper brain). The cerebrum is divided into right and left hemispheres. The sensory and motor functions of the cerebrum are *contralateral*, meaning that each hemisphere is concerned with the opposite side of the body. Each hemisphere consists of white fibrous connective tracts covered by a gray cortex of cell bodies approximately one-fourth inch in thickness. The cortex has a wrinkled appearance caused by little hills called *gyri* and valleys called *fissures,* or *sulci*. Each hemisphere is divided into four lobes, which are labeled frontal, parietal, occipital, and temporal, as depicted in Figure 3.20.

The frontal and temporal lobes are separated by the deep lateral sulcus, or *fissure of Sylvius*. The central sulcus, or *fissure of Rolando*, separates the frontal lobe from the parietal lobe. Immediately in front of the central sulcus is the **primary motor cortex,** a 2-cm-wide strip that controls voluntary motor movements. Just behind and next to the motor cortex is the somatosensory cortex, which receives sensory input from the muscles, joints, bones, and skin. Other motor and sensory functions are found in specialized regions of the cortex. Although it is easier to conceptualize the brain as having specific, localized areas with unique functions, this is not entirely accurate. There is a great deal of redundancy and diffuse organization of function such that

FIGURE 3.20

Schematic diagram of the human brain.

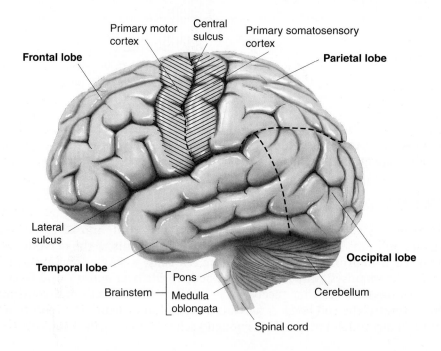

damage to a specific brain region may not completely eliminate the ability to perform that particular function.

HEMISPHERIC ASYMMETRY

Although the cerebral hemispheres are roughly symmetrical, for specialized functions such as language and speech, they are asymmetrical. In 98% of individuals, the left hemisphere is dominant for most aspects of receptive and expressive language and motor speech production. In general, all right-handers and 60 percent of left-handers are left-dominant for language, and the remainder of left-handers are right-dominant. A very small percentage of people have no apparent hemispheric dominance of language function.

The primary anatomical asymmetry in the brain is found in the left temporal lobe. Researchers have questioned whether this asymmetry is present at birth or if left hemispheric specialization for language develops as language is learned. Studies using functional magnetic resonance imaging (fMRI), a non-invasive method of assessing language laterality, have shown a strong left hemispheric language dominance of auditory comprehension abilities in children as young as 7 years of age (Balsamo et al., 2002). Other studies have found predominantly bilateral activation of auditory comprehension in children, however. Continued research is needed in this area using larger sample sizes.

SUBCORTICAL AND LOWER BRAIN STRUCTURES

The **thalamus** consists of a pair of large egg-shaped structures subdivided into topographically organized groups of nuclei (clusters of neuronal cell bodies). The thalamus is a receiving station for relaying information. Thalamic nuclei transmit motor information to muscles and receive sensory information for higher processing in the brain. Further, the thalamus may set the tone for the brain, alerting it to prepare to receive or transmit information.

The **basal ganglia** are large subcortical nuclei that regulate motor functioning and maintain posture and muscle tone. The basal ganglia modulate the activity of motor cortex, thus indirectly influencing movement. This is accomplished by direct and indirect control loops that have opposing functions. The direct pathway serves to increase or facilitate movement; the indirect pathway serves to decrease or inhibit movement. Depending on which pathway is involved, damage to basal ganglia will either result in reduced and/or slowed movement, as seen in Parkinson disease, or will result in abnormal, involuntary movements as seen in Huntington's chorea. Chorea involves quick, continuous, and purposeless movements of the head, face, tongue, and/or limbs (Duffy, 2005).

Located below the cerebrum, the **brainstem** has three longitudinal subdivisions: the midbrain, pons, and medulla, which are important for regulating respiration, chewing, swallowing, and automatic functions of the body. In addition, the brainstem processes incoming information and carries messages between the brain and the rest of the body.

The **cerebellum,** or "little brain," consists of right and left cerebellar hemispheres and a central vermis. The cerebellum is connected to many other parts of the brain and has access to much of the brain's information. The

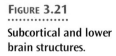

FIGURE 3.21
....
Subcortical and lower brain structures.

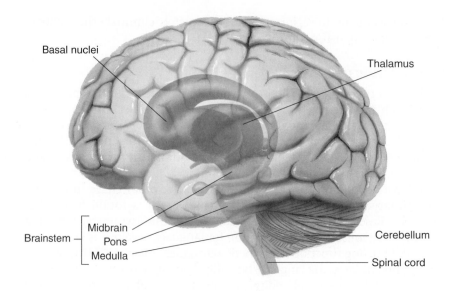

cerebellum and its connections coordinate the control of fine, complex motor activities, maintain muscle tone, and participate in motor learning. The general location of the subcortical and lower brain structures is shown in Figure 3.21.

The *spinal cord,* located within the bony spinal column, is a collection of neuronal cell bodies protected within a fatty myelin sheath. The spinal cord receives almost all of the sensory information taken in by your body, and it contains the large motor neurons that supply the muscles that move your body.

PERIPHERAL NERVOUS SYSTEM

Located outside the CNS, the **peripheral nervous system** (PNS) consists of 12 pairs of cranial nerves, most of which originate in the brainstem, and 31 pairs of spinal nerves that exit the vertebral column and travel to and from muscles of the body. By transmitting messages to muscles and receiving sensory information, the PNS helps the CNS communicate with the body.

The *cranial nerves* (Figure 3.22) are especially important for speech production. Because they are arranged vertically along the brainstem, they are referred to by Roman numerals corresponding to their vertical order. Thus number VII, the facial nerve, is seventh from the top. Twenty-two of the 31 pairs of *spinal nerves* are important for breathing for purposes of speech production, versus breathing for life that is governed by special control centers in the brainstem.

Motor Speech Control

In the process of motor speech production, first the movement plan/program, which is an organized set of motor commands that specifies all of the

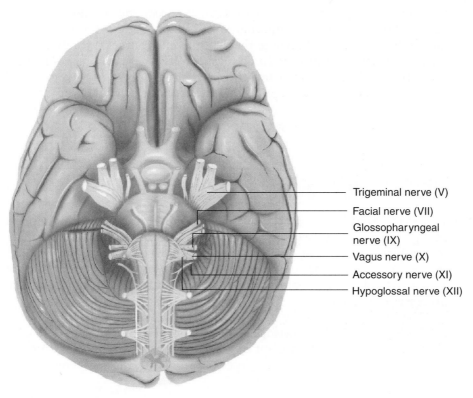

FIGURE 3.22

Cranial nerves important in speech and hearing.

Trigeminal (V): A mixed nerve with both sensory and motor functions for the jaw and tongue for speech and chewing.

Facial (VII): A mixed nerve for sensation of taste and motor control of the facial muscles important in facial expression, such as smiling, tearing, and salivation.

Glossopharyngeal (IX): A mixed nerve with sensory input from the tongue for taste and motor control of the pharynx for salivation and swallowing.

Vagus (X): A mixed nerve serving the heart, lungs, and digestive system. A sensory nerve to the larynx and throat. A motor nerve to the larynx for phonation, the soft palate for lifting, and the pharynx for swallowing.

Accessory (XI): A motor nerve controlling muscles of the pharynx, soft palate, head, and shoulders.

Hypoglossal (XII): A motor nerve controlling the muscles of tongue movement.

necessary parameters of movement (Keele, 1968), is retrieved from memory. Next, it is sent to the motor control areas; then it is transmitted with precise timing along the nerves to muscles and structures of the speech mechanism, resulting in sequences of acoustic signals that are recognized as speech sounds. Along the way, these nerve impulses are modified to ensure precise, smooth muscle movement.

Typical movement patterns are purposeful and efficient, and they are under the control of the individual, thus enabling him or her to change or modify the movement. Motor responses are initiated, changed, and coordinated on the basis of both external and internal sensory information. External sensory mechanisms detect and analyze the external environment. Internal movement feedback from muscles (proprioceptive feedback) and nerves helps us know the position and movement of body structures in space. For speech production, auditory and proprioceptive feedback help ensure proper coordination of the speech mechanism. For a comprehensive review of the motor speech production process, see Maas et al., 2008.

SUMMARY

This chapter has been a general overview of the anatomy and physiology of the speech and voice mechanism. The study of the structures that are used to produce speech and their function is extensive and complex. It is important to remember that although anatomy is static, these structures are capable of dynamic movement that can result in the unique human processes of speech.

The study of anatomy and physiology is essential for the speech-language pathologist. Knowledge and understanding of this topic will assist in the evaluation and treatment of clients whose communication disorder is the direct or indirect result of a breakdown within these systems.

THOUGHT QUESTIONS

- How might speech breathing and phonation be affected in someone who is a heavy smoker?
- How would breathing patterns be different while singing?
- You are drinking soda from a bottle. After you have taken a few sips, you blow air across the opening on the top of the bottle, and a sound is produced. After taking a few more sips, you again blow across the opening. Was the sound different the second time you blew across the top of the bottle? The bottle is a resonator. What characteristics of the resonator changed, and how did those changes influence the sound that was produced?
- How might speech and language skill deficits perhaps differ in left-handed people versus right-handed people following a stroke in the left hemisphere?

SUGGESTED READINGS

Hixon, T. (2006). *Respiratory function in singing: A primer for singers and singing teachers*. Tucson, AZ: Redington Brown.

Hixon, T., & Hoit, J. (2005). *Evaluation and management of speech breathing disorders: Principles and methods*. Tucson, AZ: Redington Brown.

Hixon, T., Weismer, G., & Hoit, J. (2008). *Preclinical speech science: Anatomy, physiology, acoustics, and perception.* San Diego, CA: Plural Publishing.

Kent, R. (1997). *The speech sciences.* San Diego, CA: Singular Publishing.

Zemlin, W. (1998). *Speech and hearing sciences anatomy and physiology* (4th ed.). Boston, MA: Allyn & Bacon.

ONLINE RESOURCES

Praat
www.praat.org
Praat: Doing Phonetics by Computer Web site has free software to download so you can perform your own spectral analyses.

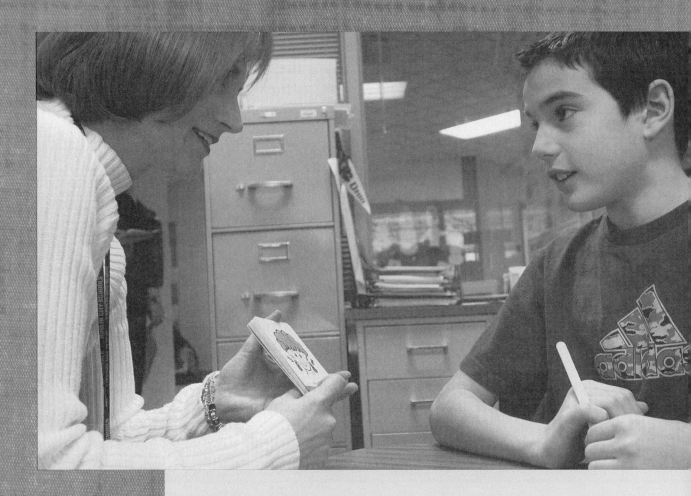

CHAPTER LEARNING GOALS

When you have finished this chapter, you should be able to:

- Describe the communication continuum of differences, dialects, and disorders

- Explain the purposes and procedures involved in assessment of communication disorders

- Explain how targets are selected for clinical remediation

- Describe some of the basic procedures in treatment and intervention

4

Assessment and Intervention

The human communication process is remarkable but not flawless. Each of us has experienced frustration at not remembering someone's name or faltering when trying to express ourselves clearly. We also know that sometimes a friend speaks to us and we don't fully understand what she or he is trying to say. The reverse happens, too, when we know that someone else misinterprets what we say. But when do these often minor annoyances constitute a problem? How do we determine that a communication disorder exists? And how do we categorize its nature? In this chapter, we provide an overview of assessment procedures. We also examine intervention principles and techniques for assisting people who have communication disorders.

DIFFERENCES, DIALECTS, DISORDERS

We learned in Chapter 2 that communication takes place within a social context. We communicate with other people. Our own culture and that of others influence the nature and success of this interaction. Ordered and disordered communication can be described only within cultural standards. It is obvious that the communication skills of a 4-year-old generally will be less sophisticated than those of a 12-year-old. Age, therefore, is one determiner of communicative proficiency. But factors such as gender, ethnicity, geographic region, language background, and socioeconomic status also contribute to the ways in which we communicate. The speech-language pathologist must recognize that variety is typical, and she or he must be able to distinguish differences from disorders.

A Communication Continuum

Everyone in Carol's family, including Carol, speaks rapidly; sometimes their words come out so fast they are hard to understand. Peter comes from a family of slow and deliberate speakers; occasionally, such a long lag time appears between Peter's words that one wonders whether he's

Age influences all aspects of communication; however, considerable variation exists within each age group.

going to complete his sentence. Carol and Peter represent different ends of the speech rate continuum. Although they are clearly not speakers you might encounter every day, you might wonder whether they are different enough to have disordered speech. To make this determination, consider the following:

1. Does the speaker feel embarrassed or uncomfortable?
2. Do listeners react negatively?
3. Is the intent of the speaker miscommunicated?

Dialects

Dialects are natural variations of a language used by all speakers of that language. As such, dialects represent language differences not disorders. Whereas languages typically, but not always, represent the political boundaries of a country or ethnic group, dialects usually represent less formal geographic distinctions. In the United States, we can usually distinguish people from Boston and Dallas by their distinctive ways of speaking. Ethnicity may also result in a dialect as in African American English. Foreign language background contributes to dialect, too. Within each region, ethnicity, and language background, additional variations exist. Not all Bostonians or African Americans share a common dialect. Similarly, speakers of Spanish (or French or any language) from different countries and regions are not identical in their communicative patterns. For example, the French of a person from Quebec is distinct from that of someone from Haiti, which is different from that of a Parisian. Women and men, too, often differ in their manner of communication, giving rise to **genderlect,** or gender-based dialect.

Everyone uses a dialect. People with a dialect that differs from yours do not have a disorder of communication. It is important to recognize that dialects are normal variations, they are not pathological.

Individuals who use a particular dialect belong to the same **speech community** and share knowledge of the communicative constraints and options in that community. Speech communities may differ from one another in specifics of vocabulary, grammar, pronunciation, rate and rhythm of speech, topics of communication, body language, communication distance, and eye contact.

Pragmatic dialect differences are not always obvious. For example, narrative or storytelling styles of schoolchildren may reflect their ethnic background. European American youngsters, like their elders, tend to build a story to its climax and then provide a resolution. Algonquin and Chinese American children typically develop a story to its high point and then stop. From the European American viewpoint, the Algonquin and Chinese tales may appear incomplete, but to someone from these cultures, this is seen as a positive technique for leaving the listener in the midst of the story (Crago et al., 1997).

In summary, in the United States, dialects are variations of Standard American English. Because we all speak some dialect, none should be considered "substandard" or "wrong." Figure 4.1 highlights a few dialect differences.

Although features can be identified as characteristic of a particular dialect, you should recognize that each dialect contains variations. For example, Latino English is spoken by people from Spain, Mexico, Puerto Rico, and many parts of South and Central America, and their linguistic patterns are not identical. In addition, individual speakers may use some or none of the features listed here. It must be emphasized that dialects are not "wrong"; they are rule-based modifications of the standard. The examples that follow are a small sample of differences based on ethnicity and language background.

SAE = Standard American English, AAE = African American English,
ME = Mandarin English, LE = Latino English.

Grammar

Past tense

(SAE) I talked to her yesterday.

(AAE) I talk to her yesterday.

(ME) I talk to her yesterday.

(LE) I talk to her yesterday.

Possession

(SAE) That is Mary's dress.

(AAE) That is Mary dress.

(ME) That is dress of Mary.

(LE) That is dress of Mary.

Nagation

(SAE) She doesn't like him.

(AAE) She don't like him.

(ME) She don't no like him.

(LE) She no like him.

Phonology

Substitutions, Omissions

(SAE) "feet" "it"

(AAE) "fee" "i-"

(ME) "fit" "eat"

(LE) "fit" "eat"

Pragmatics

Direct eye contact

(SAE)   Sign of respect and that attention is being paid

(AAE)   Used by speaker but may be considered disrespectful when used by listener

(ME)   Generally avoided

(LE)   Generally avoided

Laughter/giggling

(SAE)   Response to humor

(AAE)   Sign of friendlines

(LE)   Response to humor

FIGURE 4.1

A few examples of possible dialect differences.

Source: Based on Owens (2008) and Paul (1995).

In addition to dialect, we must consider **idiolect,** which is an individual's unique way of speaking based on an interaction of such things as age, education, personality, family, geographic background, and linguistic background. Not everyone in your hometown sounds the same. Some people use one or two aspects of a dialect, such as vocabulary or grammar, and others use different aspects such as pronunciation. Many people are bidialectical or multidialectal; they are competent in more than one dialect. They choose the dialect that is appropriate to the setting and conversational partners.

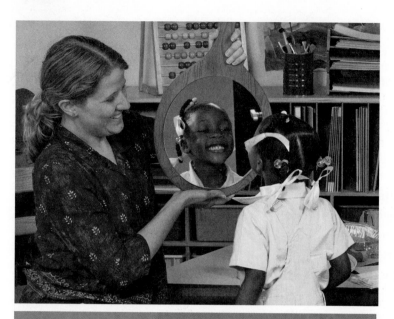

It is in the interest of young children to begin intervention services as early as possible.

Disorders

Communication disorders may affect language processing and/or transmission, that is, any aspect of speech, hearing, listening, reading, or writing. Several are listed on the ASHA Web sites at the end of the chapter. The American Speech-Language-Hearing Association (ASHA) defines a communication disorder as "an impairment in the ability to receive, send, process, and comprehend concepts or verbal, nonverbal and graphic symbol systems" (ASHA, 1993, p. 40). The exact nature and degree of impairment varies from individual to individual. It is the task of the speech-language pathologist or audiologist to describe the problem clearly and identify its extent.

Some clinicians object to the term *disorder,* especially when it is used simply to report test results that are below average. They suggest that differences make us distinct as human beings and that we should redirect our attention toward people's strengths (Miller, 1993). Although we agree, we also recognize, as do other specialists, that terminology is needed to identify people who are in need of speech, language, or hearing services, and to state that a person has an impairment, disability, or disorder should not carry with it negative stigma. It is important to recognize that an individual with a communication disorder is not a disordered person. We do not label a person as a "stutterer" or a "lisper" but rather "a person who stutters or lisps." The person is primary; the disorder is simply one aspect of the individual.

IS THERE A PROBLEM?

Not everyone is assessed for communication disorders. When there is a possibility of a problem, recognition of this precedes formal assessment. Selection for assessment may come from either referral or screening.

Specialists in communication disorders may encourage referrals from other professionals and concerned individuals by publicizing the nature of the services that they provide.

Referrals

Individuals at any age may be referred from various sources for an evaluation for a communication disorder. An infant in a hospital neonatal intensive care unit who has feeding or other oral difficulties may be referred to the speech-language pathologist (SLP) for evaluation and management of these problems.

A pediatrician may refer a toddler. Sometimes a parent, grandparent, neighbor, or friend observes that a young child is not communicating as well as others of the same age. This person might take appropriate steps so that an assessment will occur. A phone call to an area speech and hearing center, school system, rehabilitation program, or to a clinician in private practice might lead to a formal evaluation of the youngster's hearing and speech. For children enrolled in a preschool or regular school, it is common for a teacher to express a concern about a child's speech and recommend an assessment by an SLP or audiologist. ASHA offers a guide to help parents identify communication disorder (see Web site).

Adults may refer themselves if they feel they have a communication disorder. Sometimes a person might feel handicapped professionally and/or socially because of hearing or speech limitations. Family members, such as a parent or spouse, may take the initiative. Frequently, a physician refers an individual who has had an accident or a medical problem such as a stroke.

Screening

Federal legislation (see Figure 1.2) mandates that *all* children from birth to age 20 be given the opportunity to receive special services if needed. To ensure this, departments of health and welfare and departments of education throughout the country must provide a system for identifying at-risk individuals at no personal expense. Children between the ages of birth and 36 months may be brought to special centers for screening for speech, language, hearing, motor, and other functions. Older children are screened in preschools and schools.

Every state in the United States requires that hearing screening tests be given to infants at their birthing facility or as soon after birth as possible. Babies who are identified as being at risk for hearing loss are then assessed more fully, and steps toward appropriate intervention are initiated.

Some SLPs devise and use their own speech and language screening test; others use commercially available ones such as the Fluharty Speech and Language Screening Test-2 (Fluharty, 2000) or the Adolescent Language Screening Test (Morgan & Guilford, 1984). A clinician-prepared speech and language test might include speech sounds and grammatical structures attained by certain age children, comprehension of complex sentences, conceptual understanding, labeling of pictures, and estimates of voice and fluency. Such evaluations should be tested on the target populations to ensure that the items are appropriate and relevant.

DEFINING THE PROBLEM
. . . .

Assessment of communication disorders is the systematic process of obtaining information from many sources, through various means, and in different settings to verify and specify communication strengths and weaknesses, identify possible causes of problems, and make plans to address them. If a problem is identified, a speech-language pathologist may make a **diagnosis,** which distinguishes an individual's difficulties from the broad range of possible problems. Although a diagnostic report might include a label such as *dysphonia,* it should also contain a more complete description of this disorder that reflects the person's ability to communicate, variability of symptoms, severity, and possible causes (Haynes & Pindzola, 1998).

Assessment Goals

The goals of assessment are listed in Figure 4.2 and explained in the paragraphs that follow. The procedures that are used in meeting these objectives are described later in this chapter.

VERIFICATION OF COMMUNICATION PROBLEMS

A person who has been identified during screening may have a communication disorder. A screening is not a diagnostic evaluation. Screenings simply suggest which individuals should receive further evaluation.

The primary goal of diagnosis is determining exactly what is wrong. Sometimes **diagnostic therapy** is suggested. This means that the SLP will work with the client for a time and will obtain a clearer picture of the person's communication abilities and limitations in the process.

DESCRIPTION AND QUANTIFICATION OF DEFICITS AND STRENGTHS

We previously learned that communication impairments may involve hearing, speech, language, and/or processing or, more likely, some combination of these. During assessment, specifics of all of these are probed. Both the client's communicative strengths and limitations are noted. Techniques that the client uses for overcoming difficulties are observed. The SLP provides data reporting the consistency of behaviors and, where appropriate, indicates how the client compares with more typical communicators. In short, assessment must provide detailed information about all aspects of the client's communicative disabilities and abilities, recognizing the interrelatedness of speech, language, and hearing.

FIGURE 4.2
....
Goals of assessment.

Source: Based on Lund & Duchan (1993).

The communication disorders specialist is charged with answering the following questions when assessing an individual:

1. Does a communication problem exist?

2. What is the diagnosis?

3. What are the deficit areas? How consistent are they?

4. What are the individual's strengths?

5. How severe is the problem?

6. What are the probable causes of the problem?

7. What recommendations should be made?

8. What is the prognosis (likely outcome) without and with intervention?

STATEMENT OF SEVERITY

If a problem exists, the SLP will want to know how serious it is. At a general level, she or he will determine whether the disorder is profound, severe, moderate, mild, or borderline. Individuals with a profound impairment have very little functional speech communication. A person with a severe disorder would require a great deal of intervention and support. Moderate disorders also require significant treatment and accommodation. A mild or borderline communication problem might not be readily apparent to the individual himself or herself or to others; however, even subtle communication problems can have a negative impact on social, academic, and professional success. Exactly what determines a particular severity rating is related to several factors.

Published tests often suggest severity ratings depending on a client's performance scores. These must be used with caution. The clinician must be aware that there is always a range of typical communication behavior and also that a single test should not be overly relied on.

> Clinicians may differ in their judgments of the severity of a disorder. Use of objective criteria ensures more consistency in this determination.

ETIOLOGY

Etiology is the study of cause. The SLP should try to ascertain the reason(s) for the communication deficit, especially if these causes persist. Three categories of cause may be identified. A **predisposing cause** describes the underlying factor that led to the problem, for example something genetic. A **precipitating cause** is a factor that triggered the disorder, such as a stroke. A **maintaining** or **perpetuating cause** is something that keeps the problem going. In the case of Sally M. that follows, the SLP formed hypotheses concerning all three categories of etiology.

Sally M., age 7, had multiple articulation, phonological, and morphological errors in her speech. The SLP learned that Sally had frequent ear infections during her second and third years of life. The SLP hypothesized that inability to hear adequately during this period may have interfered with mastery of the sound system of English. Sally was ill so frequently that she may not have had the energy to focus on learning speech. The SLP observed that Sally's mother laughed good-naturedly at Sally's way of speaking. The SLP reported that the likely predisposing cause of Sally's communication difficulties was a tendency toward ear infections. The precipitating cause may have been the history of middle ear infections (otitis media). Possible maintaining factors were the attention and "rewards" Sally received for her immature speech.

Causality is sometimes viewed from another perspective. The terms **organic/somatogenic** and **functional/psychogenic** may also be used in describing etiology. An organic disorder has an identifiable physical cause; for example, cleft palate, cerebral palsy, and cancer of the larynx all are likely to result in communicative difficulties. The term *somatogenic* means coming form the body, and it therefore indicates a physical basis. For example, some syndromes have a genetic origin.

When no physical cause can be identified, the disorder is considered functional. Functional disorders may be due to psychogenic (psychological) factors: for example, in selective mutism, an individual has no physiological reason for not being able to speak but decides not to talk, perhaps as retaliation toward an abusive parent or fear of school (Haynes & Pindzola, 1998).

It is helpful to remember that the causes of communication problems are often elusive or idiopathic (individualistic) and sometimes we simply cannot figure out what they are. In these cases, clinicians report that the etiology is unknown. The mystery may be partly because original causes do not always persist; for example, Sally M.'s ear infections are no longer apparent at age 7. Furthermore, we have no way of knowing why Sally was especially vulnerable to getting ear infections in the first place. Finally, causality is often complex, with many factors coming together to result in the development of a particular disorder. Whether the etiology is known or not, the SLP must thoroughly describe the client's communication behavior.

THE TREATMENT PLAN

Recommendations for addressing the client's communicative deficiencies are often the most read portion of an assessment report. In making a plan, the first decision is whether intervention is warranted. If it is, then its nature must be described. Should the client be enrolled in speech and language therapy? Where? How frequent and how long should therapy sessions be? Would the client benefit more from individual or group work? What specific targets should be addressed initially? What style of therapy might be optimal? Some options include high or low structure, client or clinician directed, behavioral or cognitive, direct or indirect, pull-out or push-in, to name a few. These are described later in this chapter in the section on treatment procedures. The plan should also indicate referrals for other services such as psychological or medical evaluation. Treatment recommendations can be thought of as a "working hypothesis" (Haynes & Pindzola, 1998) that may need to be altered as intervention proceeds. Assessment continues throughout treatment in the forms of data keeping and probes of behavior.

PROGNOSIS

A **prognosis** is an informed prediction of the outcome of a disorder. For example, a parent of a 5-year-old with very disfluent speech will want to know what will happen if this is left untreated and whether therapy will prevent the child from stuttering later in life.

In communication disorders, the SLP makes a prognosis regarding whether the problem will persist if no intervention occurs and what the likely outcome is if a course of therapy or other treatment plan is followed.

Family members and clients are often eager to know the prognosis. They will ask questions such as "Will my child outgrow this problem?" or "How long will it take to correct this disorder?"

The SLP must consider the nature and severity of the disorder; the client's responsiveness to trial therapy during assessment; and the client's overall communicative, intellectual, and personal strengths and weaknesses. The client's home and school environments are also important factors that can affect the outcome.

Assessment Procedures

Assessment may take many forms. Ideally, the clinician should sample a broad variety of communication skills through multiple procedures in several settings. The focus should be on the collection of **authentic data,** that is, actual real-life information, in sufficient quantity to be able to make meaningful and accurate decisions (Damico, 1997). Several aspects of a typical evaluation are presented on the accompanying CD-ROM.

The need for use of a variety of procedures should be readily apparent. How often as a student have you said that a test did not accurately measure what you know or what you can do? The same is true for individuals with communication impairments. For example, children with attention deficit hyperactivity disorder (ADHD) perform very differently when their attentional state has been altered with medication (Sutcliffe et al., 2006). Test results are influenced by the child's attentional status. By using multiple measures and reports, the SLP or audiologist tries to obtain the most accurate description of a child's communication possible.

EVIDENCE-BASED PRACTICE

Most ASHA assessment guidelines relate to specific disorders and are described in the following chapters. Still, some general guidelines can be deduced from these evidence-based analyses. These are included in Box 4.1.

BOX 4.1
Evidence-Based Practice in Assessment of Individuals with Communication Impairments

Developmental Level

- Early identification may be especially important for young children with significant communication disorders.
- The form of communication varies with a child's age and developmental status and should be reflected in the communication features assessed.

Difference vs. Disorder

- Multilingualism and dialectal variations in the home and other care environments affect the way in which language is learned and used and should be considered in an assessment.
- Bilingual clients should be assessed in both languages in order to provide an accurate picture of speech and language strengths and weaknesses.

Format

- Significant others who interact with the client in an on-going daily basis should be included in the assessment process.

- Assessment and analysis should be multifaceted and in depth because the dividing line between typical and disordered speech and language is not always clear.
- Assessment materials and strategies should be appropriate to the culture and language of the client and family.
- The setting of the assessment should be appropriate to the developmental stage and or overall health of the client and be comfortable for both the client and significant others.
- Assessment materials and strategies should reflect the developmental level or condition of the client.

Source: New York State Department of Health. (2002). *Clinical Practice Guideline,* Publication No. 4218. Albany, NY: New York State Department of Health. Recommended by ASHA, Compendium of EBP Guidelines and Systematic Reviews. Accessed June 1, 2009 at www.asha.org/members/ebp/compendium/.

CASE HISTORY

The written **case history** provides background information that helps the SLP to prepare for an evaluation. Most speech-language pathologists require that histories, usually in the form of a questionnaire, be completed before the client's first visit. Normally, one form is tailored for adult clients, and a comparable one is for a parent or other responsible person to use with regard to a child. Case histories can also be completed with the client or reviewed with the client prior to beginning an assessment (Duffy, 2005).

Although the written case history is a valuable tool, its validity may be limited for various reasons. The respondent might not have understood all the questions. She or he might not know the answers to many questions and might guess or recall incorrectly. For example, adoptive parents may know little about their child's early life. Cultural differences also can influence the manner of response to some items (Shipley & McAfee, 1998). One study concluded that no existing self-report instruments were adequate alone for describing client communication participation (Eadie et al., 2006).

OPENING INTERVIEW

The SLP obtains background information about a client from a written case history completed by the client, parent, or significant other; an interview; and reports from other professionals.

Once the SLP has the completed case history form, additional background information is obtained through an interview. The basic purposes of the initial interview are (1) to learn more about the client that might be relevant to his or her communication and (2) to answer questions and provide reassurance and support for the client and/or family. Open-ended questions are used to encourage the respondent to provide adequate detail. In addition, the respondent must be given the opportunity to express concerns. The clinician must be sure to listen openly and nonjudgmentally. Experienced SLPs are able to guide the interview so that the objectives are met in a supportive, natural way within the allotted time frame. Sample interview questions are included in Figure 4.3.

FIGURE 4.3

Sample interview questions.

Question	*Rationale*
Has your child had any sustained or prolonged illness that included a high fever?	Sustained fevers of 104° to 105°F can result in hearing loss or cognitive injury.
In your own words, tell me what you think your child's difficulties are. (Alternative: Tell me why you're here today.)	Help parent/caregiver become invested in intervention and state his or her concern.
What does your child enjoy; what will she work for?	Identify potential reinforcers.
Do you plan on returning to Cambodia?	Assess family's motivation for learning English.
Who interacts with your child on a daily basis?	Identify potential intervention agents in the home or school.

SYSTEMATIC OBSERVATION/SAMPLING

Watching the client in more than one setting and with different people can provide considerable insight into the individual's communicative skills. One 5-year-old client stuttered severely with his gruff 60-year-old father but very little with the SLP. That's invaluable information.

Clinicians often begin their observation when the client and a family member are in the waiting room. Some children are very talkative with a parent but become silent with a stranger such as an SLP. Classroom and recess or lunchtime observations for school-age children can be revealing. Hospitalized clients should be observed with significant others when possible.

It is also important to see clients alone for a number of reasons (Duffy, 2005). Adults who have aphasia, traumatic brain injury (TBI), or other acquired neurological conditions may have very mixed emotions about performing in front of family members. In addition, an SLP may be able to coax behaviors from a client that those in the environment are unable to do.

Most clinicians also use a **speech** and/or **language sampling** technique when assessing the communication of both children and adults: Guidelines for sample collection and analysis are described in Chapter 5, "Childhood Language Impairments," and Chapter 10, "Disorders of Articulation and Phonology." Sampling adult speech is equally important. This can be accomplished while reviewing the case history with clients or asking them to explain how they spent their day or tell about their last vacation (Duffy, 2005).

HEARING SCREENING

Hearing is routinely screened in most communication evaluations. Because hearing is so important to speech, the SLP needs to ascertain that the client's hearing is adequate for speech purposes. If there is a question, the SLP would refer the client to an audiologist for an evaluation.

STRUCTURAL-FUNCTIONAL EXAMINATION

An **examination of the peripheral speech mechanism** is commonly part of the overall assessment process. The purpose is to determine that the physical structures involved in speech are not impaired and that they function adequately. During this procedure, the face, jaw, lips, teeth, tongue, pharynx, and hard and soft palates

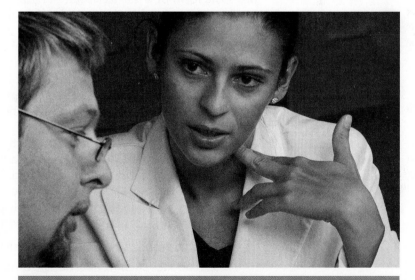

Trial theraphy is an important part of the assessment procedure.

are evaluated at rest and while the client engages in specified nonspeech and speech movements.

STANDARDIZED TESTING

Literally hundreds of published tests exist that attempt to assess either overall speech and language performance or specific components such as articulation. Most of these instruments are **norm referenced,** meaning they yield scores that are used to compare a client with a sample of similar individuals. Norm-referenced instruments must be designed and tested very carefully and the sample population controlled to include all segments of the potential population for which the test is designed. Ideally, the test has norms for bilingual populations and for children speaking different dialects of American English. Some samples also include children with impaired language skills, although this practice has been questioned because it may reduce the accuracy of the test in identifying these in identifying these populations (Peña et al., 2006).

Other published tests are **criterion referenced** and provide a systematic method for evaluating a client's strengths and weaknesses with regard to particular skills. Skilled SLPs can interpret test results to yield both norm and criterion-referenced information. Figure 4.4 contains examples of the kinds of items you would find in some published tests.

DYNAMIC ASSESSMENT

Most assessments include probing to explore the client's ability to modify behavior by producing previously misarticulated sounds, learning a language rule, reducing dysfluencies, and the like. The goal is to mesh more flexible nonstandardized approaches with more formal, structured methods found in most tests. Called **dynamic assessment,** this procedure often takes the form of a *test-teach-test* paradigm to examine the "teachability" of a communication feature. The child's potential for learning is assessed by giving small amounts of assistance and determining the difficulty for the child of performing the newly learned behavior.

Dynamic assessment rest on the concept that a child learns best when adults provide *mediated assistance* during tasks whose difficulty is just beyond the child's previous performance. The procedure involves the systematic introduction and withdrawal of prompting, such as a brief reminder to look at all pictures before choosing or providing a verbal model, to determine if and how a child's performance can be improved. While teaching, the SLP introduces a graduated amount of assistance and notes the changes in the client's responding with increasing assistance.

Mediated assistance is adult guidance in which the amount and type of assistance are individualized to suit the learner and task. Assistance might include (Justice & Ezell, 1999) the following:

- Repetition or clarification of instructions;
- Verbal cues such as questions, comments, or requests;
- Nonverbal cues such as pointing or gesturing;

Articulation Test for Children

Ask child to name the following objects:

shoe, hat, ring, letter, pencil, book, cookie, telephone, chair, scissors

Complex Phonological Naming Task

Ask client to name pictures of the following:

elephants, encyclopedia, valentine, television, telescope, library, photograph

Grammatical Understanding

Ask client to point to the correct picture when give a choice of three:

The boy is getting dressed. The boy is dressed. The boy is getting undressed.

The lady is hiding from the boy. The boy is hiding from the lady. The body and the lady are hiding.

Grammatical Production

Ask client to complete the sentence:

Clinician: This is a picture of one shoe. This is a picture of two _____.

Clinician: The boy is putting on his sock. The boys are putting on _____.

Pragmatic Language Use

Ask the client what you would say under various conditions:

A person gave you a present.

You meet a friend.

You are offered food by a friend, but you do not want any.

Functional Communication Test for Adults

The clinician must observe the client on a minimum of three occasions. On the basis of these observations, the clinician records whether the client does the following readily, with minimal assistance, with moderate assistance, with maximal assistance, or not at all:

- Refers to people by name.
- Exchanges information on the phone.
- Understands facial expressions.
- Knows what time it is.
- Expresses feelings.

FIGURE 4.4
....

Examples of types of items found on published tests.

- Direct verbal models;
- Physical guidance of a child; or
- Completion of the task with a child.

The SLP systematically explores how various mediation methods influence the child's communicative behavior in both spontaneous and planned situations to find methods that work the best (Gutierrez-Clellen, 2000).

Consolidation of Findings: Making the Diagnosis

The SLP makes a determination about a client's current functioning and the nature of the problem from multiple sources and clinical intuition.

After the speech-language pathologist has obtained information about the client from various sources, it is necessary to summarize the results and make connections between the findings. For example, background information may give insights into observed behavior. Similarly, scores from norm-based tests need to be reconciled with observations by the SLP and other important people in the client's life. The client's communicative limitations must be viewed in the context of other strengths, such as motivation and family or other support. Usually, an individual is more capable in some aspects of communication while other features are weak. For example, a child's speech might be easy to understand (readily intelligible), although he or she has a limited expressive vocabulary. The SLP must attempt to obtain a well-rounded picture of the person who is being assessed.

Closing Interview

The client and/or family will want to know the outcome of the evaluation as soon as possible. When and how this information is shared may depend on whether the setting is a hospital, private clinic, university center, or public school. In addition, each facility will establish its own set of policies.

In general, a brief conference is held immediately after the formal assessment. The SLP will probably indicate that all of the information gathered about the client has not yet been analyzed, so more complete recommendations will appear in the diagnostic report. The SLP might suggest another meeting to discuss this report.

Ethical practice requires that the SLP present the client and family with intervention options when treatment is recommended. This includes the type of intervention and potential intervention providers. Sufficient information should be provided to enable the client and/or family to make an informed choice.

Report Writing

Effective writing skills are required to accurately convey assessment information to the client, the client's family, and other professionals.

The diagnostic report is a summary of the client's history and a record of what transpired during the assessment. The implications of the findings should be clearly stated and thoughtfully justified. The report is normally the springboard for intervention and treatment. With client or parental permission the report will be sent to other professionals who will be working with the client. It is also available to the client or client's family. The report must be carefully written. If technical terms are used, they should be explained. Although speech-language pathologists may develop individual styles of writing, most reports follow a similar format and contain comparable information. Figure 4.5 presents a sample of the different aspects of a generic communication report.

SPEECH-LANGUAGE EVALUATION

FIGURE 4.5
....
Generic communication report.

Name: Date of birth:
Address: Chronological age:
Phone: Date of evaluation:
Parent or relative: Grade (for child):
Physician: Teacher (for child):
Referral: Reason for referral:
Clinician:

BACKGROUND INFORMATION EVALUATION

Hearing

Articulation/Phonology
  Intelligibility

Voice

Fluency

Language
  Test Results
      Comprehension
      Production
  Sampling

Listening

Auditory Processing
  Phonological segmentation
  Phonological blending
  Memory

Structural-Functional Examination

SUMMARY AND RECOMMENDATIONS
  Intervention targets:

_____
(SLP Signature)

INTERVENTION WITH COMMUNICATION DISORDERS
• •

Intervention for individuals with communication disorders is influenced by the nature and severity of the disorder, the age and status of the client, and environmental considerations, as well as personal and cultural characteristics of both client and clinician. Despite this, some general principles and procedures can be identified.

As mentioned in Chapter 1, ASHA has taken a proactive position stressing the need to integrate research and clinical practice (Kamhi, 2006; Katz, 2003; Ramig, 2002; Wambaugh & Bain, 2002). ASHA's Code of Ethics requires clinicians to "provide services that are based on careful, professional reasoning" (Apel & Self, 2003, p. 6). Evidence-based practices ensure that "clinicians abide by these ethical codes while best serving their clients." (Apel & Self, 2003, p.6). ASHA has established the National Center for Treatment Effectiveness in Communicative Disorders and is currently coordinating a National Institutes of Health funded effort to promote clinical research that will support EBP.

Despite the widespread acclaim for EBP, a fundamental issue confronts clinicians who wish to establish an EBP: locating relevant, germane sources of clinical evidence in a timely fashion. SLPs can use "high-yield sources" that are easily accessible via the Internet (Dollaghan, 2004; Schlosser, 2004). For example, the Agency for Healthcare Research and Quality supports a Web site (www.guideline.gov) that is a compilation of clinical evidence reviews from a large number of disciplines and a wide variety of topics.

Objectives of Intervention

Regardless of the specific nature of the problem, intervention in speech-language pathology has as its overriding goal the improvement of the client's communication skills.

1. The client should show improvement not just in a clinical setting; progress should generalize to his or her real-world environments, such as home, school, and work.
2. The client should not have to think about what has been learned; in large part, it should be **automatic.**
3. The client must be able to **self-monitor.** Although modifications should be automatic, they will still require monitoring. The client should be able to listen to and observe himself or herself and make corrections as needed without the therapist's being present.
4. The client should make optimum progress in the minimum amount of time.
5. Intervention should be sensitive to the personal and cultural characteristics of the client.

Target Selection

The assessment report should provide recommendations for long-term goals and short-term objectives for communication intervention. The clinician, however, will have to decide which specific targets should be addressed and in what sequence. The client's personal needs and the potential for generalization are most relevant in making meaningful choices. Likelihood of success and typical behavior of others of the client's age and gender might provide additional insights.

CLIENT NEEDS

The client's individual needs are paramount in target selection. For example, Johnny M. is a 6-year-old boy with numerous articulation and grammatical errors in his speech. When asked his name, he is reluctant to answer, but he may be coaxed to say, "Doddy". According to Mrs. M., people tease him about his pronunciation of his name, and this is a great source of anxiety for the child. Because of this, the phonemes /ʤ/ ("J" in Johnny) and /n/ are very important to this child and should be considered for early targeting. Similarly, Ms. K. is in the initial stages of recovery from TBI sustained in a motor vehicle accident. She produces few words and has difficulty naming common objects and people in her family. Obviously, her needs are very different from Johnny.

> Each client has individual needs. The SLP must attempt to determine which are paramount at this time and then develop a plan to meet these needs.

HOW THE TARGET WILL GENERALIZE

Generalization refers to the use of the trained target with different people in varied environmental settings and linguistic contexts. If what has been learned in therapy is in conflict with patterns found in the home environment, generalization may be difficult.

EASE OF MASTERY

A careful assessment includes diagnostic or trial therapy. In the case of Johnny M., the clinician observed that he could correctly say /n/ and "knee" when these were modeled and he was asked to repeat what he heard; in other words, Johnny was stimulable for the /n/ sound. Johnny was not successful in producing /ʤ/ even though the clinician used a variety of techniques to elicit this sound; he was not stimulable for /ʤ/. On the basis of this information, Johnny will more quickly acquire /n/ than /ʤ/. However, recent research has concluded that once learned, nonstimulable phonemes prompt greater generalization than those that were stimulable (Gierut, 1998). For this reason, both /n/ and /ʤ/ may be appropriate targets.

After probing Ms. K's naming ability, the SLP found that her client could name common objects with a carrier phrase such as "You eat with a _____" or "You wear _____." These phrases will be used initially to aid naming and then gradually faded as Ms. K comes to depend on them less.

AGE APPROPRIATENESS

Knowledge of normal development provides insights into which communication forms and functions are typical at different ages of children. For example, /n/ is generally mastered by age 2, and /ʤ/ is customarily correctly produced by age 4 (Stoel-Gammon & Dunn, 1985). This information confirms the decision to select the production of the phonemes /n/ and /ʤ/ as first objectives for Johnny.

In summary, target selection requires consideration of several variables. The clinician must make a decision that is appropriate for the particular client's needs.

Baseline Data

Formal test results during assessment differ from baseline data. During formal testing, a wide range of communicative skills are evaluated. Baseline data reveal an individual's performance level with regard to a few selected potential targets.

Before beginning a program of intervention, SLPs obtain **baseline data;** that is, they try to elicit the target behavior(s) multiple times, under multiple conditions, and record the accuracy of the client's responses. This gives them information about the client's starting point. Baselines are essential to determine the client's progress and the success of the treatment program.

Unlike a sample and standardized tests used in the initial assessment, baselines specifically probe the communication behavior that will be the focus of therapy. Let's return to Johnny M. The speech-language pathologist has decided that the phoneme /n/ is a first target. The child pronounces his name as "Doddy" and says "do" for "no" and "dife" for "knife". The SLP knows that Johnny can correctly imitate the sound /n/ and the word "knee". In baseline testing, the SLP may obtain 10 pictures of objects beginning with /n/ and 10 of objects ending with /n/. The SLP asks Johnny to name the objects. The percentage of correct /n/ productions in each of these positions is Johnny's baseline for the phoneme /n/. These data provide a starting point both for planning therapy and for measuring progress.

Behavioral Objectives

Once the clinician has obtained baseline data, short-term objectives are developed. These are the targets for each treatment session or for several sessions. A behavioral objective is a statement that specifies the target behavior in an observable and measurable way. To do this requires that the clinician identify what the client is expected to do, under what conditions, and with what degree of success. The letters ABCD might help you to remember the format for writing behavioral objectives:

A. Actor. Who is expected to do the behavior?
B. Behavior. What is the observable and measurable behavior?
C. Condition. What is the context or condition of the behavior?
D. Degree. What is the targeted degree of success?

Returning to Johnny M., the SLP has decided that she or he wants Johnny to experience early success and establishes the following as one behavioral objective for the first session:

A. Johnny
B. will produce the phoneme /n/ correctly
C. in the initial and final position of one-syllable words when modeled by the clinician
D. in 60% of the opportunities presented.

This seems a reasonable goal because Johnny was accurate in this condition 50% of the time during baseline testing.

Behavioral objectives may be used for a broad range of teaching targets. Figure 4.6 lists ten objectives written by student clinicians. Read each one to see whether it is a valid objective. Use the ABCD criteria. If the instructional objective for this task for readers of this text is 80% accuracy, did you meet it?

Clinical Elements

DIRECT TEACHING

Traditional clinical sessions begin with the SLPs explaining or reviewing the target. The amount and complexity of the explanation vary with the training target and the client's age and cognitive ability.

Behavior modification training approaches have been shown to be successful for a broad variety of communication disorders (Hegde, 1998). Behavior modification is a systematic method of changing behavior. Before training, the SLP establishes a target and collects baseline data. During training, the SLP attempts to elicit the desired response from the client by providing a **stimulus**. The client is expected to *respond*, and the

> Even young and relatively low-functioning individuals are more responsive to therapy when they understand the goals.

Which of the following is NOT a well written behavioral objective and why? (Answers are at the bottom of the test, upside down.)

1. The client will understand the words "over" and "under" when they are said to him in 90 percent of the opportunities presented.

2. The client will answer "What" questions using sentences that are 5 words in length in response to 4 of 5 questions.

3. The client will use a rate of speech of no more than 150 wpm when reading aloud from the local newspaper for 5 minutes.

4. The client will correctly name 8 of 10 farm animals when shown cards with their pictures.

5. The client will correctly use the plural form.

6. The client will appropriately respond to the clinician's greeting at the beginning of the therapy session.

7. The client will follow two-part directions given by the clinician in 90% of the opportunities presented.

8. The client will improve vocal quality while reading sentences aloud.

9. The client will distinguish between the phonemes /s/ and /z/ when produced by the clinician.

10. The client will sustain the phoneme /a/ for 20 seconds at a loudness level of 50 decibels.

Answers: 1. No, can't observe or measure "understand." 2. Yes. 3. Yes. 4. Yes. 5. No, in what situation and how often? 6. No, how often? Just today? What is meant by "appropriate"? 7. Yes. 8. No, "improve" is not measurable; also no degree is given. 9. No, degree is not given. 10. Yes.

FIGURE 4.6
....
Test yourself:
Behavioral objectives.

clinician **reinforces** this response or provides corrective feedback. The SLP records the accuracy of the client's response. After training, the SLP counts the percentage of accurate responses and determines the next target response.

INCIDENTAL TEACHING

Behavior modification follows a highly structured format and is directed by the speech-language pathologist. The SLP has a well-thought-out plan and works to guide the client through the stages required for mastery of the target.

A low-structured or more client-led approach may also be used. The SLP follows the client's lead but teaches along the way. This is referred to as **incidental teaching.** For this to be effective, planning is also necessary so that targets are reached. The SLP manipulates the environment so that communication should occur naturally. For example, imaginary play with a young child or a cooking or an art project with one who is older may serve as situations in which therapy occurs. The approach is described further in Chapter 5, "Childhood Language Impairments."

COUNSELING

In addition to direct work with the client on the communication problem, the SLP can provide a supportive environment for the client and other key people in the client's life. A person with a communication disorder may experience a host of feelings, including embarrassment, anger, depression, and inadequacy. Family members may have similar emotions regarding the client's communication and may also feel guilty, perhaps blaming themselves for the problem.

FAMILY AND ENVIRONMENTAL INVOLVEMENT

Intervention for communication disorders occurs in many settings. Broadening the base for treatment helps to ensure that what is learned in a clinical setting is transferred to a variety of real-world contexts.

An individual might spend 2 hours a week with a speech-language pathologist and 110 awake hours alone and with other people. Very young language-delayed children are sometimes bombarded with questions at home. Others may have older siblings who do the talking for them. In Johnny's case, described earlier in this chapter, it might be recommended that the younger sibling with highly unintelligible speech also receive therapy. This would benefit both youngsters.

When children are seen for speech or language therapy, SLPs often ask that a parent observe the sessions on a regular basis. Depending on the family circumstances, family members may be asked to help the child with specific activities at home to foster carryover to everyday situations. For individuals with multiple or severe handicaps, the speech-language pathologist must coordinate efforts with other specialists such as the physician, physical and occupational therapist, and psychologist.

Families and friends may learn ways of helping adults with communicative impairments. A spouse may be critical in assisting therapy for an adult who had a stroke or has a voice problem due to recent accident or illness. The SLP must recognize the significant others in the client's life, from infancy through advanced age, and engage them in productive ways. **Support groups** consisting of individuals who have similar difficulties often provide an avenue to practice what has been learned in therapy, to share feelings related to the disability, and to maintain communication skills once formal treatment has been terminated.

Whatever approaches are used, the client's interests and strengths should be utilized. For example, some individuals learn more easily when shown diagrams and pictures, whereas others profit more from a verbal approach. Some are quicker to grasp concepts; others learn more rapidly from drill. Some have families who can provide strong support; some must look elsewhere for this. Ongoing assessment helps the SLP to determine the most useful procedures for individual clients.

Measuring Effectiveness

The speech-language pathologist determines readiness for dismissal from therapy largely by assessing its effectiveness. Did the client meet the long-term goals and short-term objectives? SLP-designed **posttherapy tests** similar to those used to determine baselines are normally used to answer this question. In addition, it is essential that the client has gained a degree of *automaticity* in the use of the communication target. If he or she has to stop and think each time, overall communication will be impaired, and the targets will not have been fully mastered. Errors will occur, however, and the client should be able to *self-monitor* and self-correct when needed. If therapy has been effective, the client has been successful in *generalizing* learned skills to the out-of-clinic world. This might require the SLP to observe the client in different settings, such as home or school. More often, the SLP depends on reports from others to assess this type of generalization.

Follow-Up and Maintenance

After a client has been dismissed from therapy, the SLP must take steps to ensure that the progress that was achieved is not lost. This is done in two ways: Upon dismissal, the client or family should be encouraged to return when anyone feels a need. More reliable is the establishment of a regular follow-up schedule. The client may be contacted by telephone or letter every 6 months for a period of 2 years or so after the termination of therapy. At this time, retesting may be suggested, and **booster treatment** may be provided if needed. In **follow-up testing,** the SLP evaluates the client's communication skills to see that they are at least at dismissal level. This usually consists of a combination of conversational interaction and systematic probing of therapy targets. During booster treatment, the SLP reintroduces the therapy targets and addresses them again. Often different and abbreviated procedures are used, and the client returns to the dismissal level of accomplishment relatively quickly.

SUMMARY

Assessment of communication disorders requires an understanding of communication in context. Communication behaviors can be viewed as occurring on a continuum from typical to disordered. With each case, the SLP must decide where the demarkation is.

Dialects as a result of geography, ethnicity, foreign language background, and other factors contribute to our communicative individuality. The SLP recognizes that dialects and differences do not constitute disorders.

Referrals and screenings are the primary ways in which individuals are selected for assessment. During assessment, the SLP verifies and defines the client's problem, identifies deficits and strengths, probes causality, makes a treatment plan, and provides a prognosis for improvement. This is achieved through multiple techniques, including sampling of communicative behaviors in several settings.

Assessment and treatment function in a cyclical fashion, with one influencing the other. In many ways, an SLP is assessing the client each time the client is seen in therapy. Successful intervention often uses a team approach that involves family members as well as professionals. Provisions for follow-up ensure that the gains made in therapy are maintained. In the chapters that follow, techniques for assessment and treatment of specific communication disorders are described.

THOUGHT QUESTIONS

- What is meant by the continuum connecting communication differences, dialects, and disorders?
- What are the basic goals of communicative assessment?
- Why is it important to obtain information about a client from several sources?
- What are some differences you might expect to find as a result of systematic observation and formal testing?
- How does a speech-language pathologist decide what to target for intervention?
- How is the success of speech and language therapy determined?

SUGGESTED READINGS

Bliss, L. S. (2002). *Discourse impairments: Assessment and intervention applications.* Boston: Allyn and Bacon.

Coleman, T.J. (2000). *Clinical management of communication disorders in culturally diverse children.* Boston: Allyn and Bacon.

Hamayan, E.V., & Damico, J.S. (1991). *Limiting bias in the assessment of bilingual students.* Austin, TX: Pro-Ed.

Haynes, W.O., & Pindzola, R. H. (1998). *Diagnosis and evaluation in speech pathology* (5th ed.). Boston: Allyn and Bacon.

Klein, H.B., & Moses, N. (1999). *Intervention planning for children with communication problems: A guide for clinical practicum and professional practice* (2nd ed.). Boston: Allyn and Bacon.

Roth, F.P., & Worthington, C. K. (1996). *Treatment resource manual for speech-language pathology*. San Diego, CA: Singular.

Shipley, K. G., & McAfee, J. G. (1999). *Assessment in speech-language pathology. A resource manual* (2nd ed.). San Diego, CA: Singular.

ONLINE RESOURCES

American Speech-Language-Hearing Association

www.asha.org/research/reports/reports.htm
This is a good page on which to begin your exploration of various communication disorders and associated conditions.

www.asha.org/about/news/2008/detectdisorders.htm
Easy to read guide to help parents—and beginning students—identify possible communication disorders.

www.asha.org/practice/multicultural/readings/attitudes.htm
ASHA site has a list of several articles related to the perceptions of communication disorders.

www.asha.org/docs/html/RP1993-00208.html
ASHA site describes various classifications of communication disorders.

New York Department of Health

www.health.state.ny.us/community/infants_children/early_intervention/disorders/ch2_bkgr.htm
Thorough description of possible communication disorders assembled by experts from New York State.

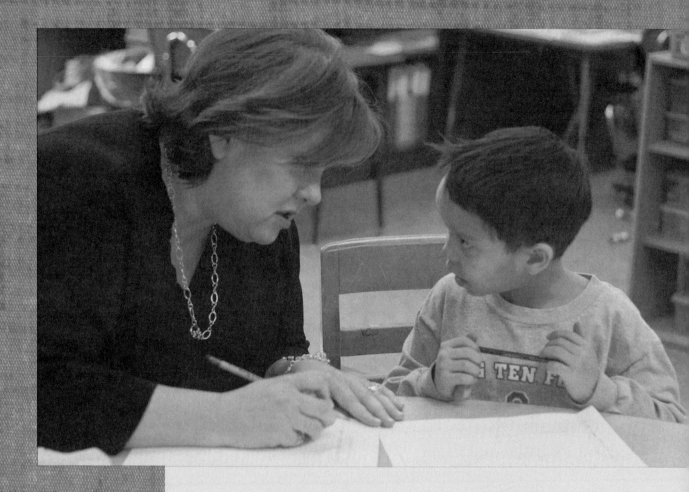

CHAPTER LEARNING GOALS

When you have finished this chapter, you should be able to:

- Characterize language impairment
- Describe the disorders associated with language impairment
- Explain the process of assessment in language impairment
- Describe the overall design of language intervention

5

Childhood Language Impairments

Language impairments are a complex group of diverse disorders and delays with a wide range of characteristics, levels of severity, and causes. Some children may exhibit disorders in which language is inappropriate, inefficient, or ineffectual; others use language that is seemingly immature.

The term **language impairment** applies to a heterogeneous group of developmental and/or acquired disorders and/or delays that are principally characterized by deficits and/or immaturities in the use of spoken or written language for comprehension and/or production purposes that may involve the form, content, and/or function of language in any combination. Case study 5.1 presents the story of one child with language impairment. Let's take this definition apart and examine it.

1. Children and adolescents with language impairment will be very different. The impairment may occur at any time within the lifespan of the individual and may vary in symptoms, manifestations, effects, and severity over time and as a consequence of context, content, and learning task.

2. The impairment may be the result of developmental abnormalities; and/or may be acquired as the result of accident, injury, or other environmental factors.

3. Deficits and/or immaturities may exist in one or more means of communication, such as listening/speech or reading/writing, and may affect receptive and/or expressive language. For example, preschoolers with language impairments are often less able to recognize and copy letters and less likely to write and draw every day, to pretend to read, and to ask questions during parental reading (Marvin & Wright, 1997). In short, young children with language impairments are at risk for literacy difficulties when they later attend school (Nathan et al., 2004).

CASE STUDY 5.1
Case Study of a Child with Language Impairment: Kassandra

Kassandra, an active 5-year-old, is an engaging child and an enthusiastic kindergartner. Born 1 month preterm and weighing only slightly over 4 pounds, she was kept in the hospital for postnatal care and observation for several weeks. The team of specialists who worked with Kassandra in the hospital recommended to her parents that she receive early intervention services, first in the home and later at a local clinic. The team was concerned because Kassandra was at risk of having later developmental problems.

By 18 months, Kassandra was not talking and the team recommended to her parents that she attend a special language-intensive preschool where she would receive both individual and group intervention services. Working together, the speech-language pathologist, developmental specialist, and classroom teacher conducted a thorough evaluation of Kassandra's early communication behaviors, motor skills, and cognitive abilities. Although Kassandra's speech and language were delayed, she appeared to have motor and cognitive abilities that were close to that of typical children.

The speech-language pathologist worked closely with both the classroom teacher and Kassandra's parents to ensure that there was consistency across different communication environments in the way the others interacted with the girl and in the communication requirements. Kassandra's program was individualized to include words and phrases for entities in her environment. Once she began to use single words, Kassandra quickly learned to combine them into longer and longer phrases. When she entered kindergarten, she demonstrated language abilities in the low normal range.

As you read the chapter, think about

- Possible explanations for Kassandra's delay.
- Possible evaluative procedures that could be used to measure Kassandra's language.
- Possible targets that the intervention team might choose to help Kassandra develop and use language.

4. One or more aspects of language—form, content, and use—may be affected. For example, as a group, children with language impairment have shorter, less elaborated sentences than typical children their age (Greenhalgh & Strong, 2001).

Box 5.1 presents an example of the somewhat scrambled language that we might find exhibited by children with language impairment. It is unclear whether most children with language impairment exhibit impairments in other areas of development as well, but language deficits persist at least through the primary school years for many children (Casby, 1997; Tomblin et al., 2003). In the classroom and even on the playground, children with language impairments, especially boys and those with severe receptive language deficits, may be reticent to speak and may lack social maturity and exhibit behavioral problems (Hart et al., 2004; Huaquing Qi & Kaiser, 2004).

Noticeably absent from our definition of impairment are language differences, such as those found in some dialectal speakers and in English language learners. Differences do not in themselves constitute language impairments and do not require clinical intervention by a speech-language pathologist, although elective intervention is possible at the client's request.

BOX 5.1
Example of Conversation with a Language-Impaired Child

Teacher: Does your family have a pet?

Child: Yeah.

Teacher: Tell me about this pet.

Child: Got a pet.

Teacher: Um-hm, tell me about the pet.

Child: Got a pet.

Teacher: Yes, and I really want to hear about him.

Child: Got with my . . . ah, go with my . . . Dad go with . . .

Teacher: Your dad walks the pet.

Child: No, me.

Teacher: Oh, you and your dad walk the pet.

Child: No, me.

Teacher: Oh, just you walk the dog.

Child: No, me.

Teacher: I'm confused.

Child: Me dog.

Teacher: Oh, it's your dog. Who walks your dog?

Child: With one of them things, you know.

Teacher: What things? Who walks your dog?

Child: With them things like this.

Teacher: Yes, you use a leash.

To guide you through this complicated topic, we'll briefly look at typical language development followed by a discussion of the major disorders associated with language impairment. Of necessity, this discussion is an overview with details left for further study.

> Theoretically, all speakers of a language should be able to communicate. Some differences are so great as to impair communication, but these differences still do not qualify as a disorder.

LANGUAGE DEVELOPMENT THROUGH THE LIFESPAN

As you already know, language is complex; thus any attempt to describe its development is, of necessity, very complicated. In the following section, we cover only the highlights of child and adolescent development and relate these to some of the disorders to be discussed later in the chapter. An outline of language development is presented in Table 5.1.

Pre-Language

Much of the first year of life is spent learning to be a communicator. Caregivers talk to newborns as if these children understand what the adults are saying. Later on, as children begin to comprehend language in limited ways, caregivers modify their style of talking to maximize comprehension and participation by the child. Listen to the caregiver-child conversations on the accompanying CD-ROM.

> Children become communicators because they are treated as if they are communicators.

TABLE 5.1

Language development through the lifespan

Age	Accomplishments
3 months	Responds vocally to partner.
8 months	Begins gesturing.
12 months	First word spoken. Words fill intentions previously signaled by gestures.
18 months	Begins combining words on the basis of word-order rules
2 years	Begins adding bound morphemes. Average length or mean length of utterance (MLU) is 1.6–2.2 morphemes.
3 years	More adultlike sentence structure. MLU is 3.0–3.3 morphemes.
4 years	Begins to change style of talking to fit conversational partner. MLU is 3.6–4.7 morphemes.
5 years	Ninety percent of language form learned.
6 years	Begins to learn visual mode of communication with writing and reading.
Adolescence	Able to participate competently in conversations and telling of narratives.
	Knows multiple meanings of words and figurative language. Uses a gender style, or genderlect, when talking.

Sources: Owens (2010).

Shortly after birth, infants become actively involved in a reciprocal process with caregivers. Infants are especially responsive to their caregivers' voices and faces. By as early as 2 weeks, infants are able to distinguish their caregivers from strangers.

Sensitive mothers vary their rate of speech based on their infants' rate of such behavior (Hane et al., 2003). To maintain attention, caregivers exaggerate their facial expressions and voice and vocalize more often. In turn, infants respond with eye contact or vocalizations. Developmental changes affect the dynamic relationship between child and caregiver behaviors and the context (Sameroff & Fiese, 1990).

Early on, infants are full partners, and their behavior is influenced by the communication behavior of their caregivers. Turn taking by adults benefits infant sound making. Infant babbling becomes more speechlike and mature, containing syllables rather than individual sounds.

Eye gaze is very important in these early dialogues. Infants are more likely to begin and to continue looking if their caregivers are looking at them. In return, the caregivers' behavior becomes more social, and play interactions begin.

During the first 3 months, caregivers' responses teach children the "signal" value of specific behaviors and infants learn a stimulus-response sequence. If they signal, by crying, for example, caregivers respond. In addition, they learn that a relatively constant stimulus or signal, such as the bottle, results in a predictable response.

By 3 to 4 months, rituals and game playing have emerged. Rituals, such as feeding and diaper changing, provide children with predictable patterns of behavior and speech. As they learn that interactions can unfold in predictable ways, they begin to form expectations of events and to participate more. Games such as "peekaboo" and "I'm gonna get you" have many of the aspects of communication. There is an exchange of turns, rules for each turn, and particular slots for words and actions. Games, like communication, are also predictable.

At about 8 to 9 months, infants develop **intentionality** in their interactions primarily through gestures. For the first time, a child considers the audience or other person when attempting a potentially communicative act. In this way, communicative behaviors, such as requesting, interacting, and attracting attention, are first fulfilled by prelinguistic communicative means and only later by language.

An intention to communicate is noted in gestures accompanied by eye contact with the child's communication partner, the use of consistent sound and intonational patterns for specific intentions, and persistent attempts to communicate. Intentional vocalizations even sound different from the "private speech" used by infants in solitary activities (Papaeliou & Trevarthen, 2006).

Initially, gestures appear without vocalizations, but the two are gradually paired. Consistent vocal patterns, dubbed **phonetically consistent forms (PCFs)** or **protowards** accompany many gestures. PCFs are a transition to words.

Around 12 months, you probably used your first meaningful word to express an intention. Real words are used with or without gestures to accomplish the functions previously filled by gestures. To develop spoken language, children must be able to store sounds, use this information for later comparison and identification, and relate these sounds to meaning.

During the first year, a child develops a perceptual framework for learning words. An infant actively learns the sound patterns of the native language. Better speech perception at 6 months of age is related to better word understanding, word production, and phrase understanding later (Tsao et al., 2004).

An infant's perceptual ability is usually restricted to its native language's speech sounds by 8 to 10 months of age. Possibly, *tuning in* to its own language sounds to comprehend requires an infant to *tune out* phonemes not in that language (Bates, 1997). Infants also attend to larger patterns, such as syllables.

These patterns play a critical role in facilitating speaking and learning word meanings (Plaut & Kello, 1999). Most words are probably comprehended based on the sound pattern, context, and nonlinguistic and paralinguistic cues.

The task of learning language and learning to represent and to symbolize is strongly related to cognitive abilities. **Representation** is the process of having one thing stand for another. For example, in play, a piece of paper might be used as a blanket for a doll. **Symbolization** is using an arbitrary symbol, such as a word or sign, to stand for something.

Games and rituals share many characteristics with conversations.

Early intentions, such as attracting attention, are established in gestures and first words fill these same functions, often with the accompanying gesture.

For example, after repeated exposure to mom's face, an infant will smile in recognition upon reexposure. Soon, the mother's voice alone will be enough to recall her image. Her voice *represents,* or stands for, her image. Later, an arbitrary symbol or word, such as *mama* or *mommy,* will be enough to recall the image or concept of mom. At about 18 months of age, the child will be able to refer to mom even though she is not present. In this very simplified explanation, the symbol has come to represent the referent or to symbolize it.

Toddler Language

By 18 months, you probably could produce approximately 50 single words and began to combine two words in predictable ways. Within a few short months, three- and four-word combinations appeared. Accompanying the increases in utterance length and vocabulary is a decrease in the use of babbling.

USE

People who are unfamiliar with young children's language often think that children either imitate all first words or use them only to name. In fact, single words are used to make requests, comments, inquiries, and more.

Words are acquired first within the intentions that the child is able to express in previously acquired gestures. Several early intentions are presented in Table 5.2. Note all the uses or intentions expressed in the conversation presented in Box 5.2.

CONTENT AND FORM

The second year is one of vocabulary growth and word combinations. Vocabulary growth is slow for the first few months but then increases rapidly. Although the ability to comprehend words develops gradually, it is

TABLE 5.2
....
Examples of early intentions of children

Intention	Example
Wanting demand	Says the name of the desired item with an insistent voice. Often accompanied by a reaching gesture.
Protesting	Says "No" or the name of the item while pushing it away, turning away, and/or making a frowning face.
Content questioning	Asks "What?," "That?," or "Wassat?" while pointing and/or looking at an item.
Verbal accompaniment	Speech accompanies some action, such as "whee-e-e" when swung or "Uh-oh" when something spills.
Greeting/farewell	Waves hi or bye with accompanying words.

Note: A fuller list can be found in Owens (2010).

BOX 5.2
Example of Toddler Language

Stacy and her mother are coloring and talking while they do. Note that the language concerns the task. Stacy's mom keeps her utterances short and cues Stacy to respond by asking questions. Stacy participates by talking about the task, often incorporating part of the previous utterance into her own.

Mom: What are you making?

Stacy: Doggie.

Mom: Are you making a doggie? Oh, that's nice, Stacy

Stacy: Where more doggie?

Mom: Is there another doggie underneath?

Stacy: Yeah.

Mom: Where? Can you find the picture? Is that what you're looking for, the picture of the doggie? Where's a doggie?

Stacy: A doggie. Color a doggie.

Mom: Okay, you color the doggie.

Stacy: Mommy color crayon.

Mom: Mommy has crayons. Mommy's coloring. What's mommy making?

Stacy: Doggie.

Mom: A doggie.

Stacy: Okay.

Mom: All right, I'll make a doggie. Is this the doggie's tail?

Stacy: Doggie's tail. More.

Mom: More doggie?

Stacy: Okay.

Mom: Can Stacy color? Hum?

Stacy: More doggie there. More doggie daddy.

Mom: More doggie daddy?

Stacy: Want a more doggie. More doggie. Put more doggie there.

Mom: Okay, you color the doggie on this page. What color's your doggie?

Stacy: Blue. Color this page, mommy.

---

highly context-dependent at first (Striano et al., 2003). Eighteen-month-olds are capable of learning new word-referent associations with as few as three exposures (Houston-Price et al., 2005). By age 2, the toddler has an expressive vocabulary of about 150 to 300 words. Two-year-olds with larger vocabularies also use a greater range of grammatical structures (McGregor, Sheng, & Smith, 2005).

Each toddler has his or her own **lexicon** or personal dictionary, with words that reflect that child's environment. In general, toddlers' definitions, based on each child's limited experience, are not the same as those of adults.

Early word combinations follow predictable word-order patterns based on semantic categories. For example, *agents,* which cause action, are placed before the *action,* which in turn precedes *objects,* which receive action. As a result, we hear *Daddy eat* and *Mommy throw,* plus *Eat cookie* and *Throw ball,* but only rarely the reverse, such as *Cookie eat.* Within a few months, working memory, where utterances are held during processing, has increased, so the child can attempt a few longer constructions such as *Daddy eat cookie* or

Adult and toddler definitions are very different, toddler definitions being based almost exclusively on experience, whereas adult ones are based more on meanings shared with others.

Throw ball me. A child's short utterances represent a complex interaction of syntactic knowledge; limited cognitive resources, especially working memory; communicative goals; and the structure of the conversation (Valian & Aubry, 2005).

Preschool Language

Language rule learning is a lengthy process that involves hypothesis testing and refinement.

For preschoolers, most communication occurs within the framework of conversations with caregivers. With increased memory, children expand their conversational skills to include recounting the past and remembering short stories. This memory and recall are aided by the child's increased language skills.

The creativity found in preschool language may reflect substitution. A high percentage of preschool children's utterances differ only slightly from utterances produced previously. For example, a child might say, "Doggies are yucky," "Kitties are yucky," "Cows are yucky," and the like (Lieven et al., 2003).

From interaction with others, children form hypotheses about the rules of language and use these to produce ever more complex language. Caregivers in each child's environment provide feedback and models for further growth, such as repeating the child's utterance in more mature form or reformulating it (Chouinard & Clark, 2003). For example in a **reformulation,** an adult might respond to "Tommy come 'morrow my birthday" with "Yes, tomorrow your cousin Tommy is coming to your birthday party with all the other kids." Through a process of further and further refinement, children's language increasingly reflects that used in their environment.

The process of language rule hypothesis building is evident in constructions such as *eated* and *goed* that are not found in adult speech but represent a rule in English. Verbs are made past tense by adding *-ed*. Unfortunately, not all verbs follow this rule.

Some children are risk takers who attempt new structures and make mistakes. Other children may make few errors because they attempt to produce new structures infrequently (Rispoli, 2005).

Use

Within conversations with caregivers, preschool children introduce topics and maintain them for an average of two to three turns. It is often easier for a preschool child to introduce a new topic than to continue an old one, as in the following example:

Child:	I got a new bike.
Partner:	What color is it?
Child:	Red.
Partner:	Did you ride it on your birthday?
Child:	Mommy saw a spider.

Within conversations, preschool children begin to consider that the listener needs to know certain information and the amount of information needed and that there is a need to change conversational style when speaking to younger children. A typical preschool conversation is presented in Box 5.3. Another example is presented on the accompanying CD-ROM.

Style of talking is also reflected in role playing and narration or story telling. Four-year-old children can tell simple sequential stories, usually about past events.

CONTENT

Children's expressive vocabularies grow to approximately 300 words by age 2, then mushroom to 900 and 1,500 at ages 3 and 4, respectively. They may comprehend two or three times that many words in context.

BOX 5.3
Example of Preschool Language

G and B are young 4-year-olds. They are playing with fire-fighter hats, dishes, and dolls. Notice how different this sample is from the toddler language in Box 5.2. Each child supports her portion of the conversation. The syntax seems adultlike, but the content is pure preschool. The rapid change of topics gives this sample a nonsensical quality. With no adult to maintain a cohesive topic structure, this is a free-for-all with only one or two turns on each topic before it shifts.

G: And I gonna wear both of these.

B: At the same time? No, I'm wearing this one.

G: I'm wearing this one.

B: And then I do this.

G: You wear this and I'll wear this.

B: Two colored cups. You drink out of this one. I drink out of the big one. I'm putting the box up there.

G: Okay, I will I have this and you have this.

B: Stay up there.

G: She doesn't look too happy.

B: Uh-oh. Why did I spill it?

G: Mine will only stand.

B: Mine sat.

G: All done with supper. What kind of spoon is this?

B: A plastic one, what else? Now it's time for me to make my own dinner.

G: Time for me too. I have to use this. My baby has to go to bed now. We have to first change their diapers.

B: No we don't.

G: Come here, look.

B: There's a button. I want something to drink.

G: Okay, I'll give you some. Look at this. Watch this. I'm gonna try and make this stand. Do you think this is a girl or a boy?

B: A boy.

G: Oh, cause the boy has the pants on and the girl has the dress on.

B: Happy birthday to you.

G: Grab everythin' up. I'm grabbing most of the doll stuff.

Words are learned quickly through a process called **fast mapping** in which the child infers the meaning from context and uses the word in a similar manner. Fuller definitions evolve over time.

In addition to single words, preschool children acquire some relational words and phrases that are used to join other words and create longer units of language. Categories of relational words include locational terms such as *in, on,* and *under;* temporal terms such as *first* and *last;* quantitative terms such as *more than;* qualitative terms such as *bigger than;* familial terms such as *brother;* and conjunctions, such as *and, if, so, but,* and *because.*

Adultlike forms of many sentences evolve during the preschool years.

In part, semantic development reflects cognitive development. For example, 4-year-olds demonstrate categorization skills that seem to indicate more advanced procedures for storage of learned information than are seen in younger children.

FORM

During the preschool years, changes in language form are very dramatic. Beginning with short, two- to four-word sentences at age 2, you probably acquired 90% of adult syntax by age 5. For English-speaking preschoolers, language becomes more complex as it becomes longer. We can describe children's language development by calculating the average, or **mean length of utterance (MLU),** in morphemes. The calculation of MLU is discussed later in this chapter. Some MLU values are presented in Table 5.1.

The simple word-order rules found in the utterances of 18- to 24-month-olds form the basis for a more elaborate grammar, and by age 3, most children's utterances contain both a subject and a verb. This basic structure is elaborated with the addition of articles, adjectives, auxiliary verbs, prepositions, pronouns, and adverbs.

In addition, adultlike negative, interrogative, and imperative sentence forms evolve. For example, the toddler negative consisting of a Negative + X form, as in *No cookie,* is modified by words such as *no, not, can't, don't,* and *won't* being placed between the subject and verb, as in *Mommy can't catch me.* Other negatives such as *wouldn't, couldn't, is not,* and *isn't* are added later.

Similarly, interrogatives or questions go from single words, such as *Doggie?* and *What?* or *Wassat?,* to more complex questions that ask *what* and *where,* followed developmentally by *who, which,* and *whose,* and finally *when, why* and *how,* and a more mature form in which the verb or auxiliary verb and subject are reversed, as in *Are you happy?* or *What are you doing?* Correct inversion of the subject and the auxiliary verb also varies with specific verbs (Rowland et al., 2005). For example, *are, have,* and *do* are more difficult for children than auxiliary verbs *is* and *has.* Repeatedly hearing caregiver questions can have a beneficial effect on a preschooler's development of adult-like questions (Valian & Casey, 2003).

By the end of preschool, children are joining two or more independent clauses together to form compound sentences. Late preschoolers can also attach dependent clauses to independent clauses to form complex sentences such as *I didn't liked the big dog that barked at grandpa last night.* These structures appear infrequently in preschool and will develop slowly and be refined throughout the school-age years.

Several bound morphemes are added during the preschool years. These include the progressive verb ending *-ing*, as in *jumping;* plural *-s*, as in *cats;* possessive *-'s* (or *-s'*), as in *mommy's;* and the past tense verb ending *-ed*, as in *talked*. As might be expected, it takes children some time to acquire the use of these morphemes, and it is not uncommon to hear words such as *eated, goed, sheeps,* and *foots.* Two samples of the speech and language of 3-year-olds is presented on the accompanying CD-ROM.

School-Age and Adolescent Language

When children begin to attend school, they start the long process of establishing their identity independent of their family. Most communication now occurs in conversations outside the home. In part, the status of adolescents within their own social grouping is determined by communication skills.

The means of communication change in school as children learn to read and write. In turn, this skill enables children to use computers and opens a whole new world of information. This development is discussed in Chapter 6.

Reading and writing development is related to **metalinguistic skills,** which enable a child to consider language in the abstract, to make judgments about its correctness, and to create verbal contexts, such as in writing. Younger children are unable to make such judgments, especially without a supporting nonlinguistic context.

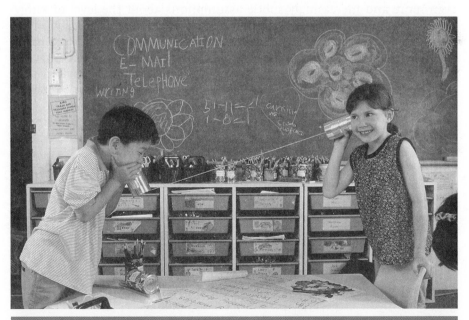

Children learn to use language through interactions with many individuals and in varying situations.

Five-year-olds use very adultlike language form, although many of the more subtle syntactic structures are missing. In addition, these children have not acquired some of the pragmatic skills that are needed to be truly effective communicators.

Over the next few years, language development slows and begins to stabilize, but it will be nonetheless significant. Many complex forms and subtle linguistic uses are learned in the adolescent period. The preschool emphasis on development of language form becomes less prominent, and semantic and pragmatic development blossoms.

Conversation continues to be the primary locus of communication, and children and adolescents learn to be more effective and efficient communicators. Adolescents consolidate their self and personal identity through peer relationships and restructured family interactions. Slang is used within the peer group to distinguish adolescents from both children and adults. Interactional lessons from the family form a basis for the deepening relationships with peers (Whitmire, 2000).

Use

Even with the development of writing, conversation is still the predominant use for language.

During the early school-age years, children's language use changes in two ways: Conversational skills continue to develop, and narratives expand and gain all the elements of mature storytelling. Children refine their conversational skills and learn effective ways to introduce new topics and to continue and to end conversations smoothly and appropriately. While in a conversation, they make relevant comments and adapt their roles and moods to fit the situation. In addition, school-age children learn to make even more and increasingly subtle assumptions about the level of knowledge of their listeners and to adjust their conversations accordingly.

Within conversation, teens demonstrate more affect and discuss topics infrequently mentioned at home. The number of turns on a topic increases greatly. Although interrupting increases, it has evolved into behaviors, such as asking pertinent questions, that serve to move the topic along (Larson & Mckinley, 1998).

Narratives, both in conversation and in writing, gain the elements needed in our culture to be considered satisfying. English literate narratives contain an introductory setting statement and a challenge or challenges that the characters overcome. Events are organized both sequentially and by cause and effect.

Content

Vocabulary continues to grow, but number of words is only the most superficial measure of semantic change. First graders have an expressive vocabulary of approximately 2,600 words but may understand as many as 8,000 root English words and possibly 14,000 when various derivations are included. Aided in school, this receptive vocabulary expands to approximately 30,000 words by sixth grade and to 60,000 words by high school.

Definitions become more dictionary-like, which means that they become less experiential or less based on individual experience and more shared, categorical, as in *An apple is a kind of fruit,* and more precise. Multiple word meanings are also acquired. The ability to provide definitions is related to the acquisition of metalinguistics (Benelli et al., 2006). The increasing size of children's vocabularies requires more precision and an organization into categories for easy retrieval.

School-age children also learn to understand and use **figurative language.** Unlike literal meanings, figurative language does not always mean what it seems to mean. For example, *idioms* are expressions that often cannot be understood literally, such as "hit the road" or "off the wall." Figurative language enriches communication, requires higher language functions of interpretion, and correlates with adolescent literacy skills (Dean Qualls et al., 2003). Some forms are not comprehended until adulthood.

FORM

Following the rapid development of language form in preschool, there is a gradual slowing, although development continues. Many forms continue to develop into adolescence.

By age 5, children use most verb tenses with common verbs and auxiliary or helping verbs, such as *would, should, must,* and *might;* possessive pronouns (*his, her, your*); and the conjunctions *and, but, if, because, when,* and *so.* They still have some difficulty with multiple auxiliary verbs, as in *should have been.* Five-year-old children also have limited use of the comparative *-er,* as in *bigger,* and superlative *-est,* as in *biggest;* relative pronouns used in complex sentences (I know *who* lives next door); gerunds (We go *fishing*); and infinitives (I want *to eat* now).

Many syntactic structures appear slowly, and children may struggle with acquisition well into the school years (Eisenberg et al., 2008). During the school years, children gradually add passive sentences, such as *The cat is chased by the dog,* in which the entity performing the action is placed at the end rather than the beginning of the sentence; reflexive pronouns, such as *myself, yourself, himself,* and *themselves;* conjunctions, such as *although* and *however* and variations of compound and complex sentences. It frequently takes the child several years of practice to gain complete control of these linguistic structures. And some, such as conjunctions, may be used correctly in speech before children fully understand the relationships expressed (Cain et al., 2005).

Morphological development focuses on derivational suffixes—word endings that change the word class, such as adding *-er* to a verb to make a noun, as in *paint/paint<u>er</u>*—and prefixes. Development of prefixes, such as *un-, ir-,* and *dis-* will continue into adulthood.

Adult Language

Language development continues through your lifespan, although at a much slower pace. Adults continue to add new words and to perfect grammatical forms, especially in the written mode. Specialized vocabulary and syntax reflect your work environment, religion, hobbies, education level, and so on. As long as you remain free of any neuropathology, you should continue to improve into old age. And you will amaze yourself with your ability to express complicated ideas with equally complex syntax.

ASSOCIATED DISORDERS AND RELATED CAUSES

Language and its use are extremely complex. It stands to reason, then, that language impairment would be even more so. So many things can go wrong at so many junctures that each child with a language impairment represents a unique set of circumstances.

In this section, we discuss several disorders in which language impairment is a significant factor. Of necessity, we discuss groups of children under different categories of disorder. Categories are helpful for discussion of shared characteristics, but categories are not the same as individuals. Each of us is unique.

The effect that any disorder has on communication and on language development varies with the severity of the disorder and the age of the client. As individuals mature, the communicative requirements change.

We will not be discussing all children with language impairment. The largest group to be excluded are individuals with hearing impairments. These individuals are discussed in Chapter 14, "Audiology and Disorder of Hearing." Children may also exhibit impairments such as aphasia or loss of language as the result of localized brain injury, discussed in Chapter 7, "Adult Language Impairments."

Mental Retardation/Intellectual Disability

The American Assiciation on Intellectual and Developmental Disabilities (AAIDD) defines intellectual disability (ID), formerly called mental retardation (MR), as consisting of the following:

- Substantial limitations in intellectual functioning;
- Significant limitations in adaptive behavior consisting of conceptual, social, and practical skills; and
- Originating before age 18 (AAIDD, 2009)

Because ID is not widely accepted yet, we use both terms interchangeably.

Accounting for approximately 2.5% of the population, people with mental retardation vary based on causality and other factors such as the amount of home support, the living environment, education, mode of communication, and age. Several Web sites at the end of the chapter provide more information on ID/MR.

Severity classifications are usually based on the level of IQ and range from mild to profound. Ranges of severity and characteristics are presented in Table 5.3. However, a rating that is based only on IQ may reveal little about overall functioning. In addition, similar IQs in individuals with different ages result in very different skill levels.

> Mental retardation means more than just a low IQ. Values such as IQ usually measure past learning only.

TABLE 5.3
....
Severities of mental retardation/developmental disability

Category	IQ Range	% of MR Population	Characteristics
Mild	52–68	89	Usually absorbed into the community where they work and live independently
Moderate	36–51	6	Capable of learning self-care skills and working within a sheltered environment; live semi-independently, with relatives, or in a community residence
Severe	20–35	3½	Capable of learning some self-care skills and are not totally dependent; often exhibit physical disabilities and deficits in speech and language
Profound	Below 20	1½	Capable of learning some basic living skills but require continual care and supervision; often exhibit severe physical and/or sensory problems

Source: From "Mental Retardation: Difference and Delay," by R. E. Owens (2010). In D. K. Bernstein and E. Tiegerman (Eds.), *Language and Communication Disorders in Children* (6th ed.). Boston: Allyn and Bacon. Reprinted with permission.

Causes of ID/MR are almost as varied as individuals. Two large categories of possible causal factors are biological and socioenvironmental. These factors are complicated by cognitive limitations that can affect the processing of incoming and outgoing information such as speech and language. Biological factors include the following:

Genetic and chromosomal abnormalities

Maternal infections during pregnancy

Toxins and chemical agents

Nutritional and metabolic causes

Gestational disorders affecting development of the fetus

Complications from pregnancy

Complications from delivery

Brain diseases

Socioenvironmental factors include a stimulation-impoverished environment, poor housing, inadequate diet, poor hygiene, and lack of medical care. The effect of each of these factors varies with each child.

Processing of information consists of four steps: attending, discriminating, organizing, and retrieving. In general, individuals with mild-moderate MR can sustain attention as well as mental-age-matched non-MR peers but have difficulty scanning and selecting stimuli to which to attend.

The ability to discriminate likenesses and differences is related to the severity of mental retardation. The more severe the mental retardation, the

> Individuals with mental retardation may process incoming sensory information differently from those without retardation.

more difficulty the person will have in discriminating. In general, individuals with MR are limited in their ability to identify relevant cues and attend to all dimensions of a task.

Organization or the categorizing of information for storage is especially challenging for individuals with ID. In short, they do not rely on strategies that link words and concepts to one another. Nor do they spontaneously rehearse information for easy retrieval.

Memory or retrieval of previously stored information is poor and operates more slowly within the population with ID/MR. Organizational deficits contribute to this performance. Humans generally retain information by rehearsal, but those with MR do not seem to use this strategy spontaneously. To some extent, memory is affected by the type of information (Kay-Raining Bird & Chapman, 1994). In general, individuals with ID have more difficulty with auditory input, especially linguistic, than with visual input.

Incoming linguistic information undergoes several types of decoding. Simultaneous synthesis occurs all at once and extracts overall meaning. Successive synthesis is more linear, occurring one at a time. Although individuals with MR exhibit some difficulty with both types, those with Down syndrome have much greater difficulty with successive processing, possibly reflecting poor auditory working memory. Working memory is the place where incoming and outgoing information is held while it is processed.

Lifespan Issues

Some newborns and infants with ID are identified early because of obvious physical factors, such as syndromes or anatomical anomalies, at-risk indicators such as low birthweight or poor physical responses, or delayed development. Intervention may begin at home or in special early intervention programs. It is best for the child if intervention begins as soon as possible. Early intervention focuses on sensorimotor skills, physical development, and social and communicative abilities. An Individualized Family Services Plan (IFSP) specifying services is written in collaboration with caregivers.

Some children with MR are not identified until age 2 or 3. These youngsters, along with those previously identified, will likely attend a special preschool. They may receive intervention services, such as physical therapy, special education, or speech-language therapy in either the home or school.

Depending on the severity of a school-age child's mental retardation, she or he may either attend a regular education class and receive special services or receive education in a self-contained, special classroom. Education and training will focus on academic skills, daily living and self-help activities, and vocational needs depending on the abilities of the child.

Only those children with the most profound MR accompanied by other disabilities are institutionalized. Generally, children who cannot reside at home live in community residences with 8 to 10 other children their age and with houseparents.

Mike, a boy with profound MR and cerebral palsy, lived at home with his parents as an infant and preschooler. As he matured and his parents aged, Mike was placed in a community residence run by the Association for

Retarded Citizens. He received daily care at this center and was able to continue his education at the same school. Most of his training involved daily living skills and use of a communication board to communicate.

In adulthood, living and working arrangements vary widely. People with milder retardation often live in the community and work competitively in minimally skilled jobs. More severely involved individuals may live with family or in community residences containing a small group of similar adults. They may work in a special workshop or be enrolled in a day treatment program in which education and training continue to be the focus.

LANGUAGE CHARACTERISTICS

Children with ID vary greatly in their communication abilities. For example, children with Down syndrome (DS) and fragile X syndrome (FXS) have moderate to severe delays in communication development in all areas of language (Roberts et al., 2001). In phonology, boys with FXS make errors similar to those of younger typically developing youth, whereas those with DS have more significant phonological differences than might be expected by delayed development alone (Roberts et al., 2005).

For many individuals with ID, language is the single most important limitation. For approximately half of the population with ID, language comprehension and/or production is even below the level of cognition. This might be indicative of cognitive processing problems that accompany MR. For example, as mentioned, those with DS exhibit auditory working memory deficits (Seung & Chapman, 2000).

In initial language development, individuals with MR follow a similar but slower developmental path than that of typically developing children. Even so, children with MR produce shorter, more immature language forms (Boudreau & Chapman, 2000). In later development, the paths begin to differ more from typical development. All areas of language exhibit some delay and disorder in children with MR.

Very few individuals with mental retardation live in large institutions. Beginning in the 1970s, a philosophy called deinstitutionalization has been responsible for the movement of individuals with MR into small community residences.

Learning Disabilities

The National Joint Committee on Learning Disabilities (1991) defines *learning disabilities (LD)* as follows:

> a generic term that refers to a heterogeneous group of disorders manifested by significant difficulties in the acquisition and use of listening, speaking, reading, writing, reasoning, or mathematical abilities. These disorders are intrinsic to the individual and are presumed to be due to *central nervous system dysfunction*. Even though a learning disability may occur concomitantly with other handicapping conditions or environmental influences, it is **not** the direct result of those conditions or influences. (p. 19)

Approximately 15% of children with LD have their major difficulty with motor learning and coordination, and more than 75% primarily have difficulty learning and using symbols (Miniutti, 1991). This latter group is said to have a **language-learning disability.**

Children with language learning disabilities have difficulty learning and using symbols for speaking, listening, reading, and writing.

Approximately 3% of all individuals have LD, but the severity varies widely. Learning disabilities affect males four times as frequently as they do females. Go to the Web sites at the end of the chapter to find more resources.

The characteristics of LD fall into six categories: motor, attention, perception, symbol, memory, and emotion. Few children exhibit all of the characteristics described. Motor difficulties may include either hyperactivity or hypoactivity. Hyperactivity or overactivity is more prevalent, especially among boys. This results in difficulty attending and concentrating for more than very short periods. Children with hypoactivity may be deficient in their sense of body movement, definition of handedness, eye-hand coordination, and space and time conceptualization.

Attentional difficulties include a short attention span, inattentiveness, and distractibility. Irrelevant stimuli may capture the child's attention, and overstimulation easily occurs. Some children become fixed on a single task or behavior and repeat it compulsively, a process called *perseveration*.

Those who have hyperactivity and attentional difficulties but do not manifest other characteristics of LD may be labeled as having **attention deficit hyperactivity disorder (ADHD).** Children with ADHD have an underlying neurological impairment in executive function that regulates behavior; as a result, they are impulsive. Although these children have difficulty using language socially and educationally, they may be missed on language testing that ignores these pragmatics aspects (Oram et al., 1999).

Perceptual difficulties of children with LD involve interpretation of incoming stimuli, although this is not a sensory disorder, such as deafness or blindness. Children with perceptual disabilities often confuse similar sounds, similar-sounding words, and similar-looking printed letters and words. In addition, children with LD may have difficulty both in determining where to focus their attention and in integrating sensory information from different sources, such as vision and hearing. Those children having particular difficulty in comprehending printed symbols or difficulty producing written symbols and may be labeled as having **dyslexia,** which is discussed in more detail in Chapter 6, "Developmental Literacy Impairments." It's estimated that as many as 80% of children with LD have some form of reading problem and that the incidence of dyslexia in the overall population may range from 5% to 17% (Sawyer, 2006).

Learning disabilities are not caused by emotional disorders; rather, the emotional problems result from misperception and from frustration.

Memory difficulties affect short-term retrieval, as in remembering directions, and long-term retrieval as in recalling names, event sequences, and words. Some children exhibit word-finding problems that result in blocks and the use of fillers ("Ah, ah, you know . . .") or circumlocutions ("Oh, it's that thing that does that stuff that goes round . . .") resembling similar behaviors in stutterers (German & Simon, 1991).

Emotional problems are usually an accompanying factor, not a causal factor. They are a reaction to the frustration that these children feel. Although most children with LD have normal intelligence, they perform poorly on language-based tasks and are told by parents or teachers that they are not trying or that they're lazy or stupid. Emotional behavior may result in children being described as aggressive, impulsive, unpredictable, withdrawn, and/or impatient. These youngsters may exhibit poor judgment, unusual fears, and/or poor adjustment to change.

The fact that LD occurs more frequently in families with a history of the disorder and in children who had a premature or difficult birth suggests possible biological causal factors. The central nervous system dysfunction mentioned in the definition may involve a breakdown along the neural pathways that connect the midbrain with the frontal cortex, an area that is responsible for attention, regulation, and planning of cognitive activity.

Although not a causal factor, socioenvironmental factors may account for at least some of the behaviors. For example, misperceptions by the child affect interactions, which influence the child's development, especially language. Language difficulties, in turn, affect the child's interactions.

Information-processing difficulties are characterized by an inability to use certain strategies or to access certain stored information. In general, children with LD exhibit poor ability to attend selectively, concentrating on inappropriate or unimportant stimuli. They have difficulty deciding on the relevant information to which to attend. As we have seen, discrimination is extremely difficult because children with LD are not sure of the relevant aspects of a stimulus that make it similar or dissimilar to another.

Information that is poorly attended to and poorly discriminated will be poorly organized. The cognitive organization of children with LD reflects this confusion. In short, the organization is too inefficient for easy retrieval, so memory is less accurate and retrieval is slower.

Lifespan Issues

As preschoolers, children with LD may exhibit little interest in language or even in books. When a child reaches school, the linguistic demands of the classroom are often well above her or his oral language abilities. The result is often academic underachievement.

Most learning disabilities are not discovered until children go to school, although some children may be enrolled in special preschool programs or may receive therapy services because of poor motor coordination, hyperactivity, or a failure to develop language typically. When they reach school with its accompanying demand for language skills, many children with LD require the services of special educators, speech-language pathologists, and reading specialists. Some children might not be identified in early grades. Very bright children may "learn" to read by memorizing word shapes rather than using phonics-based word-attack skills as discussed in Chapter 6.

Children with LD often receive special services while being included in regular classrooms. They can be successful if some adaptation, such as repeating instructions or allowing for a quiet work space, is made by the teacher to accommodate their needs. Case Study 5.2 tells the story of one child with a learning disability.

Some children with LD seem to outgrow aspects of their disability. Hyperactivity seems to fade in adolescence. Some adolescents succeed well enough to continue their education and graduate from college. We know adults with learning disabilities who are chemists, engineers, teachers, and

CASE STUDY 5.2
Personal Story of a Child with Language Learning Disabilities

Darren's language learning disability went undetected until second grade. As a preschooler, he had some difficulty with speech sounds and displayed little interest in books, letters, or drawing. His mother considered his lack of interest and his overactivity to be a "boy thing." Darren received no preschool education. In first grade, he was slow to learn to read and write, as were several of his classmates.

When Darren still seemed to be struggling in second grade, his teacher suggested an evaluation to determine whether he had a learning disability. He was evaluated by the school psychologist, a reading specialist, a special education teacher, and a speech-language pathologist. It was found that Darren's mother had received little, if any, prenatal care and that Darren was born preterm, weighing only 4 pounds, 10 ounces. After a stay in the hospital of several days, Darren went home with his mother. The rest of his preschool years were uneventful, and he remained at home with his older sister and younger brother, experiencing the occasional middle ear infection or childhood illness. Although his sister exhibits no signs of a learning disability, Darren's younger brother does exhibit hyperactivity.

At age 11, Darren is a very active child who enjoys sports, especially soccer, which he plays with his best friend Carlos. Darren has great difficulty reading and writing, and letter and word reversal and transposition are common in both. He has great difficulty sounding out new words. His speech is characterized by word retrieval problems and a limited vocabulary, peppered with "Ya know," "thing," and "one," as in "An' I got that one, ya know, that thing that goes like this."

Darren has had some difficulty behaving in school. His attention easily wanders, and he fidgets in his seat often. If he is not kept busy, he bothers the other students and keeps them from working. He finds himself in frequent fights in school, usually because he has misunderstood some comment of another student. His temper flares easily, possibly because school can be very frustrating.

Although his schoolwork has improved somewhat, he is still well behind his classmates in his ability to read, write, and work independently. This deficit, in turn, has inhibited his ability to problem-solve and to think critically in class. He continues to receive tutoring in reading and writing and to see the speech-language pathologist weekly to work on vocabulary, word retrieval, and language use skills.

speech-language pathologists, although some have lingering vestiges of LD, requiring lifelong adaptations.

Other adults continue to have difficulty. Matt received special services throughout his school years and finished high school. His language difficulties were complicated by a volatile temper and frequent misinterpretations of the communicative intentions of others. After being fired from a series of jobs, he hit on the idea of informing his new boss that he was "partially deaf" and needed all instructions and feedback repeated face to face. He no longer flies off the handle when given a simple directive by his supervisor and is gainfully employed.

LANGUAGE CHARACTERISTICS

All aspects of language, spoken and written, usually are affected in children with language-learning disabilities (Wallach & Butler, 1995). These children experience difficulty with the give-and-take of conversation and with the form and content of language. Deducing language rules is particularly difficult, resulting in delays in morphological rule acquisition and in the development of syntactic complexity. As a result, overall oral language development may be slow, and frequent communicative breakdown is possible. Word-finding problems may exist, resulting in greater time being needed to respond verbally.

Some children with LD experience disfluent speech that on the surface might seem like stuttering. Called **cluttering,** the behaviors are characterized by overuse of fillers and circumlocutions associated with word-finding difficulties, rapid speech, and word and phrase repetitions. Unlike the situation with stuttering, the child seems barely to recognize his or her disfluency, and no fear of words or speech situations seems to exist.

> Attentional, discriminatory, and memory deficits along with both receptive and expressive symbol use problems can result in many communication breakdowns.

Specific Language Impairment

Approximately 10% to 15% of middle-class U.S. children may be "late bloomers" whose early language development is delayed. Most outgrow it. Approximately half of these children continue to have problems characterized as **specific language impairment (SLI)** (Dale et al., 2003). These children are at risk for academic failure when they begin school because they will not have the basic language skills for reading and writing in first grade (Choudhury & Benasich, 2003).

Children with SLI exhibit significant limitations in language functioning that cannot be attributed to deficits in hearing, oral structure and function, general intelligence, or perception. In other words, no obvious anatomical, physical, intellectual, or perceptual cause seems to exist. Although children with SLI have typical nonverbal intelligence, they do exhibit deficits in a variety of nonverbal tasks, suggesting impaired or delayed cognitive functioning (Mainela-Arnold et al., 2006). These same children have age-appropriate visuospatial short-term and working memory, a right hemisphere function (Archibald & Gathercole, 2006).

Similar to those with LD, children with SLI exhibit language performance scores that are significantly lower than their intellectual performance scores on nonverbal tasks. The major distinction between those with LD and SLI is that those with SLI do not exhibit perceptual difficulties, the misinterpretation of incoming information.

Children with SLI are a very heterogeneous group, especially in their language skills. Because the disorder is characterized primarily by the exclusion of other disorders, some professionals doubt the very existence of the disorder (Kamhi, 1998). One study of over a thousand preschool children failed to find a distinct group corresponding to children with SLI (Dollaghan, 2004). Still, there are many children with language impairment for whom no readily identifiable causal factors exist.

As you might imagine, causal factors have been somewhat difficult to identify. Nonverbal intelligence, birth and delivery, hearing, and self-help and motor skills all seem to be within normal limits (Paul, 1991). Affecting males more than females, the oral and written language deficits of SLI appear to be cross-generational (Flax et al., 2003). There is an increased prevalence in families with a history *of speech and language problems.*

Brain imaging of children with SLI indicates brain symmetry in the left and right hemispheres unlike the usual asymmetry of left-side predominance in language processing regions (Ors et al., 2005). Further investigation using magnetic resonance imaging (MRI) suggests children with SLI exhibit different patterns of brain activation and coordination reflecting less efficient patterns of functioning, including reduced activation in the brain areas critical for communication processing (Ellis Weismer et al., 2005; Hugdahl et al., 2004). In general, children with SLI have increased integration of the parietal lobe and decreased integration of the frontal lobe on encoding and decreased integration of the parietal on decoding.

> There is no single, obvious cause for specific language impairment.

Children with SLI do exhibit some information-processing problems with certain types of incoming sensory information, with memory and problem solving (Kamhi, 1998; Weismer & Hesketh, 1996). Auditory sequential working memory and problem solving in complex reasoning tasks are affected (Kamhi et al., 1990). Limits in verbal working memory suggest that children with SLI have a limited capacity for language processing (Deevy & Leonard, 2004; Marton & Schwartz, 2003; Weismer et al., 1999).

LIFESPAN ISSUES

As preschool children, those with SLI are perceived negatively by their peers because their communication skills do not match expectations (Segebart DeThorne & Watkins, 2001). In addition, children with SLI exhibit poor social skills (Conti-Ramsden & Botting, 2004).

Many children initially thought to have SLI are later identified as having a language-learning disability. Lingering effects of SLI may result in reading difficulties that reflect difficulty with earlier language skills, such as rhyming, letter naming, and concepts related to print (Boudreau & Hedberg, 1999). In general, children with SLI exhibit slower and poorer processing of both linguistic and nonlinguistic material in elementary school (Miller et al., 2001; Weismer et al., 2000; Windsor & Hwang, 1999). Children with SLI are less successful than typical peers at initiating play interactions, thus they engage in more individual play and onlooking behaviors (Liiva & Cleave, 2005). Teachers rate these children as exhibiting more reticence and solitary-passive withdrawal (Hart et al., 2004).

Long-term data on children with SLI are sparse. Studies have indicated later academic difficulties, especially with language-based activities. For example, at age 14, children with SLI still exhibit slower response times in language tasks compared to children developing typically (Miller et al., 2006). Reticence and extreme aloneness may lead to rejection and bullying by others in middle and high school (Conti-Ramsden & Botting, 2004; Rubin et al., 2002). Many adolescents with SLI perceive themselves negatively and are less independent than their typically developing (TD) peers (Conti-Ramsden & Durkin, 2008; Jerome et al., 2002). Additional information can be found on the Web sites at the end of the chapter.

LANGUAGE CHARACTERISTICS

In general, children with SLI have difficulty (1) extracting regularities from the language around them; (2) registering different contexts for language; and (3) constructing word-referent associations for lexical growth (Connell & Stone, 1992; Kiernan et al., 1997). As a result, these youngsters experience difficulty in morphological and phonological rule formation and application and in vocabulary development (Frome Loeb & Leonard, 1991; Oetting & Morohov, 1997; Redmond, 2003). Pragmatic problems seem to result from an inability to use language forms effectively, resulting in more inappropriate utterances (Brinton et al., 1997). In addition, children with SLI have deficits in their ability to recognize the impact of and to express emotions (Brinton et al., 2007).

Both semantic and phonological deficits contribute to word-learning difficulties in children with SLI (Gray, 2004). Although word learning is difficult for children with SLI, comprehension seems to be easier than production.

Specific difficulty with grammatical markers suggests language-processing deficits in phonological working memory where words are held while processed (Corriveau et al., 2007; Montgomery & Leonard, 2006). Deficits in phonological working memory mean less capacity to store phonological information. Imagine that you have limited working memory but communication continues at a rapid rate, overwhelming and slowing the entire process. You begin to lose information as more comes in. Expressively, children with SLI may speak more slowly with frequent speech disruptions (Guo et al., 2008).

Language comprehension and processing are active processes, yet children with SLI do not appear to employ them actively. Auditory processing problems may result in difficulties with morphological inflections, such as past tense -ed, function words such as prepositions and articles (e.g., a, the), auxiliary verbs, and pronouns. Children with SLI exhibit persistent problems with morpheme use regardless of the language (Bedore & Leonard, 2001; Dromi et al., 1999; Redmond & Rice, 2001), and they are less efficient in using syntax to aid in vocabulary acquisition (Rice, Cleave, & Oetting, 2000).

Autism Spectrum and Pervasive Developmental Disorders

Autism spectrum disorder (ASD) is at the more severe end of an impairment known as **pervasive developmental disorder (PDD).** Some children with PDD may have **hyperlexia,** an inordinate interest in letters and words, characterized by early ability to read but with little comprehension. Others have **semantic-pragmatic disorder,** characterized by limited vocabulary, concrete definitions, and poor conversational skills (Aram, 1997; Snowling & Frith, 1986). A milder form of PDD, called **Aspergers syndrome (AS)** is a neurodevelopmental disorder in which cognitive, language, and self-help skills are not disordered (American Psychiatric Association, 2000), although there may be subtle language impairments, along with social interaction difficulties, restricted interests, and repetitive behaviors. Language difficulties with AS include verbosity and a pedantic speaking style.

Autism spectrum disorder is described as an impairment in reciprocal social interaction with a severely limited behavior, interest, and activity repertoire that has its onset before 30 months of age (American Psychiatric Association, 1987). It is characterized by disturbances in the following areas (Ritvo & Freeman, 1978):

- *Developmental rates and the sequence of motor, social-adaptive, and cognitive skills.* Development often proceeds in spurts and plateaus, rather than smoothly, and most areas of development are affected. Slightly more than half of the children with ASD have IQs below 50. The remainder are split evenly between IQs of 50 to 70 and IQs of 71 and above. These figures might not be accurate but rather represent our inability to test adequately.

- *Responses to sensory stimuli.* The same child may be both hypersensitive and hyposensitive in audition, vision, and tactile, motor, olfactory, and taste stimulation. The child may have preferences for routines and become extremely upset with change. In addition, the child might engage in self-stimulatory behaviors, such as hand flapping, rocking, or spinning shiny objects.

- *Speech and language, cognition, and nonverbal communication.* Individuals with ASD may be nonspeaking, minimally verbal, echolalic, or more typical in their communication.

- *Capacity to relate appropriately to people, events, and objects.* As infants, children with ASD are described as either lethargic, preferring solitude and making few demands, or highly irritable, with sleeping problems and screaming and crying. As they age, they may exhibit little affection for others, including parents, and inappropriate play behaviors, such as repeating actions inordinately. In general, the more severe the symptoms, the poorer language and overall development (Pry et al., 2005).

The primary causal factors in autism are biological. Approximately 65% of all individuals with ASD have neurological differences and 20% to 30% experience seizures. In addition, some researchers have found unusually high levels of serotonin, a neurotransmitter and natural opiate, and abnormal development of the cerebellum, which regulates incoming sensations, and of sections of the temporal lobe responsible for memory and emotions.

At least 15% of children with ASD have a genetic mutation not inherited from their parents (Sebat et al., 2007; Zhao et al., 2007). This is even higher for those with more severe forms of the disorder. Interestingly, the mutations are not similar for all children with ASD. In addition, between 2% and 6% of children with ASD also have fragile X syndrome, a genetic mutation of the X chromosome associated with ID/MR (Belmonte & Bourgerone, 2006).

 The incidence of ASD is higher among males—by a 4:1 ratio to females—and among those with a family history of autism or PDD. The family pattern suggests a genetic basis for the disorder. An audio sample of a young man with ASD is presented on the accompanying CD-ROM.

Neural studies suggest that the eye and face detection processing of children with autism may be delayed, explaining, in part, the early failure to bond with caregivers (Grice et al., 2005). Additionally, infants with autism show no difference in brain response to familiar and unfamiliar faces, supporting the notion of facial processing impairment (Dawson et al., 2002).

Differences in processing incoming information also suggest a neurological basis for ASD. Individuals with ASD experience difficulty in analyzing and integrating information. Their responding is often very overselective, resulting in a tendency to fixate on one aspect of a complex stimulus, often some irrelevant, minor detail. As a result, discrimination is difficult.

Overall processing by children with ASD has been characterized as a *gestalt* in which unanalyzed wholes are stored and later reproduced in identical fashion. The storage of unanalyzed information may account for the way in which individuals with ASD become quickly overloaded with sensory information. Storage of unanalyzed wholes also might hinder memory. It's difficult to organize information on the basis of relationships between stimuli if those stimuli remain unanalyzed. Lack of analysis would also hinder transferring or generalizing learned information from one context to another.

LIFESPAN ISSUES

At present children with ASD are identified by the time they are 2 or 3 years of age. Although early intervention (EI) is critical to maximizing outcomes for children with ASD, early indentification is often difficult. Failure to meet the following milestones may indicate need for further evaluation (see the Web sites at the end of the chapter):

- No babbling by 12 months,
- No gesturing by 12 months,
- No single words by 16 months,
- No 2-word spontaneous speech by 24 months, and
- Loss of language or social skills at any age (Filipek et al., 1999).

It may not be possible at this time to make a definitive diagnosis prior to 24 months of age (Woods & Wetherby, 2003).

School-aged children and adolescents with ASD or PDD may be included in regular education classes or be in special classes, depending on the severity of the disorder. In some children, the severity of autism or ASD lessens with age. For example, as Jeffery became a teenager, his behavior seemed to be less disruptive, and there were fewer outbursts. Although he could engage in conversation easily, he continued to become annoyed and to begin flapping his hands if more than one person spoke at a time.

People with milder forms of the disorder may be able to live on their own and hold competitive employment. For example, Dr. Temple Grandin, a woman with ASD, is employed as a college professor. Unfortunately, the vast majority of people with ASD are not so successful and require supervision and care. Many have adult life patterns similar to those of adults with MR. Case Study 5.3 presents the story of a young man with ASD.

CASE STUDY 5.3
A Young Man with Autism Spectrum Disorder (ASD)

Andrew is a 23-year-old man with high functioning autism spectrum disorder (ASD). He has a younger brother, age 16, and they both live with their parents in a suburb of a moderate-size American city. Andrew is attending the local community college for information technology (IT) and hopes to graduate this year.

When Andrew was born, he was a typical baby, according to his parents. He noticed sounds, made eye contact, nursed enthusiastically, and smiled frequently. He wasn't overly irritable or physically rigid. His muscle tone seemed appropriate, and he actively sought out noises and colorful or noise-making toys. He cried and made comfort or pleasure sounds.

Around 8 months of age, about the time when he began to gesture, Andrew seemed to change according to his mother. He withdrew, became quiet, and was less willing to interact with her in face-to-face encounters. He made fewer noises and shortly after he began to gesture, he stopped. On some occasions, he actively turned away from his parents and others and seemed to be attending totally to certain favored toys and objects. When his parents tried to interact with him, he became irritable.

Thinking it was just a phase in his development, Andrew's parents decided to give him space to develop. Andrew's pediatrician agreed. When Andrew did not begin talking at around age one, his parents took comfort in the fact that he had begun to walk. By 18 months, Andrew was still not talking, although he made high-pitched squeals when he played with selected toys. He had also ceased to explore novel objects and played while excluding his parents from his interactions. By Andrew's 2nd birthday, his parents could no longer ignore his lack of speech and took him for an evaluation at a preschool run by the Association for Retarded Citizens (ARC). Although they resisted going to this agency because to do so was to admit that there was a problem, Andrew's parents were encouraged by Andrew's maternal grandparents who accompanied the family to the evaluation. It was determined that Andrew had delayed language but no diagnostic label, such as ASD, was placed on his behavior. Andrew was enrolled in the preschool as suggested following his assessment.

Although Andrew's overall behavior improved somewhat in the next year, and he became more compliant, his communication skills improved only minimally, if at all. The ARC speech-language pathologist had begun teaching Andrew to sign because of his lack of sound play and word production. His behavior became increasingly more disruptive and resistant. Around age 3, Andrew was diagnosed as having ASD, based on his behavior and lack of communication skills.

Dissatisfied with Andrew's progress and his increasing avoidance by the other children, Andrew's parents withdrew him from the preschool and began a 2-year search for a more appropriate placement. After several unsuccessful attempts, Andrew was placed in a program using Floor Time, a play-based approach to learning for children with ASD. After a slow start, Andrew began to interact more. His sign training continued, along with attempts to teach Andrew to speak. When Andrew's brother was born, Andrew said his first spontaneous word, *baby,* accompanied by the sign. Andrew continued in the Floor Time program and in a school for other children with ASD for the next several years. Beginning slowly, speech began to replace signing.

By the time he reached middle-school age, Andrew was speaking and reading and writing at near grade level. It was decided that he should attend a regular middle school while receiving continuing services for communication and behavior control. He made few friends and now characterizes this as "a very lonely time for me."

As a community college student, Andrew achieves very good grades. He still enjoys time alone in his room at home where he explores the Internet on his laptop computer. Although his social skills have improved markedly, he is still somewhat of a loner who will respond to other students but rarely initiates communication except to request assistance. He responds best to older adults.

Andrew's plans are to acquire employment in the local IT industry and to live at home. Andrew's parents doubt that their son will be able to live on his own and seem resigned, even happy, to have him remain in their home.

Andrew is still awkward in social situations and has few acquaintances. He claims that social interactions are extremely difficult for him.

Early on, Andrew became aware that he experienced the world differently than other people. Some sounds, for example, seemed very loud while others were very low. Andrew believes that he thinks in pictures rather than in words or concepts as others seem to do. He explains that this is an advantage in dealing with IT information. He smiles when he imagines working and earning a salary.

Source: From Barron, S. (2001, September 25). A Personal Story. *The ASHA Leader, 6*(17), 5, 7, 17. © American Speech-Language-Hearing Association. Reprinted with permission.

LANGUAGE CHARACTERISTICS

Communication problems are often one of the first indicators of possible ASD. Between 25% and 60% of individuals with ASD remain nonspeaking throughout their life. Those who speak often have a wooden or robotlike voice that lacks typical intonational patterns. Many autistic children who use speech and language demonstrate some immediate or delayed echolalia, which is a whole or partial repetition of previous utterances, often with the same intonation. For example, Mickey would say little during the day but store things said to him during the day and repeat them in sequence before he went to sleep at night. In contrast, Adam would echo immediately. For some children, echolalia might either be a language-processing strategy or signal agreement with the previous utterance. Even though echolalia may be outgrown, other problems, especially those related to pragmatics, persist in the child's language. Most children with ASD who learn to talk go through a period of using echolalia (Prizant et al., 1997).

Pragmatics and semantics are affected more than language form (Lord, 1988). Syntactic errors seem to represent a lack of underlying semantic relationships. Prosodic features or suprasegmentals, such as stress, intonation, loudness, pitch, and rate, are often affected, giving the speech of children with ASD the sometimes mechanical quality mentioned. Individuals with ASD often have peculiarities and irregularities in the pragmatics of conversation. The range of intentions is often very limited and may consist solely of demands and in severe cases, unintelligible vocalizations. Some individuals incorporate entire verbal routines, called *formuli,* into their communication. For example, a child might repeat part or all of a television commercial to indicate a desire for the item that had been in the advertisement. A formula represents the person's attempt to overcome the difficulty of matching the content and form of language to the communicative context. Adults with ASD who have good language skills might still misinterpret some of the subtleties of conversation.

> Pragmatics is a continuing problem for individuals with autism, even those with seemingly typical language.

Brain Injury

Brain injury can be confused with LD, MR, or emotional disorders, although individuals with these disorders are very different. Impaired brain functioning can result from **traumatic brain injury (TBI),** cerebrovascular accident or stroke, congenital malformation, convulsive disorders, or encephalopathy, such as infection or tumors. Among children, the most common form of injury is TBI. Cerebrovascular accidents and a fuller discussion of TBI is presented in Chapter 7, "Adult Language Impairments."

Approximately a million children and adolescents in the United States have experienced TBI, which is diffuse brain damage as the result of external force, such as a blow to the head in an auto accident. Individuals with brain injury differ greatly from one another as a result of the site and extent of lesion, the age at onset, and the age of the injury. In general, the smaller the damaged area, the better the chance of recovery. Some individuals recover fully; others remain in a vegetative state. People with TBI exhibit a range of cognitive, physical, behavioral, academic, and linguistic deficits, any of which may be long term.

Cognitive deficits include difficulties in perception, memory, reasoning, and problem solving. Deficits vary and may be permanent or temporary and may partially or totally affect functioning ability. Children with TBI tend to be inattentive and easily distractible. All aspects of cognitive organization—categorizing, sequencing, abstracting, and generalization—may be affected. Children with TBI have difficulty seeing relationships, making inferences, and solving problems. They struggle to formulate goals, plan, and achieve their ends. Memory is also affected, although long-term memory before the trauma is often intact.

Psychological maladjustment or "acting out" behaviors, called *social disinhibition,* may occur in which a person is incapable of inhibiting or controlling impulsive behavior. Other characteristics of TBI may include a lack of initiative, distractibility, inability to adapt quickly, perseveration, low frustration levels, passive-aggressiveness, anxiety, depression, fear of failure, and misperception.

LIFESPAN ISSUES

After the accident, a child may be unconscious. If so, it may last only a few minutes or much longer. Upon regaining consciousness, the child usually experiences some disorientation and memory loss. Memory loss may involve only the time of the immediate accident or may be more extensive, including long-term memory. TBI may be accompanied by physical disability and personality changes.

Neural recovery over time is often unpredictable and irregular, and the variables that affect recovery of children with TBI are extremely independent. In general, a better recovery is signaled by a shorter, less severe period of unconsciousness following the injury, a shorter period of amnesia, and better posttraumatic abilities (Dennis, 1992; Russell, 1993).

The age of the injury can be an inaccurate prognosticator. In general, the older the injury, the less chance of change, although this can be complicated by the delayed onset of some deficits. For example, some neurological problems might not be manifested until later in recovery, making neural recovery unpredictable and irregular over time.

When stabilized, the child with TBI begins a long recovery process that can take years. Within the first few months, she or he might experience spontaneous recovery when large gains in ability are made.

Young children often recover quickly but experience difficulties learning new information and may exhibit severe, long-lasting problems. Older children and adolescents have more to recover from their memory but less new information to learn.

Even individuals who have made a seemingly full recovery may lack subtle cognitive and social skills. For example, although Jane had been injured in an auto accident but made a seemingly full recovery, she began to exhibit learning problems later when she attended elementary school. Unfortunately, her lack of success in school translated into disciplinary problems later on.

Although the brains of younger children are more malleable or more adaptable, this does not mean that younger children will always recover more fully. In addition to recovering the language lost, younger children may still have much language to learn, a task that is possibly made more difficult by the brain injury.

LANGUAGE CHARACTERISTICS

Language problems are evident even after mild injuries. Some deficits, especially in pragmatics, remain long after the injury even when general improvement is good. Overall, pragmatics seems to be the most disturbed aspect of language. The child may lose the central focus or topic in conversation (Chapman et al., 1997). Utterances are often lengthy, inappropriate, and off topic, and fluency is disturbed, especially if there are accompanying motor problems.

Language comprehension and higher functions such as figurative language and dual meanings are also often impaired, although language form is relatively unaffected. Semantics, especially concrete vocabulary, is also relatively undisturbed, although word retrieval, naming, and object description difficulties may be present. Narration, especially maintaining story structure and providing enough information, may also pose a problem (Chapman et al., 1997).

Neglect and Abuse

Each year in the United States, approximately 900,000 children are maltreated sufficiently for this information to be reported to the authorities (U.S. Department of Health and Human Services [DHHS], 2007). Neglect and abuse are the outward signs of a dysfunctional family, the social environment in which these children learn language.

Although neglect and abuse are rarely the direct cause of communication problems, the context in which they occur directly influences the child's development. Medical and health problems among poor Americans also can contribute, although neglect and abuse are not limited to poor families. Poor maternal health, substance abuse, poor or nonexistent pediatric services, and poor nutrition can all affect brain development and maturation.

The quality of the child-mother attachment is a more significant factor in language development than is maltreatment. Maternal attachment can be disturbed by childhood loss of a parent; death of a previous child; pregnancy and/or birth complications; family, marital, or financial problems; substance abuse; maternal age; and/or illness. The result is a lack of support for the development of meaningful communication skills.

> Lack of maternal interaction rather than outright physical abuse accounts for much of the language impairment noted among children from abusive and neglectful environments.

LIFESPAN ISSUES

The affects of childhood abuse and neglect can remain with a child for life. There might be recurring physical, psychological, and emotional problems. Many children who have been abused abuse their own children later, thereby perpetuating this pattern with all its ill effects.

LANGUAGE CHARACTERISTICS

Although all aspects of language are affected, it is in pragmatics that children who have been neglected or abused exhibit the greatest difficulties. In general, they are less talkative and have fewer conversational skills than their peers. They are less likely to volunteer information or to discuss emotions or feelings. Utterances and conversations are shorter with less complex language than nonmaltreated children (Eigsti & Cicchetti, 2004).

Fetal Alcohol Syndrome and Drug-Exposed Children

Within the last 25 years, there has been an increase in the prevalence of **fetal alcohol syndrome (FAS)** and drug-exposed children. FAS accounts for 1 in every 500 to 600 live births. Alcohol interferes with embryonic development by disrupting activation of a critical signaling molecule in the brain. Infants have a low birthweight and exhibit central nervous system problems. There is a relationship between severity of the growth deficiency and the dysmorphic features, such as the space between the eyes, and cognitive limitations (Ervalahti et al., 2007). Later, they demonstrate hyperactivity, motor problems, attention deficits, and cognitive disabilities. As a group, their mean IQ is in the borderline MR range.

The effects of drugs on the fetus vary with the drug, the manner of ingestion, and the age of the fetus (MacDonald, 1992). Crack cocaine is especially destructive because it alters the fetus's neurochemical functioning. Like infants with FAS, those who are exposed to crack have low birthweight. They also have small head circumference and are jittery and irritable (Lesar, 1992).

LIFESPAN ISSUES

Preterm babies, especially those with FAS or early drug exposure, are more likely to die during infancy and to experience developmental difficulties. The drug-exposed child's poorly coordinated behaviors and motor delays may disrupt caregiver-infant bonding (Crites et al., 1992). In addition, caregivers who are dependent on alcohol or drugs might not attend to or might reject the child. As a result, these children behave very much like children with learning disabilities. The limitations noted at birth remain with the child for life and can result in poor academic achievement and antisocial behavior.

Children with FAS and drug exposure have many learning problems similar to those of children with learning disabilities.

LANGUAGE CHARACTERISTICS

Children with FAS exhibit language problems characterized by delayed development of language, echolalia, and comprehension problems. Infants who were exposed to drugs have few infant vocalizations, inappropriate gestures, and language deficits. As preschoolers, they exhibit word-retrieval problems, short sentences, and inappropriate conversational turn taking and topic maintenance (Mentis & Lundgren, 1995). These difficulties persist and are compounded by problems with abstract meanings, multiple meanings, and temporal and spatial terms, such as *before* and *after, next* and *near, next to,* and *in front of.* Both children with FAS and those with fetal drug exposure are behind their peers in reading and other academic tasks.

Other Language Impairments

Although we've touched on some of the more prevalent language impairments, we have by no means exhausted the discussion. Other forms of language impairment include but are not limited to nonspecific language impairment (NLI), late talkers, childhood schizophrenia, selective mutism (SM), otitis media, and children who have received cochlear implants. Children with NLI have a general delay in language development, a nonverbal IQ of 86 or lower, and as in SLI, no obvious sensory or perceptual deficits, but few common characteristics (Rice et al., 2004). Although child health is an important factor among late talkers, most early language delay is environmental in origin, such as poverty and/or homelessness.

Childhood schizophrenia, a serious psychiatric illness that causes strange thinking, odd feelings, and unusual behavior, is uncommon, occurring in approximately 1 of every 14,000 children younger than 13 years of age. Approximately 55% of children and adolescents with schizophrenia have language abnormalities, including language delay especially in pragmatics (Mental Health Research Association, 2007; Nicolson et al., 2000).

Selective mutism (SM) is a relatively rare disorder in which a child does not speak in specific situations, such as school, although she or he may speak normally in others. From 0.2% to 0.7% of all children may have SM at some time with girls nearly twice as likely as boys to be affected (Bergman et al., 2002; Kristensen, 2000).

Many young children suffer from chronic otitis media. In general, the cumulative effect of recurrent otitis media can be a significant factor in delayed language development (Feldman et al., 2003).

Finally, those who receive cochlear implants develop language in a manner similar to that of typically developing children. Although those implanted later have an initial advantage of maturity that enhances language growth, this advantage seems to disappear later as children who received implants at an earlier age begin to develop spoken language at an ever-increasing rate (Ertmer et al., 2003).

Conclusion

So many disorders are associated with language impairment that they probably all have begun to look similar to you. To help your memory, Figure 5.1 presents the major characteristics of each disorder. In most cases, the child with a language impairment has other physical, cognitive, and psychological difficulties, too. In actual practice, speech-language pathologists treat each child as an individual, not as a member of a category. Of importance is each child's behavior and language features, not group characteristics.

Although this section focuses on disorders, it does not address all of the factors that may be related to language impairment. Factors such as poverty, nutrition, child and maternal health, and maternal sensitivity to and stimulation of a child are also important. For example, most children and mothers living in homeless shelters exhibit language deficits (La Paro et al., 2004; O'Neil-Pirozzi, 2003).

Disorder Most Affected	Expected Deficit Area					Language Features		
	Developmental	Cognitive	Perceptual	Affective	Unknown	Form	Content	Use
Mental retardation		X				X	X	X
Language learning disability			X			X	X	X
Specific language impairment					X	X		
Autism				X				X
Traumatic brain injury		X		X				X
Neglect and abuse	X							X

FIGURE 5.1

Summary of disorders associated with language impairment.

ASPECTS OF LANGUAGE AFFECTED

In addition to the etiological categories we have just described, language impairments can also be characterized by the language features affected. For example, a child may have difficulty with word recall and conversational initiation or possess a limited vocabulary and seemingly nonstop talking. Another child may have poor syntax and very short sentences or withdraw from conversational give-and-take. Figure 5.2 presents the most common language features associated with language impairments. A sample of a school-aged child with a language impairment is presented on the accompanying CD-ROM. In an evaluation, speech-language pathologists assess many language features to determine where to begin intervention.

ASSESSMENT

Language assessment is a process of discovery and information gathering. As we noted in Chapter 4, good clinical practice requires that the boundary between assessment and intervention be permeable. A portion of any good assessment is attempting to determine possible avenues for intervention. In turn, each intervention session should contain some assessment of the client's current skill level.

Assessment and intervention overlap and are parts of the same process

Pragmatics

Difficulty answering questions or requesting clarification

Difficulty initiating, maintaining a conversation, or securing a conversational turn

Poor flexibility in language when tailoring the message to the listener or repairing communication breakdowns

Short conversational episodes

Limited range of communication functions

Inappropriate topics and off-topic comments; ineffectual, inappropriate comments

Asocial monologues

Difficulty with stylistic variations and speaker-listener roles

Narrative difficulties

Few interactions

Semantics

Limited expressive vocabulary and slow vocabulary growth

Few or decontextualized utterances, more here-and-now; more concrete meanings

Limited variety of semantic functions

Relational term difficulty (comparative, spatial, temporal)

Figurative language and dual definition problems

Conjunction (*and, but, so, because,* etc.) confusion

Naming difficulties may reflect less rich and less elaborate semantic storage or actual retrieval difficulties

Syntax/Morphology

Short, uncomplex utterances

Rule learning difficulties

Run-on, short, or fragmented sentences

Few morphemes, especially verb endings, auxiliary verbs, pronouns, and function words (articles, prepositions)

Overreliance on word order, which takes precedence over word relationships

Difficulty with negative and passive constructions, relative clauses, contractions, and adjectival forms

Article (*a, the*) confusion

Phonology

Limited syllable structure

Fewer consonants in repertoire

Inconsistent sound production, especially as complexity increases

Comprehension

Poor discrimination of units of short duration (bound morphemes)

Impaired comprehension, especially in connected discourse such as conversations

Reliance on context to extract meaning

Wh- question confusion

Overreliance on nonlinguistic cues for meaning

FIGURE 5.2
. . . .

Most common language characteristics of children with language disorders.

Assessment should be sufficiently broad and deep so that all areas of possible concern are identified and described as accurately as possible. For example, assessment of semantics must include more than receptive understanding and expressive vocabulary size. A thorough examination might also include areas such as word learning abilities and word storage and retrieval (Brackenbury & Pye, 2005).

Referral and Screening

Referral may occur at any point in the lifespan. Some children, such as those with identifiable syndromes or those who are at risk for developing a language impairment, might be referred at birth or early infancy; others with LD might go undetected until they begin school; and those with either TBI or childhood aphasia may be of any age. Parents can be effective referral sources for children with more severe language problems, although they are less reliable in identifying mild impairment (Conti-Ramsden et al., 2006).

In a public school, the SLP may decide to test a child on the basis of results of screening testing or teacher referral. Screening tests, used to determine only the presence or absence of language problem, are routinely administered to all kindergarten and first-grade students. Screening tests must be chosen and administered very carefully. Even though a test is generally considered nonbiased, some items should be interpreted with caution because they may be problematic for children from some cultural or linguistic backgrounds (Qi et al., 2003).

Surveys and parental questionnaires are also effective diagnostic tools. They compare favorably with other language measures (Patterson, 2000; Rescorla & Alley, 2001; Thal, Jackson-Maldonado, & Acosta, 2000).

Referral and subsequent evaluation may occur within an interdisciplinary team of child specialists. The nature of many of the disorders mentioned previously may necessitate input from a pediatrician, neurologist, occupational therapist, physical therapist, developmental psychologist, special education teacher, audiologist, and speech-language pathologist. For example, an interdisciplinary assessment that includes families as active participants and collaborators has been shown to be effective with young children with ASD (Prelock et al., 2003).

> Information from referrals, questionnaires, and interviews provides needed background information from which to begin investigating for possible language impairment and determining what that impairment entails.

Case History and Interview

The case history questionnaire and interview are the first steps in a formal information-gathering process. In addition to asking the questions presented in Chapter 4, the SLP asks more specific questions relevant to language impairment. Questions relate to language development, the language environment of the home, and possible causes for language impairment. Figure 5.3 presents predictors and risk factors for language change in toddlers (Olswang et al., 1998). Possible questions are presented in Figure 5.4.

Observation

Language is heavily influenced by the context in which it occurs. It is helpful, therefore, to observe a child using language in as many contexts as possible. Although it is not always convenient to observe in multiple contexts, a school-based SLP might observe in the classroom; a clinic-based SLP might observe on a home visit, in the waiting room, or during a freeplay period between the mother and child. In all assessments, testing and sampling periods provide an additional observational period.

Predictors

Language

Production:

Small vocabulary with few verbs

Verbs mostly general-purpose, such as *want, go, got,* and *look,*

Comprehension: Six-month delay with large gap between production and comprehension

Phonology:

Few prelinguistic vocalizations and limited variety in babbling

Vowel errors and limited number of consonants

Fewer than 50% of consonants correct

Restricted syllable structure

Speech Imitation

Limited spontaneous imitations

Nonspeech

Play: Little combination of play schemes and/or little symbolic play

Gestures: Few gestures or gesture sequences

Social Skills:

Behavioral problems

Few conversational initiations

More interactions with adults than peers and difficulty gaining entrance to activities

Risk Factors

Otitis Media: Prolonged and untreated

Heritability: Family member with persistent language and learning problems

Parents

Low socioeconomic status

Directive style of interaction rather than responsive

Extreme concern

FIGURE 5.3

Predictors of and risk factors for possible language impairment in toddlers.

Source: Based on Olswang, et al. (1998).

Behaviors that are observed vary with the age of the child and the reported disorder. In addition to observing the child's communicative behavior, the SLP is also concerned with the child's interests and the caregiver's style of communicating and method of behavior control. Figure 5.5 presents some behaviors that might be observed during an assessment.

Hypotheses about the child's language impairment are formed during observation. These are either confirmed or negated during the remainder of the assessment and during intervention.

The SLP must remain focused during observation. This requires that she or he define very carefully the behaviors and/or language features that are observed and fully describe the events preceding and following them. For example, one adolescent with MR would scream, "Don't hit me" repeatedly. It was observed that this occurred when she was asked a question, but the behavior was inconsistent. It was hypothesized that the type of question influenced the response. The hypothesis was confirmed later in the assessment by careful data collection in which the type of question was modified systematically.

Language Use

Does the child . . .

Ask for information? How?

Describe things in the environment? How?

Discuss things in the past, future, or outside of the immediate context?

Make noises when playing alone?

Engage in monologues when playing?

Prefer to play alone or with others?

Express emotions or discuss feelings? How?

Request desired items? How?

Request attention? How?

Direct your attention? How?

Conversational Skills

Does the child . . .

Initiate conversations or interactions with others? What are the child's frequent topics?

Join in when others initiate?

Get your attention before saying something?

Maintain eye contact while talking?

Take turns easily while talking? Interrupt frequently? Are there long gaps between your utterances and the child's responses?

Demonstrate an expectation that you will respond when he or she speaks? What does the child do if you do not respond?

Seem confused or ask for clarification? How? How frequently?

Respond when asked to clarify? How?

Demonstrate frustration when not understood?

Relay sequential information or stories in an organized fashion so that they can be followed? Relay enough information?

Have different ways of talking to different people, such as adults and smaller children?

React more readily to certain people and situations than to others? When does the child communicate best/most?

How does the child respond when you say something? How does the child respond to others?

What emotions does the child express? How?

Are responses meaningful, mismatched, off-top, or irrelevant?

Form and Content

Does the child . . .

Know the names of common events, objects, and people in the environment?

Seem to rely on gestures, sounds, or immediate environment to be understood?

Speak in single words, phrases, or sentences? How long is a typical utterance? Does the child leave out words?

Use words such as *tomorrow, yesterday,* or *last night?*

Use verb tenses?

Put several sentences together to form complex descriptions and explanations?

Follow simple directions?

FIGURE 5.4

Possible questions for questionnaires/interviews when a language impairment is suspected.

Source: Based on Owens (2010).

With whom child communicates

Purposes for child's communication

Effectiveness of child's communication

    Obvious patterns of breakdown

Maturity of child's language

    Utterance length

    Verb usage

    Complexity

Relative amounts of initiative versus responsive communication

Relative amounts of nonsocial versus social communication

Responsiveness of caregiver

Turn allocation, relative size of child's and caregiver's turns

FIGURE 5.5

Possible behaviors to observe during an assessment of language impairment.

Few formal observational tools exist. Speech-language pathologists, recognizing the importance of observation as a vital portion of assessment, are developing reliable measures (Kaderavek & Sulzby, 1998).

Testing

After building rapport with a child, the SLP can begin testing. Tasks should be varied based on their potential effect on different children (Fagundes et al., 1998).

Although standardized, norm-referenced tests are appropriate for determining if a problem exists, they are less useful in identifying specific language deficits (Merrell & Plante, 1997). More descriptive test results allow the SLP to explore a child's strengths and weaknesses. In addition, descriptive results can provide useful information for treatment planning.

It is best to use a series of testing tasks to ensure that many features are assessed (Gray et al., 1999). One study found that a combination of tasks using children's books, such as joint story retelling, expectancy violation detection tasks in which a familiar story element is altered, and comprehension questions, were effective in identifying 96% of children with a language impairment (Skarakis-Doyle et al., 2008). At the very least, receptive and expressive aspects of language form, content, and use should be tested or sampled in some way. Some widely used tests and their characteristics are presented in Table 5.4.

Test methodology varies widely. Children may be asked to form syntactically similar sentences, to make judgments of correctness, to reconfigure scrambled sentences, or to imitate exactly what they hear. They may have to supply definitions, form sentences, or point to words named. All these tasks require different language skills. Unfamiliar tasks may unintentionally

Testing is an extraordinary situation for most children. Typical performance is more likely to be displayed in language sampling.

TABLE 5.4

Characteristics of common language tests

Test	Source	Target
Carrow Elicited Language Inventory (CELI) E. Carrow-Woodcock	DLM Teaching Resources	Identification of children with language problems; can be used to determine which specific linguistic structures may be contributing to the child's problems
Clinical Evaluation of Language Fundamentals–Preschool 2nd edition (CELF-Preschool-2) (2004) E. Wiig, W. Secord, E. Semel	Psychological Corp.	Expressive and receptive language skills: basic concept, sentence structure, word structure, naming, recalling sentence in context, linguistic concepts
Clinical Evaluation of Language Fundamentals IV (CELF-4) (2003) E. Semel, E. Wiig, W. Secord	Psychological Corp.	Expressive and receptive language skills: semantics, syntax, morphology, and memory
Fullerton Language Test for Adolescents, second edition (FTLA-2) (1986) A. R. Thorum	Consulting Psychologists Press, Inc.	Linguistic processing to identify language-impaired adolescents. Auditory synthesis, oral commands, convergent and divergent productions, syllabication, idioms, and morphological competency.
Peabody Picture Vocabulary Test, third edition (PPVT-IV) (2007) L. & L. Dunn	American Guidance Service	Receptive vocabulary
Preschool Language Scale, fourth edition (PLS-4) (2002) I. L. Zimmerman, V. Steiner, R. Pond	Psychological Corp.	Auditory comprehension and verbal ability
Test of Adolescent and Adult Language, third edition (TOAL-3) (1993) D. Hammill, V. Brown, S. Larsen, J. Wiederholt	Pro-Ed	Expressive and receptive language, semantic and syntactic skills assessed in spoken and written form
Test of Auditory Comprehension of Language–third edition (TACL-3) (1999) E. Carrow-Woodcock	Pro-Ed	Auditory comprehension of word classes and relations, grammatical relations, and elaborated sentences
Test of Early Language Development, 3rd ed. (TELD-3) (1999) W.Hresko, D. Reid, D. Hammill	Pro-Ed	Receptive and expressive language
Test of Language Development-Primary, 4th ed. (TOLD-P:4) (2008) P. Newcomer, D. Hammill	Pro-Ed	Receptive and expressive language, semantics, syntax, phonology
The Word Test 2–Adolescent (2005) L. Bowers, R. Huisingh, M. Barrett, J. Orman, C. LoGuidice	Lingui-Systems	Expressive vocabulary and semantics

TABLE 5.4
(Continued)

Age	Notes
3–8 years	Administration of the test takes 10 minutes, and scoring takes 1 hour and 30 minutes. Child's responses must be transcribed phonetically.
3–6 years	Meets PL 99–457 and PL 94–142 guidelines.
6–21 years	Provides a guideline for areas of language that are in need of further observation and testing. Takes 45 minutes to score and administer. Provides supplementary oral and written expression sections for additional information.
11–18.5 years	Standardized: provides means and standard deviation for each subset and age group. Three score breakdowns: competence level, instruction level, and frustration level.
2.5–90 years	A standard. Child points to one of four black-and-white pictures named.
0–6 years	Widely used. Wide variety of receptive and expressive tasks using pictures and toys.
12–25 years	Test requires reading and writing for some of the subtests; 1–3 hours to administer; can be administered to a group for 6 of 8 of the subtests; requires several separate booklets to administer.
K to grade 4	Individually administered, no oral response required. Child points to one of three pictures named.
2 to 7–11 years	Individually administered in about 30 minutes; normed on children from 35 states, representing U.S. population.
4 years to 8–11 years	Administered in about one hour; computer scoring is available.
12–17 years	Administration time: 25 minutes. Results: standard scores, percentile ranks, age equivalencies, no basal or ceilings. Is designed to assess a subject's facility with language and word meaning using common as well as unique contexts, surveys 6 semantic and vocabulary tasks reflective of school assignment, as well as language usage in everyday life.

Test Procedure	Example
Grammatical completion	I'm going to say a sentence with one word missing. Listen carefully, then fill in the missing word. *John has a dish and Fred has a dish. They have two _____.*
Receptive vocabulary	Look at the pictures on this page. I'm going to name one, and I want you to point to it. *Touch (Show me) the officer.*
Defining words	I'm going to say some words. I want you to tell me what each word means or use it in a sentence in a way that makes sense. For example, if I said "coin," you might respond "money made from metal" or "I put my coin in the vending machine."
Pragmatic functions	I'm going to tell you a story and ask you to imagine what the person in the story might say. *Mary lost her money and she must call home for a ride after band practice. She decides to borrow a quarter from her best friend Julie. Before practice begins, she sits down next to Julie and says _____.*
Sentence imitation	I'm going to say some sentences, and I want you to repeat exactly what I say. Let's try one. *We are going to play ball after school tomorrow.*
Parallel sentence production	Here are two pictures. I'll describe the first one, and then you describe the second one using the same type of sentence as I use. For example, for this picture I would say, "The girl is riding her bike," and for this one you would say, "The man is driving his car."
Grammatical correctness	I'm going to say a sentence, and I want you to tell if it is correct or incorrect. If it is incorrect, you must correct it. For example, if I say, "Thems is going to the dance," you would respond, "Incorrect. They are going to the dance."

FIGURE 5.6

Examples of language test tasks.

prejudice the results against the child (Peña & Quinn, 1997). Examples of language test tasks are presented in Figure 5.6.

During testing, the SLP probes the child's performance to try to identify possible effective intervention procedures. Of interest are strategies that either increase production or result in more correct production of a certain language feature (Peña et al., 2001). Sometimes called **dynamic assessment** (Olswang et al., 1990), this probing is invaluable in providing direction for subsequent intervention. Dynamic assessment and techniques that ask children to demonstrate skills that represent realistic learning demands are especially well suited for children with multicultural or bilingual backgrounds (Schraeder et al., 1999; Peña et al., 2006; Ukrainetz et al., 2000).

Test scores should be interpreted cautiously. For example, the omission of some morphological endings by bilingual children is similar to the error pattern of children with SLI (Paradis, 2005). This can lead to misdiagnosis.

In addition, children with language disorders aren't always identified by low scores (Spaulding et al., 2006). SLPs should consult test manuals carefully and select tests that are sensitive and specific to language disorders.

Sampling

If language is influenced by context, then the context of test taking should influence the language a child produces. For some, test structure decreases performance. This is especially true for young children, children from minority populations, and those with disabilities.

In addition to testing, the SLP should also engage a child in challenging conversation, so that he or she will attempt to "stretch" language abilities and in the process reveal difficulties (Hadley, 1998). These evocative techniques are especially important for children with ASD who typically do poorly on both standardized tests and spontaneous language samples (Condouris et al., 2003). A variety of discourse types, such as conversation, narration, explanation, and interview, should be included in the sample. For example, although young children engaged in freeplay produce more utterances than those telling stories, they produce more complex utterances while telling stories and in conversation (Southwood & Russell, 2004).

Typical performance may be enhanced if parents or teachers interact with the child in familiar settings. The experienced SLP can also be an excellent conversational or play partner for the child. Whenever possible, it is best to collect at least two samples of the child with different partners, locations, and activities or topics (Owens, 2010).

Samples may be either very open ended, in which topics and interactions are not defined, or more closed, in which the SLP tries to elicit specific language features. Responses vary. For example, more restrictive question-answer techniques elicit fewer complex utterances than more conversational strategies (Bradshaw et al., 1998). Narratives are especially helpful for exhibiting deficits in older children or those with TBI because of the demands on a speaker (Chapman, 1997). In addition, narratives tend to elicit a large number and variety of syntactic structures (Gummersall & Strong, 1999). With adolescents, posing peer-conflict resolution problems is an effective method for eliciting grammatically complex utterances (Nippold et al., 2007). Figure 5.7 presents two very different types of language samples.

Language samples are recorded for later transcription, and the SLP is careful to transcribe the child's exact words. MP3 players and handheld computers can be used effectively to collect language samples in situations where they are used, such as in the classroom (Olswang et al., 2006).

The transcript can be analyzed in several quantitative and qualitative ways to determine the extent and nature of the child's language difficulty. Values such as *mean length of utterance (MLU),* the average number of clauses per sentence, and the number of different words used within a given period of time can be compared to the values for typical children of the same age or developmental level (Johnston, 2001). MLU has been shown to be both a reliable and valid measure of general language development through age 10 for children with SLI (Rice et al., 2006). Samples might also

Open-Ended	*Structured*
Clinician: I'll play with this farm set, and you can too or you can pick another toy.	*Clinician:* Well, here's the puppy. What should we say to him?
	Child: Hi puppy. [GREETING]
Child: Want farm	*Clinician:* Hi Timmy. I'm hungry. We need to get someone to help us get those cookies.
Clinician: Oh, you want the farm. We can share. I wonder what should we do first.	*Child:* You help. Want cookie. [REQUESTING]
	Clinician: I wonder how I can reach it.
Child: Open door. Animals come out.	*Child:* Get chair. [HYPOTHESIZING]
Clinician: Okay.	*Clinician:* Oh, get on the chair. Should I (mumble).
Child: You be horsie and I man.	*Child:* Yeah. [DOES NOT REQUEST CLARIFICATION]
Clinician: Oh, the farmer.	*Clinician:* You want me to (mumble)?
Child: Farmerman chase horsie in barn.	*Child:* What's that? [REQUESTS CLARIFICATION]
Clinician: Oh, he did. I better run fast.	*Clinician:* Which do you want, the cookie or the chair?
Child: Man go fast in barn.	*Child:* Want cookie. No chair. [CHOICE MAKING]

FIGURE 5.7

Examples of different types of language samples.

provide information on the percent correct for a language feature, such as past tense *-ed*. More descriptive measures might be the variety of intentions expressed by the child, the number of conversational styles used, and the types of repair the child uses when the conversation breaks down (Yont et al., 2000). Being as thorough as possible, the SLP attempts to analyze the sample for all aspects of form, content, and use appropriate for the particular assessment. For example, with bilingual clients, the SLP might consider **code switching** or the movement between two languages, dialect, English proficiency, and contextual effects in addition to aspects of both languages (Gutierrez-Clellan et al., 2000).

For school-aged clients experiencing literacy difficulties, the SLP also may want to collect samples of written language (Greene, 1996). These are discussed in Chapter 6, "Developmental Literacy Impairments."

INTERVENTION

The complexity of language necessitates a multiplicity of intervention methods. Different intervention approaches target specific aspects of language and employ a variety of procedures. Within limits, we explore these diverse approaches to remediation of language impairments.

All aspects of language are interrelated. Changes in one area affect others. For example, development of the /s/ sound may affect morphological markers, such as plural *s* (*cats*) or possessive markers (*cat's*). In intervention, such changes must not be taken for granted by focusing solely on one aspect of language. Intervention goals should focus on stimulating the language acquisition process beyond the immediate target (Fey et al., 2003).

Similarly, SLPs should use a variety of intervention techniques. For example, children with ASD can improve social skills better through a combination of peer training and written cues than by either method singularly (Thiemann & Goldstein, 2004). An SLP can blend methods together to help a child be successful.

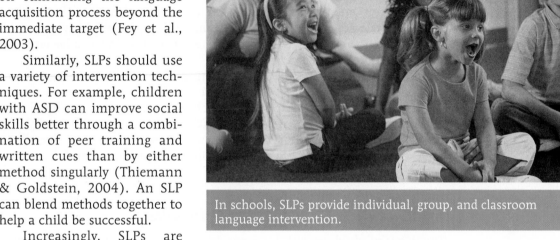

In schools, SLPs provide individual, group, and classroom language intervention.

Increasingly, SLPs are including other individuals from the child's environment in the training. Without training, day care providers fail to finely tune their language for individual children's needs (Girolametto et al., 2000). SLPs can help preschool teachers to implement intervention both through activities, such as dramatic play, art, and storybook reading, and through language instruction processes (Pence et al., 2008). When preschool staff are trained to respond to children's initiations, to engage children, to model simplified language, and to encourage peer interactions, it has a significant effect on children's language production (Girolametto et al., 2003). With the aid of the SLP, these and other care providers, such as parents, may learn how to be better language partners for children. Many successful models of the classroom collaborative model mentioned in Chapter 4 have evolved (Prelock, 2000). Even peers can serve as effective tutors or models for children with language impairments (McGregor, 2000).

Target Selection and Sequence of Training

The goal of intervention is the maximally effective use of language to accomplish communication goals within everyday interactions. Although most SLPs would agree on this overall goal, less unanimity exists on the route to achieving it. Decisions on target selection and training vary with each child and each SLP.

Using assessment results, SLPs might select different targets for the same child. A strict developmental model might suggest that a child achieve all behaviors within a given stage of language development before progressing to the next stage. A less strict developmentalist would use language acquisition knowledge as a general guide. A functional model would suggest

The criteria for target selection will vary with the child, the affected aspects of language, the child's disorder, and the needs of the environment.

that training begin at the point of communication breakdown and frustration for the child. Classroom approaches might suggest training for language used within the class. Another approach might be to begin with language features that are emerging, such as those produced correctly 10% to 50% of the time.

Decisions must also be made as to where to begin once the target is selected. Once again, the SLP must determine the point at which communication breakdown occurs. Some SLPs prefer to begin with receptive language training and progress to expressive.

Others start with expressive training. Expressive training may be bottom-up, in which one begins at the symbol level and works toward conversational goals; top-down, in which training is placed within a conversational framework; or a combination of the two. Obviously, the child's abilities are an important determiner of the method selected. To the extent possible, training should be placed within meaningful communicative contexts.

Evidence-Based Intervention Principles

The needs of children with language impairment suggest several principles that should guide intervention services. These principles, presented in Figure 5.8, recognize the need to target a child's language abilities in their

FIGURE 5.8
....
Principles of language intervention.

1. The goal of intervention should be greater facility of language use in conversation, narration, exposition, and other textual genres in hearing, speaking, reading, and writing.
2. Deficit areas are rarely, if ever, the only areas of language that should be targeted in an intervention program.
3. Select intermediate goals that stimulate a child's language acquisition processes rather than goals that focus solely on deficit areas.
4. Select specific goals of intervention based on a child's readiness and need for the targeted goals.
5. Manipulate the context to create more opportunities for the language target to occur.
6. Exploit different genres and modalities to develop appropriate contexts for intervention targets.
7. Manipulate clinical discourse so targeted areas are more noticeable and important in various contexts.
8. Systematically contrast a child's language performance with more mature adult usage by recasting a child's utterances.
9. Provide good models of easily comprehended, well-formed phrases and sentences.
10. Use a variety of verbal and nonverbal strategies to elicit and modify a child's language and to give a child practice in using language to accomplish her or his communication needs.

Note: We are deeply indebted to the fine work of Mark Fey, Steven Long, and Lizbeth Finestack (2003) on which this figure is loosely based. See Fey, M.E., Long, S.H., and Finestack, L.H. (2003). Ten Principles of Grammar Facilitation for Children with Specific Language Impairment. *American Journal of Speech-Language Pathology, 12,* 3–15.

entirety rather than to focus exclusively on one deficit area. The interrelatedness of all areas of language and the importance of communication context on the form and content of language necessitate a more holistic approach.

Throughout this text, we have stressed the importance of evidence-based practice. Although a lack of direct empirical evidence should not automatically rule out a new teaching method, it should be grounds for suspicion (Cirrin & Gillam, 2008, p. 19). Box 5.4 presents recommended practices for language disorders.

Intervention Procedures

Remember that speech-language pathologists, wherever they may work, are teaching communicative skills. A few basic tenets of good teaching behavior include, but are not limited to, the following:

- *Model the desired behavior for the client.* Modeling may include multiple exposures, called *focused stimulation,* that occur before the child is required to produce the language feature (Cleave & Fey, 1997). The need for modeling decreases as the feature is learned. Older elementary school children and adolescents may also benefit from an explanation of the targeted behavior and a rationale for why its correct use is important.

- *Cue the client to respond.* Carefully selected cues, such as the use of the word *yesterday* to signal a past-tense response, serve as aids for the client in conversation. Cues may range from very specific, such as *say, imitate,* or *point to,* to more general conversational cues, such as *I wonder what I should say now* to elicit a specific linguistic structure in context or *Maybe Carol can help us if we ask* to elicit a question.

- Cues may be either verbal or nonverbal. Verbal cues attempt to elicit the language feature by providing a linguistic framework; nonverbal cues use the context of an event to evoke the feature.

- The SLP should rate each type of cue or prompt from least to most intrusive and supportive (Timler et al., 2007). As intervention proceeds, the SLP works to minimize prompting whenever possible, so the child can become more independent.

- *Respond to the client in the form of reinforcement and/or corrective feedback.* Reinforcement varies from very direct and obvious forms, such as "Good, that was much better," to more conversational responses. Conversational responses come in many varieties, including imitating the child, imitating but expanding the child's utterance into a more mature version, replying conversationally, and asking for clarification. With some clients, especially those with vocabulary deficits, the relationship of the response to the content of the child's utterance has more effect on the child's

SLPs are teachers of language. They must plan their behaviors well to teach without overly relying on less natural strategies such as drill and the use of edible reinforcers.

BOX 5.4
Evidence-Based Practice for Childhood Language Impairments

General
- More than 200 studies report effectiveness for the vast majority of children.
- Measureable benefits accrue from intervention beginning as early as possible.

Nonsymbolic Children
- Interactive language intervention in which parents are trained to provide intervention at home is effective. Long-term and standardized measures have not been applied.

Children with Autism Spectrum Disorder
- Effective interventions are characterized by early intervention and intensive and individualized instruction.
- Methods used with children with ASD form a continuum from very structured behavioral methods stressing specific cues and reinforcers to more naturalistic play and child-based methods. Both behavioral and naturalistic approaches are effective in replacing challenging behavior with social interactions, although no method works with all children with ASD.
- Approximately two thirds of children make significant measureable gains.

Preschool
- Speech and language intervention are most effective for children with phonological or expressive vocabulary difficulties.
- No significant differences exist between interventions administered by trained parents and those administered by clinicians.
- Intervention of more than 8 weeks results in better outcomes.
- 70% of preschool children with language impairments make significant measureable gains with intervention.

School-age and Adolescent

Syntax and Morphology
- Moderately large to large effects follow use of imitation, modeling, or modeling plus evoked production strategies.

- Computerized input strategies alone have not demonstrated extensive benefit as yet.

Semantics and Vocabulary
- A real paucity of research exists on effective vocabulary instruction methods for children in early elementary grades. We do not yet have evidence on the best possible technique.
- Collaborating with teachers on large-group instruction and slowed presentation rate can positively impact vocabulary development.
- Interactive conversational reading strategies may be somewhat helpful for improving receptive and expressive vocabulary.
- There do not seem to be clear differences in outcome between the various methods used to assist children with word-finding.

Language Processing (The manner in which children attend to, perceive, discriminate, and recall sounds, syllables, words, and sentences)
- Computer intervention using modified speech stimuli or speech and language games do not improve performance.

Pragmatics and Discourse
- Direct instruction on topic initiation and group entry behaviors can yield moderately large to large effects for students with social communication deficits.
- It is possible to teach social skills to adolescents with ASD. Although several approaches have been used effectively, the data are not sufficient to identify the most effective method of intervention.

Method of Intervention
- Based on very few studies, we can tentatively conclude that preschool and early-elementary children with language impairment show greater improvement with a collaborative (teacher and SLP) teaching, classroom-based language intervention model than they do in more traditional pull-out intervention.

Sources: Based on Burgess and Turkstra (2006); Cirrin and Gillam (2008); Goldstein and Prelock (2008); Johnson and Yeates (2006); Justice and Pence (2007); Law et al. (2004); McGinty and Justice (2006); and Prelock (2008).

language than the structural input of the clinician's feedback (Girolametto et al., 1999). In other words, respond to the meaning of what the child said.

Natural reinforcers flow from the training target. The most obvious example is one in which a child obtains a desired object upon responding to the cue "What do you want?" Conversational responses are natural and reinforcing.

Corrective feedback may range from a gentle reminder to an instruction. In general, as a language feature is produced more correctly by the client, the SLP relies less on these direct forms. When a language feature is correct most of the time, conversational feedback, such as "What?" or "I don't understand," may be sufficient to cause the client to self-correct the few errors made.

- *Plan for generalization of the learned feature to the everyday use environment of the client.* SLPs can help generalization by selecting training targets that are highly likely to occur in the client's everyday communication and by including in the training elements of the everyday use environment, such as familiar locations, people, and objects. Parents are often included in the training of young children, whereas teachers may be involved in the intervention of school-age children and adolescents.

Specific examples of each teaching tenet are presented in Figure 5.9.

Effective language intervention should enhance language and social skills in real-life interactions (Timler et al., 2007). Success occurs when the newly taught language feature generalizes to a child's everyday environment.

Intervention Through the Lifespan

Targets of intervention vary with the age and functioning level of the client. An infant in an early intervention program would have different training targets than an adolescent with LD. However, an infant may be receiving some of the same training as an adolescent who has profound retardation and is functioning below age 1 year.

Early intervention, especially for children with MR and autism, can have a very positive benefit. Initial training may target presymbolic communicative skills and cognitive abilities, such as physical imitation, gestures, and receptive understanding of object names. Parents may be trained to treat their child's behaviors as having some communicative value or to interpret consistent behaviors as attempts to communicate. The SLP may attempt to establish an initial communication system using an augmentative/alternative communication system (AAC) such as gesturing, a communication board, or an electronic device. AAC is discussed in more detail in Chapter 15.

Early symbolic training may focus on vocabulary acquisition, semantic categories, word combinations, and an array of early intentions. The beneficial effects of treatment for children with delayed language extend beyond

Method	Example
Modeling	
Focused stimulation	I'll pretend to make a cake first. Watch to see if I make a mistake. I'm *putting* the eggs in the bowl and *taking* them to the table. I'm *cracking* the eggs. Now I'm *beating* the eggs. Next, I'm *sifting* the flour. I'm *adding* the flour to the eggs and *mixing* them. Now I'm *measuring* the sugar and *pouring* it into the mix....
Cuing	
Direct Verbal	
Imitation	Say "I want cookie."
Cloze	This is a _____. She should say _____.
Question	What should I say now? What's this? Which one's this?
Indirect Verbal	
Pass it on	I wonder if Joan knows the answer. How could we find the answer? [TARGET IS FORMATION OF QUESTIONS]
Nonverbal (Inherent in the activity)	Not giving child all the materials needed to complete a task. Not explaining how to accomplish an assigned task. Playing dumb.
Responding	
Direct Reinforcement	Good, I like the way you said that. Much better than the last time.
Indirect Reinforcement	
Imitation	*Child:* I go horsie. *Clinician:* I go horsie.
Expansion	*Child:* I go horsie. *Clinician:* I'm going to go on the horsie.
Extension	*Child:* I go horsie. *Clinician:* Yes, cowboys go on horses too.
Corrective Feedback	Remember, when we use a number like two, three, or more, we say /s/ on the word. Listen. One cat. Two cats.

FIGURE 5.9

Examples of teaching methods.

the trained targets into other areas of linguistic and overall development (Brand Robertson & Ellis Weismer, 1999).

Children at the preschool language level usually work on language form in both conversations and narratives. Longer utterances, bound morphemes, and early phonological processes may be intervention goals. Vocabulary will continue to be targeted.

Intervention with higher functioning children may focus on pragmatic skills in conversations and semantic targets, such as figurative language, multiple meanings, abstract terms, and more advanced relational terms. Academic skills, including summarizing a reading and different types of writing and note taking, may also be targeted. SLPs may use computerized programs to supplement more face-to-face intervention. These must be used with caution and should mesh well with the SLP's overall clinical philosophy and the child's individual needs (Gillam, 1999). Language enhancement–metalinguistics, phonology, and language use–can be infused into the curriculum (Fleming & Forester, 1997). SLPs may work with the child on both spoken and written language. It is also important for children with language impairment to learn to navigate the curriculum and to understand classroom expectations (Westby, 1997).

Language intervention doesn't end with childhood. Adolescents may continue to exhibit language impairments and be in need of services (Nippold, 2000). Adults with severe ASD or ID will most likely require continued intervention for language and communication deficits and a range of self-care, educational, and vocational needs. Individuals with LD may require additional support in postsecondary education (Downey & Snyder, 2000; Olivier et al., 2000).

SUMMARY

In this chapter, we discussed several disorders associated with language impairment. It is sometimes difficult for beginning students to remember the characteristics of the disorders related to language impairment. Refer to Figure 5.1 for the major differences.

As the definition and the many associated disorders suggest, language impairments are very complex and many faceted. We have only touched the surface in this chapter. The number of associated disorders, the language features that are affected, and the individual differences among children result in each child's language being very individualistic. It is very important to remember that each child is a unique case. Given this fact, assessment becomes the search to find and describe each child's individual language abilities. This is accomplished through referral, collection of a case history, interviews, observation, testing, and language sampling.

As a result of the assessment process and through repeated assessment probes during intervention, the speech-language pathologist attempts to find the most efficient and effective method for teaching new skills. The SLP identifies targets for intervention and trains these through a combination of techniques in various settings with the aid of additional language facilitators.

Obviously, every SLP needs thorough training and extensive experience with a variety of language impairments to serve children with these disabilities. With a firm foundation of speech and language development, speech-language pathologists take several courses in language impairment in both children and adults and complete practica with both populations.

THOUGHT QUESTIONS

- What are the characteristics of language impairment?
- What disorders are associated with language impairment? Describe each one briefly.
- What are the steps in a typical assessment in language impairment?
- What is the overall design of language intervention?

SUGGESTED READINGS

Nelson, N. W. (2010). *Language and literacy disorders: Infancy through adolescence.* Boston: Allyn and Bacon.

Owens, R. E. (2010). *Language disorders: A functional approach to assessment and intervention* (5th ed.). Boston: Allyn and Bacon.

Reed, V. A. (2005). *An introduction to children with language disorders* (3rd ed.). Boston: Allyn and Bacon.

Barnstein, D., & Tiegerman-Farber, E. (2009). *Language and communication disorders in children* (6th ed.). Boston: Allyn and Bacon.

ONLINE RESOURCES

American Speech-Language-Hearing Association
www.asha.org/publications/leader/archives/2007/070904/070904e.htm
ASHA site offers discussion on social communication intervention for adolescents with TBI.

www.asha.org/public/speech/disorders/ChildSandL.htm
ASHA site that offers descriptions of various language disorders in children.

Autism Spectrum Disorder Foundation
www.autismspectrumdisorderfoundation.org/detectingautism.html
ASD Foundation site provides some possible early warning signs.

Centers for Disease Control and Prevention
www.cdc.gov/ncbddd/autism/
Centers for Disease Control and Prevention site offering in-depth information on ASD and links to other sites.

Learning Disabilities Association
www.ldanatl.org/aboutld/professionals/index.asp
Learning Disabilities Association site with links to several others.

Merrill Center
merrill.ku.edu/IntheKnow/sciencearticles/SLIfacts.html
Merrill Center, University of Kansas site that offers more details on SLI.

National Institute of Health
www.nichd.nih.gov/health/topics/developmental_disabilities.cfm
National Institute of Child Health and Human Development site has good discussion of developmental disabilities.

National Institute of Mental Health
www.nimh.nih.gov/health/publications/autism/complete-index.shtml
National Institute of Mental Health site with in-depth information.

World Health Organization
www.searo.who.int/EN/Section1174/Section1199/Section1567/Section1825_
    8084.htm
World Health Organization (WHO) site discusses mental retardation.

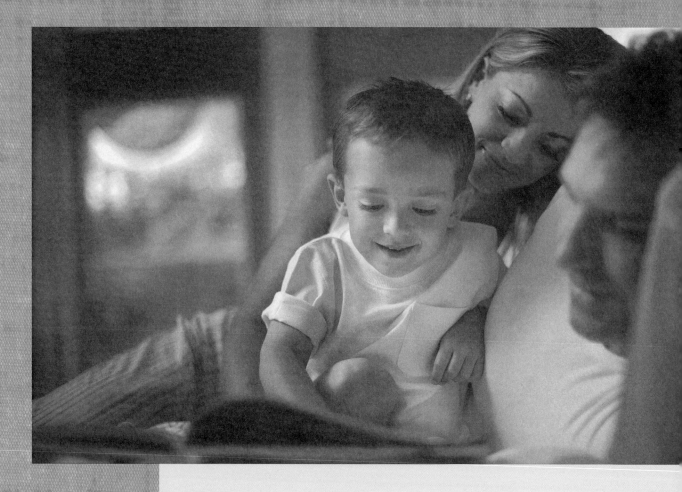

CHAPTER LEARNING GOALS

When you finish this chapter, you should be able to:

- Describe the aspects of literacy that are of concern to the SLP

- Explain how literacy develops

- Explain the deficits in literacy experienced by children with language impairment

- Describe an assessment of literacy

- Give examples of intervention for literacy

6

Developmental Literacy Impairments

Democracy is based on the premise that we are an informed people. In the beginning of the American republic, those who were best informed were literate. What does being informed mean today? Is literacy still important, and what level of proficiency is required to be a fully participating citizen? Should we be concerned when one segment of the population has deficits in literacy learning? And who is responsible for aiding these individuals? These questions go to the heart of the issue of developmental literacy impairments.

Let's begin with literacy itself. What is it? **Literacy** is the use of visual modes of communication, specifically reading and writing. The interrelatedness of aspects of literacy is illustrated by the correlation between reading and spelling ability (Bosman & van Orden, 1997; Greenberg et al., 1997; Griffith, 1991). Poor readers tend to be poor spellers (Treiman, 1997). But literacy is more than just letters and sounds. Literacy encompasses language; academics; cognitive processes, including thinking, memory, problem solving, planning, and execution; and is related to other forms of communication. Case study 6.1 presents the narrative of one child with a literacy impairment.

Although spoken and written language have much in common, they differ in very significant ways (Kamhi & Catts, 2005). Reading and writing are not just speech in print. In addition to the obvious physical difference, reading and writing lack the give-and-take of conversation, are more permanent, lack the paralinguistic features (stress, intonation, fluency, etc.) of speech, have their own vocabulary and grammar, and are processed in the brain in a different manner.

As in other forms of communication, use of literacy presupposes that the user can encode and decode, but more importantly, that he or she is able to comprehend and compose messages for others. In other words, literacy rests on a language base—and so do literacy impairments.

Many of the disorders mentioned under both childhood and adult language impairments (Chapters 5 and 7) figure prominently in literacy impairments. In fact, as high as 60% of children with language impairment

CASE STUDY 6.1
Case Study of a Child with Literacy Impairment: Juan

An athletic 7-year-old, who loves video games and riding his bike, Juan immigrated to the United States from Colombia when he was 4 years old. With three older sisters, he was the baby of the family and received plenty of attention. His mother reported that his Spanish language development was similar to that of his sisters and that she was not concerned, although her son's speech was sometimes difficult for people outside the family to understand. When the family immigrated, the children began to learn English. As the youngest, Juan learned quickly but experienced some problems with English speech sounds. He received speech and language services in kindergarten, although he was not classified as having a communication disorder.

In first grade, Juan's development of reading was fine initially, but gradually he fell more and more behind his peers. By second grade, he was nearly a year behind his classmates. The speech-language pathologist, reading speacialist, and the classroom teacher met with the parents to suggest a thorough reading diagnostic. The evaluation confirmed that Juan was reading below his age, and the reading specialist pledged to redouble her efforts. The speech-language pathologist noted Juan's especially poor performance on phonological awareness tasks and with the other team members recommended clinical intervention in this area.

Although she was unsure of the actual factors relating to Juan's difficulties, the speech-language pathologist believed that they might be related to his learning of a second language. As if to confirm this estimate, Juan quickly excelled in both phonological awareness and reading. As his phonological awareness skills improved, his speech sound production also became more accurate.

As you read the chapter, think about

- Possible explanations for Juan's reading problems.
- Possible ways in which the evaluative team could explore different aspects of reading.
- Possible explanations for Juan's success.

---

may experience difficulties with literacy (Wiig et al., 2000). Children with language impairments may be unprepared for literacy learning because they lack preliteracy skills and an oral language base. When compared to children developing typically, preschoolers and kindergarteners with language impairments may be less able to recognize and copy letters and less likely to pretend to read or write, to engage in daily preliteracy activities, or to engage adults in question-answer activities during reading and writing (Marvin & Wright, 1997).

Often, literacy impairments do not disappear as children mature (Catts et al., 1999). As adults, those who experienced literacy deficits in childhood may continue to struggle with reading and writing. One intelligent man in his 50s—known by one of the authors—has continually worked in manual labor positions because his lack of literacy skills disqualified him from managerial positions. Hopefully, with advances in intervention research, the future will see better and more evidenced-based intervention with increasingly better outcomes.

As adults, some of us may experience a neuropathology such as aphasia or progressive dementia. Whether the loss of language is sudden, as in aphasia, or more gradual, as in progressive dementia such as Alzheimer's, literacy usually is affected in some way. If there is a problem with language, there will be a problem with encoding or decoding or both.

Literacy deficits vary in complexity and severity. Maybe you are a college student with dyslexia or some other literacy problem who has been able to succeed academically by adjusting to, compensating for, or overcoming deficits in your reading or writing. The authors of this text have worked with college students who have had to overcome literacy difficulties.

Although primary responsibility for teaching reading and writing still rests with the teacher and other educational specialists, the SLP is interested in children's language deficits and the ways in which these deficits influence the acquisition of literacy. In recognition of the special skills that SLPs bring to this area, the American Speech-Language-Hearing Association (ASHA) (2001 d) recommends that SLPs play a role in literacy intervention.

As a consequence, SLPs are involved in literacy intervention from preschool through adulthood. At both the preschool and early elementary school level, speech-language pathologists focus on preventive intervention. According to ASHA, SLPs have the following responsibilities:

- Educate both teachers and parents in the oral language-literacy relationship.
- Identify children at risk.
- Make referrals to good literacy-rich programs.
- Recommend assessment and treatment in preliteracy skills when needed. (Snow et al., 1999)

Because children with language impairments are at a high risk for literacy disabilities (Lewis et al., 1998), preliteracy, reading, and writing assessment should be a portion of any thorough language evaluation when appropriate.

With older children and adults, a speech-language pathologist is concerned with improving reading and writing skills. The SLP continues to help children and adolescents develop a strong language base and addresses both reading and writing. Assessment and intervention for literacy are also a vital part of any thorough rehabilitative strategy for adults with neurological impairments (see Chapter 7, "Adult Language Impairments").

As with most communication impairments mentioned in this text, SLPs often work as part of a team, collaborating with teachers to design literacy-based programs on vocabulary, language, and thinking skills (Farber & Klein, 1999; Silliman & Wilkinson, 2004). By working with teachers, SLPs provide opportunities for children with developmental literacy impairments to use skills taught in intervention within meaningful activities in the classroom. Effective collaboration should include curriculum planning, naturalistic language facilitation, and careful teaming of personnel (Hadley et al., 2000). Other members of a literacy intervention team may include the, reading specialist, school psychologist, and parent.

In the remainder of the chapter, we discuss literacy and associated skills, disorders, assessment, and intervention, first with reading, and then writing. Most language impairments discussed in Chapter 5 also affect literacy acquisition.

> Of necessity, the concerns of SLPs will differ with the maturational level and preliteracy or literacy abilities of children.

READING

Several steps are involved in reading and reading comprehension. Both language and written context play a role in word recognition and in the ability to construct meaning from print (Gillam & Gorman, 2004).

The first step is **decoding** the printed word, which consists of breaking or segmenting a word into its component sounds and then blending them together to form a word recognizable to the reader. Words take on more meaning based on grammar and context. In addition, there is an interaction between the print of the page and linguistic and conceptual information of each reader (Whitehurst & Lonigan, 2001). We interpret based on what we know. Given these processes, it shouldn't surprise us that children with oral language impairments might have reading problems as well. Figure 6.1 is a model of this dynamic process of text interpretation.

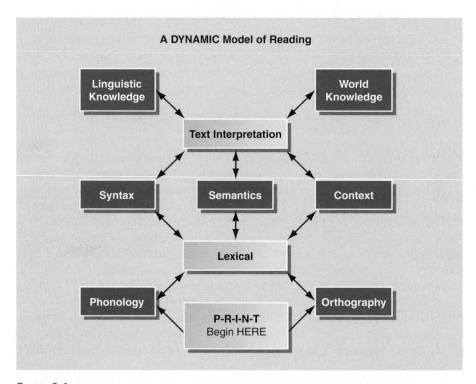

FIGURE 6.1

Reading comprehension.

Beginning with print, a reader uses the letters and speech sounds to decode words that are then recognized based on lexical or vocabulary memory. Words are combined with other words and syntax, semantics, and context are used to interpret and comprehend.

Source: Based on information from "Language and Discourse Contributions to Word Recognition and Text Interpretation," by R. B. Gillam and B. K. Gorman (2004). In E. R. Silliman and L. C. Wilkinson (Eds.), *Language and Literacy Learning in Schools* (pp. 63–97). New York: Guilford.

Obviously, comprehension requires much more than simply decoding or even interpreting a word. The active reader is concerned with self-monitoring, semantic organization, summarization, interpretation, mental imagery, connection with prior knowledge, and metacognition or knowledge about these processes, to name some of the skills involved. But let's not get ahead of ourselves; more of this later.

In summary, reading basically consists of decoding and text comprehension. Whereas phonological skills are essential for decoding, other areas of language–syntax, morphology, semantics, and pragmatics–are needed for comprehension (Nation & Norbury, 2005). The reader uses language and experience to interpret the message conveyed by the author. This may give you some idea of why language and literacy go hand in hand. Let's look briefly at two aspects of reading that are of particular interest to SLPs: phonological awareness and comprehension.

Phonological Awareness

Necessary for reading, **phonological awareness** is knowledge of the sounds and syllables and of the sound structure of words. Phonological awareness includes **phonemic awareness,** the specific ability to manipulate sounds, such as blending sounds to create new words or segmenting words into sounds. As you might guess, better phonological awareness, specifically phonemic awareness, is related to better reading skills (Cupples & Iacono, 2000; Hogan & Catts, 2004). In addition, phonological awareness skills also are the best predictor of spelling ability in elementary school (Nation & Hulme, 1997).

> Yes, it does seem easy to confuse terms. Simply put, phonological awareness is an alertness of phonology, so yes, it contains the elements of phonology.

Phonological awareness consists of many skill areas. Not all are required for reading. The auditory ability to determine a word when a phoneme or syllable is deleted (cart – t = car), **blend** or create a word from individual sounds and syllables, and to compare initial phonemes for likeness and difference are areas of phonological awareness that are particularly important for the development of reading.

Comprehension

Several levels of text comprehension exist. At the basic level, a reader is primarily concerned with decoding. Meaning is actively constructed from words and sentences and from personal meanings and experiences. Above this level is **critical literacy** in which a reader actively analyzes and synthesizes information and is able to explain the content. A reader bridges the gaps between what is written and what is meant (Caccamise & Snyder, 2005). At the highest level of **dynamic literacy,** a reader is able to interrelate content to other knowledge through both deductive and inductive reasoning. Dynamic literacy is comparing and contrasting, integrating, and using ideas for problem raising and solving (Westby, 2005).

The reader's mental representation of meaning is composed of the text and the mental model the reader creates through the comprehension

Each reader must interpret what she or he reads in light of personal experiences and knowledge. In other words, our comprehension will differ based on our own unique self.

process. Comprehension occurs as a reader combines textual material, text grammar, and the reader's world knowledge and experience (Kintsch, 1998; Sanford & Garrod, 1998).

Reading is a goal-directed activity. For example, the reader may be gathering information to be used in a problem-solving task. Knowing what to do and how to do it is called **metacognition** and two aspects are important for reading. One aspect is self-appraisal or knowledge of one's own cognitive processes. The other is **executive function** or self-regulation and includes the ability to attend; to set reasonable goals; to plan and organize to achieve each goal; to initiate, monitor, and evaluate performance in relation to the goal; and to revise plans and strategies based on feedback. As you read, you form hypotheses about the material and and predict and confirm or not confirm your predictions.

Twin studies indicate that both genetics and environment are important for reading achievement (Harlaar et al., 2008). Although genetics is important, environment seems to be a bigger factor. There is considerable overlap between language and reading achievement.

Reading Development Through the Lifespan

You may believe that literacy development begins with reading and writing instruction in school. Actually, literacy development begins much earlier and continues throughout our lives.

EMERGING LITERACY

Reading development begins within social interactions between the child and caregiver(s) at around age 1, as parents or others begin to share books with toddlers. Book sharing is usually conversational in tone with the book serving as the focus of communication. Here's an example:

Adult:	This is a book about a . . .
Child:	Bear.
Adult:	Yeah. And you found him right here. What do bears say?
Child:	Grrrrrrrr.
Adult:	Um-hm, they growl. Can you find his eye?

Reading the story is secondary to and will be included in the conversation.

As children mature, some parents engage in **dialogic reading,** an interactive method of reading picture books. When reading, adults encourage their children to become actively involved in the reading process by asking them questions and allowing them opportunities to become storytellers.

By age 3, most children in our culture are beginning to develop **print awareness.** Early print awareness consists of knowledge of the meaning and function of print, basic concepts concerning the direction print proceeds across a page and through a book, and recognition of some letters (Snow et al., 1999). Later developing skills include recognizing words as discrete units, being able to identify letters, and using terminology, such as *letter, word,* and *sentence.*

Language forms the basis for the stories children hear and tell. Children with good language skills seem to enjoy reading activities more than children with poor language and will pretend to read at an early age.

By age 4, children begin to notice phonological similarities and syllable structure in words they hear. This is the beginning of phonological awareness. Four-year-olds also appreciate both sounds and rhymes. At this age, a young child may find rhyming words very funny and may fabricate nonsense words that rhyme. Children who have been exposed to a home literacy environment and to print media have better phoneme awareness, letter knowledge, and vocabulary (Foy & Mann, 2003).

Phonological awareness may arise from a child's need to store words in his or her brain with increasingly more detailed representation. This becomes necessary as a child's vocabulary grows and there are more and more words, some very similar in sound, to store (Metsala & Walley, 1998).

Prekindergarten speech perception skills and receptive vocabulary size are good predictors of phonological awareness skills at the end of kindergarten (Rvachew, 2006). In a "literacy-rich" kindergarten environment, children begin to decode the alphabetic system and to broaden their experience with print (Snow et al., 1999). Five kindergarten variables seem to predict reading success by second grade: letter identification, sentence imitation, phonological awareness, rapid automatized naming (RAN), and maternal education level (Catts et al., 2001). RAN is the ability to name a series of items in a category quickly, such as types of clothes or food.

In general, children develop the skills associated with reading more rapidly at earlier ages than in later. Similar to what we see in language development, rapid development plateaus and is followed by slow refinement.

In first grade, children are introduced to reading instruction and learn the sound-letter correspondence called **phonics.** Words read by a child are linked with words and meanings stored in memory. Most of the child's effort goes into decoding the letters, leaving little cognitive energy for either comprehension or interpretation. This is one reason why we don't assign *War and Peace* to first graders.

Phonology (sound) and orthography (letters) are important for early reading, and grammar and meaning contribute more later. Knowledge of morphology may aid students to break words apart, recombine them, and create new words (Berninger et al., 2001).

As a child improves, reading becomes more automatic or fluent, especially for familiar words. Fluency is aided by the use of grapheme-phoneme patterns in the child's memory and by analogy, the process of relating unfamiliar words to familiar ones based on similar spelling.

By third grade, there is a shift from *learning to read to reading to learn* (Snow et al., 1999). As language continues to improve, so does comprehension with a resultant increase in reading fluency.

MATURE LITERACY

Although all reading begins with the printed word, mature readers like you use very little cognitive energy determining word pronunciation. At a higher level of processing, both language and experience are used to understand the

Establish a habit of reading now. It will serve you well as you mature.

text, which is monitored automatically to ensure that the information makes sense (Snow et al., 1999). The skilled reader then predicts the next word or phrase and glances at it to confirm the prediction. Printed words are processed quickly, automatically, and below the level of consciousness most of the time. In less than a quarter of a second, your brain retrieves all the information from a word or phrase that is needed to confirm the prediction and form another prediction of the next word or phrase. This process is presented in Figure 6.2.

Mature readers don't simply read the text; they dialogue with it. Reading is an active process in which ideas and concepts are formed and modified, details remembered and recalled, and information checked. Much of this is the unconscious process of the brain partaking of new information.

As we mature, the types and purposes of reading change, but we can continue to enjoy the process throughout our lives. Reading skill continues to be strong through adulthood as long as we exercise our ability and do not experience any neuropathologies, such as those in Chapter 7. Reading is one of the primary ways by which adults increase their vocabulary and knowledge.

Reading Problems Through the Lifespan

Public Law 107–110, the No Child Left Behind Act (NCLB) passed in 2002, states that all children in third grade, even those with disabilities, will read proficiently by 2013/2014. In short, this law requires annual testing of students in grades 3 through 8 in reading and mathematics. States that fail to meet national standards are held accountable. This law clearly emphasizes the importance of reading and of instructional and intervention methods that are *evidence based.*

Risk of reading difficulties is greatest for children with a history of problems in both articulation and in receptive and expressive language (Segebart DeThorne et al., 2006). In general, poor reading comprehenders

FIGURE 6.2
....

Model of mature reading.

Mature readers use their language skills to predict what words or phrases will appear next in the text, then momentarily glance at the print to confirm their predictions before predicting anew what will follow.

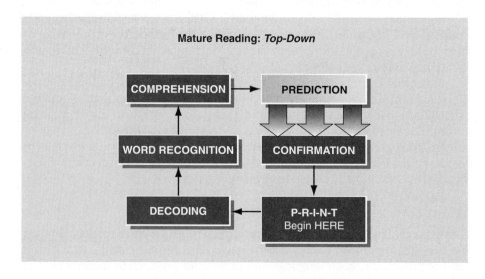

have deficits in oral language comprehension too but have normal phonological abilities. In contrast, children who are poor decoders have poor phonological abilities but little or no oral language comprehension difficulties (Catts et al., 2006). The story of a young man with learning disabilities and reading difficulties is presented in Case Study 6.2.

Children with dyslexia, mentioned in Chapter 5, have poor word recognition or decoding abilities, accompanied by problems with phonological processing. *Dyslexia,* a type of learning disability, is neurobiological in origin and characterized by difficulties with accurate and/or fluent word recognition and decoding abilities and by poor spelling (Lyon, Shaywitz, & Shaywitz, 2003). When we compare children with dyslexia to typically developing readers we find

- Comparable verbal IQ and/or listening comprehension,
- Below-average word reading,
- Well-below-average word attack or decoding skills, and
- Well-below-average phonological processing scores (Sawyer, 2006).

CASE STUDY 6.2
Justin, A Young Man with Learning Disabilities

Justin grew up in a midwestern suburb and attended public schools. He's the youngest child of four and the only male. As an adult, he's personable and friendly, works part time, and is attending the local community college. His sisters, especially the next oldest, help him with his homework when possible.

As a preschooler, Justin cared little for books. His language was slow in developing when compared to his sisters, but his parents assumed that he would be fine and that he didn't talk much because his sisters talked for him. Still, his mom enrolled him in preschool to encourage his development. He scored low on his kindergarten readiness test and, when admitted, was recommended to repeat because of a lack of pre-academic skills needed for first grade. His parents reluctantly agreed.

When he began school, Justin adjusted well, but quickly began to fall behind other children in both reading and writing. An evaluation at the end of first grade resulted in Justin's being labeled as learning disabled. It was recommended that he remain in a regular classroom with additional instruction in literacy. At home, his parents worked closely with him on his reading and written assignments.

Through most of elementary school, Justin saw a reading specialist and a speech-language pathologist several times each week. His SLP focused on Justin's language and listening skills and on his reading comprehension.

When Justin entered junior high school, he stopped seeing both the reading specialist and the speech-language therapist. Instead, it was decided by his team, including both him and his parents, that other measures would be attempted to compensate for his deficits. These included use of a word processor, recording of class lessons, and pre-preparation of lecture notes by his teachers. All through junior and senior high school, Justin met with different teachers after school for extra instruction.

When he graduated, Justin had few plans. He drifted from job to job for nearly a year before his sisters convinced him to apply to community college. Going part time, he was able to do well in his courses and has just been accepted into the physical therapy assistant major. Reading and writing are still difficult, but Justin is determined to do well and his family, especially his sisters, are extremely supportive.

Three distinct types of dyslexia have been described, including a language-based disorder that may affect comprehension and/or speech sound discrimination, a speech/motor disorder that may affect speech sound blending and motor coordination, and a visuospatial disorder that may affect letter form discrimination. The language-based disorder is the most common. Several Web sites at the end of the chapter discuss dyslexia.

Children with SLI may be similar to those with LD, exhibiting grapheme-phoneme (letter-sound) errors and syntactic, semantic, and pragmatic errors or misinterpretations when reading. Comprehension also may be impaired and may be related to a child's poor vocabulary.

Another group of children with **hyperlexia** has poor comprehension but typical or above word recognition abilities. Hyperlexia is a near-obsessive interest in letters and words found in some children with pervasive developmental disorder (PDD). Although these children appear very precocious in their reading ability, they often have poor social skills and extremely limited reading comprehension (Treffert, 2009). Many individuals with ASD have word reading skills that are more advanced than their overall reading comprehension (Church et al., 2000; Diehl et al., 2005; Smith-Myles et al, 2002, Wahlberg & Magliano, 2004).

Causal factors for literacy impairment may be extrinsic or intrinsic to an individual (Catts & Kamhi, 2005). Extrinsic factors may include experience and the manner of instruction. Intrinsic factors may include genetics, vision-based deficits, auditory processing problems, attention deficits, language impairment, and neurological problems. For example, there appear to be differences in the brains of children with dyslexia when compared to typical children (Eckert et al., 2005). Differences have been found in the temporal-parietal region (interior to the ear), in both the left and right linguistic processing areas, and in the cerebellum (near the brain stem). Neural pathways in the left temporal-parietal area of the brain are important in the development of fluent reading (Deutsch et al., 2005). These deficits in cerebellar processing are similar to those in children with fetal alcohol syndrome (FAS) (Coffin et al., 2005).

Possibly as many as seven chromosomes are involved in various aspects of the dyslexia (Grigorenko, 2005). Malformations found in the left hemisphere language processing areas and between these areas and the visual processing portions of the brain may be related to these genetic changes

For some children, reading and writing seem to be arbitrary, unfathomable processes.

(summarized in Galaburda, 2005). Possible familial links may be seen in other ways. For examples, children at high risk for reading disability have at least one parent with a significantly slower speaking rate than children at low risk for reading disability.

As might be expected given their language learning difficulties, many children with ASD have accompanying literacy impairments and uneven development of skills that are predictive of reading. In general, preschool children with ASD are severely delayed in their vocabulary relative to their nonverbal mental ages (Charman et al., 2003). In addition, oral narratives are challenging for these children (Losh & Capps, 2003; Loveland et al., 1990). As a result, children with ASD and accompanying limited verbal skills often are excluded from standard literacy curricula under the misguided assumption that they were incapable of learning to read (Colasent & Griffith, 1998; Kopenhaver & Erickson, 2003).

Similar to what we see in typically developing readers, children with LD acquire reading skills more rapidly in the initial stages then gradually slow (Skibbe et al., 2008). Even so, these children are substantially below more typical readers by fifth grade.

Phonological awareness is a beginning stage for most readers. Those with phonological disorders, especially perceptual deficits, will find phonological awareness challenging. Speech perception seems to be particularly important for the development of phonological awareness (Rvachew & Grawburg, 2006).

In attempting to read, some children with language impairments, especially those with poor phonological skills but average or above-average intelligence, may use memorized word shapes, letter names, or guessing rather than relying on decoding skills. As a result, they are unable to decode unfamiliar words. Without word attack or decoding skills, by second grade, when formal decoding instruction ends, these children begin to fail.

Most initial reading problems are related to deficient phonological processing and phonological awareness (Catts & Kamhi, 2005). Phonological awareness difficulties seem to be related to failure to analyze words into syllables and these, in turn, into smaller phonological units (Bird et al.,1995).

If a beginning reader has good phonological ability and appears to decode words well, reading comprehension problems may go unnoticed (Nation et al., 2004). Although phonics-based problems often decrease by third grade, comprehension problems persist for many children (Foster & Miller, 2007). Poor reading comprehension is associated not with phonics but with poor oral language (Nation & Frazier Norbury, 2005). For example, the majority of individuals with ASD do not become skilled readers because of their difficulties interpreting both oral and written (Lanter & Watson, 2008). If a child isn't comprehending, he or she isn't reading. Some children have difficulty interpreting written narratives because they have poor oral narrative abilities (Naremore, 2001). They may lack the story framework or linguistic skills for telling narratives.

Reading comprehension is also dependent on communication, especially social inferencing and interpersonal reasoning (Donahue & Foster,

2004). Given the low social competence of some children with language impairments, it's easy to see why this aspect of reading might be difficult (Brinton & Fujiki, 2004).

Good readers actively guide and control their reading (Anderson et al., 1985; Baker & Brown, 1984). In contrast, poor readers lack such strategies, reflecting possible deficits in executive function (Johnston & Winograd, 1985; Torgesen, 1980). They may approach reading as a random, unfathomable process. You'll recall that executive function deficit is most evident in children with TBI (Sohlberg et al., 1993; Ylvisaker & Feeney, 1995). In addition, children with ADHD and LD have been described as inattentive and impulsive, disorganized, unable to inhibit behavior, and ineffective learners, characteristics of those with impaired executive function.

As children experience repeated reading failure, they may become frustrated or passive. Lacking persistence and with low self-esteem, they may become apathetic and resigned to failure (Butkowsky & Willows, 1980). In contrast, some poor readers may become aggressive or display acting-out behaviors. All of these behaviors interfere with further learning and development (Winograd & Niquette, 1988).

In short, many children with language impairments are at risk for reading impairment (Hambly & Riddle, 2002; Miller et al., 2001; Stanovich, 1986). In general, they

- Begin with less language and may have difficulty catching up.
- Have poor comprehension skills because they lack language knowledge that would enable them to integrate what they read.
- Have poor metalinguistic skills.
- Possess linguistic processing difficulties.

When something goes wrong in the reading process, the result is reading that is less automatic and less fluent. Word decoding or text understanding may be impaired.

As mentioned, reading difficulties do not disappear. They are often related to other language problems. The ASHA Web site has links to the latest research. As adolescents, poor readers exhibit vocabulary, grammar, and verbal memory deficits when compared to typical readers (Rescorla, 2005).

Assessment of Developmental Reading

SLPs should be alert to potential reading problems among children with phonological problems or those at risk because of other diagnosed disorders such as LD, TBI, or SLI. In this section we discuss overall assessment with a more detailed discussion of assessment of phonological awareness, word recognition, comprehension, and executive function.

As mentioned in Chapter 4, assessments begin with an initial data gathering step that may include use of questionnaires, interviews, referrals, and screening testing. Figure 6.3 presents a checklist designed to identify kindergarten and first-grade school children at risk for language-based reading difficulties. No one item alone will indicate a reading problem.

Competent readers and writers approach the task with a purpose that guides their behavior

In case you've forgotten, *metalinguistics* includes the ability to consider language out of context, to make judgments about its correctness, and to understand to some extent the process of using language.

The child . . .

_____	Has difficulty remembering words or names
_____	Has problem with verbal sequences (i.e., alphabet, days of the week)
_____	Has difficulty following instructions and directions and may respond to a part rather than the whole
_____	Has difficulty remembering the words to songs and poems
_____	Requests multiple repetitions of instructions/directions with little improvement in comprehension
_____	Relies too much on context to understand what's said
_____	Has difficulty understanding questions
_____	Has difficulty understanding age-appropriate stories and making inferences, predicting outcomes, drawing conclusions
_____	Frequently mispronounces words and names
_____	Has problems saying common words with difficult sound patterns (i.e., *spaghetti, cinnamon*)
_____	Confuses similar-sounding words (i.e., the **Specific** Ocean)
_____	Combines sound patterns of similar words (i.e., **nucular** for *nuclear*)
_____	Has speech that is hesitant, contains fillers (i.e., *you know*), or words lacking specificity (i.e., *that, stuff, thing, one*)
_____	Has expressive language difficulties, such as short sentences and errors in grammar
_____	Lacks variety in vocabulary and overuses words
_____	Has difficulty giving directions or explanations
_____	Relates stories or events in a disorganized or incomplete manner
_____	Provides little specific detail when relating events
_____	Has difficulty with rules of conversation, such as turn taking, staying on topic, requesting clarification
_____	Doesn't seem to understand or enjoy rhymes
_____	Doesn't easily recognize words that begin with the same sound
_____	Has difficulty recognizing syllables
_____	Demonstrates problems learning sound-letter correspondences
_____	Doesn't engage readily in pretend play
_____	Has a history of language comprehension and/or production problems
_____	Has a family history of spoken or written language problems
_____	Has limited exposure to literacy in the home
_____	Seems to lack interest in books and shared reading activities

FIGURE 6.3
....

Checklist for early identification of language-based reading disabilities.

Source: Based on information from "The Early Identification of Language-Based Reading Disabilities," by H. W. Catts, 1997, *Language, Speech, and Hearing Services in Schools, 28,* 86–89.

Early literacy questionnaires often ask about the frequency of book reading behaviors, responses to print, language awareness, interest in letters, and early writing. Parental reports of early literacy skills of preschool children with language disorders compare favorably with professional assessments (Boudreau, 2005).

Children who read poorly may exhibit learned helplessness or have negative attitudes toward the reading process. This information can be gathered from interviews with teachers, parents, and the child and by observation within the classroom. Interview questions should include the child's perceptions of the importance of reading and difficulty with different types of reading, along with the child's self-perceptions (Wixson et al., 1984). Observation can confirm the child, teacher, and parent responses.

Collaborative reading assessment should include standardized measures, oral language samples including analysis of miscues or mistakes, and written story retelling (Gillam & Gorman, 2004). Formal testing might be accomplished by a school's reading specialist, but the SLP may wish to give selected subtests. In a more informal task, a child might be asked to read previously unread curricular materials in an attempt to assess her or his ability to function within the classroom (Nelson & Van Meter, 2002). The child's aloud reading can be recorded for later analysis of the child's miscues. Comprehension can be assessed by using questions, retelling, or paraphrasing.

PHONOLOGICAL AWARENESS

Phonological awareness assessment is multifaceted and should be accomplished within an overall assessment of reading, spelling, phonological awareness, verbal working memory, and rapid automatized naming (RAN). In addition to formal testing, the SLP can use informal assessment of rhyming, syllabication, segmentation, phoneme isolation, deletion, substitution, and blending. It is especially important to assess both segmenting and blending with school-age children.

WORD RECOGNITION

Decoding skills, especially knowledge of sound-letter correspondence, is the basis for word recognition. Of interest to the SLP will be decoding of consonant blends, long (*day*) and short (*can*) vowels, different syllable structures, and morphological affixes (*un-, dis-, -ly, -ed*).

Word recognition assessment should adhere to the following guidelines (Roth, 2004):

- Materials should be based on age and developmental appropriateness.
- Tasks should be of various types to assess different level of processing.
- Several measures should be used.
- A student's cultural and linguistic background must be considered.
- Unfamiliar test tasks may need to be demonstrated and trained.

- Reading deficits are not limited to children with emergent literacy skills.
- Observation and interpretation of test behaviors is extremely important.

Although traditional assessment procedures stress standardized testing, alternative approaches such as curriculum-based measures and dynamic assessment may be more appropriate for children with language impairment or with cultural and linguistic differences (Roth, 2004). Materials for curriculum-based assessment usually come from the local curricula and use criterion-referenced scoring, which measures a child against himself or herself over time. In this way progress is measured without reference to some abstract norm. Dynamic assessment often takes a test-teach-test format in which a child is assessed for the amount of change she or he can make during the assessment process.

Word recognition is more than just the ability to decode a word in isolation. It's important, therefore, that word recognition testing be accomplished with various clues, such as pictures or sentence forms, available to the child and with words both in isolation and within text. More important than test scores is describing a child's strengths and the strategies used.

When analyzing recorded reading data, the SLP notes all discrepancies in the recorded reading samples. All attempts at word decoding, repetitions, corrections, omitted words and morphemes, extended pauses, and dialectal usages should be noted and analyzed for possible strategies used by the child. Reading errors can be analyzed at the word level by type, such as word order is changed, word substitutions, additions, and deletions (Nelson, 1994; Nelson & Van Meter, 2002). The percentage of incorrect but linguistically acceptable words indicates the extent of a child's use of linguistic cues to predict the correct word. In addition, the SLP should note the way in which the child sounds out words (Nelson & Van Meter, 2002).

Text Comprehension

Assessing text comprehension abilities of children is complicated by the many cognitive and linguistic processes involved. At the very least, the SLP or other team members should assess a child's

- Oral language with special attention to a child's use of the more elaborate syntactic style used in literature.
- Knowledge of narrative schemes and text grammar schemes.
- Metacognition. (Westby, 2005)

Narrative schemes or the events in a story might be assessed by having a child tell a narrative from pictures or by asking questions about the pictures that relate to the organization of the story. A child's text grammar, consisting of the parts of a story, can be assessed through spontaneous narratives or by retelling previously heard narratives.

Although several norm-referenced tests measure reading comprehension, they should be supplemented by other measures of a child's ability to identify grammatical units, interpret and analyze text, make inferences, and construct meaning by combining text with personal knowledge and experience (Kamhi, 2003).

Executive Function

Whereas poor readers act as if reading is simply sounding out words rapidly and fluently, good readers expect text to make sense and to be a source for learning information. As a result, good readers read actively and with purpose, constructing mental models and organizing information as they go.

Self-regulation in reading can be assessed in many ways, including (Westby, 2004):

- Interview questions about different strategies used for different reading tasks.
- Think-alouds, or verbalizing thoughts accompanying reading.
- Error or inconsistency detection while reading.

Errors and inconsistencies can be planted in texts specifically for the assessment.

Intervention for Developmental Reading Impairment

As in several of the disorders discussed in this text, intervention for developmental literacy impairments should be a team effort. The SLP supports the efforts of all team members and the explicit instruction of the classroom teacher and reading specialist.

Team members might cooperate in an embedded/explicit model of intervention in which children participate both in literacy-rich experiences embedded in the daily curriculum and in explicit, focused, therapeutic teaching of reading (Justice & Kaderavek, 2004; Kaderavek & Justice, 2004). The literacy-rich environment might include a message board where children learn to decode an "important" message left daily by the teacher, snack activities in which sounds are embedded in snack names, recipes, music and print, book and speech sound play, rhyming pictures, and book sharing with the teacher and others (Towey et al., 2004). As little as 8 weeks of one-on-one twice-weekly 15-minute book sharing sessions in which adults read and ask both literal and inferential questions can result in gains in both types of comprehension (van Kleeck et al., 2006).

Effective instruction for reading should include sound and letter processes used in word identification, grammatical processes, and the integration of these with meaning and context (Gillam & Gorman, 2004). Training phonological (sound) and orthographic (letter) processing together seems to offer a more effective strategy than working on phonological awareness skills in isolation (Fuchs et al., 2001; Gillon, 2000).

Beginning in preschool, the SLP can increase children's print awareness with print-focused reading activities (Justice & Ezell, 2002). Print-focused strategies emphasize word concepts and alphabetic knowledge and include cues such as the following:

Show me how to hold the book so I can read.

Do I read this way or this way?

Where is the last word on the page?

How many words do you see?

Find the letter C. Whose name starts with C?

Such print-focused prompts are easy to teach, and parents have used them successfully at home with only minimal training.

Intervention for beginning readers might include a two-prong intervention model (Figure 6.4) (van Kleeck, 1995). In one part, called *meaning foundation,* the teacher or SLP guides reading for children by placing the text in context and asking questions to aid comprehension. The child learns that print contains the meaning and gains phonological awareness and letter knowledge. In a parallel thrust, called *form foundation,* phonological awareness and alphabetic knowledge are emphasized. Later reading intervention might target both linguistic and metalinguistic skills, including recognition of key words, use of all parts of the text such as the glossary and the index, and application of general learning strategies, such as graphic organizers containing photos, drawings, and print (Wallach & Butler, 1995). Now let's look at intervention for phonological awareness, word recognition, comprehension, and executive function. Check the Web sites at the end of this chapter.

Phonological Awareness

Evidence-based practice tells us that children who receive phonological awareness training have higher phonemic awareness, word attack, and word

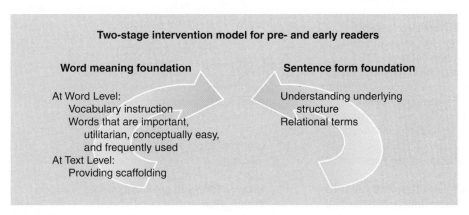

Figure 6.4
....

Two-stage intervention.

Intervention with young readers should focus on both word meaning and sentence formation.

Source: Based on information from "Emphasizing Form and Meaning Separately in Prereading and Early Reading Instruction," by A. Van Kleeck, 1995, *Topics in Language Disorders, 16*(1), pp. 27–49.

identification skills at the end of kindergarten than children who do not receive such training (Ekelman et al., 2004) Even short-term—as little as twice weekly for 6 weeks—high-quality, explicit phonemic instruction with small groups of children can be effective for most children (Koutsoftas et al., 2008). Other Evidence Based Practices are presented in Box 6.1. In addition to working with individual students, SLPs can offer phonological awareness instruction to teachers, stressing the importance of phonological awareness and its integration into the reading curriculum (Hambley & Riddle, 2002). What seems most important is that phonological awareness intervention begin before children lag too far behind others, most likely in preschool or kindergarten (Torgesen, 2000).

Whenever possible with older children, phonological awareness should be taught within meaningful text experiences, such as systematic and explicit classroom instruction, so that the emergent nature of both literacy and phonological awareness can support each other (McFadden, 1998). Phonological awareness training alone is insufficient to increase reading comprehension (Pugh & Klecan-Aker, 2004).

BOX 6.1
Evidence-Based Practice

Phonological Awareness and Metalinguistics

- We can have a moderate degree of confidence in techniques designed to improve phonological awareness in school-age children. Tasks designed to improve rhyming, sound identification, phoneme segmentation, phoneme manipulation, and grapheme-phoneme correspondence consistently yield moderately large to large effects. Similar effects can be obtained through classroom collaboration and clinician-only approaches.
- Training should be appropriate for the prereading or reading level of the child. In deciding whether to provide phonological awareness practice to older children, the SLP must consider both the nature of the reading deficit and the level of phonological awareness knowledge.
- Little is known about the appropriate length and intensity of intervention.
- Not all phonological skills are of equal importance. Segmenting and blending are critical skills needed for reading. Lower level skills are important to the extent that they facilitate subsequent development of segmenting and blending. This said, we have not identified the skill level for these two that is needed before word decoding instruction should begin.
- Some tasks are easier than others:
  - Consonants are easier to segment than vowels.
  - Initial sounds are easier to segment than final sounds.
  - Shorter words are easier to segment than longer words.
  - It's easier to segment an initial sound in a consonant-vowel-consonant (CVC) word than in a CCV word.
- Highly effective intervention is contingent on adult responses to child errors. In short, adult responses should consider the reason for the child's error and the learning level and facilitate a correct response.
- Teaching is enhanced when SLPs anticipate the types of errors that a child is likely to make and plan scaffolding or guiding strategies to elicit correct responses.

Sources: Based on Cirrin and Gillam (2008); Schuele and Boudreau (2008).

Within intervention, the SLP can address both segmentation (*cat → c-a-t*) and blending (*c-a-t → cat*), working at the syllable and phoneme levels. In general, programs focusing on one or two phonological awareness skills yield better results than those that try to teach with a broader focus (National Reading Panel, 2000). It's best if the SLP teaches skills that will directly impact the child's performance of an everyday task.

Intervention can begin with syllable and sound recognition and identification and be both receptive and expressive. Next, the SLP can move to syllable segmentation and blending (*stapler → stap-ler → stapler*) and, finally, to phoneme segmentation and blending (cat → *c-a-t → cat*). In general, segmentation is easier for most children than blending.

The concept of syllables can be introduced as naturally occurring "beats" in a word. Multisensory approaches are also helpful and can make the training interesting. Clapping hands or drum beats can be used to help children recognize and identify syllables. Other

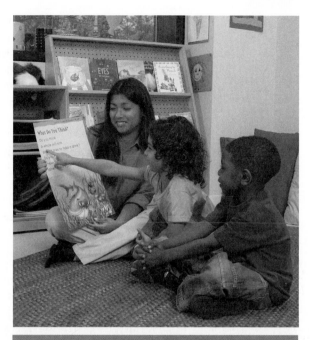

Literacy-rich environments are critical for children with literacy impairments.

examples include dropping objects into cans, stacking toys, playing hopscotch, or taking turns in any number of child games during auditory recognition training.

Phoneme intervention might progress from recognition of a target sound in isolation, through identification when paired with other sounds, to sounds in syllables, then words (Gerber & Klein, 2004). It is best to work with one or two sounds at a time. Memory can be aided by pairing sounds with real objects or pictures and finally with printed letters and words.

Word Recognition

The goals of intervention for word recognition are

- To teach phonemic decoding skills, resulting in accurate and fluent reading of new words.
- To develop a rich vocabulary of sight words.
- To improve reading comprehension (Torgesen et al., 2005).

Success in the last two depends on achievement of the first. Teaching decoding skills can result in gains, followed by increases in reading accuracy, fluency, and comprehension (Torgesen, 2005). Support for learning can be provided by encouragement and positive feedback and by breaking tasks into smaller steps or by giving a child as much direction as necessary to complete the task successfully.

Context can be used to help children predict words in text. Intervention might begin with obvious words, such as *I took my umbrella because it looked like _____*. Training can then move to more ambiguous choices and the use of other strategies that include morphological and orthographic cues, such as *Let's have _____ for lunch* followed by *Let's have p _____ for lunch* or *Let's have p _____ s for lunch.*

TEXT COMPREHENSION

Comprehension relies on many different aspects of processing. As mentioned, when we read, our knowledge and experience blend with the information on the page to form a mental representation of the meaning (Kintsch, 1998). The active reader makes inferences from the text and past knowledge and experience that bridge these gaps.

Children who lack internalized story frameworks necessary for interpreting narratives might begin intervention with telling stories (Naremore, 2001). Intervention can progress to oral then written narrative interpretation (Boudreau & Larson, 2004). Storybook reading can be divided into before, during, and after reading activities to aid comprehension. Postreading might include creating story organizers, retelling, and creating variations of the narrative. Narratives can also be divided into story parts and recombined.

Similarly, comprehension by children with LD and dyslexia who read with difficulty can be improved by also focusing on before, during, and after reading strategies (Vaughn & Klingner, 2004). Through prereading techniques such as establishing the content and setting the scene or context, establishing relationships, and discussing unfamiliar vocabulary and concepts, an SLP or teacher can assist students in constructing meaning from what they read. Activation of prior knowledge can improve comprehension, especially for children with LD (Carr & Thompson, 1996; Dole et al., 1996).

Comprehension may also be enhanced by teaching children the more explicit and precise language style found in written communication (Westby, 2005). This style can be taught through tasks in which children must follow very explicit oral instructions to be successful or tasks in which contextual cues, such as objects or pictures, are present. Literate vocabularies can be enhanced through prereading activities that focus on the words to be encountered and through use of visual or verbal memory aids. Complex grammar may be taught through books with familiar stories or books in which the grammar becomes increasingly complex.

Adult strategies should differ according to when they are used in the reading process. For example, prior to reading, semantic strategies, such as giving definitions or synonyms for key words, reduce reading miscues or errors. Graphophonemic strategies are more effective during reading (Kouri et al., 2006). Graphophonemic strategies include encouraging a child to "sound out" a word, calling a child's attention to phonetic regularities, or asking a child to identify initial or final sounds or consonant blends.

During reading, SLPs can facilitate comprehension through instruction, questions, visual and verbal cues, explanations and comments (Crowe, 2003). Using a conversational style, the adult provides cues and feedback as oral group reading occurs. It's important that questions reflect the level of comprehension targeted for each child. This semantic strategy should be accompanied by direct vocabulary instruction (Ehren, 2006).

Ideally, students will internalize comprehension strategies and use them as they read actively. Active strategies might include the following:

- Using context to analyze word meaning,
- Activating prior knowledge,
- Rereading difficult passages,
- Self-questioning to help frame key ideas,
- Analyzing text structures to determine type of reading,
- Visualizing content,
- Paraphrasing in one's own words, and
- Summarizing (Ehren, 2005, 2006; Pressley & Hilden, 2004).

These strategies can be used along with the monitoring in which a reader actively decides if a reading passage makes sense and if not what to do about it. Good readers recognize when they have not comprehended a written passage and therefore rereading it.

When we analyze children's eye movements of typical readers, we find that their eyes are bounding ahead and back, trying to check the accuracy of words within the surrounding meaning. Children with reading impairments can be taught to use this information to determine word meaning (Owens & Kim, 2007).

At another level, comprehension includes a social dialogue with the authors and characters. Comprehension training should also include discussion of the author's goals, and the feelings and motivations of characters (Donahue & Foster, 2004). Knowledge of the text can be used to predict a character's behavior within a narrative.

EXECUTIVE FUNCTION

Specific areas of executive function that might be targeted in intervention include working memory, self-directed speech (*How can I figure out the meaning of this word?*), and problem solving (Westby, 2004). Just teaching strategies is not enough. The SLP and classroom teacher must help each child achieve independent and appropriate use of these strategies.

Of importance for more advanced readers is *distancing* or moving away from dependence on the text and toward independent thinking about the text. This can be accomplished by questions that move from answers explicitly stated in the text (*What did she do next?*) to ones in which the question is generated by something in the text but the answer is generated from the student's knowledge (*could she have solved the problem differently?*).

WRITING

As with all modes of communication, writing is a social act. Just like a speaker, the writer must consider the audience, but because the audience is not present when the writing occurs, writing demands more cognitive resources for planning and execution than does speaking (Golder & Coirier, 1994; Graham & Harris, 1996, 1997; Scott, 1999).

In short, writing is using knowledge and new ideas combined with language knowledge to create text (Kintsch, 1998). It's a complex process that includes generating ideas, organizing, and planning, acting on that plan, revising, and monitoring based on self-feedback (Scott, 1999). Writing involves motor, cognitive, linguistic, affective, and executive processes.

Writing is more abstract and **decontextualized** than conversation and requires internal knowledge of different writing forms, such as narratives and expository writing. Decontextualized means outside of a conversational context. When you write, the entire context is contained in the writing. You create the context with your language rather than having the context created by your conversational partners.

There are several aspects to the writing process (Berninger, 2000):

- Handwriting, word-processing, text-messaging
- Spelling
- Executive function
- Text construction or going from ideas to written texts
- Memory

As mentioned previously, executive function is self-regulation and includes attending, goal setting, planning, and the like. Memory provides ideas for content and language symbols and rules to guide the formation of that content and is used for word recognition and storage of ideas as they are worked and reworked. As you can see, writing is a very complicated process. Let's look more closely at spelling and then writing development and impairment, followed by assessment and intervention.

Spelling

Spelling of most words is self-taught using a trial-and-error approach. It is estimated that only 4,000 words are explicitly taught in elementary school. Rather, classroom teachers focus on strategies and regularities that children can use to determine word spelling.

Good spellers use a variety of strategies and actively search words for patterns and consistency (Hughes & Searle, 1997). More specifically, mature spellers, like you, rely on memory; on spelling and reading experience; phonological, semantic, and morphological knowledge; orthographic or letter knowledge and mental grapheme representations; and analogy (Apel & Masterson, 2001). Semantic knowledge is concerned with the interrelationship of spelling and meaning, whereas morphological knowledge is knowing the internal structure of words, affixes (*un-, dis-, -ly, -ment*),

Your brain doesn't store words letter-by-letter; rather it stores them by more useful units. For example, *stand* is probably stored as *st-and*, which enables you to spell *land, band, hand, bland, strand*, and so on.

and the derivation of words (*happy, unhappily*). Mental grapheme representations are best exhibited when you ask yourself "Does that word look right?" Your representations are formed through repeated exposure to words in print. Finally, through analogy, the speller tries to spell an unfamiliar word using prior knowledge of words that sound the same.

Spelling competes with other aspects of writing for limited cognitive energy. Excessive energy expended at this level comes at the cost to higher language functions. As a result, poor spellers generally produce poorer, shorter texts.

Writing Development Through the Lifespan

Writing and speaking development are interdependent and parallel, and many aspects of language overlap both modes. In turn, writing development includes development of several previously mentioned interdependent processes. For example, reading level matched typically developing children and those with Down syndrome (DS) both exhibit oral narratives that are longer and more complex than written narratives. Among the children with DS, vocabulary comprehension was the best predictor of narrative skills (Kay-Raining Bird et al., 2008).

EMERGING LITERACY

Initially, children treat writing and speaking as two separate systems. Three-year-olds, for example, will "write" in their own way—usually scribbling—but don't yet realize that writing represents sounds. The story may be contained in an accompanying drawing. By age 4, some real letters of the parent language may be included.

As with reading, in early writing, children expend a great deal of cognitive energy on the mechanics, such as sound-letter associations and letter forming. Gradually, spelling, like reading, becomes more accurate and fluent or automatic.

For a few years, the spoken and written systems converge and children write in the same manner as they speak, although speech is more complex. Around age 9 or 10, talking and speaking become differentiated as children become increasingly literate. Writing slowly overtakes speech as written sentences become longer and more complex than speaking. Children display increasing awareness of the audience through their use of syntax, vocabulary, textual themes, and attitude. Some language forms are used almost exclusively in either speech or writing, such as using *and* to begin many sentences in speech but only rarely in writing.

MATURE LITERACY

In a phase not achieved by all writers, speaking and writing become consciously separate. The syntactic and semantics are consciously recognized as somewhat different and the writer has great flexibility of style. You may or may not have achieved this phase yet. If you find yourself using an enlarged vocabulary when writing or pondering how sentences flow from one to the next, then you are probably there. As with reading, practice results in improvement that should continue throughout the lifespan. In general, the writing of adults as compared to adolescents contains longer, more complex sentences and uses more abstract nouns, such as *longevity* and *kindness*, and more metalinguistic and metacognitive words, such as *reflect* and *disagree* (Nippold et al., 2005).

Writing consists of handwriting, word processing, or text messaging; spelling; executive function; text construction or going from ideas to written texts; and memory. Let's discuss, in that order, the ones of particular interest to speech-language pathologists.

SPELLING

Spelling development is a long, slow process. As mentioned, initial *preliterate* attempts at spelling consist mostly of scribbles and drawing with an occasional letter thrown in. Later children use some phoneme-grapheme knowledge along with letter names. For example, *bee* might be spelled as *B*. Gradually, they become aware of conventional spelling and are able to analyze a word into sounds and letters, although vowels will be difficult for some time. As mentioned earlier, mature spellers are able to call on multiple learning strategies and different types of knowledge (Rittle-Johnson & Siegler, 1999; Treiman & Cassar, 1997; Varnhagen et al., 1997).

As knowledge of the alphabetic system emerges, the child slowly connects letters and sounds and devises a system called "invented spelling" in which the names of letters may be used in spelling, as in *SKP* for *escape* or *LFT* for *elephant* (Henderson, 1990). One letter may represent a sound grouping, as in **set** for **street**. Because children lack full knowledge of the phoneme-grapheme system, they have difficulty separating words into phonemes (Treiman, 1993).

As spelling becomes more sophisticated, children learn about spacing, sequencing, various ways to represent phonemes, and the morpheme-grapheme relationship (Henderson, 1990). The parallel development of reading aids this process.

Children who possess full knowledge of the alphabetic system of letters and sounds can segment words into phonemes and know the conventional phoneme-grapheme correspondences. As children begin to recognize more regularities and consolidate the alphabetic system, they becomes more efficient spellers (Ehri, 2000). Increased memory capacity for these regularities is at the heart of spelling ability.

Many vowel representations, phonological variations, such as *later-latter*, and morphophonemic variations, such as *sign-signal*, will take several years to acquire (Treiman, 1993). Gradually, children learn about consonant doubling (la**dd**er) stressed and unstressed syllables (**report-re**port**), and root words and derivations (*add-addition*).

Most spellers shift from a purely phonological strategy to a mixed one between second and fifth grade (Goswami, 1988; Lennox & Siegel, 1996). As words and strategies are stored in long-term memory and access becomes fluent, the load on cognitive capacity is lessened and can be focused on other writing tasks.

Adults spell in several ways, letter-by-letter, by syllable, and by sub-syllable unit, such as *ck*, used for *back, stick,* and *rock* but never in *ckar* (car). The method used seems to vary with the task. Next time you're word processing, notice if your spelling is conscious and letter-by-letter.

EXECUTIVE FUNCTION

It is not until early adulthood—about where most of you are right now—that writers develop the cognitive processes and executive functions needed for mature writing (Berninger, 2000; Ylvisaker & DeBonis, 2000). It takes this long because of the protracted period of anatomical and physiological development of your brain's frontal lobe where executive function is housed.

Until adolescence, young writers need adult guidance in planning and revising their writing. By junior high school, teens are capable of revising all aspects of writing. Improved long-term memory results in improved overall compositional quality (Berninger et al., 1994).

TEXT GENERATION

Once children begin to produce true spelling, they begin to generate text. In first grade, text may consist of only a single sentence, as in *My dog is old.* Early compositions often lack cohesion and use structures repeatedly, as in the following:

> *I like school. I like gym. I like recess. I like art.*

Mature writers use more variety for dramatic effect. The facts and events characteristic of early writing evolve into use of judgments and opinions, parenthetical expressions, qualifications, contrasts, and generalizations (Berninger, 2000).

Initially, compositions lack coherence and organization. Later, ideas may relate to a central idea or consist of a list of sequential events. Written narratives or stories emerge first, followed by expository texts. Expository writing, the writing of the classroom, is of several genres: procedural, as in explaining how to do something; descriptive; opinion; cause-and-effect; and compare-and-contrast. Essays need to include at least a unifying topic sentence, comments referenced to the topic, and elaborations on the comments.

By adolescence, expository writing has greatly increased in overall length, mean length of utterance, relative clause production, and use of literate words that transition between thoughts, abstract nouns, and metalinguistic/metacognitive verbs (Nippold et al., 2005). Literate words include *however, finally,* and *personally;* abstract nouns are words such as *kindness, loyalty,* and *peace;* and metalinguistic and metacognitive verbs include *think, reflect,* and *persuade.*

Writing Problems Through the Lifespan

Children with language deficits often have writing deficits too. Unfortunately, their writing difficulties may remain through the lifespan, and the gap between their writing abilities and that of children developing typically widens.

Children with LD may have difficulties with all aspects of the writing process (Graham et al., 1991; McFadden & Gillam, 1996; Roth et al., 1991; Troia et al., 1999; Vallecorsa & Garriss, 1990; Wong, 2000). Writing problems associated with dyslexia are characterized by spelling errors, word omissions and substitutions, punctuation errors, agrammatical sentences, and a lack of organization. A sample of the writing of a child with LD is presented in Figure 6.5. Because they have little knowledge of the writing process, these children fail to plan and make few substantive revisions. They are easily discouraged and may devote very little time on a given task. Clarity and organization are forsaken for spelling, handwriting, and punctuation, leaving little cognitive capacity for text generation. In the process, meaning suffers.

DEFICITS IN SPELLING

Poor spellers view spelling as arbitrary, random, and seemingly unlearnable (Hughes & Searle, 1997). Misspellings are characterized by omission of syllables, morphological markers such as plural "s," and letters; letter substitutions; and confusion of homonyms such as *to/too/two*. Even adults, especially those with LD, often cite spelling as their primary area of concern (Blalock & Johnson, 1987).

Usually, deficits in spelling represent poor phonological processing and poor knowledge and use of phoneme-grapheme information. Although most spellers shift to greater use of analogy between second and fifth grade, poor spellers tend to rely on visual matching skills and phoneme position rules as compensation for their limited knowledge of sound-letter correspondences (Kamhi & Hinton, 2000).

DEFICITS IN EXECUTIVE FUNCTION

When you write, you begin with ideas. Your ideas are converted into language. At this point, executive function becomes important.

FIGURE 6.5
....

Sample writing of an 11-year-old child with dyslexia.

Dear mom and dad, How are you? I am fine. Today we went . . .

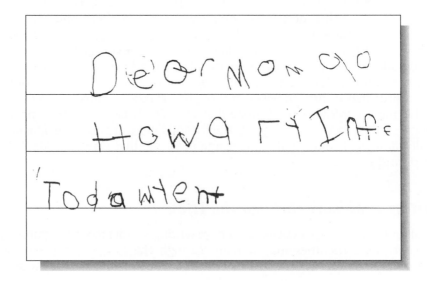

When executive function or self-regulation is impaired, communication and even problem-solving abilities are diminished, especially in complex linguistic tasks, such as writing. Lacking self-regulation, some children with LD follow a writing strategy of putting on paper whatever comes to mind with little thought to planning. They produce and elaborate little, revise ineffectively and with seeming indifference to their intended audience, detect errors poorly, and experience difficulty executing intended changes (Graham & Harris, 1999). Planning is difficult because of language formulation difficulties.

One adult professional with LD, known to the authors, uses different templates for his reports in which he fills in the blanks. Otherwise, the task of planning, writing, and revising a report would overwhelm his executive abilities. Until he and his spouse devised the templates, he would call from work at the end of each day to be talked through the report writing process.

DEFICITS IN TEXT GENERATION

In narrative writing as in storytelling, children with language impairment may lack mature internalized story models or be unable to visualize the words even from their own spoken narratives (Graves et al., 1990; Montague et al., 1991; Roth et al., 1991; Vallecorsa & Garriss, 1990). When compared to the narratives of chronological age-matched peers with typical language, the narratives of children with LD contained shorter, less complex sentences (Scott & Windsor, 2000). As a result, both the oral and written narratives often are shorter with fewer episodes, contain fewer details, and fail to consider the needs of the listener.

Expository writing tasks follow a format, such as statement of a problem, examination of several factors, and a conclusion. Children with language impairment have difficulty with these writing tasks and approach them with seemingly little thought or planning. The results are often extremely short, poorly organized, and containing numerous errors of grammar, punctuation, and spelling. There is often little revision. In addition, children with LD have substantial difficulty with morphological endings, such as regular past tense and regular plurals, even when they demonstrated accuracy with these units in their speech (Windsor et al., 2000).

Just as the poor reader expends all his or her energy in decoding, the poor writer becomes bogged down in the mechanics of the writing and spelling process. Both leave the poor reader or writer with little energy for higher cognitive functions such as comprehension or text generation, respectively.

Assessment of Developmental Writing

The best writing samples are actual writing from varying contexts. One method of assessing writing in the classroom is through the use of portfolios of children's writing (Paratore, 1995). A portfolio is a collection of meaningful writing collaboratively selected by the child, the SLP, and the teacher that contains samples of the child's writing over time, thus enabling the child to demonstrate progress. The wide variety helps to increase the validity of the sample. Items in a portfolio may include SLP or teacher observation notes, work samples, and first drafts of writing samples, such as journal entries, and projects/papers, final drafts of the same, and peer and teacher evaluations.

Executive function is very difficult to assess without some task to accomplish, thus the context is very important.

Narratives are best for young elementary school children (Nelson, 1998). Older elementary school children or adolescents can provide expository writing samples.

Executive function is best measured within actual writing tasks as part of an overall writing assessment rather than separate from functional communication tasks. Samples should be written in ink to allow for analysis of revisions. It's helpful to allow children to plan and to write drafts. All notes and plans should be collected along with the finished product and added to the portfolio mentioned previously.

Whenever possible, the SLP, teacher, or an instructional aide can observe the writing process for evidence of planning and organizing, drafting, writing, revising, and editing. Added information can be obtained if children read their paper aloud while being recorded. This procedure aids the SLP or teacher in interpreting garbled or poorly spelled words.

Writing can be analyzed on several levels, including textual, linguistic, and orthographic (spelling). At a textual level, the SLP can note length, any indication of the amount of effort, overall quality, and structure or the way in which comments support the topic (Berninger, 2000). Of interest are the total number of words, clauses, and sentences, as well as the structural complexity as measured in words/clause and clauses/sentence. Writing conventions, such as capitalization and punctuation, plus the use of sentences and paragraphs, should be noted.

ASSESSMENT OF SPELLING

Spelling deficits are very complex and can be difficult to describe. Collection should be of sufficient quantity to allow for a broad-based analysis. Spelling deficits should be assessed through both dictation and connected writing such as that in a child's portfolio (Masterson & Apel, 2000). Standardized tests should also be included and can be administered by a classroom teacher, writing specialist, or school psychologist. Informal assessments should include several phoneme-grapheme variations, such as single consonants in various positions in words, consonant blends (*str-*), morphological inflections (*-est*, *dis-*), diphthongs, digraphs (two letters for one sound, as in ch" and "sh"), and complex morphological derivations.

Single-word spelling does not measure a child's ability in a real communicative context (Moats, 1995). Connected writing, such as that found in a portfolio, can offer samples closer to actual practice.

Descriptive analysis should focus on patterns evident in the child's spelling (Bear et al., 2000). Of interest are the most frequent and the lowest level patterns. Figure 6.6 presents a possible analysis system that suggests several possible intervention strategies.

ASSESSMENT OF TEXT GENERATION

SLPs and teachers can assess a child's writing using the papers assembled in his or her portfolio. Analysis may include the total number of words and the number of different words. This is an overall measure of a child's vocabulary and flexibility in its use. Other measures might include the maturity of the words used, clause and sentence length, and coherence. Narratives and

FIGURE 6.6
....
Examples of language-based spelling analysis.

Phonological: Segmenting, blending, and phonemic awareness

Omission of internal and unstressed phonemes and cluster reduction

> Stop → SOP   Sand → SAD

Syllable deletion

> Elephant → ELFANT

Letter reversal (most common with liquids and nasals)

> Sing → SIGN

Orthographic: Sound-symbol relationship (/k/ = k, c, ck, cc, ch, q, x), letter combinations, letter and positional patterns, and grapheme representations

Letter sound confusion

> Cash → CAS

Nonallowable letter sequences

> Dry → JRIE   Queen → KWEN

Possible spellings that violate location-pattern rules

> Chip → TCHIP   Corn → CKORN

Different spellings on repeated attempts (no cognitive representation or graphemic representation of word)

Morphological: Inflectional (-ed, -ing, -s) and derivational (un-, dis-, -er, -ist, -ment) morphemes, relationship of root word and inflected or derived form

More difficult if a form has more than one meaning (fast**er**, teach**er**), multiple pronunciations (walk**ed**, jogg**ed**, collid**ed**), and both phonological and orthographic properties are changed when inflected or derived (*ascend* and *ascension*).

Semantic: Effect of spelling on meaning

Homophone confusions

> Won → ONE   They're → THER   Which → WITCH

expository writing can be analyzed for the presence or absence of elements of both. For example, does a narrative include a setting statement of *who, what, when, where?*

Intervention for Developmental Writing Impairment

Intervention for writing may involve both general training and more specific and explicit techniques for both narrative and expository forms. To learn to write, you must write, so intervention needs to focus on the actual writing process.

SPELLING

Spelling intervention should be integrated into real writing and reading within the classroom. Words are the vehicles for teaching spelling principles

(Berninger et al., 1998). Ideally, intervention can occur when a child is actually writing and can be reminded of alphabetic and orthographic principles (Scott, 2000). Spelling can be taught within teaching of general executive function in which the child is taught to proofread, correct, and edit.

The way children spell is indicative of the way they read (Templeton, 2004). This would suggest that spelling intervention should also be integrated with reading to enable a child to learn and to use word knowledge.

Words selected for intervention should be individualized for each child and reflect the curriculum, the child's desires, words attempted but in error, and error patterns (Bear et al., 2004; Graham et al., 1994). Spelling strategies can be discussed with the child using the data from the SLP's analysis. The goal is to learn strategies of spelling and rules rather than specific words. For example, if the child's errors are primarily morphologic (see Figure 6.6), the SLP can target root words and the influence of various morphemes through morpheme finding and word building tasks. Intervention focusing on increasing awareness of the morphological structure of words with particular attention to the orthographic rules that apply when suffixes are added can significantly increase both spelling and reading accuracy and generalize to new words (Kirk & Gillon, 2008). In contrast, if the child's errors are orthographic, the SLP can teach rules through key words, demonstrating alternative spellings and acceptable and unacceptable sound-letter combinations.

> The SLP should not be teaching this week's spelling words from class. SLPs target spelling strategies, not individual words.

Children with LD benefit from multisensory input such as pictures, objects, or actions (Graham, 1999). Several multisensory techniques have been proposed in which the child may complete any of several steps, including listening to the SLP say and spell the word, saying the word aloud while looking at it or touching it, writing it while saying it, checking spelling, saying the letters in sequence, tracing the word while saying it, closing his or her eyes and visualizing the word, and rewriting the word and checking or comparing the spelling (Berninger et al., 1998; Graham & Freeman, 1986; Horn, 1954).

Word analysis and sorting tasks or placing words into groups can be used (Scott, 2000). Sorting tasks will differ based on the targeted error patterns found in the child's misspellings. Pairs of words that differ on the bases of these patterns, such as *pint-pit*, *meant-meat*, and *bunt-but*, can be used to demonstrate the consequences of misspelling (Masterson & Crede, 1999). For example, word meaning could be used to help the child note the difference between *head* and *hid*. Other contrasting words might include *dead-did*, *read-rid*, and *lead-lid*. The SLP should begin with known, frequently used words and gradually introduce less frequently used and unknown words to facilitate generalization. Different spelling/meaning patterns might provide clues to the meaning and spelling of unfamiliar ones (Templeton, 2003). For example, a child might be helped to see the relationship between *evaluate* and *evaluation*. Some principles for word study and spelling intervention are included in Figure 6.7.

Use of computers alone aids spelling somewhat. Although use of word processing can encourage editing in children, spell checkers, as you know, are not foolproof, and a child may learn little in the process. In general, spell checkers miss words in which the misspelling has inadvertently produced another word. Suggested spelling may also confuse the

Focus on what students are "using but confusing" in their spelling rather than beginning with focusing on what a child doesn't know.

Step back and consolidate learning before moving forward.

Use words students know and can read, so that one literacy aspect influences another.

Compare words "that do" have the spelling feature, such as silent "e" with words "that don't", as in *dime-dim*, *tone-ton*, and *cube-cub*.

Help a child look at words in many ways through sorting tasks that include sound, sight, and meaning.

Begin with obvious contrasts first; ones that are easy to hear or clearly demonstrate a rule.

Don't hide exceptions, rather deal with them, because they will enhance generalization.

Avoid rules until a child has learned enough examples to see the rule clearly.

Work for sorting and spelling fluency.

Glean words from a child's writing and reading, and then return to meaningful tasks and texts.

FIGURE 6.7
....
Principles for guiding spelling intervention.

Source: Based on information from *Words Their Way: Word Study With Phonics, Vocabulary, and Spelling Instruction* (3rd ed.), by D. R. Bear, M. Invernizzi, S. Templeton, and F. Johnston, 2004, Upper Saddle River, NJ: Merrill/Prentice Hall.

child with poor word attack skills. In addition, suggested spellings may be far afield if the original word is seriously misspelled. Spell checkers help only 37% of the time for children with LD, a lower percentage than found among children developing typically (MacArthur et al., 1996).

If children with literacy impairments are taught to spell phonetically when unsure of the correct spelling, spell checkers generate more correct suggestions. Proofing and editing on a hard copy also seems to increase the number of correctly spelled words (McNaughton et al., 1997).

Use of Internet searches can foster spelling learning because correct spelling is needed to complete searches successfully.

Word prediction programs reduce spelling errors of children with language impairment by over half, although the user must get the initial letters correct for the program to work effectively (Newell et al., 1992). It's important that a word prediction program's vocabulary match the writing task. Several programs can incorporate word frequency or various topics (MacArthur, 1999; Zhang et al., 1995).

EXECUTIVE FUNCTION

Executive function can be targeted within the writing process using a goal-plan-do-review format (Ylvisaker & Feeney, 1995; Ylvisaker & Szekeres, 1989; Ylvisaker et al., 1998). The SLP can provide external support to enable children to experience some level of success (Ylvisaker & DeBonis, 2000).

Intervention can begin by allowing children to select their own topics. This increases motivation and shifts the focus to ideas. In the planning phase, the SLP and child can brainstorm ideas for inclusion in the writing

(Troia et al., 1999). Drawings and ideational maps or "spider diagrams" can help. It is also helpful for the child to focus on the potential audience. The SLP can ask questions such as the following (Graham & Harris, 1999):

Who will read this paper?

What do the readers know?

What do the readers need to know?

Why are you writing?

The SLP and child may prefer to use computers as an assistive technology for writing (MacArthur, 2000). Software, such as *Inspiration* (Inspiration Software, 1997), can aid text generation, and the result is easily modifiable by the child or teacher. Children with LD who receive training in executive function along with word processing make greater gains in the quality of their writing than children instructed only in executive function or word processing alone (MacArthur & Graham, 1987; MacArthur et al., 1995; Vace, 1987).

Grammar checkers miss many errors, especially if there are multiple spelling errors. In addition, the child may be unable to figure out just what the error is. Speech recognition software allows a child to compose by dictation, but the software can not overcome oral language difficulties, although these can be moderated with the additional use of grammar checkers.

NARRATIVE TEXT GENERATION

For some children, narrative writing intervention may need to begin at the oral narrative level (Naremore, 2001). They may need to learn to tell common event sequences, such as getting ready for school, and helped to include all the elements of a narrative, called a **story grammar.**

Children with language and writing impairments may not realize that they know a narrative or how to get it started. Story swapping with peers, spin-offs from reading or real life, draw-tell-write methods, or topic selection from a prepared list can all be used to facilitate this process (Tattershall, 2004). Once a topic is selected, a child can be encouraged to write one statement, then another and another by SLP questions such as "And then what happened?" A child can be guided by narrative-enhancing questions from the classroom teacher or SLP and by pictures that outline the story events.

During the writing process, the SLP or classroom teacher can guide a child's writing through the use of brainstorming of ideas, story guides, prompts, and acronyms to aid a child. Story guides are questions that help the student construct the narrative; prompts are story beginning and ending phrases (Graves et al., 1990; Montague et al., 1991; Thomas et al., 1984). Acronyms, such as SPACE for *setting, problem, action*, and *consequent events*, can also act as prompts for guiding writing (Harris & Graham, 1996). Children can be encouraged to write more with verbal prompts such as "Tell me more". Feelings and motivations can be encouraged with pictures and questions such as "How do you think she felt?" (Roth, 2000).

Written narration may require explicit instruction in story grammar or structure. Story maps using pictures or story frames may be necessary initially. Story maps may be pictures that highlight a narrative's main events.

Story frames (Fowler, 1982) are written starters for each main story element. The child completes the sentence and continues with that portion of the narrative. Cards or checklists can also be used to remind the child of story grammar elements (Graves et al., 1990; Montague et al., 1991).

EXPOSITORY TEXT GENERATION

Procedures for intervention with expository writing may include collaborative planning and guidance by SLP/teacher and peer input; individual, independent writing; conferencing with the SLP/teacher and peers; individual, independent revising; and final editing (Van Meter et al., 2004; Wong, 2000). Collaborative planning is important. Children should think aloud and solicit opinions. Such brainstorming often provides a child with alternative views.

One promising method of teaching expository text writing is called Em-POWER, which treats writing as a problem-solving task involving six steps: **E**valuate, **M**ake a **P**lan, **O**rganize, **W**ork, **E**valuate, and **R**ework (Englert et al., 1988). In addition, research has indicated that certain strategies, presented in Figure 6.8 are especially effective with children with LLD (Singer & Bashir, 2004).

Once a topic is selected and discussed in small groups, with a peer, and/or with the SLP, the SLP can give the child a planning sheet to help organize her or his thoughts. After the child has completed the sheet, the SLP can help the child organize the information. This is a great time to challenge and help a child clarify views and prepare for independent writing.

Include other students in a supportive environment.

Place training within a literacy-rich environement.

Provide extensive modeling.

Teach

Writing explicitly and systematically.
Various types of writing.
Planning and organizing strategies

Use

Verbal prompts to support self-regulation.
A variety of strategies to address different needs.
Graphics for display and as a means of storing test-relevant information, such as words, grammar, and ideas.

Move from oral to written forms by integrating the two.

Provide ample opportunity for communication and language to develop.

Collaborate with teachers in mentoring students to write.

Ensure the seamless integration of language intervention and classroom instruction and learning.

FIGURE 6.8
....

Strategies for teaching expository writing.

Source: Based on information from "EmPOWER, A Strategy of Teaching Students with Language Learning Disabilities How to Write Expository Text" by B. D. Singer and A. S.Bashir (2004). In E. R. Silliman and L. C. Wilkinson (Eds.), *Language and Literacy Learning in Schools* (pp. 239–272). New York: Guilford.

FIGURE **6.9**
·············
Sample prompts for opinion writing.

Sources: Based on Wong (2000); Wong et al. (1996).

Section of Paper	*Examples*
Introduction	In my opinion . . .
	I believe . . .
	From my point of view, . . .
	I disagree with . . .
	Supporting words: first, second, finally, for example, most importants is . . . , consider, think about, remember.
Counter Opinion	Although . . .
	However, . . .
	On the other hand, . . .
	To the contrary, . . .
	Even though . . .
Conclusion	In conclusion, . . .
	After considering both sides, . . .
	To summarize, . . .

Writing, even independent writing, can be fostered through the use of a prompt card containing key words for each major section of the paper (Wong et al., 1996). Figure 6.9 presents some sample prompts.

After a child has completed the paper, he or she can conference with peers for feedback while the SLP mediates. The child then revises the paper based on this feedback.

At each stage in the process, a child can record progress on a checklist that provides a model for the writing process. The checklist can also motivate a child as she or he notes progress.

SUMMARY

Although many aspects of literacy impairment clearly are the domain of the classroom teacher and reading specialist, some justifiably belong in the speech-language pathologist's realm. Working with a team, the SLP helps the child obtain language-based skills upon which literacy is based. This is a natural extension of the SLP's concern for language in all modes of communication, something you will note in Chapter 7, "Adult Language Impairments."

THOUGHT QUESTIONS

- How do reading and writing differ?
- Briefly explain the development of both reading and writing.

- How are language and literacy impairments related?
- How would you assess for literacy impairment?
- Suggest some intervention methods for literacy impairments.

SUGGESTED READINGS

Catts, H. W., & Kamhi, A. G. (2005). *Language and reading disabilities* (2nd ed.). Boston: Allyn and Bacon.

McGee, L. M., & Richgels, D. J. (2004). *Literacy's beginnings: Supporting young readers and writers* (4th ed.). Boston: Allyn and Bacon.

Nelson, N. W. (2010). *Language and literacy disorders: Infancy through adolescence.* Boston: Allyn and Bacon.

Sanders, M. (2001). *Understanding dyslexia and the reading process: A guide for educators and parents.* Boston: Allyn and Bacon.

ONLINE RESOURCES

American Speech-Language-Hearing Association
www.asha.org/publications/leader/archives/2007/070904/070904f.htm
ASHA site has discussion of neurobiology and reading.

search.asha.org/query.html?col=journals&qt=dyslexia&charset=iso-8859-1
ASHA search site has links to research article abstracts.

Bright Solutions for Dyslexia

www.dys-add.com/define.html
Bright Solutions for Dyslexia site has several definitions and offers teaching tips. Students should be aware this is a commercial site.

Dyslexia Teacher

www.dyslexia-teacher.com/
Dyslexia Teacher site offers worldwide resources and links.

Learning Disabilities Association of America
www.ldaamerica.org/aboutld/parents/ld_basics/dyslexia.asp
Learning Disabilities Association of America site has a brief checklist of symptoms for parents.

Mayoclinic
www.mayoclinic.com/health/dyslexia/DS00224
Mayo Clinic site covers signs, symptoms, causes, and treatment of this most common reading disability.

Medicinenet
www.medicinenet.com/dyslexia/article.htm
Medicinenet site offers detailed description of dyslexia.

WETA
www.ldonline.org/article/16282
Public service station WETA site has International Dyslexia Association's Dyslexia Basics.

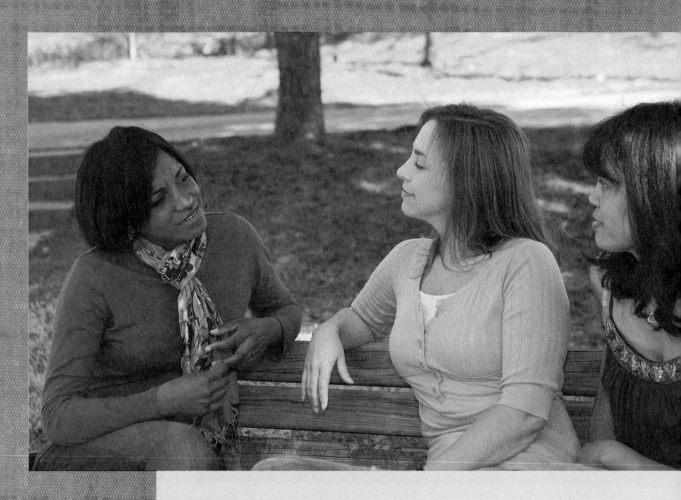

CHAPTER LEARNING GOALS

When you have finished this chapter, you should be able to:

- Differentiate between aphasia, right hemisphere damage, traumatic brain injury, and dementia

- List the concomitant or accompanying deficits that occur with aphasia

- Explain the different types of aphasia and stroke

7

Adult Language Impairments

Many language impairments found in childhood continue into the adult years. Mental retardation, autism, and learning disability do not disappear, although they may change or their effect on language may alter. Other language impairments may lessen or disappear, such as specific language impairment.

This chapter is not about those impairments. Rather, this chapter focuses on language disorders that occur or develop during adulthood (see Case Study 7.1). Specifically, we discuss aphasia, right hemisphere damage, traumatic brain injury, and degenerative neurological conditions. We describe language problems related to interruption of blood supply to the brain, direct destruction of neural tissue, or a pathological process. This will be your introduction, and, of necessity, it will only scratch the surface. Although the speech-language pathologist is concerned primarily with communication, the disorders described in this chapter require an understanding of the medical conditions from which they originate.

In this chapter, we explore adult language and four neurological impairments that affect it. Within each impairment we discuss characteristics, causes, lifespan issues, and assessment and intervention for language deficits.

Space precludes examining all possible neurological disorders. For example, we will not be discussing impairments such as chronic schizophrenia, which typically affects pragmatic aspects of language, such as turn-taking, topic selection, and intentions (Meilijson et al., 2004).

LANGUAGE DEVELOPMENT THROUGH THE LIFESPAN

By adulthood, speech and language have matured and adults are able to communicate in a variety of modes, using not only speech and language, but paralinguistic and nonlinguistic signals effectively. A subtle pause or shift in word emphasis can signal vast differences of meaning in speech. Reading and writing are also essential communication tools.

CASE STUDY 7.1
Case Study of an Adult with Language Impairment: Marsha

A single mom, Marsha has been the sole breadwinner in her family for several years. Two of her three children are grown and her youngest is in high school. With no high school diploma, Marsha has had to work in sales or house-keeping jobs to make ends meet. Most recently, she has been a sales associate in the women's fashions section of a large department store.

Nearly a year ago, Marsha awoke one morning with a very strong headache. Although she felt somewhat unsteady on her feet, she determined that she should go to work anyway. Her right leg became weak as she walked to the bus stop and she collapsed before she had reached her destination.

She awoke in the hospital several hours later, confused and disoriented. She tried to talk with the staff and with her family but seemed unable to comprehend their speech and to form replies. Her medical team, consisting of her physician, a neurologist, the speech-language pathologist, a physical therapist, and an occupational therapist, recommended that Marsha be released from the hospital after 1 week and that she receive services in a rehabilitation center. Both of her older children were eager to help.

The speech-language pathologist worked with Marsha and her family on strengthening Marsha's comprehension and production of language and on her speech. Her intervention services were comprehensive and involved both physical and occupational therapy as well. To date Marsha has recovered much of her speech and language. Some speech sounds are slightly slurred and she still has some lingering word retrieval difficulties. She was able to return to her job and is able to communicate well.

As you read the chapter, think about

- Possible causes of Marsha's stroke.
- Possible ways in which the team could coordinate services and work together.
- Possible problems Marsha might still experience at work.

Language and communication should continue to develop throughout one's life.

Unless debilitated in some way through accident, disease, or disorder, adults continue to refine their communication abilities throughout their lives. Writing and speaking abilities continue to improve with use, new words are added to vocabularies, and new styles of talking are acquired.

Language development proceeds slowly throughout adulthood. Even people with delayed development, such as individuals with MR, experience continued but slowed language growth.

Use

Adult language use is extremely flexible because of the variety of language forms, the large size of the vocabulary, and the breadth of language uses.

Through the use of various communication techniques, competent adults can influence others, impart information, and make their needs known. Some adults are even capable of oratory on a par with that of a Winston Churchill or a Martin Luther King, which can call up the heroic and the unselfish in others.

Compared to children, adults are very effective communicators and skilled conversationalists who have a variety of styles of talking from formal to casual. Styles require modification not only in the manner of talking, but also in the topics introduced and the vocabulary used. As the Little Prince noted when talking with adults (Saint-Exupéry, 1968):

> I would talk . . . about bridge, and golf, and politics, and neckties. And the grown-up would be greatly pleased to have met such a sensible man.

Competent adult communicators quickly sense their role in an interaction and adjust their language and speech accordingly. For example, some people are addressed as *sir* and some as *honey*, and adults do well not to confuse the two. Communication may vary from direct, as in *Turn up the heat*, to indirect, as in *Do you feel a chill?* The goal is the same, but the linguistic methodology is very different.

The number of communicative intentions increases gradually so that adults are able to hypothesize, to cajole, to inspire, to entice, to pun, and so on. The skilled speaker knows how to fulfill these intentions and when to use them.

Although adults continue to refine both their writing and reading ability, these changes are not dramatic. In general, the writing of adults as compared to adolescents is longer with longer, more complex sentences (Nippold, Ward-Lonergan, et al., 2005).

Adult narratives improve steadily into middle age and the early senior years (Marini et al., 2005). Abilities decrease after the late 70s. Those over 75 have less flexibility and ease with word retrieval and make more language form errors.

Content

Adults continue to add to their personal vocabularies and most use between 30,000 and 60,000 words expressively. Receptive vocabularies are even larger. Specialized vocabularies develop for work, religion, hobbies, and social and interest groups. Some words fade from the language and are used less frequently while new words are added. For example, you no longer *dial* a telephone number. Multiple definitions and figurative meanings are also expanded.

Typical seniors experience some deficits in the accuracy and speed of word retrieval and naming (Nicholas et al., 1997). When compared to younger adults, seniors use more indefinite words, such as *thing* and *one* in place of specific names (Cooper, 1990). These deficits reflect accompanying deficits in working memory and, in turn, they affect ability to produce grammatically complex sentences (Kemper et al., 2001).

Form

Within language form, adults continue to acquire prefixes (un-, pre-, dis-), morphophonemic contrasts (*real*, *reality*), and infrequently used irregular verbs. Conversations become more cohesive through more effective use of linguistic devices, such as pronouns, articles, verb tenses, and aspect (which, for example, allows us to talk about the past from the vantage point of the future, as in *Tomorrow, I'll look back and say, "That was a great picnic"*). In general, written language is more complex than spoken language.

The length and syntactic complexity of oral sentences increases into early adulthood and stabilizes in middle age (Nippold, Hesketh, et al., 2005). As mentioned, older seniors experience a decline in complex sentence production that seems related to word retrieval problems.

With aging, there is a decline in both oral and written language comprehension, understanding syntactically complex sentences, and inferencing (Nicholas et al., 1998).

APHASIA

Aphasia means literally "without language," a feature that describes the most severe varieties of this impairment. The aphasic population is extremely diverse. Although aphasia results from localized brain damage, the exact locations and the resultant severity and type of aphasia are not a perfect match. Nor does all brain damage result in aphasia. Damage to the brain may result in loss of motor or sensory function, impaired memory, and poor judgment while leaving language intact. Although mildly aphasic individuals may have language that is similar to that of typical elderly persons, individuals with aphasia usually exhibit greater deficits in expressive language and overall efficiency of communication (Ross & Wertz, 2003).

It is estimated that over one million Americans have aphasia. Over 200 individuals—primarily adults—become aphasic in the United States each day. For these people, language has suddenly become a jumble of strange and seemingly unfamiliar words that they are unable to comprehend and/or produce. Most of you, regardless of whether your chosen profession is speech-language pathology, are likely to have some experience with aphasia through a relative, friend, neighbor, or possibly firsthand. Several excellent Web sites at the end of the chapter offer more insight into aphasia.

Many severities and varieties of aphasia exist. Problems in two areas, auditory comprehension and word retrieval, seem to be common to varying degrees in all. Word retrieval difficulties suggest that memory may also be impaired in some way. Aphasia is not the result of a motor speech impairment, dementia, or the deterioration of intelligence.

Aphasia may affect listening, speaking, reading, and/or writing as well as specific language functions such as naming. Related language functions such as arithmetic, gesturing, telling time, counting money, or interpreting environmental noises such as a dog's bark may also be difficult. Given the great variation possible, it may be better to think of aphasia as a general term that represents several syndromes.

Expressive deficits may include reduced vocabulary, either omission or addition of words, stereotypic utterances, either delayed and reduced output of speech or hyperfluent speech, and word substitutions. Each of these characteristics is an example of a deeper language-processing problem. **Hyperfluent speech,** very rapid speech with few pauses, may be incoherent, inefficient, and pragmatically inappropriate.

It is rare that brain injury is so precise as to affect only language. Other related areas of cognitive function and motor behaviors may also suffer damage.

Language comprehension deficits, whether spoken or written, involve the impaired interpretation of incoming linguistic information. Although individuals with aphasia may have normal hearing and vision, difficulty comes in the interpretation or the ability to make sense of the incoming signal.

Severity may range from individuals with a few intelligible words and little comprehension to those with very high-level subtle linguistic deficits that are barely discernible in normal conversation. Severity is related to several variables, including the cause of the disorder, the location and extent of the brain injury, the age of the injury, and the age and general health of the client. Differences in individual brains may account for different aphasic characteristics and for the lack of similar characteristics when similar areas of the brain are injured.

Although individuals with aphasia differ greatly, several patterns of behavior exist that enable us to categorize the disorder into numerous types or *syndromes*. Although categories of the disorder describe certain similarities among individuals with aphasia, they do not adequately characterize any one individual. Speech-language pathologists and other professionals, such as neurologists and psychiatrists, must thoroughly assess each individual and describe individual strengths and weaknesses.

Other neurogenic disorders—those that affect the central nervous system—such as apraxia or dysarthria often exist along with aphasia, and these complicate classification. Apraxia and dysarthria are discussed in Chapter 12. Individuals with aphasia may also experience seizures and depression. Depression is also a common condition in neurological disorders.

This is an appropriate place to stress that it is extremely difficult to identify the exact spot where language and speech reside in the brain. Language is a complex process performed by many different areas of the brain (Bates, 1997). For example, position emission tomography (PET), a brain-imaging technique, has identified several regions of the brain that are active during speech sound processing (Poeppel, 1996). The number and location of activated regions differ across individuals and with the task, the type of input and output, amount and kind of memory required, the relative difficulty, attention level, and other simultaneous tasks.

Although there is little evidence of a unitary language processing area, some areas do seem to be more important than others, especially the frontal and temporal regions of the left hemisphere. These areas are more active than other regions in both perception and production.

As best we can, we'll try to identify the areas of the brain affected by the disorders being discussed. These are presented in Figure 7.1. You'll want to refer back to this figure as we proceed.

Concomitant or Accompanying Deficits

Physical and psychosocial problems may accompany aphasia and be traced to the same cause. Physical impairments may include hemiparesis, hemiplegia, and hemisensory impairment. **Hemiparesis** is a weakness on one side of the body in which strength and control are greatly reduced. In contrast,

Hemi means "half," as in "hemisphere."

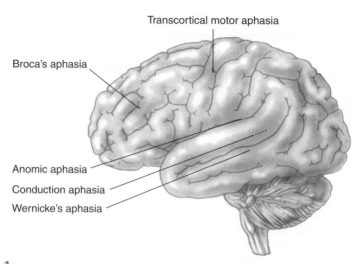

Transcortical motor aphasia

Broca's aphasia

Anomic aphasia

Conduction aphasia

Wernicke's aphasia

FIGURE 7.1

Brain schematic showing probable location of selected aphasias.

Some aphasias are not shown because their possible location is believed to be well below the surface. These include transcortical sensory aphasia, subcortical aphasia, and global aphasia.

hemiplegia is paralysis on one side. Finally, **hemisensory impairment** may accompany either and is a loss of the ability to perceive sensory information. The client may complain of cold, numbness, or tingling on the affected side and may be unable to sense pain or touch.

Visual processing deficits may affect communication. Individuals with deep lesions in the left hemisphere interior to the ear and across the top of the brain may experience blindness in the right visual field of each eye. Called **hemianopsia,** this condition will affect the individual's ability to read.

When paresis, or paralysis, and/or sensory impairment involve the neck and face, the client may have difficulty chewing or swallowing. There may be accompanying drooling or gagging. This condition, known as **dysphagia,** is also the concern of speech-language pathologists and is addressed in Chapter 13.

In addition, brain damage may result in seizure disorder or epilepsy seen in approximately 20% of aphasic adults. Seizures may be of the tonic-clonic type, which result in periods of unconsciousness, or the *petit mal* and psychomotor type, in which the client may lose motor control but remain conscious. The discussion of aphasia is complicated and uses terminology that might be unfamiliar to you. As we discuss each, try to think of it as an extreme form of some behaviors that you already manifest. For example, occasionally, we all have difficulty recalling a name or remembering a word. In its extreme form, we call this *anomia.* Some of the more common terms are listed here with a brief description.

TABLE 7.1

Examples of the expressive language deficits in the speech of adults with aphasia

Deficit	Characteristic	Example
Agrammatism	Omission of unstressed words; telegraphic speech	Take dog walk. Go home. Make instant coffee, watch T.V.
Anomia	Difficulty naming entities	It's a . . . a . . . thing . . . that thing that you do that with . . . you know, that thing for doing stuff with.
Jargon	Meaningless or irrelevant speech with typical intonational patterns	We went for the cookies to laugh in the elephants, didn't we?
Neologism	Novel word	Cow juice and cookies, that's what I like, especially mixed up chocolate (*chocolate milkshake*).
Paraphasia	Word and phoneme substitutions	I need the pen . . . pen . . . pencil and the sheet . . . peeper . . . peeper sheet to color on.
Verbal stereotype	An expression repeated over and over	I see, I see, I see, I see.

Examples of these expressive deficits of adults with aphasia are presented in Table 7.1 and Figure 7.2.

Agnosia: A sensory deficit accompanying some aphasias that makes it difficult for the client to understand incoming sensory information. The disorder may be specific to auditory or visual information.

Agrammatism: Omission of grammatical elements. Individuals with aphasia may omit short, unstressed words, such as articles or prepositions. They may also omit morphological endings, such as the plural -*s* or past-tense -*ed*.

Agraphia: Difficulty writing. Writing may be full of mistakes and poorly formed. Clients may be unable to write what they are able to say. Agrammatism, jargon, and neologisms may be present in written language as well as in spoken.

Alexia: Reading problems. Clients may be unable to recognize even common words they use in their speech and writing. Paraphasia and neologisms may also be present.

Anomia: Difficulty naming entities. Clients may struggle greatly. Individuals who have recovered from aphasia report that they knew

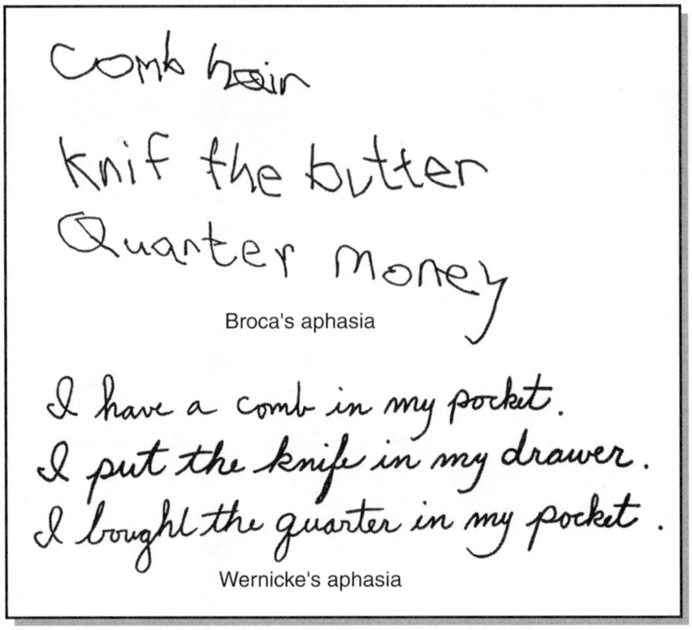

FIGURE 7.2
....

Examples of the expressive
language deficits in the
writing of adults with
aphasia.

Comb hair

knif the butter

Quarter money

Broca's aphasia

I have a comb in my pocket.
I put the knife in my drawer.
I bought the quarter in my pocket.

Wernicke's aphasia

what they wanted to say but could not locate the appropriate word.
An incorrect response may continue to be produced even when the
client recognizes that it is incorrect.

Jargon: Meaningless or irrelevant speech with typical intonational patterns. Responses are often long and syntactically correct although
containing nonsense. Jargon may contain neologisms.

Neologism: A novel word. Some individuals with aphasia may create
novel words that do not exist in their language, using these words
quite confidently.

Paraphasia: Word substitutions found in clients who may talk fluently
and grammatically. Associations to the intended word may be based
on meaning, such as saying *truck* for *car*; on similar sound, such as
tar for *car*; or on some other relationship.

Verbal stereotype: An expression repeated over and over. One young man
responded to every question with "I know," occasionally stringing it
together to form "I know I know I know." Sometimes the expression is
an obscene word or expletive or a neologism. One Mother Superior,
seen in the clinic, continually uttered the same obscene word with great
gusto, to her total embarrassment but seeming inability to stop.

Types of Aphasia

Aphasias can be classified into two large categories based on the ease of producing speech: **fluent aphasia** and **nonfluent aphasia.** In turn, these can
be subdivided. The most common types of aphasia and their characteristics
are presented in Table 7.2.

TABLE 7.2
....
Characteristics of fluent and nonfluent aphasias

Aphasia Type	Speech Production	Speech Comprehension	Speech Characteristics	Reading Comprehension	Naming	Speech Repetition
Wernicke's	Fluent or hyperfluent	Impaired to poor	Verbal paraphasia, jargon	Impaired	Impaired to poor	Impaired to poor
Anomic	Fluent	Mild to moderately impaired	Word retrieval and misnaming good syntax and articulation	Good	Severely impaired in both speech and writing	Good
Conduction	Fluent	Mildly impaired to good	Paraphasia and incorrect ordering with frequent self-correction attempts, good articulation and syntax	Good	Usually impaired	Poor
Transcortical Sensory	Fluent	Poor	Paraphasia, possible perseveration	Impaired to poor	Severely impaired	Unimpaired
Broca's	Nonfluent	Relatively good	Short sentences, agrammatism; slow, labored, with articulation and phonological errors	Unimpaired to poor	Poor	Poor
Transcortical	Nonfluent	Mildly impaired	Impaired, labored, difficulty initiating, syntactic errors	Unimpaired to poor	Impaired	Good
Global	Nonfluent	Poor, limited to single words or short phrases	Limited spontaneous ability of a few words or stereotypes	Poor	Poor	Poor, limited to single words or short phrases

FLUENT APHASIAS

The fluent aphasias are characterized by word substitutions, neologisms, and often verbose verbal output. Lesions in fluent aphasia tend to be found in the posterior portions of the left hemisphere.

Adults with fluent aphasia have typical rate, intonation, pauses, and stress patterns.

Wernicke's Aphasia   As a fluent aphasia, **Wernicke's aphasia** is characterized by rapid-fire strings of sentences with little pause for acknowledgment or turn-taking. Individuals are often unaware of their difficulties. Content may seem a jumble and may be incoherent or incomprehensible although fluent and well articulated. Characteristics include the following:

1. Fluent or hyperfluent speech
2. Poor auditory and visual comprehension
3. Verbal paraphasia or unintended words and neologisms
4. Sentences formed by strings of unrelated words, called jargon
5. Mild to severe impairment in naming and imitative speech

Intonational patterns and sound-combination patterns are maintained.

Poor comprehension extends to reading as well as listening. In addition, poor auditory comprehension affects verbal repetition. The client might not be able to repeat back what was said to him or her. Further, clients may demonstrate reduced ability to comprehend their own speech as well as that of others.

Damage in Wernicke's aphasia is near Wernicke's area in the posterior portions of the left temporal lobe (interior to the left ear). The following is an example of the speech of a client with Wernicke's aphasia:

> I love to go for rides in the car. Cars are expensive these days. Everything's expensive. Even groceries. When I was a child you could spend five dollars and get a whole wagon full. I had a little red wagon. My brother and I would ride down the hill by our house. My brother served in World War II. He moved away after the war. There was so little housing available. My house is a split-level.

An audio sample of a person with Wernicke's aphasia is presented on the accompanying CD-ROM.

Anomic Aphasia   As the name suggests, **anomic aphasia** is characterized by naming difficulties. Most aspects of speech are normal with the exception of word retrieval. Other characteristics include the following:

1. Severe anomia in both speech and writing
2. Fluent spontaneous speech marred by word retrieval difficulties
3. Mild to moderate auditory comprehension problems

Names may be unavailable, or entities may be misnamed with both related and nonrelated words. Imitated or repetitive language is less affected.

Brain damage seems to be at the convergence of the parietal-temporal-occipital cortex (above and posterior to the left ear). Memory difficulties are evident. The following is an example of the speech of a client with anomic aphasia:

> It was very good. We had a bird . . . a big thing with feathers and . . . a bird . . . a turkey stuffed . . . turkey with stuffing and that stuff . . . you know . . .

and that stuff, that berry stuff . . . that stuff . . . berries, berries . . . cranberry stuffing . . . stuffing and cranberries . . . and gravy on things . . . smashed things . . . Oh, darn, smashed potatoes.

Conduction Aphasia   Like the other fluent aphasias, **conduction aphasia** is characterized by conversation that is abundant and quick, although filled with paraphasia. Characteristics include the following:

1. Anomia
2. Only mild impairment of auditory comprehension, if any
3. Extremely poor repetitive or imitative speech
4. Paraphasia or the inappropriate use of words formed by the addition of sounds and incorrect ordering of sounds or by substituting related words

Paraphasia may be severe enough to make the individual's speech incomprehensible. Given the good comprehension skills of many individuals with conduction aphasia, self-correction attempts are frequent, although the client may be unable to benefit from the verbal cues of others.

Damage may be deep below the brain surface between areas where language is formulated and speech programmed. The following is an example of the speech of a client with conduction aphasia:

We went to me girl, my girl . . . oh, a little girl's palace . . . no, daughter's palace, not a castle, but a pal . . . place . . . home for a sivit . . . and he . . . visit and she made a cook, cook a made . . . a cake.

Transcortical Sensory Aphasia   The rarest of the fluent aphasias, **transcortical sensory aphasia,** is characterized by conversation and spontaneous speech as fluent as in Wernicke's aphasia, but filled with word errors. Characteristics include the following:

1. Unimpaired ability to repeat or imitate words phrases, and sentences
2. Verbal paraphasia or word substitutions
3. Lack of nouns and severe anomia
4. Poor auditory comprehension

The unimpaired imitative ability may be perseverative or may become so persistent as to seem echolalic. Echolalic speech is characterized by an immediate or delayed whole or partial repetition of the speech of another speaker. Brain damage seems to isolate language areas from other areas of cortical control.

Subcortical Aphasia   Although its existence had been hypothesized, **subcortical aphasia** could not be confirmed until the advent of neuro-imaging techniques.

Lesions occur deep in the brain without involvement of the cerebral cortex. Characteristics include the following:

1. Fluent expressive speech
2. Paraphasia and neologisms
3. Repetition unaffected
4. Auditory and reading comprehension relatively unaffected
5. Cognitive deficits and reduced vigilance

Additional language characteristics may include word-finding difficulties, perseveration, and nonimitative speech. Other characteristics, including dysarthria, have been related to specific sites in the basal ganglia (Kirshner, 1995).

Nonfluent Aphasias

Nonfluent aphasia is characterized by slow, labored speech and struggle to retrieve words and form sentences. In general, the site of lesion is in or near the frontal lobe.

Adults with nonfluent aphasia have slow rate, less intonation, inappropriately placed and abnormally long pauses, and less varied stress patterns than typical speakers.

Broca's Aphasia   **Broca's aphasia** is associated with damage to the anterior or forward parts of the frontal lobe of the left cerebral hemisphere, centered in Broca's area, which is responsible for both motor planning and working memory. The most common traits are the following:

1. Short sentences with agrammatism in which auxiliary or helping verbs, the verb *to be*, prepositions, articles, and morphological endings are omitted
2. Anomia
3. Problems with imitation of speech because of overall speech problems
4. Slow, labored speech and writing
5. Articulation and phonological errors

Auditory comprehension seems unimpaired, although careful testing may reveal subtle deficits in understanding.

The following is an example of the speech of a client with Broca's aphasia:

Foam, foam, phone, damn, phone . . . not ude . . . phone not ude . . . ude . . . ude . . . use . . . can't ude . . . no foam can ude.

Transcortical Motor Aphasia   This is the nonfluent counterpart of transcortical sensory aphasia. Individuals with **transcortical motor aphasia** may have difficulty initiating speech or writing. Characteristics of this syndrome include the following:

1. Impaired speech, especially in conversation
2. Good verbal imitative abilities
3. Mildly impaired auditory comprehension

Severely impaired speech is characteristic of damage to the motor cortex, although the areas that are affected may go well below the surface of the brain.

Global or Mixed Aphasia   As the name implies, **global or mixed aphasia** is characterized by profound language impairment in all modalities. It is considered the most severely debilitating form of aphasia. Other characteristics include the following:

1. Limited spontaneous expressive ability of a few words or stereotypes, such as overlearned utterances or emotional responses
2. Imitative speech and naming affected
3. Auditory and visual comprehension limited to single words or short phrases

Global aphasia has both the auditory comprehension problems found in some fluent aphasias and the labored speech of nonfluent aphasias.

These symptoms are associated with a large, deep lesion in an area below the brain's surface. Often, both the anterior speech and posterior language areas of the left hemisphere are involved.

ADDITIONAL TYPES OF APHASIA

Not all aphasias can be neatly classified within the fluent-nonfluent system. Other aphasias may affect primarily one communication modality, such as writing. Examples of these specific aphasias include the following:

Alexia with agraphia: Reading and writing impairment

Alexia without agraphia: Reading impairment with no accompanying writing difficulty

Pure agraphia: Severe writing disorder

Pure word deafness: Lack of auditory comprehension with error-free spontaneous speech

Crossed aphasia: Aphasia accompanying right hemisphere damage

Aphasia classification and its relation to the location of lesions are controversial issues and areas of continued study.

Causes of Aphasia

The onset of aphasia is rapid. Usually, it occurs in people who have no former history of speech and language difficulties. The lesion or injury leaves an area of the brain unable to function as it had just moments before.

The most common cause of aphasia is a **stroke** or **cerebrovascular accident,** the third leading cause of death in the United States. Strokes affect half a million Americans annually. Seventy percent of these are over 65 years of age (Stroke Center, 2005). Although strokes are rare in children, infants suffer strokes at a rate similar to elderly adults (Lee et al., 2005). The

Stroke is caused by an interruption of the blood supply to the brain.

National Aphasia Association estimates that as a result of strokes, approximately 100,000 people become aphasic each year.

Strokes are of two basic types: ischemic and hemorrhagic. More common **ischemic strokes** result from a complete or partial blockage (occlusion) of the arteries transporting blood to the brain as in cerebral arteriosclerosis, embolism, and thrombosis. **Cerebral arteriosclerosis** is a thickening of the walls of cerebral arteries in which elasticity is lost or reduced, the walls become weakened, and blood flow is restricted. The resulting ischemia, or reduction of oxygen, may be temporary or may cause permanent damage through the death of brain tissue. An **embolism** is an obstruction to blood flow caused by a blood clot, fatty materials, or an air bubble. The obstruction may travel through the circulatory system until it blocks the flow of blood in a small artery. For example, a clot may form in the heart or the large arteries of the chest, break off, and become an embolus. As in cerebral arteriosclerosis, blockage results in a lack of oxygen-carrying blood, depriving brain cells of needed oxygen. Similarly, a **thrombosis** also blocks blood flow. In this case, plaque buildup or a blood clot is formed on site and does not travel. The result is the same.

Some individuals experience a **transient ischemic attack** (TIA), sometimes called a mini-stroke, a temporary condition whose symptoms mirror those of a stroke. A TIA occurs when blood flow to some portion of the brain is blocked or reduced. After a short interval, the symptoms decrease as blood flow returns. TIAs should be taken seriously because they can be a warning sign of increased likelihood of a stroke occurring in the future.

A **hemorrhagic stroke** is one in which the weakened arterial walls burst under pressure, as occurs with an aneurysm or arteriovenous malformation. An **aneurysm** is a saclike bulging in a weakened artery wall. The thin wall may rupture, causing a cerebral hemorrhage. Most aneurysms occur in the meninges, the layered membranes surrounding the brain, and blood flowing into this space can damage the brain or in serious cases, cause death.

Arteriovenous malformation is rare and consists of a poorly formed tangle of arteries and veins that may occur in a highly viscous organ such as the brain. Malformed arterial walls may be weak and give way under pressure.

Patterns of recovery differ with the type of stroke. Often, with ischemic stroke, there is a noticeable improvement within the first weeks after the injury. Recovery slows after 3 months. In contrast, the results of hemorrhagic strokes are usually more severe after injury. The period of most rapid recovery is at the end of the first month and into the second as swelling lessens and injured neurons regain functioning.

Damage from stroke may occur in any part of the brain. In all right-handed individuals and in some left-handed ones, injury to left hemisphere language areas produces aphasia. Injury to the right hemisphere results in aphasia in only a small percentage of cases, usually left-handed individuals whose right hemisphere is more important for language.

Aphasia-like symptoms also may be noted with head injury, neural infections, degenerative neurological disorders, and tumors. In most of these cases, however, other cortical areas are also affected, resulting in clinically different disorders.

The results of a stroke are further complicated by the prestroke storage patterns for language.

One syndrome, **primary progressive aphasia**, should be mentioned here. Primary progressive aphasia is a degenerative disorder of language, with preservation of other mental functions and of activities of daily living. The disorder, which takes at least 2 years to develop, is not dementia or loss of cognitive functioning, and many individuals with primary progressive aphasia can take care of themselves, some even remaining employed. Over its course, the disorder progresses from primarily a motor speech disorder to a near-total inability to speak, although comprehension remains relatively preserved.

The human brain is extremely complex. Categorizing the types of aphasias that we have discussed helps to bring some understanding to the subject of brain disorders but may have little practical clinical value. Each client presents unique characteristics. It is all the more important, therefore, that speech-language pathologists describe each client's abilities and disabilities carefully and clearly.

Lifespan Issues

Although children and adolescents can experience aphasia, especially accompanying brain tumors, most victims are adults in middle age and beyond who previously lived healthy productive lives. The risk of stroke is increased if the individual has a history of smoking, alcohol use, poor diet, lack of exercise, high blood pressure, high cholesterol, diabetes, obesity, and TIAs or previous strokes. Usually, the onset of symptoms is rapid when the cause is vascular, but it can take months or years to become evident with tumor or degenerative disease. These patterns are presented in Figure 7.3.

In the most common situation, the individual suffers an ischemic stroke, depriving the brain of a needed supply of oxygenated blood. First

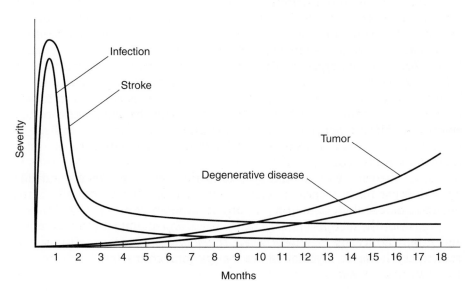

FIGURE 7.3

Severity of symptoms by neurological condition. Individuals will differ in severity and path of the disorder.

Source: Based on information from *Introduction to Neurogenic Communication Disorders* (5th ed.), by R. H. Brookshire, 1997, St. Louis, MO: Mosby-Year Book.

indications may be loss of consciousness, headache, weak or immobile limbs, and/or slurred speech. This condition *may* be either temporary in which function returns quickly or more permanent. Some individuals may experience a series of TIAs spaced over a period of years before they become alarmed. Some TIAs go undetected by the individual.

Usually, the individual is rushed to the hospital. Approximately a third of individuals die from the stroke or shortly thereafter. For those who survive, there may be a period of unconsciousness, followed by disorientation. Deep long-lasting periods of unconsciousness or coma are associated with poorer eventual recovery.

For the individual who has experienced a stroke, language is probably not his or her immediate or central concern. Initial reaction may be fear or anxiety. The patient and the family are focused on survival and may be fearful of another stroke. For most individuals, this is a novel situation, and they are unaware of how possible limitations will affect their future. As chronic effects settle in, the individual begins to focus on the physical and language complications. This can lead to frustration and depression. The mother of one of the authors refused to participate in physical therapy in this stage. The newly aphasic patient may not be ready to receive factual information about his or her condition or structured intervention.

Likewise, families of individuals with aphasia are often frightened and confused. Because no one prepares in advance for stroke, families are usually ill informed. In other words, the patient and family are in crisis.

Most individuals remain in acute care for only a few days until their condition stabilizes. Following this, an individual may receive a variety of care depending on the severity of the stroke. These include rehabilitative hospitalization, outpatient rehabilitation, or nursing home care. Most return home but with some impairment.

Although intervention services may occur for years, most individuals receive services for at least the first several months. In addition to neuromuscular deficits and seizures, the individual with aphasia may exhibit behavior changes, including perseveration, disinhibition, and emotional problems depending on the site of the lesion. *Perseveration* is the repetition of inappropriate responses in which the client may become fixed on a single task or behavior and repeat it. *Disinhibition* is a seeming inability to inhibit certain asocial or inappropriate behaviors, such as touching others. Finally, brain damage may contribute to exaggerated swings in emotion in which the emotion is appropriate but the magnitude and the suddenness of the emotional shift are not. Emotional behavior must be considered in light of the extreme frustration experienced by some individuals with aphasia. Depression is also common.

Given the variety of possible symptoms following a stroke, the individual will most likely receive services from a team of professionals. Team members may include a neurologist, physical therapist, occupational therapist, nutritionist, speech-language pathologist, and audiologist. Life changes and family concerns may necessitate the services of a counseling social worker, psychologist, psychiatrist, and/or pastoral counselor.

Immediately after the incident, neurological functioning is most severely affected. Within days, the body's natural recovery process begins. As swelling is reduced, injured cells may recover and begin to function normally. Adjacent areas of the brain that shared brain functions with the injured area may begin to play a larger role. The course and extent of this recovery process are difficult to predict, but the rate is fastest during the first few weeks and months after the stroke, then slows, and usually ceases after 6 months. During this process, the entire syndrome that the client presents may change and most certainly will lessen in severity. The most frequent linguistic gains are in auditory comprehension (Kertesz & McCabe, 1997). In general, less severely affected individuals, those who are younger, in general good health, and left-handed, recover from aphasia better and faster than those who are more severe, older, in poor health, and right-handed.

Most individuals experience some type of **spontaneous recovery,** a natural restorative process. In general, individuals who experience ischemic strokes begin spontaneous recovery earlier than those who experience intracerebral hemorrhage but improve less rapidly (Nicholas et al., 1993). Although the anatomical and physiological basis for the spontaneous recovery of language is not well understood, maximum improvement is seen in the first 3 months. This immediate physiological restitution may be complemented by reorganization of brain function in the later stages of recovery. Neuroimaging studies show use of left hemisphere structures that were previously involved in language function and use of similar regions in the right hemisphere with a corresponding shift in some language functioning to the right (Pataraia et al., 2004; Price et al., 1998, Thompson, 2004; Weiller et al., 1995).

With or without spontaneous recovery, assessment and intervention begin as soon as the client's individual condition permits. Clients who are most responsive are probably the best candidates for intervention services. A general rule is that the earlier the treatment, the better the rate of recovery, but clients do not all recover similarly (Robey, 1994, 1998). The SLP's first goal is to determine the feasibility of clinical intervention. Although it is not possible to predict accurately how much gain will be the result of spontaneous recovery and how much the outcome of intervention, the SLP attempts to determine which clients will benefit most from clinical intervention (Marshall, 1997).

Loss of the ability to use language efficiently changes the social role of each individual with aphasia and can result in social isolation. This situation is complicated by the often incorrect assumption that cognitive abilities are also damaged. In addition, inability to communicate may cause the affected individual to become dependent on others for the simplest of daily tasks. Family roles and responsibilities may also change. Wives, husbands, and children may have to take on new responsibilities. If the individual supported the family prior to the incident, there may be economic problems in addition to medical ones. Case Study 7.2 presents the story of one individual with aphasia.

Communication is so entwined in our social interactions and in our very definition of who we are that the effects of aphasia reach well beyond speech and language.

CASE STUDY 7.2
Personal Story of an Adult with Aphasia

When Mr. W. was 55 years of age, he looked fitter than most men 10 years his junior. Having earned a master's degree in labor relations from Cornell University, Mr. W. was employed for many years as a labor mediator by the small city in which he lived. Mr. W. was viewed as cheerful by his circle of friends, primarily fellow hikers with whom he explored mountain trails almost every Saturday.

Although Mr. W. had been rugged and capable of vigorous outdoor activity, he knew that he had high blood pressure, and he was taking medication under a doctor's care. Mr. W. was rarely ill, and he had been hospitalized only once, for acute appendicitis, before his stroke.

One Sunday afternoon, Mr. W. decided to lie down after a 4-hour cross-country ski outing. He had a bad headache, and he hoped that a short rest would relieve it before a dinner date with skiing buddies. When he awoke from his nap, he got up to go to the bathroom but collapsed. His friends were concerned when he failed to meet them. They phoned and got no answer, so someone went to his home. Mr. W. was found on the floor, breathing but unconscious. He had suffered a cerebrovascular accident (CVA), or stroke.

Mr. W. was taken to the emergency room of the local hospital. When he became conscious, he was disoriented, did not seem to understand what was said to him, and was unable to speak. The right side of his body was partially paralyzed. The medical report stated that he had "sustained a left CVA that resulted in right hemiplegia and aphasia." He remained hospitalized for 6 weeks. In addition to the attending neurologist and family physician, Mr. W. was seen by a speech-language pathologist and a physical therapist. The SLP performed an initial bedside assessment and counseled family members and friends. The SLP's initial report stated that "Mr. W. presented with severe expressive/receptive aphasia characterized by severe oral motor apraxia and a severe auditory comprehension deficit with moderate to severe reading comprehension deficits for single words."

When Mr. W. was discharged from the hospital, he moved in with his sister and her family. He was cared for largely by family and friends, and he was taken for medical appointments and twice-weekly physical and speech-language therapy. Early goals were simple auditory comprehension requiring yes/no head nods as responses, and the expression of needs such as "eat."

Two years after the stroke, Mr. W. was able to walk with a walker. Family members reported that they could understand approximately 85% of his intentional speech. Strangers could understand only about 20%. He used gestures and largely unintelligible sounds to express himself. Mr. W.'s ability to comprehend language had improved dramatically, and he was now able to follow directions that contained three critical elements ("put the pencil on top of the card and then put it back"). Friends reported that he often seemed agitated, but he apparently liked their visits. Because Mr. W. had always enjoyed being outdoors, his friends frequently took him for short walks. Family members said that they tried to sing together on a regular basis and that Mr. W. joined in to the extent that he was able.

Recently, Mr. W. was evaluated for augmentative/alternative communication. He has received an electronic voice output system and is being taught how to use it. He will never be able to speak normally, but this device should greatly facilitate his ability to communicate.

Assessment for Aphasia

Assessment and intervention may begin in the hospital and continue as outpatient service. Successful intervention is a team effort. The relative importance of each specialist will change as the client recovers. In addition, a spouse, other family member, or close friend may be a critical participant in the recuperative process.

Before beginning any intervention, it is necessary to complete a thorough assessment of each client's abilities and deficits. This process may continue in several stages as the client stabilizes and experiences **spontaneous recovery.**

The assessment procedures outlined in Chapter 4 provide a model. Especially important are the client's medical history, the interview with the client and family, the oral peripheral examination, the hearing testing, and direct speech and language testing. The medical history can reveal information about general health and previous cerebrovascular incidents. In addition, current neurological reports and medical progress notes provide valuable information on present and changing status.

In addition to collecting data during the interview, it will be necessary for the SLP to provide information. The client may be disoriented and need reassurance. Family members will have many questions regarding recovery, family dynamics, income, medical expenses, and the like. Often a social worker will address these issues also. It is important for families to know the extent of the injuries and to have a realistic appraisal of recovery with and without professional assistance. Although it is unethical to promise a "cure," the SLP should give the family an honest estimate of expected progress.

Counseling with the family by team members will be ongoing. The family and client may need professional counseling to cope with the enormous changes that have occurred in their lives.

Careful observation throughout is essential, especially shortly after the incident, when more formal testing is not possible. It is important to observe the client's general speech and language behavior and to listen and observe what is communicated and how. Observing spontaneous language use can give the SLP important information on the nature and extent of the disorder (Davis, 1993; Helm-Estabrooks & Albert, 1991).

A thorough oral peripheral examination is important because of the potential for either neuromuscular paralysis or weakness. Speech disorders such as apraxia and dysarthria frequently are associated with aphasia and should be described or ruled out. See Chapter 12, "Neurogenic Speech Disorders," for a fuller discussion.

Possible hearing loss must also be ascertained, especially given the older age of most individuals with aphasia. It is important to separate hearing loss from comprehension deficits.

Initial speech and language testing is often at the patient's bedside and is confounded by spontaneous recovery that decreases the need for extensive formal testing (Marshall, 1997). Instead, the SLP administers informal probes of the patient's language strengths and weaknesses. More formal testing is usually postponed until the patient has maintained a stable level on simple language tasks for at least several days. Simple tasks are administered at least once daily in a short 15-minute time frame (Holland & Fridriksson, 2001). The SLP notes subtle changes in the patient's behavior. It's important not to tire the patient because fatigue can have a negative effect on communicative ability. Figure 7.4 presents a sample of some of the tasks involved in a bedside assessment.

SLPs should expect some improvement in some areas over just a few days. Positive changes should be reinforced and pointed out to the patient and family.

Comprehensive testing of clients with aphasia should include at least the two input modalities of vision and audition and the three output modalities of speech, writing, and gestures.

FIGURE 7.4
....
Possible components
of an informal bedside
evaluation.

Source: Based on Holland and
Fridriksson (2001).

Memory: Once introduced, names can be used to assess verbal memory on subsequent visits.

Reading: Ask the patient to read get-well cards.

Writing: Observe patient studying and filling in a hospital menu.

Word retrieval and writing: Provide writing impements and ask patients to write a few words, such as the names of their children.

Memory and more complex language: Ask the patient to identify the person who sent each greeting card.

Naming: Ask patient to name a few common objects around the room.

Auditory comprehension: Note how client responds during conversation.

Auditory comprehension and working memory: Have patient follow a few simple commands.

Automatic language: Ask the patient to count or say the alphabet or days of the week.

Pragmatics: Note greeting and leave-taking; make a few simple mistakes, such as calling the patient by the wrong name, and observe the response; ask absurd questions (e.g., "Do helicopters eat their young?"); and take careful note of the conversational repairs, turn-taking behavior, and general appropriateness of the conversation structure.

More formal speech and language testing and sampling phases should assess overall communication skills as well as receptive and expressive language within all modalities–reading, writing, auditory comprehension, expressive language, and gestures and nonlinguistic communication–and across all five aspects of language: pragmatics, semantics, syntax, morphology, and phonology. With higher functioning clients, the SLP will want to assess higher language skills such as verbal reasoning and analogies, figurative language, categorization, and explanations of complex tasks. Table 7.3 is an overview of the areas that ASHA recommends be evaluated in a functional assessment of communication abilities.

Several standardized tests are available for assessing specific language skills. Figure 7.5 presents some frequently used aphasia batteries. Formal tests must be selected carefully, given the varying range and scope of different instruments. Overall test construction varies from those that view aphasia as a multimodality disorder, such as the *Minnesota Test of Differential Diagnosis of Aphasia* (Schuell, 1972) and the *Porch Index of Communicative Abilities* (Porch, 1981), to those that consider performance in each modality to be somewhat distinct and describe different syndromes, such as the *Boston Diagnostic Aphasia Examination* (Goodglass & Kaplan, 1983a). Some measures, such as the *Functional Communication Profile* (Sarno, 1969) and *Communication Abilities in Daily Living* (Holland, 1980), follow neither model and attempt to describe the client's communicative abilities in daily living tasks. Most tests include picture or object naming,

TABLE 7.3

ASHA recommendations for a functional assessment of communicative abilities with adults with aphasia

Assessment Domains	Behaviors
Social communication	Use names of familiar people
	Express agreement and disagreement
	Request information
	Exchange information on the telephone
	Answer yes/no questions
	Follow directions
	Understand facial expressions and tone of voice
	Understand nonliteral meaning and intent
	Understand conversations in noisy surroundings
	Understand TV and radio
	Participate in conversations
	Recognize and correct communication errors
Communication of basic needs	Recognize familiar faces and voices
	Make strong likes and dislikes known
	Express feelings
	Request help
	Make needs and wants known
	Respond in an emergency
Reading, writing, number concepts	Understand simple signs
	Use reference materials
	Follow written directions
	Understand printed material
	Print, write, and type name
	Complete forms
	Write messages
	Understand signs with numbers
	Make money transactions
	Understand units of measure
Daily planning	Tell time
	Dial telephone numbers
	Keep scheduled appointments
	Use a calendar
	Follow a map

Source: Information from American Speech-Language-Hearing Association. (1994). *Functional assessment of communicative skills for adults (FACS)*. Washington, DC: Author.

FIGURE 7.5
....

Frequently used aphasia batteries.

Aphasia Assessment Battery

Boston Diagnostic Aphasia Exam (Goodglass & Kaplan, 1983a)

Boston Naming Test (Goodglass & Kaplan, 1983b)

Communication Abilities in Daily Living (Holland, 1980)

Minnesota Test of Differential Diagnosis of Aphasia (Schuell, 1972)

Porch Index of Communicative Abilities (Porch, 1981)

Western Aphasia Battery (Kertesz & McCabe, 1982)

pointing to pictures named, automatic language, repeating sentences, describing pictures and answering questions, reading and answering questions and/or drawing conclusions, and writing. It is important for the SLP to remain flexible and to continue to probe the client's behavior for the duration of intervention, especially as behaviors change.

Interpretation of client behavior during testing is extremely important. It is critical, for example, whether the client failed to respond because she or he could not retrieve the answer or because she or he did not comprehend the verbal cue.

Most test tasks involve decision making or problem solving, the endpoints of several cognitive and linguistic processes. Subcomponents of the process are not assessed individually. *Online* assessment, which measures effects at various points within the process, may be more sensitive to individual client strengths and weaknesses (Shapiro et al., 1998). To date, most online analysis is limited to research, but such procedures are slowly being adapted for clinical use.

Because most individuals with aphasia have some residual communication impairment, the goal of intervention is to maximize communication effectiveness in the face of this impairment.

Intervention

The overall goal of intervention is to aid in the recovery of language and to provide strategies to compensate for persistent language deficits (Rosenbek et al., 1989). Individual intervention goals are determined by the results of the assessment and by the desires of both the client and family. Goals will be individualized according to the type and severity of the aphasia and upon the individual needs of each client. Ideally, the goals are mutually acceptable to the client, family, and SLP. All members of the team coordinate their efforts to strengthen treatment received from others. Some guidelines for working with individuals with aphasia are presented in Figure 7.6.

Intervention approaches reflect the SLP's theoretical position on aphasia plus a strong does of practical knowledge regarding the most effective techniques. Each clinician must decide whether to work on underlying skills, such as memory and auditory comprehension, or to begin with specific skill deficits, such as naming. If the SLP decides that the client's brain needs help to reorganize, he or she may choose cross-modality training, such as reading aloud while tracing the letters with one's finger.

Treat the client in an age-appropriate manner.

Keep your own language simple, clear, and unambiguous and control for length and complexity.

Adjust your language and the speed of production for the processing capabilities of the client.

Use everyday items and tasks and involve the family.

Use repetition and familiar routines, situations, and responses to facilitate learning.

Structure tasks to improve performance and adjust the amount of structure just enough to support the client's efforts but not foster dependency.

Provide a context to supportive the client's language processing.

Increase the demands made on the client gradually based on the client's abilities.

Teach the client to use his or her strengths to compensate for weaknesses.

FIGURE 7.6

Guidelines for intervention with individuals with aphasia.

The SLP can also take advantage of cross-modality generalization in which skills trained in one modality generalize to another. For example, some individuals with agrammatism benefit from comprehension training more than production training (Jacobs & Thompson, 2000). Comprehension training seems to generalize to comprehension and production. Similarly, generalization occurs across linguistically related structures and from more complex structures to less complex ones (Thompson et al., 2003).

There is very little data on the effects of treatment during the early phases of recovery. Although the focus of early aphasia management often consists of providing support, prevention, and education rather than on structured language therapy (Marshall, 1997), many individuals benefit from less directive, more counseling-oriented treatment (Holland & Fridriksson, 2001).

In both initial and follow-on intervention, conversational techniques can provide language therapy and therapeutic support, especially in the early stages of intervention (Holland & Fridriksson, 2001). Within a therapeutic conversation, the client carries as much of the "communication burden" as possible. Mindful of small improvements by the client, the SLP revises the demands made of the client. In short sessions using conversation, the SLP reassures, explains what's happening to the client, and points out positive changes. As clients progress, the SLP provides less support and provides a variety of communication contexts and experiences.

Another method of intervention is to have the client attempt to access the language in the left hemisphere by "bridging" from the right. This might be attempted by teaching the client to gesture or sign and simultaneously attempt to say the names of familiar objects. It is reasoned that gestures or signs, being visuospatial in nature, are stored in part in the right hemisphere. Another method, called *melodic intonational therapy* (Sparks et al., 1974;

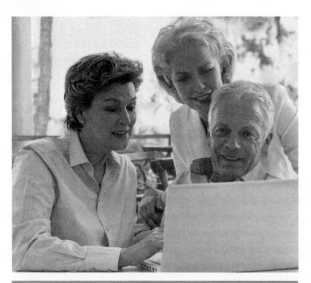

Speech and language services are part of a team approach to intervention.

Sparks & Holland, 1976), uses the client's usually intact right hemisphere ability to sing or produce intonational patterns. Words and phrases are taught by using different patterns of rhythm and melody. In either example, the signs or the intonational patterns are gradually faded as the client begins spontaneously to produce the targeted words and phrases without their aid.

As in many areas of language intervention, unanimity on cross-hemispheric treatment methods does not exist. Many SLPs prefer to remediate language deficits by more direct multimodality stimulation of the affected cognitive processes (Heiss et al., 1999; Peach, 2001; Warburton et al., 1999). The goal is reactivation of speech areas in the dominant hemisphere.

Sign, gesture, or some other form of augmentative/alternative communication may become the primary communicative modality for clients who possess profoundly impaired language and/or speech disorders. Communication boards or electronic forms of communication may be appropriate for those who also have neuromuscular impairments. Amerind, or American Indian signs, may also be useful because many require only one hand and are easily guessable by others. See Chapter 15. "Augmentative and Alternative Communication."

Intervention might also focus on cognitive abilities, such as memory and attention, in addition to more linguistic targets (Murray et al., 1997, 1998). Clinician-assisted training may also be supplemented by more minimally assisted training, such as computer-provided reading tasks including visual matching and reading comprehension (Katz & Wertz, 1997).

The adaptive capacity of the central nervous system, or *plasticity*, holds promise for individuals with aphasia. Data strongly suggest that neurons and other brain cells have the ability to alter their structure and function in response to a variety of pressures, including training. Plasticity may be the key to helping damaged brains relearn lost behavior through intervention. Much more research is needed to translate from clinical research and practice (Kleim & Jones, 2008).

Assuming that the family is amenable, it may be beneficial to involve them in the communication training program under the SLP's guidance. The familiar atmosphere of the home and the objects, actions, and people in it can provide a context that can facilitate a client's recovery and strengthen his or her relearned communicative behaviors. It is important for professionals to remember that the beneficial involvement of the family must not be at their emotional expense. Family members must not be made to feel guilt if the client progresses little.

Augmentative/alternative communication may become the primary mode of communication or may be used as a facilitative tool to access verbal language.

Volunteers can also be trained to support the conversational attempts of individuals with aphasia (Kagan et al., 2001). These individuals need to acknowledge and respond to a client's interactive behaviors. This feedback can affect motivation and performance and is an essential part of intervention (Simmons-Mackie et al., 1999).

Evidence-Based Practice

Although we can conclude from the myriad of studies on intervention with individuals with aphasia that behavioral intervention promotes recovery, we cannot definitively say which intervention methods are best for the various forms of aphasia (Raymer et al., 2008). What we can say is that failure to participate in intervention has an adverse effect on recovery. Other EBP findings are presented in Box 7.1.

BOX 7.1
Evidence-Based Practice for Individuals with Aphasia

Overall Methods of Intervention

- Individuals with aphasia significantly benefit from the services of SLPs over those who receive no intervention. At least 80% make measurable progress affecting both the quantity and quality of language.
- Behavioral intervention promotes language recovery. In general, aphasia treatment is effective compared with spontaneous recovery alone.
- The most effective forms of intervention for different forms of aphasia and different language behaviors have not been thoroughly evaluated. Most evaluative studies use test performance rather than than investigate the effect of aphasia treatment for functional use of communication. More research is needed in how stroke recovery factors, such as lesion size and location, age, and type of language deficit, influence treatment, especially neural reorganization.

Specific Techniques

- Although timing of intervention after the injury is critical, the optimal interval before beginning intense intervention is unknown. In general, we can say that treatment within the first 3 months is maximally beneficial, but that later treatment can also improve language ability and use.
- Repetition is important for maintaining changes in brain function and physiology.

- Although more intense intervention (9 or more hours/week) yields better results, the optimal amount is unknown. In chronic aphasia, there is modest evidence for more intensive treatment. Of particular interest is *Constraint-induced language therapy* (CILT) (Pulvermuller et al., 2001). CILT involves (1) requiring the patient to use verbal language while limiting or constraining all other use channels and (2) massed practice or a high-intensity treatment schedule of 3 to 4 hours daily for 2 weeks. The effects are similar to other intensive treatments that do not employ the use of constraint (Cherny et al., 2008).
- Training complex language material results in improvements in less complex, untrained language when the trained and untrained material are linguistically related. Training simple material has little effect on learning of more complex material.

Generalization

- Research results on the generalization of treatment effects to untrained language behaviors are mixed.
- Generalization is most likely to occur to a language feature that is similar to one that is trained, such as generalization to untrained sentences that are syntactically related to trained sentences.

Source: Based on DeRuyter et al. (2008); Raymer et al. (2008).

Conclusion

Aphasia is a complex impairment varying in scope and extent across individuals. In addition, clients may have other impairments, such as paralysis, as a result of their injury. Only a careful description of individual abilities and deficits in each specific modality of communication will enable the SLP to plan and carry out effective intervention. The individual variation in symptoms and severity, the team approach to intervention, and the possibility of spontaneous recovery complicate our efforts to measure intervention effectiveness and offer opportunities for those of you interested in research.

RIGHT HEMISPHERE DAMAGE

The term **right hemisphere damage (RHD)** refers to a group of deficits that result from injury the right hemisphere of the brain, the nondominant hemisphere for nearly all language functions. Deficits may be neuromuscular, perceptual, and linguistic. In addition, individuals may exhibit unusual behaviors. One client would regularly take a shower with his clothes on and try to go outside nude. Families report personality and mood changes including indifference and apathy. Even less-involved clients can have unrealistic estimates of their own condition and prognosis. An apparent lack of concern may actually mask a client's confusion.

Less information exists on RHD than on damage to the left hemisphere, although approximately half the individuals who have suffered stroke have right hemisphere involvement. The communication disorders that clients with RHD experience are not language based. Rather, a combination of cognitive deficits results in the communication problem. As a result, the efficiency, effectiveness, and accuracy of communication are affected.

The role of the right hemisphere in language processing has not been explored as much as that of the left. Linguistic information is processed on the left, and nonlinguistic and paralinguistic information is analyzed on the right. In general, the right plays a role in some aspects of pragmatics, including the perception and expression of emotion, understanding jokes, irony and figurative language, and producing and comprehending coherent discourse. The right hemisphere also plays a greater role in processing emotion in nonverbal contexts. Although there is greater activation in the left hemisphere during both reception and production, some right hemisphere involvement also occurs (Fridriksson et al., 2009).

The right hemisphere also plays a role in semantic processing. Let's take a look at sentence processing for a moment. In the sentence "Ann bumped into Kathy and she fell over," the person who fell is in doubt. If we measure brain activity using event-related potentials (ERPs), a measure of the electrical activity generated by the brain, we find that the right hemisphere is much more involved in processing sentences such as this as the brain attempts to clarify the meaning (Streb et al., 2004).

Approximately 4% of the population are either right hemisphere dominant for language or have bilateral language processing. If these individuals become aphasic as a result of left-hemisphere damage, they usually experience milder impairment and quicker recovery than those who are left-hemisphere dominant. The role of the right hemisphere is unclear in the recovery of left-dominant individuals with aphasia.

Characteristics

Deficits in RHD are not as obvious as those that result from left hemisphere damage. The most common include the following (Meyers, 1999):

1. Neglect of all information from the left side
2. Unrealistic denial of illness or limb involvement
3. Impaired judgment and selfmonitoring
4. Lack of motivation
5. Inattention

For a more detailed list, see Dr. McCaffrey's Web site listed at the end of the chapter.

Deficits may be very subtle but can have a great effect on everyday life. Although these deficits may seem nonlinguistic in nature, they can have a great effect on communication (Meyers, 1999; Tompkins, 1995).

Disturbances can be grouped into attentional, visuospatial, and communicative. Attentional disturbances are characterized by client's lack of response to information coming from the left side of the body. This phenomenon is exhibited in the drawings of individuals with mild RHD who may omit all or provide few left-side details. Figure 7.7 shows an example of

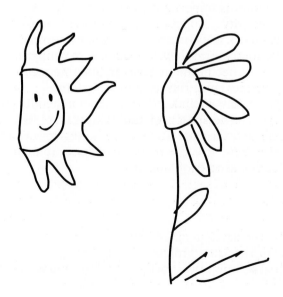

FIGURE 7.7

Drawings of an individual with mild RHD that demonstrate left side neglect.

About half of individuals with RHD have communication impairments.

left-side neglect in a drawing. More severely impaired individuals may even refuse to look to the left side.

Visuospatial deficits may include poor visual discrimination and poor scanning and tracking. The client may have difficulty recognizing familiar faces, remembering familiar routes, and reading maps. Some clients fail to recognize family members.

Communication impairments can be divided into linguistic and paralinguistic deficits. Linguistic difficulties occur in both reception and expression. Of the various aspects of language, pragmatics seems to be the most impaired. For example, topic maintenance, appreciation of the communication situation, and determination of listener needs are impaired. In general, the expressive language of individuals with RHD is characterized as tangential to the topic and more egocentric. There are also extremes of verbosity or paucity of speech (Lehman Blake, 2006).

Clients with RHD may exhibit poor auditory and visual comprehension of complex information and limited word discrimination and visual word recognition. They may also incorrectly interpret complex information, possibly because of a tendency to respond to superficial qualities of stimuli and not to observe relationships among them. In general, individuals with RHD fail to suppress irrelevant or inappropriate information, which in turn affects comprehension (Tompkins et al., 2000). In addition, clients may fail to make use of other contextual, paralinguistic, and nonlinguistic cues (Meyers, 1999). Contextual information may be misinterpreted and the client may fail to integrate sensory information.

Understanding may be very concrete with literal interpretation of humor, indirect requests, and common figurative expressions, such as *hit the roof.* In indirect requests, the speaker does not state his or her request or demand directly. For example, a speaker might say, *I think I'll get my sweater* when meaning *Please turn up the heat.*

Clients with RHD also exhibit poor judgment in determining which incoming information is important and which is not. A similar pattern of difficulty with selectivity is noted in expressive use of language. Clients may include unnecessary, irrelevant, repetitious, and unrelated information, seemingly unable to organize their language in meaningful ways or to present it efficiently. Other problem areas include naming, repetition, and writing, especially letter substitutions and omissions.

Paralinguistic deficits include difficulty comprehending and producing emotional language. The speech of individuals with RHD lacks normal rhythm or prosody and the emphasis used to express joy or sadness, anger or delight. Called *aprosodia*, it is the reduced ability or inability to produce or comprehend affective aspects of language.

Assessment

As with aphasia, the assessment of individuals with RHD is a team effort involving many of the same professionals and diagnostic tasks. The SLP is interested in visual scanning and tracking, auditory and visual comprehension of words and sentences, direction following, response to emotion, naming and describing pictures, and writing. For example, the client may be asked to recreate patterns with blocks or to find two objects or pictures that are the same; to recall words or sentences heard, seen in print, or both; and to describe a picture accurately enough for the SLP to recreate it. Sampling and observational data are essential in assessing the client's pragmatic abilities in conversational contexts.

Portions of aphasia batteries, standardized tests for RHD, and nonstandardized procedures may be used in the assessment. Standardized batteries include the *Right Hemisphere Language Battery* (Bryan, 1989) and the *Mini Inventory of Right Brain Injury* (Pimental & Kingsbury, 1989). Tasks include reading and writing, affective language, and figurative language. The *Rehabilitation Institute of Chicago Evaluation* (RICE) *of Communicative Problems in Right–Hemisphere Dysfunction* (Burns et al., 1985) is a nonstandard testing procedure that includes interviewing, observation, and ratings of the client's behavior along with testing of communication.

Intervention

Intervention often begins with visual and auditory recognition. These skills are essential before progressing to more complex tasks, such as naming, describing, reading, and writing. Self-monitoring and paralinguistics are introduced, and the complexity of the content is gradually increased. Despite increasing knowledge about the deficits of individuals with RHD, knowledge about how to treat them is lacking (Lehman Blake, 2007). In the face of this lack of EBP, SLPs are left to select intervention based on theories of brain function or to modify methods used for other brain disorders with similar deficits. What we do know is presented in Box 7.2.

> Because of the diffuse effects on behavior seen in RHD, we know less about the treatment of these patients.

BOX 7.2
Evidence-Based Practice for Individuals with Right Hemisphere Damage

General

- Cognitive rehabilitation intervention has positive effects on attention, functional communication, memory, and problem solving.
- Approximately 70% to 80% of clients who receive SLP intervention services make significant measurable improvements in communication.

- Communication intervention services as part of a broader interdisciplinary approach including physical, emotional, vocational, and communication, plus family education and support, resulted in greater independence in daily living and return to modified work programs.

Source: Based on Lehman Blake and Tompkins (2008).

Clients are helped to respond appropriately to common communicative initiations and to track increasingly complex information in conversations. Beginning with questions from the SLP that require precise information, the client learns to make responses that come to the point. These questions become more open-ended as the client learns to make off-topic responses less frequently. Similarly, time restraints may limit conversational turns to keep the client from rambling.

Sequencing tasks and explanations of common multistep actions, such as making coffee, will be introduced to help the client organize linguistic content and make relevant contributions. Cues such as objects or pictures may be used initially to aid organization.

Finally, within conversations, the SLP will help the client to synthesize these many skills. Visual and verbal cues may aid in turn taking. Important nonlinguistic markers such as eye contact, body language, and gestures may be targeted. Topic maintenance and relevant conversational contributions are stressed.

TRAUMATIC BRAIN INJURY (TBI)

A traumatic brain injury (TBI) is a disruption in the normal functioning caused by a blow or jolt to the head or a penetrating head injury. The leading causes are falls (28%), motor vehicle/traffic crashes (20%), other blows to the head often from sports (19%), and assaults (11%) (National Center for Injury Prevention and Control, 2009). Falls mostly affect the very young and the very old. The two age groups at highest risk for TBI are 0- to 4-year-olds and 15- to 19-year-olds. The increase in motor vehicles, motorcycles, and off-road vehicles is directly related to the increase in TBI among teens and young adults. Another disturbing increase is the rise in attempted homicides and gun-related injuries, especially in urban areas. The authors have seen adult clients with TBI as the result of automobile, motorcycle, and bicycle collisions; falls; violent crime; and failed suicide attempts involving firearms.

Annually, approximately 1.4 million people sustain TBI in the United States (National Center for Injury Prevention and Control, 2009). Most are treated in emergency rooms and released, but 50,000 die and 235,000 require longer hospitalization. Motor vehicle accidents result in the greatest number of hospitalizations. The number of people with TBI who do not seek medical treatment or care is unknown. It's estimated that as a result of TBI at least 5.3 million Americans, approximately 2% of the U.S. population, currently have a long-term or lifelong need for help to perform daily living activities. Males are about twice as likely as females to sustain a TBI. The statistics tell a chilling story but do not begin to explain the pain and suffering or the long struggle to recover. Case Study 7.3 presents the personal story of one young man with TBI.

In addition, the National Institute of Neurological Disorders and Stroke Web site listed at the end of the chapter provides links to further your inquiry.

You will recall from our discussion of language disorders in children that, unlike stroke, which injures a specific area of the brain, TBI is a diffuse

CASE STUDY 7.3
Personal Story of a Young Man with TBI

His family called him Felipe, but he preferred to use the more Americanized nickname "Chip" that his friends had given him. He was excited to be leaving home for college. Thoughts of being on his own thrilled him with endless possibilities. Even though he was only a freshman, he planned to live with some older friends in their off-campus apartment.

A few weeks after school began, Felipe decided to hitch-hike home to surprise his mother, who missed him a great deal. He stuck out his thumb early on Friday afternoon but never made it home. After his first ride, he bought a soda and began to thumb anew. Shortly afterward, he was struck in the head by the mirror on a pickup truck. Luckily, Felipe was carrying identification in his backpack, and his family was alerted shortly after he was admitted to the hospital.

When he regained consciousness, a few hours after the accident, Felipe was extremely disoriented. He made no attempt to speak and was very lethargic. Although he seemed to recognize his family, he made no attempt to communicate with them. Over the next few weeks, his condition slowly stabilized. Physicians were initially concerned about swelling in the area of the injury. There was evidence of some internal bleeding, but it was not a major problem.

Once the swelling began to recede, Felipe's abilities slowly returned. He began to recall the names of family members and common objects. Walking was extremely difficult because of paralysis on the right side of his body. He dropped out of college and remained at home, where he received intervention services. As an outpatient, he was seen by the speech-language pathologist, physical therapist, and occupational therapist.

After a year's absence from school, Felipe returned and was able to be successful with some adaptations, such as the use of a tape recorder and extra time for completing written tests. He retains a slight limp in his right leg and some minimal weakness in his right arm. His language and speech skills have returned, although he has some mild word-finding difficulties. His cognitive abilities are more concrete than those he had before the accident, and problem-solving tasks require a greater effort. All indications are that he will be successful in his academic pursuits, although his physical and cognitive limitations will continue to affect him.

injury to the entire brain; it is nonfocused. Damage may result from bruising and laceration of the brain caused by forceful contact with the relatively rough inner surfaces of the skull and from secondary **edema** or swelling due to increased fluid, which can lead to increased pressure; infection; hypoxia (oxygen deprivation); intracranial pressure from tissue swelling; **infarction,** or death of tissue deprived of blood supply; and **hematoma,** or focal bleeding (Sohlberg & Mateer, 1989). Aphasia-like symptoms are rare, but linguistic impairments related to cognitive damage are not. In addition, the individual with TBI may have sensory, motor, behavioral, and affective disabilities. Neuromuscular impairments may include epilepsy, hemisensory impairment, and hemiparesis or hemiplegia. The symptoms and the life changes that result can be profound.

Characteristics

The behavioral characteristics of adults with TBI are similar to those of children who are similarly injured. Adults with TBI are a heterogeneous group with a diverse collection of physical, cognitive, communicative, and psychosocial deficits. Usually, the most devastating aspect is an inability to resume interests and daily living tasks to the level that existed before the injury. Some clients exhibit near total dependence on others. Cognitive difficulties may be evident in orientation, memory, attention, reasoning and problem solving, and executive function, which is the planning, execution, and self-monitoring of goal-directed behavior (Sohlberg & Mateer, 1989).

Language may be affected in 3 of 4 individuals with TBI (McKinlay et al., 1981). The two most commonly reported symptoms for TBI are anomia and impaired comprehension (Coelho, 1997).

As with children, the most disturbed language area and that with the most pervasive problems is pragmatics (Sohlberg & Mateer, 1989). Most published tests target language form and content and may miss pragmatic deficits that are evident in conversation. Pragmatic impairments result from the inability to inhibit behavior and from errors of judgment. The result may be rambling speech and incoherence, as manifested by off-topic and irrelevant comments and inability to maintain a topic, and by poor turn-taking skills, such as frequent interruption of others. In addition, communication may be marked by poor affective or emotional language abilities and inappropriate laughter and swearing.

Deficits are not limited to language and may include speech, voice, and swallowing difficulties. Approximately a third of all individuals with TBI exhibit dysarthria, a disorder resulting from weakness or incoordination of the muscles that control speech production (Sarno et al., 1986) (see Chapter 12). Language deficits reflect underlying disruptions in information-processing, problem-solving, and reasoning abilities. In addition, psychosocial and personality changes may include disinhibition or impulsivity, poor organization and social judgment, and either withdrawal or aggressiveness. Physical signs may include difficulty walking, poor coordination, and vision problems. A more complete list of the possible outcomes of TBI is presented in Figure 7.8.

Severity seems to be related to initial levels of consciousness and post-traumatic amnesia. Consciousness levels can be classified along a continuum from extended states of unconsciousness or coma, in which the body responds only minimally to external stimuli, to consciousness with disorientation, stupor, and lethargy. Amnesia, or memory loss, is a frequent result of TBI. The duration of both coma and amnesia has been used successfully, but not infallibly, as a predictor of severity and prognosis. In general, the shorter both are, the less severe the resultant deficits of TBI and the better the potential outcome.

Lifespan Issues

Most adults with TBI are young and have experienced an auto or motorcycle accident. Imagine that you, a college student, are riding in a friend's car. The next thing that you remember is waking in the hospital, dazed, disoriented, and unaware of your surroundings. You may have language or other impairments that will change your life forever or at least for the immediate future.

Cognition	Emotion/Personality
Inattentive	Aggression/withdrawal
Disoriented	Apathy and indifference
Poor memory	Denial
Poor problem-solving abilities	Depression
Language, Speech, and Oral Mechanism	Disinhibition and impulsivity
	Impatience
Dysphagia	Phobias
Dysarthria	Socially inappropriate behavior and comments
Possible mutism	
Pragmatic difficulties (talks better than can communicate)	Suspiciousness and anxiety
Confused language–irrelevance, confabulation or casual unfocused chatting, circumlocution, off-topic comments, lack of logical sequencing, and misnaming	

FIGURE 7.8
....
Possible outcomes of TBI.

Several stages of recovery exist, and clinical intervention varies with each. Most individuals will not reach full recovery and some residual deficits will most likely remain. Initially, the individual may be nonresponsive to stimuli and need total assistance in a hospital setting.

When the individual does begin to respond, his or her behavior may not reflect the varying nature of the stimuli. In other words, the patient may persist with a response although the situation has changed. Responses may be delayed. Vocalizations may seem purposeless.

Gradually, the individual begins to respond differently to different stimuli and to recognize familiar individuals. Response to commands is still often inconsistent.

As the client becomes more alert, he or she may seem confused or agitated. Short-term memory and goal-directed behaviors may be poor. Although able to sit and walk, these behaviors are performed without purpose. Subject to violent mood swings, the individual may have incoherent, inappropriate, or emotional language. Although the individual still needs rehabilitative hospital care, he or she has recovered enough to move from intensive care.

As agitation fades and language continues to return, the individual can remain alert for short periods of time and hold brief conversations if strong external cues are used. There are still periods of nonpurposeful behavior. Short-term memory is still severely impaired. With structure, the patient can perform learned tasks but is unable to learn new behaviors.

As the individual continues to improve, he or she needs less assistance. Able to attend for up to 30 minutes with redirection, the individual is aware of the appropriate responses to self, family, and basic needs, which become more goal-directed. Relearned tasks exhibit some carryover, although new learning does not. Language is used appropriately only in highly familiar contexts.

Gradually, the individual becomes oriented to persons and place. Time is still confusing and the individual demonstrates only superficial understanding of his or her condition. Usually in outpatient status, the individual is able to learn and carry over this learning to other tasks and to monitor his or her own behavior with minimal assistance. Still unable to recognize inappropriate social behavior, the client is often uncooperative, unrealistic in his or her expectations, and unaware of the needs and feelings of others.

As the individual gains more of an understanding of his or her condition and is able to plan and initiate routine tasks, frustration may build, and he or she may become depressed, argumentative, irritable, or overly dependent or independent. Living at home and possibly having returned to work, the individual may be able to concentrate for an hour even with distractions, to recall past and present events, and to learn new tasks with only minimal assistance.

Increasing abilities may not reduce the individual's low tolerance for frustration, although behavioral responses may be less. In the later stages of recovery, the individual can shift between tasks for up to 2 hours and initiate and carry out familiar tasks. Able to acknowledge his or her impairment, the client is able to consider the consequences of his or her actions and to recognize the needs and feeling of others.

Finally, the individual may be able to consistently act in a socially appropriate manner, to respond appropriately to others, and to plan, initiate, and complete both familiar and unfamiliar tasks. Periodic depression may occur and irritability may reappear with illness, inability to perform a task, and in emotional situations.

The individual with TBI may face a long period of rehabilitation. Even those who have made a near-full recovery will have some lingering deficits, especially in pragmatics. The authors have worked with college students with TBI who were able to gain their degrees with only minimal adaptations.

Assessment

The SLP is a member of an interdisciplinary team of rehabilitation specialists who collaborate in assessment of and intervention with persons with TBI (Ylvisaker, 1994). As such, the SLP is responsible for assessing all aspects of communication, cognitive-communicative functioning, and swallowing.

Unlike individuals with aphasia, those with TBI progress through recognizable stages of recovery. Assessment must be ongoing and varies with each stage. Neurological, psychiatric, and psychological reports will aid in the planning of both assessment and intervention. Observation can aid the SLP in deciding which areas to probe, especially in determining pragmatic deficits that may be missed in formal testing.

To date, few comprehensive tools exist for assessment of language skills in individuals with TBI. Many SLPs working with this population have compiled a series of individual tests for aspects of both language and cognition. These tests are often portions of larger test batteries. Language testing must be comprehensive. Tests that emphasize language form and content may fail to adequately assess pragmatics, thus underestimating the extent of the language impairment.

Sampling is essential because pragmatic behavior that varies across communicative contexts cannot be adequately assessed in a testing context alone (Starch & Falltrick, 1990). Sampling contexts should include functional activities, such as talking on the phone or grocery shopping, in natural environments, such as the home. Sampling should occur within a discourse unit, a series of related linguistic units that convey a message (Coelho et al., 1995).

Intervention

With or without intervention, the pattern of recovery for individuals with TBI is predictable. Unlike those with focal damage such as a stroke, who progress smoothly, those with TBI recover in a plateau fashion characterized by periods of little or no change interspersed with periods of rapid improvement. After a period of unconsciousness, the person often responds indiscriminately and seemingly without purpose. Attention may be fleeting, and overall level of arousal may fluctuate. The client is often hyperresponsive to stimuli and easily irritated and agitated. Clients may become very emotional and exhibit shouting, biting, and repetitive, stereotypic movements such as rocking. With recovery, clients become more clear thinking, and their behavior becomes more purposeful, although restlessness and irritability may persist.

As the client becomes more oriented in place and time, he or she is better able to respond to simple requests, although attention span is short and distractibility high. Memory and abstract reasoning may continue to be a problem even as the client becomes better able to manage daily living and to begin to function independently.

Intervention for cognitive-communicative deficits with individuals with TBI is called **cognitive rehabilitation,** a treatment regimen designed to increase functional abilities for everyday life by improving the capacity to process incoming information. The two primary approaches are restorative and compensatory (Ben-Yishay & Diller, 1993). The restorative approach attempts to rebuild neural circuitry and function through repetitive activities, while the compensatory approach concedes that some functions will not be recovered and develops alternatives. Restorative techniques might include classification tasks and word associations. In contrast, compensatory strategies to improve memory might include focused attending and rehearsal of new information. Traditionally, restorative strategies are

Cognitive rehabilitation promotes independent functioning in daily life by focusing on specific cognitive processes such as memory and language processing.

attempted first and may include rehearsal and encoding strategies and the use of memory aids (Hutchinson & Marquardt, 1997). Compensatory methods are typically used when the restorative attempts have failed. Slowly, professionals are recognizing that compensatory strategies aid in restorative development, and both methods are being used simultaneously (Coelho, 1997).

The SLP is responsible for designing and implementing treatment programs to decrease the effects of impairment. Evidince-based practices are presented in Box 7.3. In addition to providing direct intervention, the SLP helps to identify functional supports, such as memory logs, and work adjustments that aid in successful independent living.

Intervention programs vary depending on the stage of recovery. During the early stages, intervention focuses on orientation, sensorimotor stimulation, and recognition of familiar people and common objects and events. Early intervention results in shorter rehabilitation and higher levels of cognitive functioning (Mackay et al., 1992).

In the middle stages, training becomes more structured and formal. The goals are to reduce confusion and improve memory and goal-directed behavior. Much of the training involves increasing the client's orientation to the everyday world. Consistency and routines are important in orientation training. The SLP may target active listening and auditory comprehension and following directions with increasingly more complex information. Word definitions, descriptions of entities and events, and classification of objects and words are also targeted. Conversational speech training is also attempted. For example, one SLP, recognizing that the act of taking a conversational turn is too difficult for some clients, begins by using a beanbag or other object, which is passed back and forth to signal turn changes. Over time, the object is replaced with subtle nonverbal signals, such as eye contact.

During the late stages of recovery, the goal is client independence. Targets include comprehension of complex information and directions and conversational and social skills. The SLP helps the client to explore alternative

BOX 7.3
Evidence-Based Practice for Individuals with Traumatic Brain Injury

General

- The most effective interventions are those that are tailored to the individual client's unique needs and situation. Those receiving communication intervention make gains in cognitive communication, activities, and social participation.
- Those receiving communication services are discharged with higher levels of cognitive functioning

and in greater percentages to home versus long-term care.
- Better than 80% make significant measureable gains in memory, attention, and pragmatics.

Source: Based on Coelho et al. (2008).

strategies for word recall, memory, and problem solving. Conversational problem-solving tasks are also targeted, along with self-inhibition and self-monitoring. Real-world contexts are emphasized, especially those that are potentially confusing or emotional.

DEMENTIA
· ·

We live in a youth-oriented culture. Commercial images lead to the stereotype of older people with deteriorated bodies and minds. Although physical decline with age is inevitable, intellectual capacity is frequently unimpaired. Fewer than 15% of the elderly experience dementia, and as many as 20% of these positively respond to treatment (Shekim, 1990). The incidence of dementia is increasing rapidly as the percentage of the U.S. population over age 65 increases. It is estimated that as high as 48% of new admissions to long-term care facilities have a diagnosis of dementia (Magaziner et al., 2000).

> Dementia is an impairment of intellect and cognition.

Dementia is an umbrella term for a group of both pathological conditions and syndromes. It is acquired and is characterized by intellectual decline due to neurogenic causes. Memory is the most obvious function affected (American Psychiatric Association, 1994). Additional deficits include poor reasoning or judgment, impaired abstract thinking, inability to attend to relevant information, impaired communication, and personality changes.

Dementia can be divided into cortical and subcortical types based on patterns of neurophysiological impairment (Cummings & Benson, 1992). The characteristics of cortical dementias, such as Alzheimer's and Pick's diseases, resemble those of focal impairments such as aphasia and RHD. These include visuospatial deficits, memory problems, judgment and abstract thinking disturbances, and language deficits in naming, reading and writing, and auditory comprehension. Alzheimer's disease accounts for 60% to 80% of all dementia cases, or 5.3 million adults in the United States (Alzheimer's Association, 2009).

Subcortical dementias may accompany multiple sclerosis, AIDS-related encephalopathy, and Parkinson's and Huntington's diseases. A slow, progressive deterioration of cognitive functioning occurs with deficits in memory, problem solving, language, and neuromuscular control. Those disorders that involve neuromuscular functioning, such as Parkinson, will be discussed in Chapter 9, "The Voice and Voice Disorders," and Chapter 12, "Neurogenic Speech Disorders."

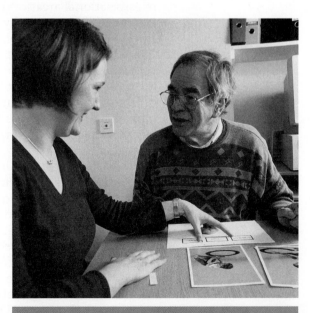

With dementia, language is affected by deficits in memory.

The language functions that most depend on memory seem to be primarily affected by dementia. A significant decline is noted in naming and word retrieval. Language form–phonology, morphology, and syntax–is generally less disordered, although syntax may be less coherent than before as the client struggles with anomia. As a consequence, conversations may lack coherence and may be filled with repetitions, stereotypic utterances, false starts, verbal repairs, jargon, neologisms, and the use of phrases such as *that one* and *you know* (Shekim & LaPointe, 1984). One client would repeat "I know" several times.

Alzheimer's Disease

Alzheimer's is characterized by microscopic changes in the neurons of the cerebral cortex.

Alzheimer's disease (AD) is a cortical pathology that affects approximately 13% of individuals over age 65 and possibly as high as 50% of those over age 85 (Alzheimer's Association, 2009). Given the aging U.S. population, the prevalence of Alzheimer's disease will increase 50% by 2030 unless science finds a way to slow the progression of the disease or prevent it. A heterogeneous population, individuals with AD may be primarily impaired in memory, language, or visuospatial skills (DeSanti, 1997). Alzheimer's is twice as common in women as in men primarily because women tend to live longer.

The cause of AD is unknown but may be a combination of genetic and environmental factors. The neuropathology is characterized by the presence of twisted neurofilaments in the cytoplasm of neurons that deteriorate cell functioning. These tangles are most pronounced in the temporal lobe and in associational areas of the brain (see Figure 7.9). Nerve fibers degenerate, resulting in brain atrophy that may decrease brain weight as much as 20%, especially in the temporal, frontal, and parietal lobes (Kemper, 1984; Koo & Price, 1993). Other physical changes include extensive damage to the hippocampus, located on the interior portion of the temporal lobes (interior to the ears) and formation of senile plaques within the cortex that affect nerve cell interactive functioning. A variation of the APOE gene found in all humans greatly increases the likelihood of developing AD. Environmental risk factors include head trauma, heart and circulatory problems, poor overall health, and diabetes.

Mild dementia may be characterized by name recall difficulties, occasional disorientation, and memory loss. Memory problems are the most obvious changes. Retention of newly learned information is most impaired (Convit et al., 1995). Long-term memory is unimpaired initially but deteriorates as the disease progresses.

Language is not affected in all individuals initially. Early problems involve word finding, off-topic comments, and comprehension. At these early stages, deficits are mostly pragmatic and semantic-conceptual in nature, and syntax is relatively unaffected compared to that of elderly individuals not affected by AD (Kavé & Levy, 2003).

Later characteristics include paraphasia (word substitution) and delayed responding. In more severe stages, expressive and receptive

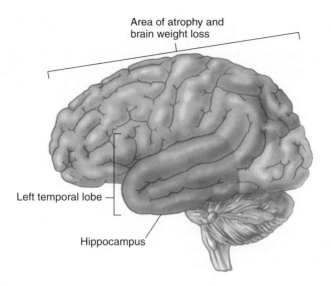

Area of atrophy and
brain weight loss

Left temporal lobe

Hippocampus

FIGURE 7.9
. . . .
Alzheimer's disease.

There may be as much as a 20% loss in brain weight in the frontal, parietal, and temporal lobes as the brain atrophies. This is accompanied by nerve tangles in the left temporal lobe, including language processing areas, and in the hippocampus located on the interior portion of the temporal lobe.

vocabulary and complex sentence production become reduced; pronoun confusion, topic digression, and inability to return to and to shift topic are more pronounced; and writing and reading errors occur (Mentis et al., 1995). In its most severe form, the language of individuals with AD is characterized by naming errors and the use of generic words (*this, that*), syntactic errors, minimal comprehension, jargon, echolalia, or mutism (DeSanti, 1997). As might be expected, increased severity results in more conversational breakdowns (Orange et al., 1996).

All areas of communication, including writing, are affected. Writing impairment may arise at several different steps in the process, including planning, sequencing, and organization at the letter, word, sentence, and narrative levels (Neils-Strunjas et al., 2006). Deficits may include misspelling, poor narrative organization, content word errors and perseveration or repetition of words or ideas, grammatical errors, and reduced syntactic complexity. Writing problems reflect general language deficits as well as deficits in working memory, attention, and motor control.

LIFESPAN ISSUES

AD is a genetic disorder that lies in hiding, although early screening is possible in some cases. Both genetic and environmental factors seem to be important. Often the person who will be afflicted with the disease is unaware and/or ignores early signs. At present there are no cures, but some early drug therapies seem to lessen the effects.

In the early stages, the individual experiences memory loss, especially of new information. The individual experiences word retrieval problems and some difficulty with higher language functions, such as humor and analogies. The individual may seem indifferent and initiate little communication. Able to live at home, the individual can become an increasing burden on an elderly spouse or on adult children with families of their own.

As the disease progresses, memory loss increases with the effect that vocabulary decreases. Comprehension is reduced. Language production may be reduced to ritualistic or high-usage phrases accompanied by poor topic maintenance and repair of errors, frequent repetition and word retrieval problems, and insensitivity to conversational partners. Irritability and restlessness may increase. The individual may be able to live at home with visiting nurse care to help with daily living routines.

In the most advanced stages of the disease, all intellectual functions including memory are severely impaired and almost all individuals reside in nursing homes. Language may be meaningless or the individual may be mute or echolalic. Most clients cannot recall the names of loved ones and may undergo radical personality changes. Motor function is also severely impaired and the individual needs total care.

Assessment

Definitive diagnosis of AD is difficult in the early stages of the disease. Use of neuroimaging techniques may help in early identification, especially for specific protein buildup in the brain (DeKosky, 2008). Pupil dilation tests may also indicate the presence of the disease in the early stages. Finally, computer-based assessments, such as the Computerized Assessment of Mild Cognitive Impairment (CAMCI), are being developed and tested. These measures usually test attention, recognition, and recall of both words and pictures.

Working as a member of a diagnostic team, SLPs usually help identify changes in language performance that may signal intellectual deterioration and aspects of behavior amenable to change (Hopper, 2005). The results of this assessment may help differentiate AD from other neuropathologies.

Genetic history and general and neurological health data are important elements in the assessment process. Observation of the individual in different communication environments is also important. In the early stages, dementia may be confused with other disorders, such as depression. The progressive nature of the disorder makes it imperative that the SLP remain current on the changing condition and learning ability of a client.

Although few language tests for this population exist, the *Arizona Battery for Communicative Disorders of Dementia* (Bayles & Kazniak, 1987) has been specifically designed to assess the retrieval, perceptual, and linguistic deficits common to dementia. Cognitive-communicative strengths may be measured using the *Functional Linguistic Communication Inventory*

(Bayles & Tomoeda, 1994), assessment of the client's ability to participate in the give-and-take of daily communication in a number of areas.

Writing assessment is important because decline in written language may precede other cognitive and spoken language deficits (Kavrie & Neils-Strunjas, 2002). Functional writing tasks, such as writing a letter, are one of the earliest affected areas of linguistic performance.

Several scales exist for rating the severity of a client's loss. Of particular importance are the memory deficits that are common (Azuma & Bayles, 1997). In addition, many assessment batteries that are used with individuals with aphasia can be helpful in evaluating the communication skills of persons with dementia. Detailed understanding of a client's strengths and weaknesses is essential for helping family members choose the most effective communicative strategies (Causino Lamar et al., 1994).

INTERVENTION

Intervention with those with progressive disorders can sometimes feel like trying to hold back the tide. Decline is inevitable, given the present state of our knowledge. That does not mean that we do nothing. Quite the contrary, clinical intervention by an SLP can help to maintain the client at her or his highest level of performance and help others to maximize the client's participation in conversational interactions. It is imperative, therefore, that the SLP emphasize the use of intact cognitive abilities to compensate for deficient ones (Hopper, 2005). The ASHA Web site defines the role of the SLP with clients with dementia.

Intervention is not undertaken in isolation. As in the other disorders discussed in this chapter, the SLP is a member of a team. Professionals consult with one another and with the client and family on the best course of action.

The SLP may target memory or word retrieval by working on word associations and categories, auditory attending and comprehension in conversational contexts, coherent verbal responses, and formation of longer, more complex utterances with the help of memory aids. Family members can be helped to keep conversations focused on the present, to validate the client's comments, to reduce distractions and limit the number of participants, and to foster comprehension and participation by slowing the rate and decreasing the complexity of their utterances, using nonlinguistic cues and yes/no response questions (Shekim, 1990; Small & Perry, 2005). Interactive strategies that result in the least communication breakdown include eliminating distractions, speaking in simple sentences, and employing yes/no questions (Small et al., 2003). Relatively intact reading and visual memory can be used to facilitate verbal memory (Hopper, 2005).

New drug and gene therapies and bioengineering techniques hold the promise that many of the diseases that cause dementia may one day be controllable. At present, intervention that stimulates cognitive processes combined with pharmacological approaches that increase certain neural chemicals important for memory is best. Embryonic stem cells may also be used to someday regenerate brain tissue.

Appropriate and effective intervention requires that the SLP understand what the family of the client is experiencing.

SUMMARY

Aphasia, right hemisphere damage, traumatic brain damage and dementia result in very different types of language impairment. Aphasia, the result of a focal brain injury, most likely a stroke, may result in a wide variety of impairments that may affect one or more modalities of communication, although comprehension, speech, and naming are usually impaired. Stroke is also the primary cause of right hemisphere injury. Comprehension and production of paralinguistics and complex linguistic structures are affected. Pragmatics is the most affected aspect of language. This is also true for traumatic brain injury, which, in contrast to the previous two, is a nonfocused rather than a focal injury. Finally, dementia, particularly that caused by Alzheimer's disease, is a degenerative disease. Word-finding difficulties, off-topic comments, and comprehension deficits are the most common characteristics.

In the adult language impairments discussed, the SLP functions as a member of a multidisciplinary collaborative team. The role of the SLP includes assessment of communicative abilities and their implication of other cognitive deficits, swallowing, and associated neurological disorders. Other responsibilities include treatment planning and programming, direct intervention services, interdisciplinary consultation, and family training and counseling. Intervention usually focuses on retrieval of language skills and on compensatory strategies.

THOUGHT QUESTIONS

- What are the major differences between aphasia, right hemisphere injury, traumatic brain injury, and dementia?
- What are the concomitant or accompanying deficits found with aphasia?
- What are the two main types of aphasia and the characteristics of each?
- Describe the different types of stroke or CVA.

SUGGESTED READINGS

Brookshire, R. H. (2007). *Introduction to neurogenic communication disorders* (7th ed.). Boston: Elsevier.

Davis, G. B. (2007). *Aphasiology: Disorders and clinical practice* (2nd ed.). Boston: Allyn and Bacon.

Martin, N., Thompson, C., & Worrall, L. (2007). *Aphasia rehabilitation: The impairment and its consequences*. San Diego: Plural.

ONLINE RESOURCES

American Speech-Language-Hearing Association
www.asha.org/docs/html/PS2005-00118.html
ASHA site describes the role of SLPs with clients with dementia.

www.asha.org/docs/html/PS2005-00110.html
ASHA site describes the role of SLPs with clients who have cognitive-communication disorders.

www.asha.org/docs/html/KS2005-00078.html
ASHA position paper on the knowledge and skills needed by SLPs working with clients who have cognitive-communication disorders.

www.asha.org/public/speech/disorders/RightBrainDamage.html
ASHA site presents a description of right-hemisphere damage for the general public.

California State University at Chico
www.csuchico.edu/~pmccaffrey//syllabi/SPPA336/336unit13.html
Professor Patrick McCaffrey, California State University at Chico, has a detailed description of the characteristics and diagnosis of right-hemisphere damage.

National Aphasia Association
www.aphasia.org/
National Aphasia Association has links to several useful sites.

National Institute of Deafness and Other Communication Disorders
www.nidcd.nih.gov/health/voice/aphasia.htm
National Institute of Deafness and Other Communication Disorders site has an in-depth description of aphasia.

National Institute of Neurological Disorders and Stroke
www.ninds.nih.gov/disorders/tbi/tbi.htm
National Institute of Neurological Disorders and Stroke Web site has description of traumatic brain injury with links to several useful sites.

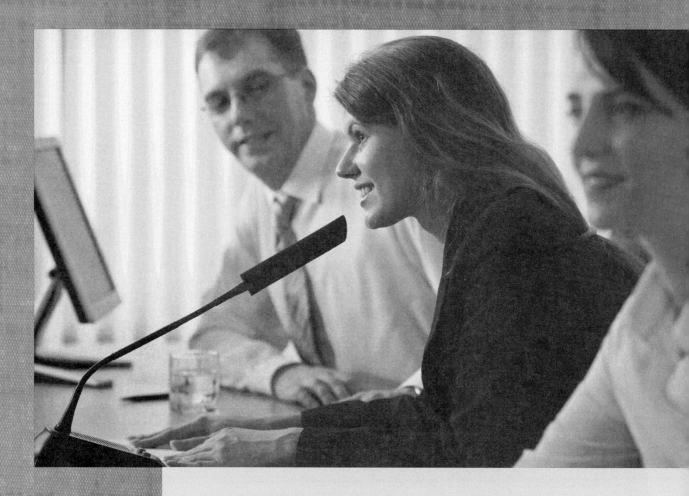

CHAPTER LEARNING GOALS

When you have finished this chapter, you should be able to:

- Describe differences between fluent and stuttered speech

- Describe the onset and development of stuttering

- Describe the major etiological theories and conceptual models of stuttering

- Describe the important components involved in the evaluations of stuttering

- Describe evidence-based treatment approaches and techniques that are effective for children and adults who stutter

Fluency Disorders

8

Fluent speech is the consistent ability to move the speech production apparatus in an effortless, smooth, and rapid manner resulting in a continuous, uninterrupted forward flow of speech. Several conditions that adversely affect speech and language production can also disrupt the fluency of speech. Dysarthria, apraxia, cerebral palsy, and some forms of aphasia affect the fluency of speech. These disorders and their effects on speech and language production are discussed in Chapters 7 and 12 of this book. The focus of this chapter is on a disorder of speech called "developmental stuttering." Developmental stuttering, or simply "stuttering," primarily influences the speaker's ability to produce fluent speech. Stuttered speech is characterized by involuntary repetitions of sounds and syllables (e.g., b-b-b-ball), sound prolongations (e.g., mmmmm-mommy), and broken words (e.g., b—oy). All three of these interruptions are considered to be stuttering behaviors, and they have a negative impact on the speaker's ability to produce fluent speech. Case Study 8.1 provides an example of a young child with developmental stuttering.

In this chapter, we define stuttering and discuss how stuttering begins and develops as a disorder, paying particular attention to how stuttered speech differs from fluent speech. Consideration is given to some of the major theories regarding stuttering, the clinical diagnosis of stuttering, and, finally, evidence-based treatment practices. As you begin reading this chapter, consider carefully the thoughts of the late Charles Van Riper, a pioneer in the treatment of stuttering. His words set the tone for this chapter. In the dedication to his 1992 book entitled *The Nature of Stuttering,* Van Riper wrote:

> To the ancient birch tree to whom, when I was a youth and it was a sapling, I swore an oath to find the cause and cure of the stuttering that afflicted me and so many others. Though I have failed and we have both grown old I did my utmost and am content. Others will take up my quest. (dedication page)

CASE STUDY 8.1
Case Study of a Child with Stuttering: Tamara

Mrs. Fisher brought her 4-year-old daughter, Tamara, to the speech and hearing clinic at a nearby university. In an interview with the clinic's director, Mrs. Fisher explained that when Tamara was about $3\frac{1}{2}$ years old she had trouble starting to speak because she repeated the first sounds and syllables at the beginning of each utterance like "C-c-c-can I have some ice cream?" or "Ba-ba-ba-ba-baseball is boring." This difficulty lasted about 2 weeks, and then it went away as abruptly as it began. Tamara's speech was free of such disruptions for the next 6 months. Mrs. Fisher further explained that about 2 weeks prior to her visit to the clinic, Tamara's speech interruptions reappeared. And, she showed great concern when she told the clinic director that in addition to repeating sounds and syllables at the beginning of utterances she was holding or prolonging sounds at numerous places in her utterances like "I-I-I-I want to sssssssssit over there."

The clinic director observed Mrs. Fisher and her daughter interacting with one another in an adjoining room via a one-way mirror. The clinic director observed that Mrs. Fisher spoke at a very rapid rate and that she tended to use complex sentence structures when she spoke to her daughter. A formal evaluation of Tamara's speech revealed that she produced an average of 15 instances of stuttering per 100 words spoken, she would frequently lose eye contact with the examiner, and she scored 30 points on the *Stuttering Prediction Instrument*. Based on these findings, it was recommended that Tamara be seen in direct therapy two times per week and that Mrs. Fisher be given instruction regarding reducing her speaking rate and sentence complexity.

Following 4 months of the start of direct intervention and parental instruction, her disfluent behaviors were markedly reduced, falling well within normal limits. And Tamara's mother had learned to slow her speaking rate and speak in relatively simple sentence structure when she conversed with her daughter.

As you read this chapter, think about

- The nature of the speech interruptions Tamara had developed.
- The developmental course of Tamara's disfluent behaviors.
- Why the clinic director recommended direct therapy for Tamara and instruction for her mother to reduce her speaking rate and linguistic complexity.

Dr. Charles Van Riper was a distinguished professor of speech-language pathology for many years at Western Michigan University. Dr. Van Riper learned to control his stuttering and spent most of his life searching for the cause and cure of stuttering. Therapy techniques that he developed are still in use today.

Many people have indeed taken up Van Riper's quest to find the cause of stuttering and a cure for it, but neither has been discovered. The cause of stuttering is elusive, and our understanding of stuttering is incomplete, despite its long and diverse history. Stuttering has been part of the human condition for all recorded time. Clay tablets found in Mesopotamia dating from centuries before the birth of Christ record the disorder, hieroglyphics from the 20th century B.C. depict stuttering, and poems written in China more than 2,500 years ago allude to stuttering (cf. Van Riper, 1992). Stuttering affects people worldwide. Physicist Sir Isaac Newton, author W. Somerset Maugham (*Of Human Bondage*), and statesman Winston Churchill stuttered. Performers James Earl Jones, Carly Simon, Marilyn Monroe, and Bruce Willis stuttered. Stuttering is insensitive to race, creed, color, intellect, and virtually any other attribute that could be used to distinguish one human being from another.

The number of adults who report that they had stuttered at some time in their life is 5% (Andrews et al., 1983; Conture & Guitar, 1993). However, this 5% incidence rate includes the high percentage of children who naturally recover from the disorder before the age of 6 (Conture, 1996). Relatively new information indicates that 65% to 75% of children will recover from stuttering within the first 2 years after its onset and 85% will recover within the next few years. Given a recovery rate of about 85% (i.e., more than 4 of 5 children), the 5% lifetime incidence percentage reduces down to about a 1% incidence (Conture, 1996; Yairi & Ambrose, 1992a; Yairi & Ambrose, 2004; Yairi et al., 1993). It is not well understood why some children naturally recover from stuttering and others do not. For example, females appear to recover from stuttering more frequently than males.

The prevalence of stuttering is determined by ascertaining the number of cases in a given population (usually school-age children) during a given period of time. Research findings of many studies conducted in various regions around the United States suggest an average prevalence rate of 0.97% for school-age children (Bloodstein, 1995). This figure is consistent with the 1% incidence estimate and with prevalence estimates from European and Near East countries. The prevalence of stuttering is stable from the first to the ninth grade with a precipitous decline in stuttering during grades 10, 11, and 12.

Stuttering affects more males than females, the reported sex ratio differences ranging from 2.3 to 1 to 3.0 to 1. This difference has been attributed to differences in the physical maturation rates of boys and girls and to differences in speech and language development, but genetic factors may also be involved.

Stuttering has a high degree of familial incidence. Fifty percent of people who stutter report that they have a relative who stuttered at some time in his or her life. Fifteen percent of first-degree relatives (parents, sisters, and brothers) of people who stutter are current or recovered stutterers. This threefold increase over the reported 5% lifetime incidence for the general population is genetically significant. (Felsenfeld, 1997; Felsenfeld et al., 2000; Kidd, 1984). Additionally, if one twin stutters, there is a high probability that the other twin will stutter, and the rate of concordance (both twins exhibiting the disorder) is higher for monozygotic twins (genetically identical) than for dizygotic (fraternal) twins.

Recent genetic research has indicated that stuttering may be linked to a specific single gene, although the location and nature of such a gene is unknown (Ambrose et al., 1993; Shugart et al., 2004). Continued genetic research will ultimately play a role in our understanding of stuttering, but the actual contributions of such research "remain over the horizon" (Felsenfeld, 1997, p. 20).

FLUENT SPEECH VERSUS STUTTERING

Anyone who has listened carefully to a young child speak can attest to the fact that the flow of most children's speech is not continuously forward and uninterrupted. Children exhibit many hesitations, revisions, and interruptions in their utterances. Children are not born as fluent speakers. Fluency requires some degree of physical maturation and language experience, but it does not develop linearly as the child matures. Longitudinal research indicates that children around 25 months of age are more fluent than they will be at 29 months and at 37 months of age (Yairi, 1981, 1982). There is a gradual increase in disfluent speech behaviors beginning around 2 years of age that peaks around the third birthday. Fluency then improves after age 3, and the types of disfluency change.

Normal Disfluencies

The type of disfluency exhibited by the normally developing child changes between the ages of 25 and 37 months. At approximately 2 years of age, typical disfluencies are whole-word repetitions (I-I-I want a cookie), interjections (Can we-uhm-go now?), and syllable repetitions (I like ba-baseball). Revisions such as "He can't–he won't play baseball" are the dominant disfluency type when the child is approximately 3 years old (Yairi, 1982). Normal disfluencies persist throughout the course of one's life, but they do not tend to adversely affect the continuous forward flow of speech. Normally fluent speakers frequently interrupt the forward flow of speech by repeating whole multisyllablic words (I really-really like hockey), interjecting a word or phrase (He will, uhhhhh, you know, not like that idea), repeating a phrase (Will you, will you please stop that), or revising a sentence (She can't–She didn't do that).

> Some parenthetical interjections or asides that are common interruptions in adult speech are devices that help to maintain listener interest. An example of a parenthetical interjection is "When John slipped on the stairs—like Mary slipped in the same spot last week—he broke his ankle."

Stuttered Disfluencies

What is stuttering and how is it different from normally fluent and normally disfluent speech? These are not simple questions, and there are no simple answers. Consider the words of English literary genius Samuel Johnson (1709–1784) when he mused about poetry: "Sir, what is poetry? Why, sir, it is much easier to say what it is not" (Gregory, 1981, p. 416). We might say the same about stuttering.

The issue of what stuttering is and how to define it lies at the center of some unresolved issues (Ingham & Cordes, 1997). Can clinicians determine reliably if and when stuttering has occurred? Do normal disfluencies and stuttered disfluencies lie along the same continuum or are they categorically different behavioral events? There are no absolute answers to these questions. At present, no universally accepted definition of stuttering exists. However, a reasonable framework from which one can begin to distinguish between normal disfluencies and those that are likely to be regarded as stuttered disfluencies has been proposed:[1]

> Speech, like many other human behaviors, is occasionally produced by speakers with hesitations, interruptions, prolongations and repetitions. These disruptions in . . . ongoing speech behavior are termed *disfluency* and the frequency, duration, type, severity and so forth of these speech disfluencies

[1]See also Guitar's (2006) definition of stuttering.

vary greatly from person to person and from speaking situation to speaking situation. Some speech disfluencies, particularly those which involve within-word disruptions (such as sound or syllable repetitions), are most apt to be classified or judged by listeners as *stuttering*. (Conture, 1990a, p. 2)

Specifically, stuttering or stuttered speech involves audible or silent repetitions and prolongations (Andrews et al., 1983). Tense pauses and hesitations within and between words may also be regarded as stuttering. Within-word and some between-word disfluencies are believed to be the cardinal, universal features of stuttering (see Table 8.1 for specific examples).

In young children, however, there continues to be some debate about when speech disfluencies constitute stuttering behaviors. Some studies have shown that children who are considered to be stutterers produce many more part-word repetitions and prolongations than do children considered to be nonstutterers. Other studies have found that children presenting with the same type and severity of disfluencies were considered to be nonstutterers. These conflicting findings may relate to the notion of a "perceptual threshold" for stuttering (Martin & Haroldson, 1981). Disfluencies that are likely to be regarded as instances of stuttering include monosyllabic whole-word repetitions (he-he-he-he-hit me), sound repetitions (p-p-p-p-pail), syllable repetitions (ba-ba-ba-ba-baseball), audible prolongations

TABLE 8.1

Types of within-word (stuttered) and between-word (normal) speech disfluencies

Disfluency Type	Within-Word	Between-Word	Examples
Sound/syllable repetitions	X		He's a b-b-b-boy. G-g-g-g-go away. Yes, puh-puh-please.
Sound prolongation	X		Ssssssee me swing! T--oronto is cool.
Broken word	X		Base-(pause)-ball.
Monosyllablic whole-word repetitions	X	X	I-I-I-hit the ball. It's my-my-my-turn.
Multisyllabic whole-word repetitions		X	I'm going-going home.
Phrase repetition/ interjection		X	She hit–she hit me. I like, uh, ya know, big boats.
Revisions		X	He went, he came back.

Source: Based on Conture (1990b).

(sssssss-snow), and inaudible prolongations (g----irl). Examples of stuttered speech can be heard and seen on the book's CD-ROM.

More than one type of within-word disfluency may be present in a given disruption that interferes with the forward flow of speech. Consider the following disfluent production of the word "mommy" that contains elements of both sound repetition and an audible prolongation: "m-m-m-mmmommy" (Yaruss, 1997). Such productions, called "clustered disfluencies," are quite common in the speech of young children who stutter. Some researchers have suggested that the presence of clustered disfluencies may indicate incipient stuttering (stuttering that is just beginning) and that they may help to differentiate children who stutter from children who do not stutter.

Other behaviors may accompany instances of speech disfluency. Such behaviors that occur concomitantly with stuttered disfluencies are called *secondary characteristics,* or accessory behaviors, and are widely varied and idiosyncratic. Some common secondary characteristics include blinking of the eyes; facial grimacing; facial tension; and exaggerated movements of the head, shoulders, and arms. Interjected speech fragments that are superfluous to the utterance are also considered to be secondary characteristics, particularly when they occur in conjunction with a disfluency. An example of an interjected speech fragment is the superfluous phrase "that is to say" in the utterance "I met her in T-T-T-T, that is to say, I met her in Toronto." An example of secondary characteristics can be viewed on the book's CD-ROM.

The speaker may have adopted these behaviors in an effort to minimize stuttering (Bloodstein, 1995). The person who stutters discovers through trial and error that some action (e.g., bodily movements) momentarily distracts from the act of speaking and that action appears to help terminate or avoid an instance of stuttering. Behaviors such as eye blinking, however, soon lose their apparent power to reduce stuttering, and the individual is forced to replace the ineffective behavior with a new behavior, such as shrugging the shoulders, to reduce stuttering. Unfortunately, the eye blinking behavior may have become so strongly habituated that it will remain permanently associated with a person's stuttering. How do these cardinal stuttering behaviors and secondary characteristics develop and how do they change over the course of an individual's life?

THE ONSET AND DEVELOPMENT OF STUTTERING THROUGH THE LIFESPAN

Although stuttering can develop at any age, the most common form of stuttering begins in the preschool years and is called **developmental stuttering.** Developmental stuttering is contrasted with the second form of stuttering, called **neurogenic stuttering,** which is typically associated with neurological disease or trauma. Neurogenic stuttering differs from the more common developmental stuttering in several ways.

Disfluencies associated with developmental stuttering usually occur on content words (e.g., nouns, verbs), whereas disfluencies associated with neurogenic stuttering can occur on function words (e.g., conjunctions, prepositions) and content words. People who have developmental stuttering frequently exhibit secondary characteristics and anxiety about speaking, whereas neurogenic stutterers do not. Also, developmental stuttering tends to occur on the initial syllables of words, whereas neurogenic stuttering can be more widely dispersed throughout the utterance (Ringo & Dietrich, 1995). Unlike developmental stuttering, there are no clear differences in stuttering frequency across speaking tasks (i.e., word imitation versus connected speech). Finally, neurogenic stutterers do not improve (i.e., adapt) with repeated readings or singing like developmental stutterers (Duffy, 2005). We will focus primarily on developmental stuttering at this point.

It is generally accepted that the onset of developmental stuttering occurs between the ages of 2 and 5 and that 75% of the risk of developing stuttering occurs before the child is $3\frac{1}{2}$ years old (Yairi, 1983, 2004; Yairi & Ambrose, 1992a, 1992b, 2004). The onset of stuttering is gradual for the majority of children who develop the condition, with stuttering severity increasing as the child grows older. When stuttering develops in a gradual manner, some general trends regarding stuttering behaviors, reactions to stuttering, and conditions that seem to promote stuttering can be observed. We will outline some of these developmental trends (Bloodstein, 1995). Not all children exactly follow this developmental framework of stuttering, but it generally does capture the onset and progression of the disorder. This developmental framework is divided into four phases that have a sequential relationship to each other.

Phase 1 corresponds to the preschool years, roughly between the ages of 2 and 6. During phase 1, periods of stuttering are followed by periods of relative fluency. The episodic nature of stuttering is an indication that stuttering is in its most rudimentary form. The child may stutter for weeks at a time between long interludes of normally fluent speech. The child tends to stutter most when he or she is upset or excited, and in conditions of communicative pressure, such as when a parent forces a child to recite in front of friends or relatives. Sound and syllable repetitions are the dominant feature, but there is also a tendency to repeat whole words. Stuttering tends to occur at the beginnings of sentences, clauses, and phrases on both content words (e.g., nouns, verbs) and function words (e.g., articles, prepositions, etc.) unlike more advanced forms of stuttering, in which disfluencies are generally confined to content words. Finally, during phase 1, most children are unaware of the interruptions in their speech or not bothered by them.

Phase 2 represents a progression of the disorder and is associated with children of elementary school age. In phase 2, stuttering is essentially chronic, or habitual, with few intervals of fluent speech. The child has developed a self-concept as a person who stutters and will refer to himself or herself in that way. Stuttering in phase 2 occurs primarily on content words with much less tendency to stutter only on the initial words of sentences and phrases. Stuttering is more widely dispersed throughout the child's utterances. Stuttering in phase 2 also increases under conditions of excitement.

Phase 3 is associated with individuals who can range in age from about 8 years to young adulthood. Stuttering in phase 3 seems to be in response to specific situations such as speaking to strangers, speaking in front of groups, or talking on the telephone. Certain words are regarded as more difficult than others, and the person who stutters attempts to avoid such words by using word substitutions and circumlocutions. An example of a word substitution is "I want a ni-ni-ni–five cents"; the individual substitutes "five cents" for the originally intended word "nickel." Circumlocutions are roundabout or indirect ways of speaking. A circumlocution used to avoid the term "fire truck" in a child's request for a toy might take on the following form "I want a—ya know—red thing—sirens and ladders—truck for my birthday." Despite the

TABLE 8.2

Summary of Bloodstein's four phases of the onset and development of stuttering

Phase	Age	Highlights
One	2–6 years	Stuttering is episodic.
		Most stuttering occurs when the child is upset or excited.
		Sound/syllable repetitions are the dominant speech feature.
		Child seems unaware of the stuttering.
Two	Elementary school age	Stuttering is chronic.
		Stuttering occurs on content words (nouns, verbs).
		Child regards himself or herself as a stutterer.
Three	8 years to adulthood	Stuttering is situational (speaking on the telephone, speaking to large groups).
		Certain words are regarded as more difficult than others.
		Circumlocutions and word substitutions are frequent.
Four	8 years to adulthood	Stuttering is at its apex of development.
		There is fearful anticipation of stuttering.
		Certain sounds, words, and speaking situations are avoided.
		Increased circumlocutions and word substitutions are present.

individual's awareness of stuttering, he or she will generally present little evidence of fear or embarrassment and will not avoid specific speaking situations.

In phase 4, the apex of development, stuttering is in its most advanced form. A primary characteristic of phase 4 is vivid and fearful anticipation of stuttering. Certain sounds, words, and speaking situations are feared and avoided, word substitutions and circumlocutions are frequent, and there is evidence of embarrassment. Stuttered words may have associated audible vocal tension and rising pitch, which can be seen on the book's CD-ROM. These phases are summarized in Table 8.2. See Case Study 8.2 for the personal story of a young man whose fear of speaking prevented him from eating his favorite food.

Stuttering does not always develop gradually. For some individuals, when stuttering is first diagnosed in young children, the symptoms appear to be very advanced and secondary characteristics may be present (Van Riper, 1982; Yairi, 2004; Yairi & Ambrose, 1992a, 1992b, 2004; Yairi et al., 1993). The onset may be a distinct and sudden event for as high as 36% of children, and the stuttering behaviors may be considered to be moderate to severe (Yairi & Ambrose, 1992a). More research is needed on the onset and development of stuttering and the factors that underlie persistence and natural recovery.

CASE STUDY 8.2
Personal Story of a Young Man with Stuttering

Geoff was a teenage boy who was first seen at the speech and hearing clinic on his 13th birthday. His parents explained, during an initial interview, that Geoff had begun stuttering when he was around 3 years old. They further explained that the stuttering would come and go, and he would sometimes have fluent periods that lasted 2 months. Although the parents were concerned about Geoff's stuttering behaviors, they thought that he would outgrow the stuttering. This belief was reinforced by his long periods of fluency.

Geoff was evaluated by an SLP. Formal tests of stuttering placed him as a severe stutterer, most of his stuttering behaviors taking the form of long sound prolongations. Geoff told the SLP that his grades in school were falling because he would not speak in class and that he didn't like to interact with his classmates because they "always make fun of the way I talk." He also reported that there were certain words that he could not say without stuttering severely.

The SLP recommended that Geoff enroll in therapy twice a week for a trial period of 6 months. The parents and Geoff agreed. He made good progress during this trial period and stayed in therapy for an additional 4 months. At the end of 10 months of therapy, he was dismissed, exhibiting good control over his stuttering.

Two months later, he and his mother came back to the clinic for a reevaluation of his fluency skills. During the reevaluation, Geoff told the SLP that he was happy with his new speech because he could say any word he wanted without stuttering. He told the SLP that he loved to go to McDonald's or Burger King to eat cheeseburgers and french fries. But before therapy, if he had to place his own order, he wouldn't order the french fries because he knew he would stutter on the word "french." He went without the fries more times than he cared to recall. Nowadays, Geoff is enjoying his cheeseburgers *with* the french fries that he orders himself. According to Geoff, that makes him the "happiest kid on the planet."

THE EFFECTS OF STUTTERING THROUGH THE LIFESPAN

Stuttering almost always has its onset in early childhood. Research conducted at the University of Illinois indicates that in 68% of the children studied, stuttering onset occurred by 36 months of age and in 95% of the children studied by 48 months of age (Yairi, 2004; Yairi & Ambrose, 2004). Although the prevalence of stuttering (the number of persons in the population who stutter) is 1%, research indicates that "the magnitude of the problem is much larger among young children" (Yairi & Ambrose, 2004, p. 5). To put the effects of stuttering throughout the lifespan in perspective, however, we briefly discuss the model developed by the World Health Organization.

From within the context of this model, stuttering is considered to be a *handicap* or a *handicapping condition*. Specifically, a handicap comprises "the disadvantages that result from reactions to the audible and visible events of a person's stuttering, including those of the person who stutters" (Conture, 1996, p. S20). Both informal and formal observations suggest that stuttering has a negative effect on a wide variety of daily life activities, especially in three main venues of life, school, work, and social interactions. Children may withdraw and refuse to communicate orally in school, adults may select professions that require little or no oral communication, and both children and adults may avoid social contact because of a fear of speaking.

Let us first consider the negative impact stuttering can have on a child's school performance. Stutterers, on the whole, are poorer in educational adjustment than normal speakers. This conclusion is based on the amount of retention in grade at school. On average, children who stutter are delayed about half a year or half a grade level. Schoolchildren who stutter are older than their classmates who do not stutter, a finding suggesting that children who stutter are more likely to be held back in school. If so, timely and appropriate treatment should be expected to improve the academic performance of children who stutter (Bloodstein, 1995; Conture, 1996). An additional concern is children's vulnerability to being bullied. School-age children who stutter were significantly more likely to be bullied and/or teased than their peers who do not stutter (Blood & Blood, 2004).

The educational and personal disadvantages stuttering may pose on a young person do not end when the child leaves school. Stuttering can also have a negative impact in the workplace and is a vocationally handicapping condition because employers view it as a disorder that decreases employability and opportunities for promotion (Hurst & Cooper, 1983). Despite this view, when an employee who stutters seeks treatment, there is an attendant improvement in the employer's perception of the employee (Craig & Calvert, 1991). This enhanced perception is reflected by increased numbers of job promotions among employees who sought treatment and were successful in maintaining fluency following treatment.

Stuttering's potential effects on an individual's social interactions and quality of life are not well understood. Clinical observations suggest that successfully treated individuals, particularly adults, experience an improvement in their social interactions, but the nature and significance of these changes in social behavior are not well documented (Conture, 1996). However, considerable research has indicated that people who stutter do not as a group exhibit consistent, recognized patterns of psychoneurotic disturbance, but mild forms of social maladjustment are frequently reported (Bloodstein, 1995). Further research is needed to determine whether and to what extent stuttering treatment influences psychosocial adjustment (Conture, 1996).

THEORIES AND CONCEPTUALIZATIONS OF STUTTERING

An examination of some of the more prominent etiological theories of stuttering will provide you with an appreciation of the various models that have influenced stuttering research and treatment for over 80 years. Additionally, various aspects of some of the theories we consider are implicitly present in contemporary stuttering research and treatment. Etiological theories of stuttering can be classified into three categories: organic, behavioral, and psychological.

Organic Theory

Organic theories propose an actual physical cause for stuttering. Speculations about a physical cause for stuttering date back to the writings of Aristotle, who suggested that stuttering was a disconnection between the mind and the body and that the muscles of the tongue could not follow the commands of the brain (Rieber & Wollock, 1977). Many organic theories have been proposed since Aristotle's writings, but they have all failed in one manner or another to explain stuttering satisfactorily. For example, the *theory of cerebral dominance* or the "handedness theory" proposed by Samuel Orton and Lee Travis in the 1930s (Bloodstein, 1995) assumed that when neither cerebral hemisphere was dominant, both would send competing neural impulses to their respective muscles of speech, resulting in a discoordination between the right and left halves of the speech musculature. This discoordination was believed to result in stuttering. A renewed interest in this theory has come about due to recent findings from brain-imaging studies that have revealed structural and functional differences in the brains of adults with chronic developmental stuttering.

Current brain-imaging research may facilitate the development of a comprehensive neurophysiological model for both fluent and stuttered speech that could lead to new stuttering prevention and treatment methods (Brown et al., 2005; c.f., Ingham et al., 2003).

Well-controlled experimental investigations over the past 30 years have consistently demonstrated the robust and immediate effects of behavioral modification techniques such as rewarding fluent speech and correcting stuttered speech.

Behavioral Theory

Behavioral theories assert that stuttering is a learned response to conditions external to the individual. A prominent behavioral theory, the *diagnosogenic* theory, was developed by Wendell Johnson during the 1940s and 1950s. According to this theory, stuttering began in the parent's ear, not in the child's mouth. Overly concerned parents would react to the child's normal speech hesitations and repetitions with negative statements admonishing the child to speak more slowly and not to stutter. Such parental behaviors made the child anxious about speaking, and the child's anxiety fostered further hesitations and repetitions.

Not only is there no evidence to support this theory, there is evidence to the contrary. Studies have shown that the process of natural recovery may actually be due in part to parents explicitly telling their child to slow down, stop and start again, or think before speaking when their child is stuttering (e.g., Langford & Cooper, 1974; Martin & Lindamood, 1986).

Psychological Theory

Psychological theory contends that stuttering is a neurotic symptom with ties to unconscious needs and internal conflicts, treated most appropriately by psychotherapy. Some psychological theories regard people who stutter as individuals with neuroses; other theories regard stuttering as a phobic manifestation. However, research indicates that psychotherapy is not an effective method for the treatment of stuttering. Some people who stutter may indeed have neuroses, but psychological theory has yet to provide a cogent explanation for the underlying cause of stuttering or its onset and development.

Current Conceptual Models of Stuttering

The *covert repair hypothesis*, based on a language production model, assumes that stuttering is a reaction to some flaw in the speech production plan (Postma & Kolk, 1993). Speakers have the capability of monitoring their speech as it is being formulated and detecting errors in the speech plan. People who stutter have poorly developed phonological encoding skills that cause them to introduce errors into their speech plan. If there are more errors in the speech plan, there will be more occasions for error correction. Stuttering is not the error. Rather, stuttering is a "normal" repair reaction to an abnormal phonetic plan.

Another conceptualization of stuttering is the *demands and capacities model* (DCM) (Starkweather, 1987, 1997). This model asserts that stuttering develops when the environmental demands placed on a child to produce fluent speech exceed the child's physical and learned capacities. The child's capacity for fluent speech depends on a balance of motor skills, language production skills, emotional maturity, and cognitive development. Children who stutter presumably lack one or more of these capacities for fluent speech. Parents of a child who lacks the required motor skills for fluency might talk rapidly; rapid rates of speech may put a time pressure on the child that exceeds his or her motoric ability to respond. Other parents might insist on the use of advanced language structures that are in excess of the child's language development. In every case of stuttering within the DCM, there is an imbalance between the environmental demands that are placed on the child and the child's capacity for fluent speech.

The DCM is not a theory of stuttering, and it does not suggest a cause for stuttering. Rather, the DCM is a useful tool that helps clinicians to understand the dynamics of forces that contribute to the development of stuttering. Therapeutically, the DCM provides useful guidelines for understanding what capacities a child may lack for fluent speech production and the elements of the child's environment that may be challenging those capacities.

One more theoretical construct regarding stuttering is worthy of mention. The EXPLAN model (Howell, 2004) is an account of the production of spontaneous speech that applies to both fluent speakers and speakers who stutter. In this model, speech planning (PLAN) is the linguistic process of language formulation, and execution (EX) is the motor activity related to production of the language formulation. Although some theoretical accounts of stuttering have placed the primary site of disruption in the language formulation phase and other accounts have placed the primary site at the instructions sent to the motor system, the EXPLAN model posits that stuttering results from a failure in normal interactions between the PLAN and EX processes (Howell, 2004). Fluency failures occur when linguistic plans are sent too slowly to the motor system.

Alternatively, computer simulation models of speech production have been programmed to simulate stuttering, providing evidence for a disrupted speech motor control system in individuals who stutter (c.f. Max et al., 2004). These scientifically sophisticated models may further our understanding of the basic nature of stuttering and of stuttering treatment.

THERAPEUTIC TECHNIQUES USED WITH YOUNG CHILDREN

When parents are concerned that a child is stuttering, it is the speech-language pathologist's (SLP) responsibility to determine whether there should be concern and, if so, to plan an appropriate course of action. Two important components of the evaluation of a child suspected of stuttering are observations of the child speaking and a detailed parental interview (see Figure 8.1 for some common questions for parents with a disfluent child).

The Evaluation of Stuttering

The primary component of the stuttering evaluation is a detailed analysis of the child's speech behaviors. The SLP determines the average number of

Introduction

Why are you here today?

Tell us (me) about your child's problem.

General Development

Tell us (me) about your child's development from birth to present

How does this compare with his or her siblings?

Family History

Do any other family members have speech, hearing, or language problems?

Did they receive speech therapy?

Speech/Language Development

When did your child say his or her first words?

When did your child say his or her first phrases and sentences?

History/Description of the Problem

Describe your child's speaking problems.

When did the problem start?

What was your reaction? Did you bring the problem to your child's attention?

Can you describe your child's stuttering when it first began?

Has it changed over time?

Does your child lose eye contact when talking to you?

Does your child have excessive body movements when talking?

Does he or she avoid speaking situations?

Have you done anything to help your child stop stuttering?

Family Interactions

What do you and your child do when you spend time together?

What kind of things do you do as a family?

How do you handle sibling hostilities?

Wrap Up

If you could wish for three things for your child, what would you wish for?

FIGURE 8.1
....

Common questions for parents of a disfluent child.

Source: Based on Conture (1990b).

each type of disfluency the child produces (e.g., within-word repetitions, sound prolongations). Three or more within-word disfluencies per 100 words spoken may indicate that the child has a fluency problem (Conture, 1990b). The percentage of the total disfluency that each type of disfluency contributes is another important evaluative measure. For example, if the child produces 10 disfluencies per 100 words spoken and 6 of them are sound prolongations, then 60% of all the disfluencies are sound prolongations. A high percentage of sound prolongations may indicate a chronic fluency problem. The SLP will also measure the duration of several disfluencies. Longer durations and/or multiple sound or syllable repetitions may represent an increase in the severity of the stuttering problem. See the Web site link at the end of the chapter to measure syllables stuttered.

Standardized tests such as the *Stuttering Prediction Instrument* (SPI; Riley & Riley, 1981) may also be used in the fluency evaluation. The SPI yields a numerical score based on a number of stuttering-related behaviors such as the duration of disfluencies and stuttering frequency. The numerical score is converted to a verbal stuttering severity rating. Finally, the SLP will record the types of secondary symptoms that the child presents. A wide assortment of secondary symptoms may indicate a progression of the disorder.

The SLP's decision to recommend therapy is not based on any single behavior or test result. Therapy may be recommended if two or more of the following behaviors are observed:

1. Sound prolongations constitute more than 25% of the total disfluencies produced by the child.
2. Instances of sound or syllable repetitions or sound prolongations on the first syllables of words during iterative speech tasks (e.g., iterative productions of pa-ta-ka, pa-ta-ka, pa-ta-ka).
3. Loss of eye contact on more than 50% of the child's utterances.
4. A score of 18 or more on the SPI (Conture, 1990b).
5. At least one adult expressing concern about the child's speech fluency skills (Chang et al., 2002)

Indirect and Direct Stuttering Intervention

If the SLP determines that the child has a stuttering problem or a high probability of developing stuttering, therapeutic intervention is indicated. In general, two broad intervention strategies can be used with young children who stutter: indirect therapy and direct therapy. Indirect approaches are considered viable for children who are just beginning to stutter and whose stuttering is fairly mild. Direct approaches are typically reserved for children who have been stuttering for at least a year and whose stuttering is moderate to severe.

An indirect approach does not explicitly try to modify or change the child's speech fluency, focusing instead on the child, the child's parents, and the child's environment. Important aspects of indirect therapy are information sharing and teaching parents to provide a slow, relaxed speech model for the child. Play-oriented activities that encourage slow and relaxed speech are the central component of such intervention. There is no explicit discussion about the child's fluent or stuttering speaking behaviors. The goal of indirect therapy is to facilitate fluency through environmental manipulation.

Direct approaches involve explicit and direct attempts to modify the child's speech and speech-related behaviors. In direct therapy, concepts such as "hard" and "easy" speech are introduced. Hard speech is rapid and relatively tense (such as a tense sound prolongation of /s/ in sssssssssss-snake), whereas easy speech is slow and relaxed. The terms "hard" and "easy" are simple and carry little negative connotation for the child. Children are taught to identify both types of speech by first monitoring their recorded utterances and later by identifying these types of speech in their ongoing productions. Once the child is able to identify hard and easy speech segments accurately and reliably, the SLP teaches the child strategies that will help him or her increase easy speech and change from hard speech to easy speech when required. The therapeutic sequence of identification followed by identification/modification forms the core elements of many strategies for children and adults.

THERAPEUTIC TECHNIQUES USED WITH OLDER CHILDREN AND ADULTS WHO STUTTER

Individuals who continue to stutter into their teenage years and beyond will likely have many negative reactions to speaking situations that may affect their social lives and vocational goals. Many of these individuals will have had previous unsuccessful speech therapy and perhaps other forms of remediation to combat the fluency problem. The adult who stutters "brings a complexity of attitudes, experiences, and coping attempts to the therapeutic process, and these must be dealt with directly or indirectly" (Gelfer, 1996, p. 160).

The primary focus of this section is on therapeutic techniques used to manage adulthood stuttering. In particular, we explore direct techniques that are used to establish fluency. Changing certain aspects of one's speaking behavior is of fundamental importance in stuttering intervention and is often a source of confusion among clinicians who treat adults who stutter (Sommers & Caruso, 1995).

Therapeutic techniques designed to modify stuttering behaviors are classified generally into two broad categories: *fluency-shaping techniques* and *stuttering modification techniques*. When used properly, both techniques have a powerful effect in reducing stuttering. Fluency-shaping techniques involve changing the overall speech timing patterns of the individual in an effort to reduce or eliminate stuttering. This is typically accomplished by lengthening the duration of sounds and words and greatly slowing down the overall rate of speech. Stuttering modification techniques involve changing only the stuttering behaviors. This is typically accomplished by lengthening the duration of or in some way modifying only the speech segment on which the stuttering is occurring. Treatment programs for stuttering often combine these two approaches (Guitar, 2006). See Prins and Ingham (2009) for a historical, evidence-based perspective of fluency-shaping and stuttering modification treatments.

> Delayed auditory feedback systems use a microphone and earphones. A person wearing the earphones speaks into the microphone, which transmits the speech to a device that electronically delays sending the speech to the earphones. If the delay were set at 250 milliseconds (or $\frac{1}{4}$ second) the speaker would hear his or her utterance $\frac{1}{4}$ of a second after it was uttered. Delaying the auditory feedback causes the speaker to reduce the rate of speaking.

Fluency-Shaping Techniques

Reducing speech rate, known as **prolonged speech,** is one of the most powerful ways to reduce or eliminate stuttering. Prolonged speech may be a specific therapeutic goal, or it may involve use of various techniques that serve to reduce speaking rate and increase fluency. The term *prolonged speech* arose from research conducted in the 1960s regarding the effects of delayed auditory feedback (DAF) on speech production. DAF is a condition in which a speaker hears his or her own speech after an instrumental delay of some finite period of time, such as 250 or 500 milliseconds. When a person speaks under DAF, his or her speech is slowed involuntarily because the duration of syllables is prolonged. For example, when people who stutter speak under conditions of DAF, speaking rates decrease dramatically and the longer the delay, the slower the speech. This slowing of speech rate under DAF conditions is accompanied by a substantial decrease in stuttering.

When DAF is used clinically to prolong speech, the feedback delay is set to promote speaking rates of about 30 to 60 syllables per minute. During this initial phase, the person who stutters is taught to prolong the duration of each syllable but not to increase the duration of pauses between syllables (Boburg & Kully, 1995; Max & Caruso, 1997). This prolonged speech pattern is systematically altered over the course of intervention by adjusting the DAF times to reduce the magnitude of syllable prolongation while maintaining fluent speech. Speech rates ranging from 120 to 200 syllables per minute are typical targets for the termination of therapy. An example of DAF-facilitated prolonged speech can be seen on the book's CD-ROM.

Behavioral techniques that serve not only to reduce speech rate but also reduce physical tension in the speech musculature before and during occurrences of stuttering, promoting smooth speech, are *light articulatory contacts* and *gentle voicing onsets* (GVOs). The therapeutic use of light articulatory contacts involves instructing the speaker to use less tension in the articulators, particularly during production of stop consonants (/p/, /b/, /t/, /d/, /k/, and /g/) that involve a complete constriction of the vocal tract (Max & Caruso, 1997). Reducing articulatory tension is believed to prevent occurrence of prolonged articulatory postures that interfere with smooth articulatory transitions from sound to sound. Light touches promote continuity and ease of articulation by preventing excessive pressure and tension in the articulators (Boburg & Kully, 1995).

Gentle voicing onsets are a cardinal feature of many therapy programs, and they are known by many different names, such as Fluency Initiation of Gestures (FIGS) (Cooper, 1984). The basic characteristic of GVOs is a tension-free onset of voicing that gradually builds in intensity. One can appreciate the dynamics of this technique by initiating production of the vowel /a/ in a whisper, gradually engaging the vocal folds such that the vowel is produced with a breathy voice quality, and finally increasing the vowel's intensity. GVOs are typically learned in a hierarchical fashion beginning with vowel production, followed by syllable productions, and then word productions.

Another clinical rate reduction technique that has an ameliorative effect on stuttering is called pausing/phrasing, which is designed to lengthen naturally occurring pauses (clause and sentence boundaries) and to add pauses between other words or phrases. Additionally, pausing/phrasing techniques may attempt to limit utterance length to 2 to 5 syllables. A formal stuttering treatment known as the *Gradual Increase in Length and Complexity of Utterance* program (Ryan, 1974) capitalizes on the underlying principles of pausing/phrasing techniques and has been found to be effective in reducing or eliminating stuttering, particularly in school-age children.

Another powerful fluency-shaping therapeutic intervention consistently found to reduce or eliminate stuttering is response-contingent stimulation (RCS). RCS procedures have their origins in learning theory and are based on B. F. Skinner's behavioral (operant) conditioning paradigm. Operant conditioning results in the association between a behavior

> People who stutter frequently use excessive articulator pressure when producing sounds. They may, for example, press the tongue very hard on the roof of the mouth during the production of /t/ and /d/ sounds. Teaching the individual to reduce such pressure, or make light articulatory contacts, promotes fluency.

(response) and the stimulus that follows (consequence), and thus determines the future occurrence of that behavior.

Skinner's system of behavioral modification is the basis for response-contingent time-out from speaking (RCTO), which requires the individual to pause briefly from speaking after a stuttering behavior has occurred. This pause or cessation from speaking serves as the consequence for stuttering. Research has consistently shown its positive effects on reducing stuttering frequency to zero or near-zero levels. Adolescents and adults who stutter have also been taught to self-administer a time-out from speaking immediately after a self-identified instance of stuttering (Hewat et al., 2006; James, 1981a). The mechanism underlying the success of RCTO remains elusive, however.

Response contingent procedures have been especially effective as a behavioral treatment for young children who stutter when administered by parents in the child's everyday environment. In long-term treatment outcome trials, the *Lidcombe program* has been shown to be highly effective in decreasing stuttering to zero or near-zero levels for 2 to 7 years following treatment (Lincoln & Onslow, 1997). The Lidcombe program is a parent-administered treatment in which positive reinforcement is provided to the child for stutter-free speech, and a correction is used following stuttering (i.e., the child is asked to repeat the stuttered word(s) correctly). Praise and reinforcement for fluent speech is provided by parents five times more often than requests for correction of stuttered speech. Learn more about the Lidcombe program on the Web site listed at the end of the chapter.

Stuttering Modification Techniques

Unlike the fluency-shaping approach that seeks to reduce or eliminate stuttering by teaching the individual who stutters to speak in a way that prevents stuttering, the stuttering modification approach teaches the person who stutters to react to his or her stuttering calmly, without unnecessary effort or struggle (Prins & Ingham, 2009). Stuttering modification procedures were born out of Charles Van Riper's conceptualization of stuttering as a disruption in speech timing causing fluency breakdowns, as well as the triggering of negative reactions to such breakdowns. As such, three techniques developed by Van Riper not only work to modify speech timing, but also to modify abnormal reactions to stuttering (Prins & Ingham, 2009). They are known as *cancellations, pull-outs,* and *preparatory sets.*

These three techniques are introduced therapeutically in sequential order, beginning with stuttering cancellation. During the cancellation phase of therapy, an individual is required to complete the word that was stuttered and pause deliberately following the production of that stuttered word. The individual pauses for a minimum of 3 seconds and then reproduces the stuttered word in slow motion. This ostensibly provides practice with the motoric integration and speech timing movements that are required for a fluent production of that word. When the individual reaches a criterion level of cancellation proficiency, he or she will move to the second technique, known as pull-outs.

During the pull-out phase of therapy, the individual does not wait until after the stuttered word is completed to correct the inappropriate behavior. Rather, the individual modifies the stuttered word during the actual occurrence of the stuttering. This modification involves slowing down the sequential movements of the syllable or word when stuttering occurs in a fashion similar to the slowed and exaggerated movements that were learned in the cancellation phase of therapy. In essence, the individual is modifying the stuttering online, "pulling out" of the stuttering behavior and completing it with a more fluent production of the intended word. Once again, when the individual reaches a criterion level of proficiency, he or she will move to the last stage, known as preparatory sets.

Preparatory sets involve using the slow-motion speech strategies that were learned during the first two phases of therapy, not as a response to an occurrence of stuttering, but in anticipation of stuttering. A person who stutters typically knows when and on what word a stuttering will occur. When an individual anticipates a stuttering, he or she will start preparing to use the newly learned fluency producing strategies before the word is attempted. The goal of this phase of therapy is to initiate the word in a more fluent manner even though the individual is producing consecutive speech movements and transitions in a slowed manner.

Selecting Intervention Techniques

The SLP's selection of a specific management technique depends on many factors, including the severity of the stuttering problem, the motivation and specific needs of the person who stutters, and the SLP's knowledge of the specific techniques available. Careful and detailed observation of an individual's stuttering behaviors before initiating treatment and during the treatment process is an essential component of successful clinical management. Such observation will assist the SLP in "selecting, combining, and modifying available techniques in order to teach the client how to alter timing and tension aspects of his or her speech movements" (Max & Caruso, 1997, p. 50). In short, a one-size-fits-all clinical program does not and should not exist. Inherent differences among individuals within the stuttering population prohibit the use of inflexible clinical protocols that cannot be modified to meet the individual's needs.

THE EFFECTIVENESS OF STUTTERING INTERVENTION THROUGH THE LIFESPAN

Determining how effective stuttering treatment is depends largely on how "effectiveness" is defined. This is a complex issue. However, a "treatment for stuttering might be considered *effective* if it resulted in the individual's being able to speak with disfluencies within normal limits whenever and to whomever he or she chose, without undue concern or worry about speaking" (Conture, 1996, p. S20). The treatment of stuttering differs across an individual's lifespan in terms of frequency and nature of therapy, and rates of recovery. Therefore, the review of treatment efficacy is probably best considered relative to four age groups: preschoolers, school-age children, teenagers, and adults. Review of the published research in stuttering intervention provides support for use of several treatment approaches and/or techniques. These are briefly reviewed in Box 8.1.

BOX 8.1
Evidence-Based Practices for Individuals with Stuttering

General

- Individuals who stutter can benefit from intervention by an SLP at any time during their lifespan.
- Treatments with the greatest efficacy for reducing stuttering in older children and adults include those that change the rate of speech and tension during speaking.
- Comprehensive approaches focusing on the individual's attitude toward speaking and on addressing the negative impact of stuttering on one's life are reported by clients as being of more benefit than those approaches that just focus on speech alone.
- Between 60% and 80% of clients who participate in stuttering treatment make significant improvement.

Specific Behavioral Treatment Approaches or Techniques

- The long-term effectiveness of the parent-administered behavioral intervention, the Lidcombe program, is well established, particularly for preschool children. Parents are taught to praise their child's fluent speech by saying, "Good job, that was nice and smooth", and correct stuttered speech by saying "Oops, that was bumpy, can you say _____ again" in a 5:1 ratio of positive reinforcement to stuttering correction.
- A program of gradual increase in length and complexity of utterances, called GILCO, in which a child progresses from one-word stutter-free responses to 5 minutes of stutter-free speech during reading, monologue speaking, and conversation has been found to be highly effective with older children.
- Prolonged speech techniques (e.g., light articulatory contacts, gentle voicing onsets) have been found to be highly effective with older children and adults, particularly when taught in the context of a structured program with opportunities for daily practice. No one technique has been found to be effective on its own, however.
- Response-contingent time-out from speaking is based on behavioral (operant) conditioning and involves the individual pausing briefly from speaking immediately after a stuttering event. This procedure is highly effective in reducing stuttering in adolescents and adults. Usually, the SLP tells the individual to stop speaking after an instance of stuttering; however, individuals can be taught to self-deliver a time-out from speaking following a self-identified stuttering moment.

Source: Based on Bothe et al. (2006); Conture and Yaruss (2009); Craig et al. (1996); Hewat et al. (2006); James, 1981a; Onslow et al. (2003); Ryan (1974).

Efficacy of Intervention with Preschool-Age Children

In general, the findings of most recent studies are quite encouraging and indicate the potential benefits of early diagnosis and treatment of stuttering. As many as 91% of preschool children who had been in a stuttering treatment program maintained their fluent speech 5 years after their initial evaluation (Fosnot, 1993). Among preschool-age children enrolled in a parent-conducted therapy program, all maintained their fluent speech 7 years after dismissal from treatment (Lincoln & Onslow, 1997). In another study, 100% of 45 preschool-age children who stuttered had maintained fluent speech 2 years following dismissal from treatment (Gottwald & Starkweather, 1995).

Efficacy of Intervention with School-Age Children

One noteworthy study of stuttering treatment effectiveness used four different treatment approaches with school-age children and reported an average 60% post-treatment improvement (Ryan & Van Kirk Ryan, 1983). Even better results were found in another study in which 96% of the school-age children enrolled in two treatment programs maintained fluent speech 14 months after treatment (Ryan & Van Kirk Ryan, 1995).

The findings of nine investigations of the effectiveness of stuttering treatment involving 160 school-age children are mildly encouraging. The findings of these studies indicated a 61% average (range of 33% to over 90%) decrease in stuttering frequency and/or stuttering severity across the nine studies. As with the stuttering treatment efficacy findings among preschool-age children, these studies suggest cautious optimism (Conture, 1996).

Efficacy of Intervention with Adolescents and Adults

Teenagers who stutter can be difficult to manage clinically, and little information is available regarding specific therapy programs for this age group (Daly et al., 1995; Schwartz, 1993). In sharp contrast, many reports of treatment outcomes for the adult who stutters are available. A wide variety of adult stuttering treatment techniques have been investigated, ranging from operant conditioning techniques to drug therapies. Collectively, these studies suggest a 60% to 80% improvement rate regardless of the therapeutic technique that was used.

In summary, stuttering intervention across all age groups results in an average improvement for about 70% of all cases, with preschool-age children improving more quickly and easily than people who have a longer history with stuttering. The clinical research that we have considered indicates that effective treatment of stuttering is increasingly able to improve the daily life of people who stutter by increasing their ability to communicate whenever and with whomever they choose without undue concern about speaking.

SUMMARY

Stuttering is a handicapping condition primarily characterized by sound and syllable repetitions and sound prolongations that interrupt the smooth forward flow of speech. Stuttering is a universal problem that affects males more than females. In most cases, stuttering appears between the ages of 2 to 4 years, and as the disorder progresses, it increases in severity. Stuttering can adversely affect an individual's school performance, employment, and social interactions. The treatment of stuttering is most effective when it is initiated in early childhood, although treatment at any age can reduce stuttering.

A number of theories–organic, behavioral, and psychological–attempt to account for the onset and development of stuttering, but its cause is unknown. Solving the riddle of stuttering will undoubtedly require expertise from many specialists including SLPs, neurolinguists, geneticists, and medical specialists. Perhaps one of you reading this text will find your own birch tree and take up Van Riper's quest to find the cause and a cure for stuttering.

THOUGHT QUESTIONS

- In what ways could a parent's speech pattern influence the speech pattern of his or her child? Do you think mothers and fathers exhibit different speech patterns with their children?
- What kinds of jobs require a great deal of speaking? Do you think people who stutter avoid such jobs?
- If the motor speech control system is affected in people who stutter, do you think they may also have generalized motor difficulties (e.g., incoordination)?

SUGGESTED READINGS

Bloodstein, O. (1995). *A handbook on stuttering.* San Diego, CA: Singular.

Bothe, A., Davidow, J., Bramlett, R., & Ingham, R. (2006). Stuttering treatment research 1970–2005: I. Systematic review incorporating trial quality assessment of behavioral, cognitive, and related approaches. *American Journal of Speech-Language Pathology, 15,* 321–341.

Guitar, G. (2006). *Stuttering: An integrated approach to its nature and treatment.* Philadelphia: Lippincott Williams & Wilkins.

Onslow, M., Packman, A., & Harrison, E. (2003). *The Lidcombe program of early stuttering intervention: A clinician's guide.* Austin, TX: Pro-Ed.

Prins, D., & Ingham, R. (2009). Evidence-based treatment and stuttering—historical perspective. *Journal of Speech, Language, and Hearing Research, 52,* 254–263.

ONLINE RESOURCES

Lidcombe

www3.fhs.usyd.edu.au/asrcwww/treatment/lidcombe.htm

The Lidcombe site has the latest instruction manual for the program.

University of California, Santa Barbara

www.speech.ucsb.edu/roger.htm

At the University of California, Santa Barbara, Web site, you can download the free stuttering measurement system (SMS) software to measure the percentage of syllables stuttered.

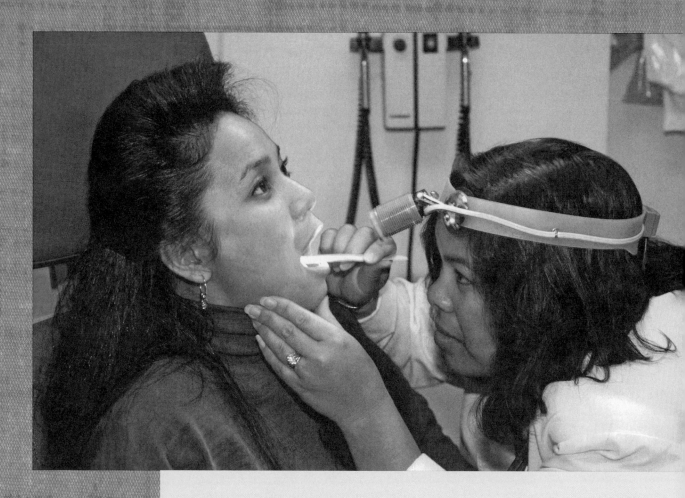

CHAPTER LEARNING GOALS

When you have finished this chapter, you should be able to:

- Explain the normal phonation process

- Describe the perceptual signs of a voice disorder

- Describe voice disorders that are associated with vocal misuse or abuse, medical or physical conditions, and psychological or stress conditions

- Describe the major goals of voice therapy and effective voice treatment approaches and techniques

9

The Voice and Voice Disorders

Voice is our primary means of expression and is an essential feature of the uniquely human attribute known as speech (Boone & McFarlane, 2000; Colton & Casper, 1996; Titze, 1994). Your voice reflects gender, personality, personal habits, age, and the general condition of health. Research has shown that certain characteristics of the voice reflect various personality dimensions, and these vocal characteristics correlate well with standardized tests of personality (Colton & Casper, 1990; Markel, et al., 1964). Your voice is an emotional outlet that mirrors your moods, attitudes, and general feelings. Expressions of anger can be achieved by shouting, and expressions of affection can be achieved by speaking softly; these types of vocal expression have great potential to evoke emotional responses from a listener. Evoking emotional responses from listeners through controlled vocal expression is key to a successful operatic performance. Dramatic actors achieve pathos through deliberate and controlled vocal expression. The evocative nature of vocal expressions, however, is hardly limited to stage performances. We constantly vary the tone of our voices to achieve some specific meaning or intention. Your voice is a powerful tool that delivers a message and simultaneously adds to the meaning of that message (Colton & Casper, 1990).

In Chapter 3, we discussed the basic concepts related to normal voice production. We extend some of these basic concepts in this chapter with a discussion of how one changes the pitch and loudness of the voice. Next, we discuss voice disorders associated with vocal misuse and hyperfunction, abnormal medical and physical conditions, and psychological and stress conditions in children and adults. Finally, assessment, treatment, treatment efficacy issues, and evidence-based practices are discussed. See Case Study 9.1 for an example of a voice disorder due to laryngeal pathology.

VOCAL PITCH AND THE PITCH-CHANGING MECHANISM

You are probably aware that the relative pitch of your voice depends somewhat on your sex and age. *Pitch* of the voice is the perceptual counterpart to fundamental frequency associated with the speed of vocal fold vibration. As

CASE STUDY 9.1
Case Study of a Young Man with a Voice Disorder: Jonathan

Jonathan, a 20-year-old college student, was seen at the university medical center's speech-language pathology department on a Monday late in October. Jonathan, an avid college football fan, attended all his school's home games. He had attended the home football game that was held the Saturday before he reported to the speech-language pathology department. Jonathan reported that he was yelling loudly during much of Saturday's game until his voice became weak. He further reported that when he woke on Sunday morning it felt like there was something stuck in his throat. As he spoke, the SLP noted that his voice quality was very hoarse and excessively breathy.

The SLP referred him to the otolaryngology department of the medical center. There, an otolaryngologist examined Jonathan's vocal folds using a flexible fiberoptic endoscope. The otolaryngologist reported that Jonathan had a large unilateral sessile polyp on his right vocal fold, and she recommended that the polyp be removed surgically. It was further recommended that following the removal of the polyp Jonathan should be scheduled for voice therapy.

One month following surgery, he began attending voice therapy. The principal focus of therapeutic intervention was to educate him regarding conditions that are detrimental to vocal fold tissue and to educate him regarding proper vocal hygiene. Jonathan remains an avid football fan, but he uses his voice in a healthy fashion when he attends games.

As you read this chapter, think about the following:

- Why the SLP referred Jonathan to the otolaryngologist.
- Why Jonathan required voice therapy following the polyp's removal.
- What possible strategies Jonathan was taught to promote vocal hygiene.

During one complete vibratory cycle of vocal fold vibration, the vocal folds move from a closed or adducted position to an open or abducted position and back to the closed position.

the speed of vocal fold vibration increases, the perceived pitch of the voice increases. As we discussed in Chapter 3, the speed at which the vocal folds vibrate is called the fundamental frequency of the voice. Frequency is measured in **hertz (Hz),** or the number of complete vibrations per second. The fundamental frequency of the voice varies considerably during speaking, but each individual speaker has an average fundamental frequency, or *habitual pitch*. Each individual also has a particularly suitable pitch level known as the **optimal pitch level,** which is largely determined by vocal fold structure. For example, on average, adult men have fundamental frequencies of around 130 Hz (the vocal folds open and close 130 times per second), whereas adult women have fundamental frequencies around 250 Hz. Therefore, the perceived pitch of male voices is, on average, lower than the perceived pitch of female voices. The fundamental frequency of young children's voices can be as high as 500 Hz, resulting in a very high-pitched voice. The difference in vocal fundamental frequency (and resulting vocal pitch) among men, women, and children is due largely to the structure of the vocal folds themselves.

At birth, the infant larynx is positioned relatively high in the neck, at about the level of the third cervical vertebra. The epiglottis is in contact with the soft palate. The elevated laryngeal position allows the infant to breathe while nursing and reduces the risk of choking (Kent, 1997; Zemlin, 1998).

The infant larynx begins to descend in the neck shortly after birth, reaching the level of the sixth cervical vertebra by about 5 years of age. Laryngeal descent continues until the larynx reaches the level of the seventh cervical vertebra between 15 and 20 years of age.

At birth, the vocal folds are approximately 3 mm long for both sexes. The growth rate of the vocal folds is approximately 0.4 mm/year in females and 0.7 mm/year in males, but this difference in growth rate does not result in appreciable average pitch differences between boys and girls (Titze, 1994). Males and females have similar fundamental frequencies until about 12 years of age. During puberty, however, male vocal folds rapidly increase in length by about 10 mm and, importantly, they also thicken. The increase in vocal fold length and thickness during the pubertal period results in a large drop in the male's vocal fundamental frequency. In comparison, female vocal folds lengthen by approximately 4 mm during puberty with no significant thickening of the folds. Female fundamental frequency drops only about three musical tones during puberty. Postpubertal vocal fold length ranges from 17 mm to 20 mm in males and from 12.5 mm to 17 mm in females (Zemlin, 1998). In general, because of their larger structure, male vocal folds vibrate with a lower fundamental frequency than female vocal folds, resulting in a lower-pitched male voice. The structural changes of the vocal folds and the relationship to vocal fundamental frequency are summarized in Table 9.1.

Although individuals have a habitual speaking frequency (average pitch), the frequency of the voice constantly varies during speech production. A monotonous or **monotone** voice is the result of not varying the habitual speaking frequency during speech production. People who use a monotone voice are not terribly interesting to listen to, and listeners quickly

TABLE 9.1

Summary of laryngeal development and fundamental frequency characteristics through the lifespan

Time	Structural Development	Fundamental Frequency
Birth	Larynx positioned high in the neck; vocal fold length is 3 mm	Average is about 400 Hz; unstable
4 years	Little sex difference in vocal fold length until about 10 years	Stable from 4 to 10 years with little sex influence
Puberty	10 mm increase in vocal fold length for males; 4 mm increase for females	One octave decrease for males; decreases three musical tones for females
Adulthood	Vocal fold length is 20 mm in men; vocal fold length is 17 mm in women	Males' average is 130 Hz; females' average is 250 Hz

Source: Based on Kent (1997).

lose interest in what is being said. Varying the pitch of the voice also has linguistic significance. Consider these two sentences:

Tom has a dog.

Tom has a dog?

The words in these two sentences are identical, but the sentences' meanings are quite different. "Tom has a dog" is a statement of fact (a declarative), whereas "Tom has a dog?" is a question (an interrogative). Say those two sentences out loud, paying particular attention to what happens to your pitch at the end of each sentence. For the declarative, the pitch of your voice will decrease or fall off as you are saying the word "dog." In contrast, for the interrogative, the pitch of your voice will increase when you are saying the word "dog."

How does one change the pitch of the voice? Modifications in the length and tension of the vocal folds are necessary to produce pitch change. Lengthening and tensing the vocal folds via intrinsic muscle contraction will increase the pitch of the voice, whereas relaxing these muscles will decrease pitch. Check out the National Center for Voice and Speech Web site listed at the end of this chapter for an in-depth look at pitch and loudness control.

VOCAL LOUDNESS AND THE LOUDNESS-CHANGING MECHANISM

Like changing the pitch of the voice, changing vocal loudness is also necessary for adequate communication. Vocal loudness is the perceptual correlate of intensity, which is measured in **decibels (dB).** In general, as vocal intensity increases, the perceived loudness of the voice increases. The loudness of normal conversational speech, such as conversations at the dinner table, averages around 60 dB. Changes in vocal intensity require the vocal folds to stay together longer during the closed phase of vibration, but alveolar pressure is the major determinant of vocal intensity (Kent, 1997; Zemlin, 1998). As discussed in Chapter 3, alveolar pressure is the pressure placed on the inferior aspects of the vocal folds by the lungs. Every time alveolar pressure doubles, there is an 8 to 12 dB increase in vocal intensity. The *Guinness Book of World Records* reports that the loudest scream ever recorded was produced at 123.2 dB, and a man named Anthony Fieldhouse won the World Shouting contest with a yell that was registered at 112.4 dB (Kent, 1997). Unless you are a record seeker, this kind of behavior is not recommended, as we see later in the chapter.

Disorders of Voice

Disordered voice production involves deviations in voice quality, pitch, loudness, and flexibility that may signify illness and/or interfere with communication (Aronson, 1990). Voice disorders can affect people of any age. It is estimated that approximately 3% to 6% of school-age children and 3% to 9% of adults in the United States have a voice disorder. In the adult population, men are more commonly affected than women (Ramig & Verdolini, 1998).

Data from the National Center for Voice and Speech (Ramig & Verdolini, 1998) suggest that approximately 3% of the working population in the United States have occupations (e.g., police, air, traffic controllers, pilots) in which use of their voice is necessary for public safety. More recently, data have shown that "approximately 10 percent of the workforce in the United States would be classified as heavy occupational voice users" (Roy, 2005, p. 8). For example, schoolteachers have a higher prevalence of voice disorders than nonteaching adults (11.0% versus 6.2%) (Roy et al., 2004). It is clear that the occurrence of voice disorders in adults is "potentially one of great magnitude from a health, as well as economic standpoint" (Laguaite, 1972, p. 151).

Unlike voice disorders in children, which are usually related to vocal misuse or abuse and in most cases are temporary, adult voice disorders are quite varied. Perceptual signs of a voice disorder are related to specific characteristics of a person's voice, which can be evaluated by a clinician. Clinically, perceptual signs in conjunction with a person's case history serve as the initial benchmarks in the differential diagnosis of a voice disorder. Perceptual signs of voice can be divided into five broad categories: pitch, loudness, quality, nonphonatory behaviors, and aphonia, or the absence of phonation (Colton & Casper, 1996).

Disorders of Vocal Pitch

As we stated earlier in this chapter, pitch is the perceptual correlate of fundamental frequency. Three aspects of pitch may suggest a voice disorder. The first is **monopitch.** A monopitch voice lacks normal inflectional variation and, in some instances, the ability to change pitch voluntarily. Monopitch may be a sign of a neurological impairment or a psychiatric disability, or it may simply reflect the person's personality. **Inappropriate pitch** refers to the voice that is judged to be outside the normal range of pitch for age and/or sex. A vocal pitch that is too high may indicate underdevelopment of the larynx, whereas a vocal pitch that is excessively low may be related to endocrinological problems such as hypothyroidism. It is also possible that a vocal pitch that is excessively high or low may be related to personal preference or habit.

Pitch breaks are sudden uncontrolled upward or downward changes in pitch. Pitch breaks are common among young men who are going through puberty, but this condition usually resolves itself over time. Certain types of laryngeal pathologies and/or abnormal neurological conditions can be related to pitch breaks.

Disorders of Vocal Loudness

Loudness is the perceptual correlate of vocal intensity. Two aspects related to vocal loudness may indicate a voice disorder. The first is **monoloudness.** A monoloud voice lacks normal variations of intensity that occur during speech, and there may be an inability to change vocal loudness voluntarily. Monoloudness may be a reflection of neurological impairment or psychiatric disability or merely a habit associated with the person's personality. **Loudness variations** are extreme variations in vocal intensity in which the voice is either too soft or too loud for the particular speaking situation. The inability to control vocal loudness may reflect a loss of neural control of the respiratory or laryngeal mechanism. Psychological problems may also contribute to abnormal variations in vocal loudness.

Disorders of Vocal Quality

Several perceptual characteristics of the voice are related to vocal quality. *Hoarseness/roughness* is the first. A hoarse/rough voice lacks clarity, and the voice is noisy. Pathologies that affect vocal fold vibration can result in a hoarse/rough vocal quality. Some of these pathologies are discussed later in this chapter. A hoarse/rough voice can also be a temporary condition that results from minor forms of vocal misuse or abuse that produce vocal fold swelling called edema.

Some research suggests that normal female voices are perceived to be more breathy than normal male voices. Research also suggests that young women use more air than young men to produce a syllable.

Breathiness is the perception of audible air escaping through the glottis during phonation. Excessive airflow through the glottis usually indicates inadequate glottal closure during vocal fold vibration. The inability to close the glottis during vocal fold vibration may be related to the presence of a lesion on the vocal folds that prevents closure or some form of neurological impairment.

Tremor involves variations in the pitch and loudness of the voice that are not under voluntary control. **Vocal tremor** is usually an indication of a loss of central nervous system control over the laryngeal mechanism. **Strain and struggle** behaviors are related to difficulties initiating and maintaining voice. During speech production, the voice fades in and out, and actual voice stoppages may occur. Strain and struggle behaviors are usually related to neurological impairment, but psychological problems may also cause them.

Nonphonatory Vocal Disorders

Stridor is noisy breathing or involuntary sound that accompanies inspiration and expiration. Stridor is indicative of a narrowing somewhere in the airway. Stridor is always abnormal and serious because its presence represents a blockage of the airway.

Excessive throat clearing, a frequent accompaniment to many voice disorders, is an attempt to clear mucus from the vocal folds. Although throat clearing is a normal behavior, it is considered abnormal when it occurs with excessive frequency.

Consistent aphonia is the persistent absence of voice and perceived as whispering. Aphonia may be related to vocal fold paralysis, disorders of the central nervous system, or psychological problems. **Episodic aphonia** is uncontrolled, unpredictable aphonic breaks in voice that can last for a

FIGURE 9.1
....

Perceptual signs of voice disorders.

Source: Based on Colton and Casper (1990).

I. Pitch

  A. Monopitch

  B. Inappropriate pitch

  C. Pitch breaks

II. Loudness

  A. Monoloudness

  B. Inappropriate loudness
     (soft, loud, uncontrolled)

III. Quality

  A. Hoarseness/roughness

  B. Breathiness

  C. Tremor

  D. Strain/struggle

IV. Nonphonatory Behaviors

  A. Stridor

  B. Excessive throat clearing

V. Aphonia

  A. Consistent

  B. Episodic

fraction of a second or longer. Central nervous system disorders and psychological problems can contribute to episodic aphonia. The perceptual signs of voice disorders are summarized in Figure 9.1.

Before we turn our attention to specific voice disorders, note that many of the perceptual signs of voice disorders can be objectively quantified with clinical instruments that are readily available to the SLP (Behrman & Orlikoff, 1997). Briefly, quantitative assessments of the voice are easily made by using specially designed computer hardware and software. Kay Elemetrics, for example, manufactures a computer-based instrument called the VisiPitch (see Figure 9.2). It is a user-friendly instrument that permits

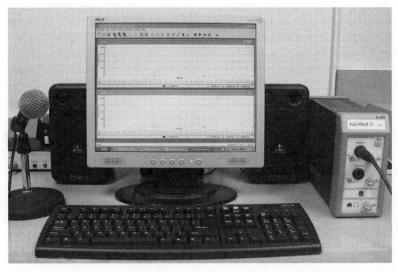

FIGURE 9.2
....
Kay Elemetrics VisiPitch.

numerous objective assessments of the physical correlates of pitch, loudness, and hoarseness/roughness. Objective assessments are valuable for diagnostic purposes as well as monitoring improvements during voice therapy. VisiPitch operations can be seen on the book's CD-ROM.

Instruments are also available that measure airflow and air volume exchanges during phonation that can be used to objectively assess vocal breathiness. These instruments can be interfaced with specially designed computer hardware and software for vocal assessment. Normative data exist for many objective correlates that are related to the perceptual signs of voice disorders (see, e.g., Baken & Orlikoff, 2000).

Three general etiologies of voice disorders are vocal misuse or abuse (functional) conditions, medical or physical (organic) conditions, and psychological or stress conditions (Ramig, 1994). The exact etiology of a specific voice disorder is not always easy to determine, and some voice disorders may have multiple causes. With this caution in mind, we use these three general etiologies to examine some of the more common disorders of voice.

Voice Disorders Associated with Vocal Misuse or Abuse

Vocal misuse and abuse are frequently claimed to contribute to structural damage of vocal fold tissue, which in turn affects vocal fold vibratory behavior. Although there is a fine distinction between vocal misuse and abuse, vocal abuse is considered to be the harsher of the two with a greater risk of injuring vocal fold tissue (Colton & Casper, 1996). Conditions and behaviors that are considered to be vocal misuse and abuse are listed in Table 9.2 and discussed below.

Vocal nodules are a common vocal fold pathology that is secondary to vocal misuse/abuse. Nodules are localized growths on the vocal folds resulting from frequent, hard vocal fold collisions that occur, for example, during yelling or shouting (Colton & Casper, 1996; Gray et al., 1987). They are generally bilateral (appearing on both vocal folds), although they can appear on only one vocal fold (see Figure 9.3). Nodules are soft and pliable early in their formation. Over time, however, they become hard and fibrous, interfering greatly with vocal fold vibration. Nodules usually appear at the juncture of the anterior one third and posterior two thirds of the vocal folds where contact is greatest. Nodules occur more frequently in adult women, particularly those

TABLE 9.2

Common conditions and behaviors considered to be misuse or abuse of the voice

Misuse	Abuse
Abrupt voicing onsets	Screaming or yelling
High laryngeal position	Excessive use of alcohol
Lack of pitch variability	Excessive throat clearing and coughing

Source: Adapted from Colton and Casper (1990).

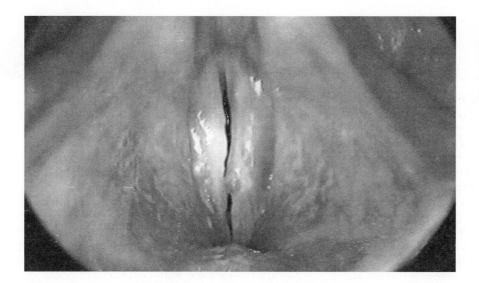

FIGURE 9.3

Unilateral vocal fold nodule. (Photograph courtesy of Robert Orlikoff, Ph.D., West Virginia University)

between 20 and 50 years of age. However, children who are prone to excessive loud talking or screaming may also develop vocal nodules; in this age group, they are more likely to develop in boys (Colton & Casper, 1996).

The primary perceptual voice symptoms of vocal nodules are hoarseness and breathiness. People who have vocal nodules may complain of soreness in the throat and an inability to use the upper third of their pitch range. Newly formed nodules are often treated with vocal rest (no talking). To prevent their return, however, people with vocal nodules need to alter the vocal behaviors that produced the nodules. Consulting an SLP for voice therapy and education is usually recommended. Longstanding nodules may require surgical removal followed by voice therapy designed to eliminate vocally abusive behaviors. See Case Study 9.2 for the personal story of a college music student with nodules that were effectively treated with therapy and vocal rest. A voice sample of a woman with bilateral vocal nodules can be heard on the book's CD-ROM.

Contact ulcers are reddened ulcerations that develop on the posterior surface of the vocal folds in the region of the arytenoid cartilages. Contact ulcers, like vocal nodules, are usually bilateral, but unlike nodules, they can be painful. Pain is usually unilateral, and it may radiate into the ear. It was once believed that contact ulcers, which occur predominantly in men older than 40 years, resulted from forceful and aggressive speaking behaviors (Colton & Casper, 1996; Titze, 1994). Contemporary thought, however, suggests that the regurgitation of stomach acids into the esophagus and throat (gastric reflux) during sleep may be an important predisposing condition for the development of contact ulcers. Stomach acids irritate vocal fold tissue, promoting excessive throat clearing, which is abusive to the tissue and causes the ulcerations (Colton & Casper, 1996).

The primary voice symptoms of contact ulcers are vocal hoarseness and breathiness. Throat clearing and vocal fatigue accompany the disorder. Although some individuals claim that contact ulcers can be treated

CASE STUDY 9.2
Personal Story of a College Woman with Vocal Nodules

Jessica, a music major, decided to pledge a sorority in the fall semester of her sophomore year. A talented vocal performer, Jessica had aspirations to teach singing and to perform professionally. During the fall semester, her course work was demanding, requiring several vocal performances and long hours of rehearsal. Pledging turned out to be demanding vocally also. Jessica was talking excessively all day long and well into the night, in addition to shouting loudly at sorority events.

During the fifth week of the semester, Jessica noted that her voice fatigued easily, she sounded hoarse, and she could not reach some of the high notes required in her singing. Her voice teacher suggested that she be evaluated at the university's speech and hearing clinic in an effort to determine the cause of her diminished vocal capacity. A perceptual and instrumental evaluation of Jessica's voice was performed by two graduate students enrolled in the university's communication disorders program. The findings of this evaluation suggested the possibility of vocal nodules. During the consultation after the evaluation, the supervising professor and the two graduate students explained their findings to Jessica

and told her that she needed to be examined by an otolaryngologist before they could proceed further. Otolaryngologic examination is required to confirm or disconfirm the presence of nodules, and speech language pathologists are required ethically to ensure that such an examination has been performed before they initiate therapy.

The otolaryngologic examination confirmed the presence of newly formed bilateral vocal nodules. Her physician prescribed complete vocal rest for a week followed by voice therapy. Jessica enrolled in voice therapy at the university for 6 weeks. Vocal hygiene was stressed during therapy sessions. Jessica was examined by her otolaryngologist at the end of week 6 of therapy. Her vocal nodules were significantly reduced in size and were no longer adversely affecting her voice.

Jessica completed her academic semester and sorority pledging successfully, graduated 2 years later, and went on to graduate school at the Juilliard School of Music in New York City. She maintains contact with the university's speech clinic and reports that she continues to practice good vocal hygiene.

effectively with voice therapy (e.g., Boone & McFarlane, 2000), others suggest that successful treatment is questionable and not well documented. Quite frequently, contact ulcers reappear after surgical removal; therefore, managing gastric reflux with medication prior to surgical intervention has been suggested (Catten et al., 1998). A voice sample of a man with contact ulcers can be heard on the book's CD-ROM.

Vocal polyps, like vocal nodules, are caused by trauma to the vocal folds associated with vocal misuse or abuse. Polyps develop when blood vessels in the vocal folds rupture and swell, developing fluid-filled lesions. Polyps tend to be unilateral, larger than nodules, vascular, and prone to hemorrhage (Colton & Casper, 1996). Unlike vocal nodules, polyps can result from a single traumatic incident such as yelling at a sporting event.

Two general types of polyps have been identified: sessile and pedunculated (Colton & Casper, 1996; Titze, 1994). A **sessile** (closely adhering or attached to vocal fold tissue) **polyp** (see Figure 9.4) can cover up to two thirds of the vocal fold. A **pedunculated polyp** appears to be attached to the vocal fold by means of a stalk and can be found on the free margins of the vocal folds as well as on the upper and lower surfaces of the folds.

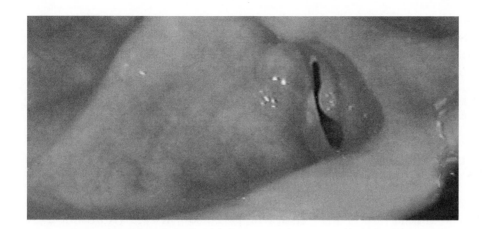

FIGURE 9.4

Sessile polyp. (Photograph courtesy of Robert Orlikoff, Ph.D., West Virginia University)

Hoarseness, breathiness, and roughness are the typical vocal symptoms, and individuals who have a vocal polyp may report the sensation of something in the throat. The combination of surgical removal of the polyp and voice therapy to eliminate vocal misuse or abuse is effective in treating this condition (Ramig, 1994).

Acute and **chronic laryngitis** are inflammation of the vocal folds that can result from exposure to noxious agents (tobacco smoke, alcohol, etc.), allergies, or vocal abuse (Colton & Casper, 1996). Acute laryngitis is a temporary swelling of the vocal folds that can result in vocal hoarseness.

Chronic laryngitis is the result of vocal abuse during periods of acute laryngitis, and it can lead to serious deterioration of vocal fold tissue. The vocal folds appear thickened, swollen, and reddened because of excessive fluid retention and dilated blood vessels in the vocal folds. If chronic laryngitis persists, a marked atrophy (wasting away of tissue) of the vocal folds will occur. The vocal folds become dry and sticky, resulting in a persistent cough, and the individual reports frequent throat aches (Boone & McFarlane, 2000). The voice symptoms of chronic laryngitis range from mild hoarseness to near aphonia. Surgery and subsequent voice therapy are usually both necessary to treat chronic laryngitis effectively.

Voice Disorders Associated with Medical or Physical Conditions

The second major group of voice disorders is those caused by central nervous system (CNS) disorders, organic disease, or laryngeal trauma. A number of the conditions discussed in this section of the chapter have a general deleterious impact on bodily functions. We focus primarily on how these conditions affect voice production.

Disorders of the CNS can result in speech and voice disorders that are characterized by muscle weakness, discoordination, tremor, or paralysis. Generally called *dysarthrias,* most involve generalized neurological damage resulting in complex patterns of speech and voice symptoms. It is useful to broadly separate CNS disorders that affect the voice into two categories: those that result in **hypoadduction,** or reduced vocal adduction, and those that result in **hyperadduction,** or increased adduction (Ramig, 1994).[1] These categories are related generally to the anatomical location of CNS lesions or disease. CNS disorders are discussed in more detail in Chapter 12, "Neurogenic Speech Disorders."

Voice Disorders Associated with Hypoadduction

Parkinson disease is a CNS disease that results in vocal fold hypoadduction. Muscle rigidity, tremor, and an overall slowness of movement, or hypokinesia, are characteristics of Parkinson disease (Aronson, 1990; Colton & Casper, 1996). Facial appearance is unemotional and sometimes referred to as masklike. The voice symptoms associated with Parkinson disease include monopitch, monoloudness, harshness, and breathiness (Duffy, 2005).

Parkinson disease is a serious medical condition treated aggressively with a variety of drugs. Although such neuropharmacological treatments have a positive effect on limb movement, speech and voice symptoms are not consistently improved. Intensive voice therapy aimed at improving vocal fold adduction has been successful in improving vocal loudness and speech intelligibility (e.g., Ramig et al., 2001). A voice sample of a man with Parkinson disease can be heard on the book's CD-ROM.

The recurrent branch of the vagus nerve was severed frequently in the early days of open heart surgery, resulting in postoperative aphonia. Improved surgical procedures have minimized this problem, although the risk still exists.

Unilateral and bilateral **vocal fold paralysis** is another common hypoadductory disorder that can result from CNS damage. The **recurrent branch** of the 10th cranial nerve (vagus) is the nerve supply for most of the laryngeal muscles associated with voice production. This nerve leaves the brain stem and travels down into the chest cavity, loops around the heart's aorta, and then courses upward, inserting into the larynx from below. Damage to this nerve can occur through injuries to the head, neck, or chest; from viral infections; and sometimes during neck or chest surgery. If the recurrent laryngeal nerve is damaged on one side, unilateral vocal fold paralysis results. If it is damaged on both sides, bilateral vocal fold paralysis results.

The voice symptoms of unilateral vocal fold paralysis include a hoarse, weak, and breathy voice quality. The paralyzed vocal fold is flaccid (limp or weak) in comparison to the nonparalyzed vocal fold. Therefore, the two vocal folds vibrate at different speeds, resulting in **diplophonia,** the perception of two vocal frequencies. The voice is very weak or totally absent in cases of bilateral vocal fold paralysis. If nerve regeneration and improved function are not observed within 6 months after the injury, surgical treatment may be required to facilitate vocal fold closure. Collagen or Teflon can sometimes be injected surgically into a paralyzed vocal fold to

---

[1]Ramig (1994) also proposes a third category, called phonatory instability, which is characterized by involuntary variations of pitch and loudness.

build up its mass. Vocal fold implantation helps to promote vocal fold contact. Voice therapy after surgery aims at increasing vocal fold closure and vocal loudness. Three examples of vocal fold paralysis can be heard on the book's CD-ROM.

Voice Disorders Associated with Hyperadduction

Spastic dysarthria is a neurological motor speech disturbance that results in vocal fold hyperadduction. It is caused by bilateral damage to the brain usually as a result of strokes, brain injuries, or multiple sclerosis. People with bilateral damage who have spastic dysarthria also have great difficulty swallowing and speaking. These individuals may also exhibit emotional lability or break into fits of crying or laughing for no apparent reason. Such behaviors appear to be uncontrolled. Prominent voice symptoms of spastic dysarthria include harshness, pitch breaks, and a strained or strangled voice quality (Duffy, 2005). These symptoms are all characteristic of vocal fold hyperadduction.

Another neurological disorder associated with hyperadduction of the vocal folds is called **spasmodic dysphonia** (SD). SD occurs with equal incidence in men and women, and the average age of onset is 45 to 50 years of age. For years, SD was believed to be a psychological voice disturbance resulting from stress, anxiety, or emotional trauma. We know now that SD can be neurological, psychological, or idiopathic (of unknown etiology). Psychological or **psychogenic** voice disturbances are discussed later in this chapter. SD of neurological origin results from an abnormal adductor laryngospasm that causes a strained, effortful, tight voice and intermittent voice stoppages. SD is often associated with voice tremor that is best heard during prolongation of the /a/ vowel. Botulinum toxin injection into specific laryngeal muscles causing incomplete paralysis is the preferred method of treatment for neurological or idiopathic SD (Duffy, 2005). A voice sample of a woman with SD can be heard on the book's CD-ROM.

Other Conditions that Affect Voice Production

A number of other conditions unrelated to CNS disorders can affect the larynx and, in turn, voice production. **Laryngeal papillomas** are small wartlike growths that cover the vocal folds and the interior aspects of the larynx. These lesions are caused by a papovavirus and are common in children younger than 6 years (Boone & McFarlane, 2000; Colton & Casper, 1996). Papillomas are noncancerous, but they can obstruct the airway, hindering breathing. Children with the disorder exhibit stridor during inhalation and may be aphonic (Wilson, 1987). Papillomas must be surgically removed, but they have a strong tendency to reappear, requiring multiple operations that may damage vocal fold tissue.

Congenital laryngeal webbing is present at birth. Congenital webs typically form on the anterior aspects of the vocal folds and can interfere

Botulinum toxin (Botox) is one of the most poisonous substances known. It is produced by bacteria found in contaminated meat products. When ingested, it causes paralysis of muscles in the body, including the respiratory muscles that regulate breathing, and can lead to death. However, in small doses injected into localized areas, Botox has been found to be a safe and effective way to weaken or paralyze selected muscles temporarily for medical and cosmetic reasons including reducing abnormal muscle contractions, managing pain, and reducing the appearance of wrinkles.

Over 75% of people who are diagnosed with cancer of the larynx are or were heavy cigarette smokers. Particles in tobacco smoke are a major irritant to vocal fold tissue.

with breathing. Laryngeal webbing must be removed surgically. Webs may produce a high-pitched, hoarse voice quality.

Laryngeal cancer is the most serious organic disorder of the voice; it has been linked to cigarette smoking and the excessive use of alcohol. One of the early signs of laryngeal cancer is persistent hoarseness in the absence of colds or allergies (Ramig, 1994). Once cancer is diagnosed, it is frequently necessary to remove the entire larynx to prevent the spread of the cancer to other parts of the body. When the larynx is removed surgically, the trachea is repositioned to form a stoma (mouthlike opening) on the anterior aspect of the throat for breathing purposes. Two voice samples of a man and a woman with laryngeal cancer can be heard on the book's CD-ROM.

Removal of the larynx requires alternate methods of producing voice. Some alaryngeal (without larynx) speakers use a technique called **esophageal speech,** which uses the esophagus as a vibratory source. Essentially, these individuals learn to speak using "burps" as a substitute for actual voice production. Some individuals are incapable of producing esophageal speech. Several prosthetic devices are available to produce an alternative form of voicing for these alaryngeal speakers. One such device is a battery-powered **electrolarynx.** The electrolarynx has a vibrating diaphragm that is placed on the lateral aspects of the neck. This vibration excites the air in the vocal tract and thus serves as an alternate form of voicing. Some alaryngeal speakers may be candidates for devices that are inserted through a surgical opening in the throat. A device called a **tracheoesophageal shunt (TEP)** directs air from the trachea into the esophagus, allowing the speaker to use respiratory air and a muscle of the esophagus, the cricopharyngeous muscle, for voice production (Ramig, 1994). This device enhances esophageal speech. Voice samples of a man and a woman using a TEP can be heard on the book's CD-ROM. Other augmentative and alternative communication systems are available (see Chapter 15).

Trauma can damage the nerve supply to the larynx or cause structural damage to laryngeal cartilages and vocal folds. For example, a condition associated with surgical intubation of the larynx (respiratory tube placed between the vocal folds) is called **granuloma** (see Figure 9.5).

The severity of this condition is directly related to the size of the tube and the length of time it is in place between the vocal folds (Titze, 1994). Granulomas are ruptured capillaries covered with epithelial tissue (Colton & Casper, 1996). The preferred treatment for granuloma is surgical removal followed by voice therapy.

Voice Disorders Associated with Psychological or Stress Conditions

Your voice involuntarily responds to emotional changes. Strong emotional reactions such as extreme sadness, fear, anger, or happiness are reflected by your voice. When experiencing strong emotions, you might not be able to control your voice.

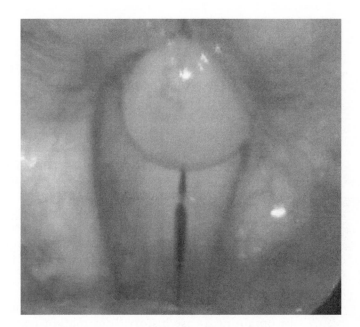

FIGURE 9.5

Granuloma. (Photograph courtesy of Robert Orlikoff, Ph.D., West Virginia University)

Strong emotions, when they are suppressed, can cause *psychogenic* voice disorders. Psychogenic voice disorders that are the result of psychological suppression of emotion are called **conversion disorders** because the person is converting emotional conflicts into physical symptoms. In these cases, the vocal folds are structurally normal, and they function normally for nonspeech behaviors. One type of vocal conversion disorder is called **conversion aphonia.** People who suffer from conversion aphonia whisper to produce voice. Although these individuals are capable of coughing and clearing the throat, indicating the capability of glottal closure, they do not approximate the vocal folds for speech production. In many cases, people with conversion aphonia believe they have a physical condition that prevents them from using their voice (Duffy, 2005).

It is believed that conversion aphonias develop out of a desire to avoid some type of personal conflict or unpleasant situation in the person's life (Duffy, 2005). Conversion aphonia is not a common condition, and it will likely persist until the person is willing to resolve the emotional conflict. People with deep-rooted psychological problems may require psychotherapy or psychiatric treatment.

THE VOICE EVALUATION AND INTERVENTION

Evaluation and treatment of voice disorders requires a multidisciplinary team approach. The specific nature of the disorder determines the precise composition of the team. At the very least, however, the team needs to comprise an otolaryngologist and an SLP.

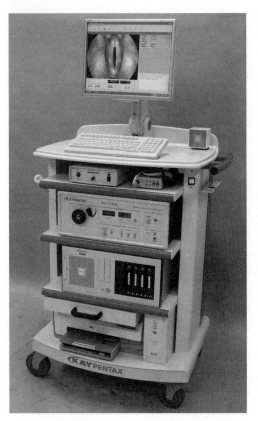

FIGURE 9.6
....

An endoscope. (Courtesy of KayPENTAX)

Fiber optics are specially constructed flexible, tubular-shaped rods of glass that conduct light in only one direction. In an endoscope, small fiber optics transmit light from a source to illuminate an object, and a larger fiber optic transmits light from the illuminated object to a camera lens or viewing instrument.

The Voice Evaluation

The first step in the evaluation of any suspected voice disorder is an examination performed by an otolaryngologist. The otolaryngologic examination provides information about vocal fold tissue damage, presence of nodules, polyps, or other abnormal growths. A direct examination of the vocal folds and other laryngeal structures is essential to determine whether the voice disorder has an organic basis. The otolaryngologist makes direct observation of the laryngeal structures using laryngeal mirrors (similar to the mirror used by a dentist) or with an **endoscope.** An endoscope (see Figure 9.6) is basically a lens coupled with a light source. The light source[2] illuminates the larynx, and laryngeal structures are viewed through the lens. Biopsies of vocal fold tissue may be taken if laryngeal cancer is suspected.

The SLP's role in the voice evaluation typically begins by obtaining a case history. Information regarding the nature of the voice disorder, how it affects daily life activities, the developmental history and duration of the disorder, the person's social and vocational use of the voice, and his or her overall physical and psychological condition are important areas of interest in taking a case history (Colton & Casper, 1996).

A perceptual evaluation is also conducted to describe the pitch, loudness, and voice quality characteristics of the voice. In some clinical situations, detailed acoustic and physiological data regarding vocal function are collected and compared to normative data. The data obtained by the otolaryngologist and the SLP are considered collectively, and a therapeutic plan is recommended.

Intervention for Voice Disorders Associated with Vocal Misuse or Abuse

Treatment of any voice disorder may involve behavioral voice therapy, surgical intervention, psychological or psychiatric counseling, drug treatments, or various combinations of these. Treatment protocol decisions are based on the specific needs of the individual and the established clinical efficacy of the treatment (Ramig, 1994). Voice therapy is frequently the clinical method of choice for voice disorders that have resulted from vocal misuse or abuse.

When voice therapy is the primary treatment method, the SLP works toward several goals: (1) restore the vocal fold tissue to a healthy condition,

[2]The light source can be a stroboscopic light that flashes light rapidly in synchrony with vocal fold vibration.

FIGURE 9.7
....
Behaviors that promote good vocal hygiene.

Drink plenty of fluids, especially water.	Avoid loud, dry, or smoky environments.
Limit the intake of caffeine.	Do not use "unnatural" voices, such as imitating cartoon characters.
Limit the intake of alcoholic beverages.	Practice vocal rest.
Avoid tobacco products.	Avoid excessive throat clearing and coughing.
Avoid yelling and screaming.	
Speak at a comfortable loudness level; don't "push" your voice.	

(2) regain clear and full vocal function, (3) identify and eliminate behaviors that are abusive to the voice, and (4) establish improved vocal habits (Colton & Casper, 1996). Figure 9.7 lists some suggestions for good **vocal hygiene** that the SLP might recommend during a counseling session. When voice therapy is a secondary treatment method, as after the surgical removal of vocal nodules or polyps, the SLP works toward these goals: restore healthy vocal function, help the individual discover the "best" voice of which he or she is capable, and make environmental changes as necessary (Colton & Casper, 1996).

The SLP uses a number of therapeutic techniques in an effort to reach the goals just outlined: breathing and relaxation exercises, soft glottal attacks (initiation of voice with a whisper), reducing vocal loudness, and a variety of other techniques that facilitate healthy use of the voice. The therapeutic process may also involve discussions regarding personal concerns, and it is important that the SLP listen in nonjudgmental fashion. It is also essential that the SLP provide support and encouragement that will help an individual accept a changed or restored voice (Colton & Casper, 1996).

Intervention for Voice Disorders Associated with Medical or Physical Conditions

Treatment of voice disorders associated with disease processes does not focus on elimination of the disorder (such as reducing the size of a nodule) or on precipitating conditions (frequent yelling at sporting events), but rather on assisting the individual to achieve the best voice possible or on establishing alternative manners to produce voice. For example, voice disorders associated with neurological problems are usually not the primary disability. Therefore, direct treatment of voice disorders associated with certain types of neurological disease may be a secondary concern to the SLP's treatment of related disabilities such as apraxia, aphasia, or dysphagia (Colton & Casper, 1996).

If voice therapy is indicated, the overriding therapeutic goal is to assist the individual to produce the best voice possible to remain communicatively functional in vocational and social settings. Additionally, the SLP can be helpful in assessing the effects of medications or surgery on voice production. Some of the specific techniques that the SLP uses to establish the best voice possible include increasing respiratory function for speech, changing speaking rate, and changing the overall prosody of speech. It is essential that the SLP recognize the limitations of voice therapy for certain medical or physical conditions and help the individual to achieve the best possible means of communication (Colton & Casper, 1996).

Intervention for Voice Disorders Associated with Psychological or Stress Conditions

Treatment of voice disorders associated with psychological or stress conditions can be effective if the SLP succeeds in convincing the individual that there is nothing wrong physically with his or her voice. Individuals who have recognized conditions of stress or emotional conflict in their life and the relation of this stress to their voice problem are the best candidates for voice therapy. These individuals want the ability to use their voice again, and the SLP can help the patient see how his or her psychosocial history may have contributed to the voice problem (Duffy, 2005).

A recommended therapeutic technique for voice disorders associated with psychological or stress conditions (conversion aphonia) begins by having the individual initiate voice from a grunt to a sigh to a prolonged sound, then to a syllable or word (e.g., "uh-huh"). Such techniques provide solid evidence to the individual that he or she is physically capable of normal voice production (Boone & McFarlane, 2000; Duffy, 2005).

For many individuals with conversion aphonia or dysphonia, voice can return to normal in minutes or over several sessions with the help of the SLP. For these individuals, in fact, psychiatric referral is often not needed after successful treatment by the SLP (c.f. Duffy, 2005).

Efficacy of Voice Therapy

Assessing the efficacy of the treatment of voice disorders is complex because of the variety of conditions that produce voice disorders; varying severity levels of specific types of voice disorders; the variety and combinations of behavioral, pharmacological, and surgical treatments available; and the manner in which treatment efficacy is defined. Despite these complexities, clinical and experimental data suggest a general clinical effectiveness. In particular, voice disorders associated with vocal misuse or abuse, including those with structural tissue damage, some voice disorders associated with medical or physical conditions like Parkinson disease, and voice disorders associated with psychological or stress conditions, respond reasonably well to treatment. See Box 9.1 for specific approaches and techniques that have been shown to be effective.

BOX 9.1
Evidence-Based Practices for Individuals with Voice Disorders

General intervention with laryngeal-based voice disorders

- SLP administered voice intervention is effective when medical intervention, such as surgery, is not warranted.
- For some types of laryngeal pathology, SLP voice intervention may be as effective or more effective than medical intervention.
- In general, treatment pre- and postsurgery results in better outcomes.

Specific behavioral treatment approaches or techniques

- Systematic programs of vocal rest, such as the *Voice Use Reduction Program,* provide specific guidelines on when and how much the voice can be used during a particular day or week, and in which communicative situations, with voice use progressively increasing as the voice improves. Such programs are effective in improving voice disorders associated with vocal abuse and misuse.
- Vocal function exercises (e.g., pitch glides, sustained low or high pitches) are effective in treating psychogenic voice disorders, as well as voice disorders associated with laryngeal hyperfunction by lowering the larynx and facilitating production of a more relaxed voice.
- The *Yawn-Sigh* technique also effectively lowers the larynx and opens the glottis, thereby decreasing laryngeal strain and facilitating ease of phonation.

This technique is suggested for individuals with laryngeal pathology associated with vocal hyperfunction (e.g., vocal nodules).

- Vocal hygiene programs, which involve educating individuals about voice production, and identifying and providing alternatives to vocally abusive behaviors (e.g., yelling, excessive throat clearing), are somewhat effective in eliminating or preventing these behaviors that can often lead to laryngeal pathology. Patient adherence is a critical variable, however. Classroom-based vocal hygiene programs may also prove useful for young children but require age-appropriate materials and teaching aids.
- An intensive treatment focused on increasing loudness, the *Lee Silverman Voice Treatment (LSVT)*, has repeatedly shown to improve voice production in both children and adults with neurological diseases (e.g., cerebral palsy, Parkinson disease, and multiple sclerosis). Therapy entails practicing using a louder voice while saying /a/, producing functional sentences, and producing utterances of increasing complexity four times per week for 4 weeks.

Source: Based on Behrman et al. (2008); Boone and McFarlane (1993); Elliott et al. (1997); Fox et al. (2002, 2006); Pindzola (1993); Ramig and Verdolini (2009); Roy et al. (2001); Sabol et al. (1995); and van der Merwe (2004).

SUMMARY

The human larynx is a versatile instrument that, in addition to its primary biological function of protecting the lower airways from invasion of foreign substances, serves as the primary sound generator for spoken communication. The human voice reflects one's personality, general state of health and age, and emotional condition. Vocal function changes in predictable ways as one matures. The infant's crying to satisfy some particular need soon gives way to more purposeful communication designed to control his or her environment. Most adults have full control over their voices and are capable of a wide assortment of differentiated vocalizations that convey meaning, attitude, and emotion.

Disorders of the voice affect a substantial number of people in the United States. These disorders can range from relatively uncomplicated abnormalities such as vocal hoarseness resulting from yelling excessively at a sporting event to life-threatening cancer of the larynx. Voice disorders vary in both etiology and severity, and the specific method of treatment in large measure is dictated by the etiology and severity of the disorder.

SLPs play a pivotal role in the treatment of voice disorders, but effective and ethical intervention demands a team approach. In many instances, surgical intervention followed by voice therapy is the treatment protocol of choice; in other instances, voice therapy may precede surgery, perhaps rendering surgery unnecessary. Dealing effectively with individuals with voice disorders requires detailed and specific knowledge about normal and abnormal laryngeal functioning. Because many voice disorders respond well to techniques used by SLPs, it can be a rewarding and exciting clinical endeavor.

THOUGHT QUESTIONS

- Do you think there is such a thing as a "voiceprint" similar to a person's fingerprint?
- If you were prescribed a specified period of vocal rest, how would your daily life activities be affected? Could you comply with this treatment approach?
- What materials or activities might you use to implement a program of vocal hygiene successfully with young children?

SUGGESTED READINGS

Colton, R. H., & Casper, J. K. (1996). *Understanding voice problems: A physiological perspective for diagnosis and treatment* (2nd ed.). Baltimore: Williams & Wilkins.

Hollien, H. (2002). *Forensic voice identification.* San Diego, CA: Academic Press.

The entire issue of the *Language, Speech, and Hearing Services in Schools, 35*(4) (2004) is devoted to the assessment and treatment of children with voice disorders.

Titze, I. R. (1994). *Principles of voice production.* Englewood Cliffs, NJ: Prentice Hall.

ONLINE RESOURCES

National Center for Voice and Speech
www.ncvs.org/ncvs/tutorials/voiceprod/index.html
The National Center for Voice and Speech site has free voice production tutorials and computer simulation models of vocal fold vibration.

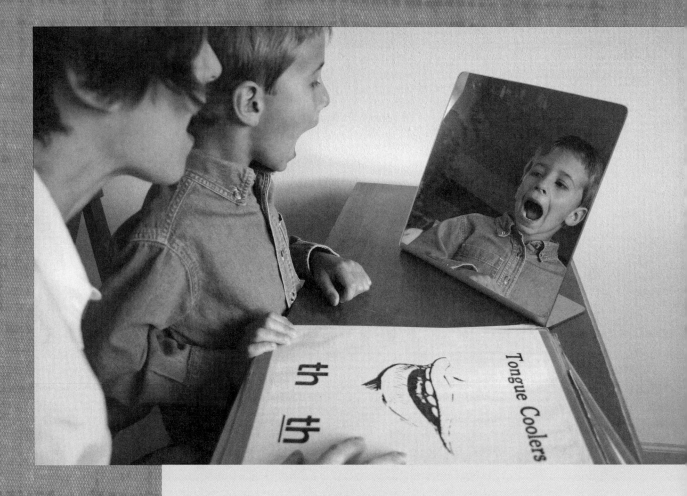

CHAPTER LEARNING GOALS

When you have finished this chapter, you should be able to:

- Describe the nature of speech sounds and the relationship between phonology and articulation

- Describe the correlates and causes of disorders of articulation and phonology

- Explain the procedures for assessing speech-sound disorders

- Describe the approaches and techniques for treatment of articulatory and phonological disorders and the supporting evidence available

10

Disorders of Articulation and Phonology

Although the written alphabet we use contains 26 letters, spoken English has 41 to 43 different speech sounds. In this chapter, we are concerned primarily with speech sounds, or phonemes, which are combined to form spoken words, phrases, and sentences. For example, the word "cat" contains three phonemes [kæt]. Note that phonemes and letters are not the same. The word "that" also has three phonemes [ðæt]. Phonemes are generally written between two slashes, as in /p/; transcribed phonemic combinations such as words are often transcribed between brackets as in [ðæt]. Some phonemes are universal and found in all languages; other phonemes are used in only a few languages. For example, the tongue clicks used in some African languages are not used as phonemes in English. In general, the more phonemes two languages have in common, the more similar the languages sound. The phonemic symbols for standard American English speech sounds are shown in Table 10.1.

In addition to phonemes, which are the building blocks of speech, *phonotactic* rules exist that specify acceptable sequences and locations. For example, the "ks" combination is never used at the beginning of an English word, but it is fine at the end in words such as "books" [bʊks]. Many Polish and Russian names are difficult for English speakers to pronounce because these Slavic languages permit consonant combinations that are not found in English.

Each phoneme is really a family of related sounds and may be said with some variation but still be considered that particular phoneme. These variations are called **allophones.** Compare the "p" in the words "pot" and "spot." When "p" is at the beginning of a word and followed by a vowel it is pronounced with a little puff of air (**aspiration**), but in most regions of the United States, when "p" is immediately preceded by "s," it is not aspirated.

TABLE 10.1

Phonemic symbols for standard American English speech sounds

Consonants				Vowels			
Phoneme	Example	Phoneme	Example	Phoneme	Example	Phoneme	Example
/p/	pan	/ʃ/	shed	/i/	eat	/ɔ/	sauce
/b/	boot	/ʒ/	measure	/ɪ/	pit	/ɑ/	father
/t/	tall	/h/	high	/e/	cake		
/d/	down	/tʃ/	chop	/ɛ/	bed	Diphthongs	
/k/	kite	/dʒ/	jump	/æ/	at	Phoneme	Example
/g/	go	/m/	mat	/ʌ/	cup	/aɪ/	ice
/f/	fan	/n/	noon	/ə/	above	/aʊ/	cow
/v/	vase	/ŋ/	ring	/ɝ/	bird	/ɔɪ/	toy
/θ/	thumb	/l/	lamb	/ɚ/	paper		
/ð/	then	/w/	wit	/u/	you		
/s/	sun	/j/	yellow	/ʊ/	would		
/z/	zoo	/r/	rod	/o/	no		

Allophonic variations contribute to regional and foreign dialects. The examples given in the text do not apply to all English speakers.

Still, we recognize both as /p/. If the wrong allophone is used, the spoken words do not sound right.

We begin our discussion of articulation and phonology with information about how sounds are produced and classified. We examine the distinction between articulation and phonology, then we go on to describe development of speech and impairments that may be related to articulatory and phonological disorders. The second half of the chapter is devoted to assessment and treatment. Case Study 10.1 describes a child diagnosed with impaired speech sound production skills who was successfully treated by the speech-language pathologist.

UNDERSTANDING SPEECH SOUNDS

All spoken languages have vowels and consonants. The intelligibility of the utterance is determined largely by the consonants, whereas the sound energy comes primarily from the vowels.

Phonemes are often categorized as either **vowel** or **consonant.** Very generally, vowels are produced with a relatively open or unobstructed vocal tract, and consonants are made with some degree of constriction.

Consonant phonemes may be classified according to which articulators are used (place of articulation), how the sound is made (manner of production), and whether they occur with laryngeal vibration (voicing). Vowels are normally described according to tongue and lip position and relative degree of tension in these articulators. In addition, the concept of **distinctive features** is sometimes used to describe both vowels and consonants. These methods of characterizing phonemes are described in the next few pages.

CASE STUDY 10.1
Case Study of a Child with an Articulation Disorder: Kee

Although his grandparents are somewhat recent immigrants, Kee was born in the United States and speaks only English. Thoroughly acculturated, he loves baseball and pizza. Now in fifth grade, Kee has no remnants of the articulation problem he experienced as a younger child.

Kee's parents became concerned about his speech when he was a preschooler. Unsure who to ask, they inquired of the family physician, who told them that it was normal for children to have speech sound problems, and they shouldn't worry. Reassured, they made no further inquiries.

In kindergarten, Kee was identified as a child with a possible speech problem and his parents agreed to further testing by the speech-language pathologist. He determined that Kee had difficulty with both the "s" and "sh"

sounds and to a lesser extent with the "z," demonstrating a frontal lisp on all three. Prognosis was good because Kee produced the "s" and "sh" correctly 12% and 19% of the time, respectively, and the "z" 42% of the time.

Kee received speech-language pathology services in school twice per week beginning in kindergarten. In the middle of second grade he was dismissed from therapy because of satisfactory progress.

As you read the chapter, think about

- Possible explanations for Kee's difficulties.
- Possible ways Kee's speech-language pathologist may have gathered diagnostic data.
- Possible intervention methods that may have contributed to Kee's progress.

Classification of Consonants by Place and Manner

As we mentioned, consonants are characterized by constriction somewhere along the vocal tract. This point of contact or constriction is used to classify consonants. Consonants in which constriction is made with both lips are called **bilabial,** meaning "two lips." **Labiodental** consonants are made with the bottom lip and upper teeth in contact. **Interdental** consonants are produced with the tongue between the teeth and are sometimes called **linguadental. Alveolar** sounds are made when the tongue tip is touching the alveolar or upper gum ridge. In **palatal** consonants, the center of the tongue is near the hard palate. The rear of the tongue approaches the velum or soft palate in the production of **velar** consonants. When the constriction occurs at the level of the vocal folds, the phonemes produced are called **glottal.**

Consonants may be *voiced or voiceless,* that is, produced with or without laryngeal vibration. **Obstruents,** in which airflow is blocked or obstructed, include stops, fricatives, and affricates. In the production of **stops,** air pressure is built up behind the point of constriction, momentarily stopped, and then released, as in the /p/ sound. **Fricatives** are nonresonants that are made with a narrow passageway for the air to pass through, creating a frictionlike sound. **Affricates** begin as stops and then are released as fricatives. **Resonants** are the **nasals** and **approximants.** The special characteristic of nasals is that they are produced with resonance in the nasal cavity. Approximants include **glides** and **liquids.** Glides occur when the articulatory posture changes gradually from consonant to vowel. Liquids include /l/ and /r/.

TABLE 10.2

Classification of American English consonants by manner and place of production

Manner	Place Bilabial VL V*	Labio-dental VL V*	Inter-dental VL V*	Alveolar VL V*	Palatal VL V*	Velar VL V*	Glottal VL V*
Nonresonants							
Stops	p b			t d		k g	
Fricatives		f v	θ ð	s z	ʃ ʒ		h
Affricates					tʃ ʤ		
Resonants							
Nasal	m			n		ŋ	
Approximants							
Glides	w				j	w	
Liquids				l	ɹ		

*VL = voiceless; V = voiced.

Source: Adapted from *Fundamentals of Phonetics: A Practical Guide for Students,* by L. H. Small, 1999. Boston: Allyn and Bacon. Used with permission.

Table 10.2 depicts the classification of consonants by manner and place of production.

Classification of Vowels by Tongue and Lip Position and Tension

Vowels are produced by resonating the exhaled air within the oral cavity. The exact sound that is made depends on which part of the tongue is elevated (front, center, or back), its relative height (high, mid, or low), and the amount of tension (tense or lax) in the articulators. Whether the lips are rounded (pursed) or retracted (pulled back into a sort of smile) also influences the sound that is produced. Figure 10.1 is a diagram of American

FIGURE 10.1

Classification of American English vowels by height and frontness/backness of tongue.

Source: Adapted from Shriberg & Kent (1995) and Yavas (1998).

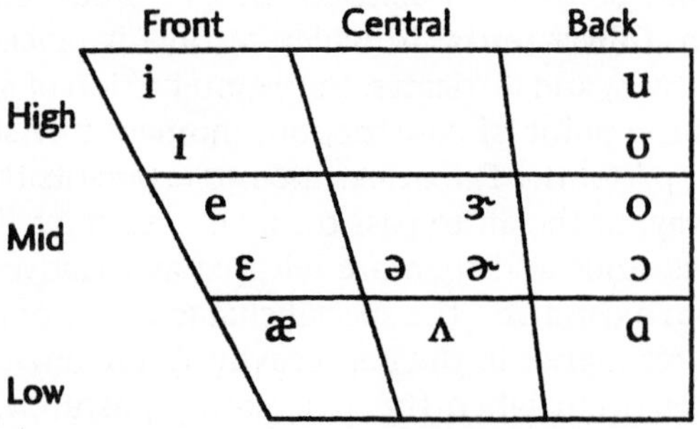

English vowels. In the figure, the higher vowel of the front and back paired vowels and /ɝ/ are relatively tense; all other vowels are lax. High and mid back vowels and the back central vowels are produced with the lips somewhat rounded. All other English vowels are unrounded. All English vowels are normally voiced and not nasal. Exceptions occur when you whisper and when nasal resonance occurs for any number of reasons including proximity to a nasal phoneme, such as /m/ or /n/.

When two vowels are said in close proximity, they produce a special type of phoneme called a **diphthong.** In English, the vowels in the words "sigh," "now," and "boy" are diphthongs. "Sigh" contains /aɪ/, "now" has /aʊ/, and "boy" contains /ɔɪ/. To see animations with sounds, along with step-by-step descriptions of all the sounds in American English, go to the University of Iowa Web site listed at the end of the chapter.

Distinctive Feature Analysis

In an attempt to provide a system for describing phonemes found in all languages, linguists identified the components of individual sounds and called these distinctive features. Each phoneme can then be theoretically identified by the presence or absence of each of these features (Chomsky & Halle, 1968). For example, three English phonemes (/m/, /n/, and /ŋ/) are produced with nasal resonance. They are considered + nasal. All other English phonemes are − nasal. To further distinguish among the nasal phonemes, we might note that /m/ and /n/ are produced with obstruction in the front portion of the mouth; they are + anterior, whereas /ŋ/ is − anterior. The phonemes /m/ and /n/ can be differentiated on the basis of the distinctive feature "distributed." If the constriction extends for some distance along the direction of the airflow, it is + distributed. In the example we are using, /m/ is considered + distributed; /n/ is − distributed.

The concept of distinctive feature analysis has been helpful in finding patterns of speech-sound errors and thereby facilitating their correction. Figure 10.2 contains brief definitions and examples of some of the more commonly used distinctive features.

SPEECH-SOUND DEVELOPMENT THROUGH THE LIFESPAN

Although you gained early control of most of the muscles needed for speech, it took you longer to perfect their movement and to learn to produce all the sounds of American English. Even so, most children can produce English speech sounds by early elementary school.

Pre-Speech

Although newborns produce predominantly reflexive sounds, such as fussing and crying, and vegetative sounds, such as burping and swallowing, both

Anterior:	Sounds produced with an obstruction in the front portion of the mouth—specifically, labials, dentals, and alveolars
	Examples of + anterior: /m, p, b, f, v, θ, ð, n, t, d/
Consonantal:	Sounds produced with obstruction in the oral cavity—specifically, obstruents and nasals
	Examples of + consonantal: /s, z, t, d, m, n, r, l/
	Examples of − consonantal: /æ, i, e, o, u/
Continuant:	Sounds in which the air may flow without interruption—specifically, fricatives, glides, liquids, vowels.
	Examples of + continuant: /f, v, s, z, h, j, r, l, i, e, o, u/
	Examples of − continuant: /p, t, k, b, d, g/
Distributed:	Consonants produced with a constriction that extends a relatively long distance along the direction of airflow
	Examples of + distributed: /m, p, b, ʃ, ʒ, tʃ, ʤ/
Nasal:	Phonemes produced with a lowered soft palate
	Examples of + nasal: /m, n, ŋ/
Sonorant:	Sounds produced with a relatively open vocal tract, such that spontaneous voicing is possible—specifically, vowels, nasals, liquids, glides
	Examples of + sonorant: /æ, o, m, n, l, r, w, j/
	Examples of − sonorant: /p, b, t, d, k, g, ʃ, tʃ
Strident:	Sounds in which the airstream is constricted in such a way as to produce a high-intensity noise
	Examples of + strident: /s, z, f, v/
	Examples of − strident /p, b, i, e, o/
Syllabic:	Sounds that serve as the nucleus of a syllable—specifically vowels, syllabic liquids, syllabic nasals
	Examples of + syllabic: [bʌ tn̠] as in "button"
	Examples of − syllabic: the /b/ and /t/ in "button."
Voiced:	Sounds produced with vocal fold vibration—specifically all vowels, nasals, glides, voiced consonants
	Examples of + voice: /i, e, o, m, n, j, w, b, d, g, z, v/
	Examples of − voice: /p, t, k, s, f/

FIGURE 10.2
. . . .

Definitions and examples of some common distinctive features.

Source: Based on Chomsky & Halle (1968).

decrease with maturation. This disappearance is related to the rapid rate of brain growth and to myelination. **Myelination** is the development of a protective myelin sheath or sleeve around the cranial nerves. Myelination is not completed until adulthood.

Initially, newborns cry on both inhalation and exhalation. The expiration phase—a more efficient sound production source—gradually increases. Crying helps children to become accustomed to air flow across the vocal folds and to modifying their breathing patterns. Because speech sounds originate at the level of the larynx, this early stimulation is necessary. However, noncrying vocalizations are far more important in the development of speech.

Noncrying sounds usually accompany feeding or are produced in response to smiling or talking by the caregivers. These noncrying vowellike sounds contain some *phonation* or vibration at the larynx, but the child has insufficient ability to produce full speech sounds.

By 2 months of age, infants develop nondistress sounds called either "gooing" or "cooing." During gooing, infants produce back consonant sounds similar to /g/ and /k/ and middle and back vowel sounds, such as /ʌ/ and /ʊ/, with incomplete resonance.

By 3 months of age, infants vocalize in response to the speech of others. Infants are most responsive if their caregivers respond to them.

At 5 months, infants are able to imitate the tone and pitch signals of their caregivers. Most infant imitative and nonimitative vocalizations are single-syllable units of consonant-vowel (CV) or vowel-consonant (VC) construction. These sound units that begin around 4 months are called **babbling.**

With maturity, longer sequences and prolonged individual sounds evolve. Children produce increasingly more complex combinations. Sounds are now more like adult speech sounds. As muscle control moves to the front of the oral cavity, we see strong tongue projection in 4- to 6-month-olds. Initially, back consonants predominate in babbling, but by 6 months, labial or lip sounds, such as /m/ and /p/, are produced more frequently.

Babbling is random sound play, and even deaf infants babble. During babbling, infants experiment with sound production. With age, children's babbling increasingly reflects the syllable structure and intonation of the caregivers' speech.

At about 6 or 7 months, infants' babbling begins to change to **reduplicated babbling,** which contains strings of consonant-vowel syllable repetitions or self-imitations (CV-CV-CV), such as "ma-ma-ma." Hearing ability appears to be very important. Children with deafness continue to babble, but the range of consonants decreases, and few reduplicated strings are produced.

The consonant-vowel (CV) syllable becomes one of the predominant building blocks in first words.

In contrast to babbling, reduplicated babbling more closely approximates mature speech in its resonant quality and timing. The child is beginning to adapt the speech patterns of the environment. Regardless of the language, infants' vocalizations and later first words have similar phonological patterns. For example, stops (/p, b, t, d, k, g/), nasals (/m, n, ŋ/), and approximants (/w, j/) constitute approximately 80% of the consonants in infant vocalizations and in the first 50 words of Spanish-, Korean-, and English-speaking children.

The period from 8 to 12 months has been called the *echolalic* stage. **Echolalia** is speech that is an imitation of some other speaker. At first, children imitate only those sounds they have produced spontaneously on their own.

Gradually, infants begin to use imitation to expand and modify their repertoire of speech sounds. At about the same time, they begin using gestures, with or without vocalizations, to communicate. Speech during this period is characterized by **variegated babbling,** in which adjacent and successive syllables in the string are purposely not identical.

In the second half of the first year, children begin to recognize recurring patterns of sounds within specific situations. The child may even produce sounds in these situations. For example, the child might begin to say "M-m-m" during feeding if this sound is modeled for him or her. In response to caregiver conversations, infants may begin to experiment with *jargon,* long strings of syllables with adultlike intonation.

Many speech sounds develop sound-meaning relationships. Called phonetically consistent forms (PCFs), these sound patterns function as protowords or "words" for the infant (Dore et al., 1976). The infant has noticed that adults consistently use certain sound patterns to refer to the same things in the environment.

> PCFs are the child's first attempt at consistent use of a sound to represent or "stand for" something else.

Word production depends on sound grouping and sound variation. Children adopt a problem-solving or trial-and-error approach to word production. The resultant speech is a complex interaction of the ease of production and perception of the target syllable and its member sounds.

Toddler Speech

At around 12 months of age, you probably produced your first recognizable word. Sometimes a child's word is easily recognizable to others, but some words may be modified by the child for ease of speaking.

When faced with a difficult word, children adopt similar strategies. Armed with the consonant-vowel (CV) structures of babbling and the CV-CV-CV strings of reduplicated babbling, children attempt to pronounce the adult words they encounter. It is not surprising, therefore, that many words are reduced to variations of a CV structure or other simplification. These adaptations, called phonological processes, are presented in Table 10.3.

Toddlers often omit final consonants, resulting in a CVC word being produced as CV, as in *cake* pronounced as *ca*. It is also possible that children will add an additional vowel to form the CV-CV *cake-a*. Multisyllable words may be reduced to one or two syllables, or the syllables may be repeated. For example, *telephone* might become *tephone,* and *baby* might be modified to *bebe*. If the syllables are not duplicated, only the consonants may be, as in *doggie* becoming *goggie*. Consonant blends might be shortened to single consonants, as in *stop* becoming *top*. Finally, one type of sound might be substituted for another. For example, all initial consonants in words might be pronounced as the same consonant, as in, *Go bye-bye* becoming *Bo bye-bye*.

TABLE 10.3

Phonological processes of young children

Process	Explanation	Example
Final Consonant Deletion	Reduces CVC structure to more familiar CV	*Cat* becomes *ca* *Carrot* becomes *cara* CVCVC → CVCV
Weak Syllable Deletion	Reduces number of syllables to conform to the child's ability to produce multisyllable words	*Telephone* becomes *tephone* *Vacation* becomes *cation*
Reduplication	Syllables in multisyllable words repeat	*Baby* becomes *bebe* *Mommy* becomes *mama*
Consonant Cluster Reduction	Reduces CCV+ structures to the more familiar CV	*Tree* becomes *te* *Stay* becomes *tay*
Assimilation	One consonant becomes like another, although the vowel is usually not affected	*Doggie* becomes *goggie*
Stopping	Fricatives (/f/, /v/, /s/, /z/, and others) are replaced by stops (/b/, /p/, /d/, /t/, /g/, /k/)	*Face* becomes *pace* *This* becomes *dis*
Fronting	Velars are replaced with more anteriorly produced sounds	*go* becomes *do* *ring* becomes *rin*

Preschool Speech

Most of the phonological processes described for toddlers have disappeared by age 4. Consonant blends consisting of two or more adjacent consonants, as in "strong," continue to be difficult for some children, and simplification strategies, resulting in "tong," may continue into early elementary school. Children who experience continuing phonological difficulties may persist in the use of more immature phonological processes.

Children continue to master new speech sounds throughout the preschool period. The acquisition process is a gradual one and depends on the individual sound, its location in words, its frequency of use, and its proximity to other speech sounds. A sound may be produced correctly in single words but not in connected speech.

Development of individual sounds depends on the location in words, frequency of use, and the influence of other speech sounds.

We can make a few generalizations about speech-sound acquisition by young children:

1. Phoneme acquisition is a gradual process.
2. Vowels are easier to master than consonants. Usually, English vowels are acquired by age 3, whereas some consonants may not be mastered until age 7 or 8.
3. Many sounds are first acquired in the initial position in words.
4. Consonant clusters (*consider*) and blends (*street*) are not mastered until age 7 or 8, although some clusters appear as early as age 4.
5. Some sounds are easier than others and are acquired first by most children. As a group, stops (/p, b, t, d, g, k/) and nasals (/m, n, ŋ/) are acquired first.
6. Much individual difference exists.

This information is presented in Figure 10.3. Children with neuromuscular problems, sensory deficits, perceptual problems, or poor learning skills are going to have difficulty acquiring all the sounds of the language.

School-Age Speech

By early elementary school, your phonological system probably resembled that of adults. A few children will still have difficulty with multiple consonant blends, such as *str* and *sts,* as in *street* and *beasts,* respectively.

Other developments such as **morphophonemic contrasts**—changes in pronunciation as a result of morphological changes—will take several years to master, some extending into adulthood. For example, in the verb *derive,* the second vowel is a long "i," transcribed phonetically as /aɪ/. When we change *derive* to the noun *derivative,* the second vowel is changed to sound like the "i" in *give,* transcribed as /ɪ/. Other contrasts were mentioned in Chapter 2.

Five-year-olds still have difficulty with a few consonant sounds and with consonant blends. Six-year-olds have acquired most English speech sounds. By age 8, children have acquired consonant blends, such as *str, sl,* and *dr.*

FIGURE 10.3
....
Mastery of English speech sounds.

Sources: Compiled from Olmsted (1971); Prather et al., (1975); Sanders (1972).

Ages by which most children have acquired speech sounds in all positions. Vowels are not included because they are usually mastered by age 2–3 years.	
Age 2	p, h, n, b, k
Age 3	m, w, g, f, d
Age 4	t, ʃ ("sh"), j ("y")
Age 5	s, v, ŋ ("ng"), r, l, tʃ ("ch"), z, ʤ ("j")
Age 6	θ ("th" in "<u>th</u>in"), ð ("th" in "<u>th</u>e"), ʒ ("zh" in "mea<u>s</u>ure")
Age 8	Consonant blends and clusters

Phonology and Articulation

The correct use of speech sounds within a language requires knowledge of the sounds of the language and the rules that govern their production and combination, called *phonology*. Speech also requires neuromotor coordination to actually say sounds, words, and sentences; termed *articulation*. To help you understand this distinction, visualize learning a new language such as French. You will be exposed to new words and sound combinations and begin to grasp the nature of that language's sound system or phonology. But you must also be able to form the words with your lips, tongue, and so on. You might find this very difficult because your neuromotor pathways have been trained to make English words; the inability to coordinate your muscles to produce the words correctly is a problem of articulation.

Phonological impairments are disorders of conceptualization or language rules. Remember that phonology is concerned with classes of sounds and sound patterns within words. For example, English has both open and closed syllables at the end of words. An **open syllable** is one that ends in a vowel—for example, "hi"; a **closed syllable** ends in a consonant ("hat"). A child who uses only open syllables and deletes all final consonants would be exhibiting a disorder of phonology. In this example, the child would say "hi" correctly but produce "hat" as "ha."

Articulation impairments are disorders of production. A child whose only speech error is incorrect production of the /s/ phoneme has a disorder of articulation. Disorders of articulation are typically characterized as

- Substitutions
- Omissions
- Distortions
- Additions

Substitutions occur when one phoneme is replaced with another. For example, a person who says "shair" for "chair" would be substituting "sh" for "ch." An omission is the deletion of a phoneme, as in "chai" for "chair." Distortions occur when a nonstandard form of the phoneme is used. An example of an addition would be "ch<u>uh</u>-air" for "chair." Some individuals have disorders of both phonology and articulation. We talk more about specific patterns and types of errors later in this chapter.

ASSOCIATED DISORDERS AND RELATED CAUSES

The causes of phonological and articulatory disorders in most children are not readily identifiable. In these cases, when no cause is known, it may be termed a *functional disorder*. Recognizing the limited usefulness of this concept, researchers have directed their attention to **correlates,** or related factors. Correlation means that two or more things occur together but one does not necessarily cause the other(s). Nevertheless, correlates may offer some clues to causality that should prompt further research. Figure 10.4

> The distinction between phonology and articulation is often difficult to understand. Articulation refers to the actual production of speech sounds; phonology is knowledge of speech sounds within a language and the ways in which they are combined.

> Most children with disordered articulation and phonology do not exhibit an identifiable physical reason for the problem.

FIGURE 10.4
....
Possible correlates of
phonological and
articulatory
impairments.

Hearing loss

History of otitis media during the first few years of life

Diminished speech-sound perception and discrimination ability

Atypical tooth alignment and missing teeth

Impaired oral-motor skills

Eating problems

Tongue thrust swallow after 6 years of age

Neuromotor disabilities

Mental retardation

Language difficulties

Male sex

Family history of speech delay

Low maternal education

lists some correlates of phonological impairment. In the next few sections, we describe the characteristics associated with a few well-established correlates of phonological and articulatory impairment. Data from long-term studies suggest that more persistent problems may be related to motor-speech deficits (Flipsen, 2003).

Developmental Impairment in Children

Language and speech learning is not easy. Words are composed of phonemes that are typically acquired gradually by 8 years of age. Many children with articulation and phonological difficulties exhibit a developmental impairment in speech-sound production with no readily identifiable corollary factors. Figure 10.3 lists the consonants that are typically mastered at various ages. When a child's speech is delayed, you would expect that he or she is not producing the phonemes expected at that age. Other children may be idiosyncratic in their phoneme use. Some researchers identify these children as "disordered" in their development. This dichotomy is a difficult one, however, because of the wide range of behaviors in young children (Howell & Dean, 1994; Stoel-Gammon & Dunn, 1985).

PHONOLOGICAL IMPAIRMENTS

Phonological processes involve more than individual phonemes. Final consonant deletion can involve any consonant, as when the target "Give him the book" is produced as "Gi- hi- the boo." Many children exhibit multiple processes.

As previously mentioned, children's phonological and phonotactic simplifications are called phonological patterns or processes (Table 10.3). The average age of diagnosis of a phonological disorder is 4 years, 2 months (Shriberg & Kwiatkowski, 1994), although the roots of these problems may present much earlier. Case Study 10.2 describes a young girl who demonstrates the unusual phonological process of *backing*.

CASE STUDY 10.2
Personal Story of a Child with a Phonological Disorder

Brandi was just over 3 years of age when she was first brought to the University Speech and Hearing Center by her mother, Mrs. A. Brandi had been identified in a preschool screening program as needing further evaluation. Mrs. A. noted that Brandi mispronounced many words and could not be understood by people outside of the family, Brandi's 5-year-old brother frequently interpreted Brandi's speech so that others could understand her. Examination at the center revealed that Brandi had normal hearing and physical structure for speech. Her receptive and expressive language skills were above average in all areas but phonology. Brandi was diagnosed with a moderate-to-severe phonological disorder of unknown cause, and therapy was recommended.

An example of Brandi's speech at the beginning of therapy is as follows:

Target: Stop playing with my toy.

Brandi: Kop payin' wid my koy.

Because of her young age and her high spirits, therapy was presented through structured play activities. By the end of 3 months, she frequently self-corrected in the clinical setting. At the end of a year of therapy, Brandi's mother reported that her daughter was self-correcting at home. As a result, her speech intelligibility improved dramatically, even to unfamilar listeners.

LIFESPAN ISSUES

By age 6, 75% of children outgrow their speech-sound errors; by age 9, most of these children will have normalized their errors (Shriberg, 1997). Speech therapy can help children correct speech-sound errors more quickly, however. A small percentage of children will continue to have residual sound errors, possibly throughout their lives. These often involve substitution or distortion of /r/, /s/, /z/ and/or/ /l/. Such errors may have a negative impact on the individual's academic and professional accomplishments as well as on personal relationships. Although speech-sound production can be modified at any stage of life, old habits become more firmly entrenched, so change can be more difficult.

Language Impairments

Children who have language impairments, as described in Chapter 5, may also be impaired in their production of the sounds of the language. It has been estimated that a general impairment in expressive language is present in about 60% of children who are difficult to understand and who have multiple speech-sound errors (Shriberg & Kwiatkowsi, 1994; Tyler & Watterson, 1991). These children have more complicated problems than those of youngsters with isolated phonological or articulatory deficiencies.

SPEECH CHARACTERISTICS

The speech-sound productions of children with language learning disabilities are similar to those with developmental impairments, although complex syllable structures may be especially challenging (Orsolini et al., 2001). Children with language learning difficulties are also more likely to exhibit phonological errors that affect morpheme production (Owen et al., 2001). Speech-sound errors may increase also when they produce longer, more complex sentences.

LIFESPAN ISSUES

Although many individuals with language learning difficulties have normal or near-normal intelligence, speech-sound disorders may have a deleterious effect on the acquisition of reading and writing skills. Learning to read requires a knowledge and awareness of sounds, and how sounds combine to form syllables, words, and sentences (i.e., phonological awareness skills). Children with language learning deficits and phonological disorders may have poor phonological awareness skills (Larrivee & Catts, 1999; Peterson et al., 2009) and are at greater risk for reading and writing difficulties. This may require support and the use of various strategies to achieve their full potential (Owens, 2010).

Hearing Impairments

Because hearing is the primary way in which we acquire the speech sounds of a language, it is no surprise that individuals with hearing impairments may have disordered articulation and phonology. Not only are those with hearing loss limited in their ability to hear others, but their ability to monitor their own speech production may be inadequate. It must be recognized that phonology will not be impaired alone, but all parameters of speech, including voice quality, pitch, rate, and rhythm, will similarly be affected.

SPEECH CHARACTERISTICS

Although the specifics vary, in general, the more severe a person's hearing loss, the less intelligible his or her speech is likely to be (Wolk & Schildroth, 1986). Although an exact relationship between type and degree of hearing impairment and speech cannot be made, certain patterns are frequently observed (Bernthal et al., 2009). Speech-sound errors produced by deaf children are provided in Table 10.4.

Children who have a history of frequent bouts of **otitis media** (middle ear infections), resulting in transient conductive hearing loss, are at risk for developing phonological and articulation disorders. (Bankson & Bernthal, 1998a). Common errors are presented in Table 10.5

LIFESPAN ISSUES

The age at onset and the degree and type of hearing impairment influence the nature of the articulation and phonological disability. Individuals who are born deaf or with severe hearing impairment typically have poorer speech than those who lose hearing later in life. Speech deteriorates over

TABLE 10.4
....

Typical speech-sound errors in children who are deaf

Sound Substitution Pattern	Examples
Voiced for voiceless sounds	"see" → "zee" [zi]
	"can" → "gan" [gæn]
Nasal for oral consonants	"dog" → "nong" [nɔŋ]
Sounds with easy tactile perception for those difficult to perceive	"run" → "wun" [wʌn]
Tense vowels for lax vowels	"sick" → "seek" [sik]
Diphthongs for vowels	"miss" → "mice" [maɪs]
Vowels for diphthongs	"child" → "chilled" [tʃɪld]

Sources: Based on Bankson & Bernthal (1998a) and Calvert (1982).

time, however, for those who are initially hearing and become hard-of-hearing or deaf after they have learned to talk. Accuracy of speech-sound production can be enhanced by the use of hearing aids (for individuals with some hearing) and appropriate training. (See Chapter 14, "Audiology and Disorders of Hearing.") Even the best speech of many adults with deafness is nearly unintelligible to others.

TABLE 10.5
....

Phonological processes often observed in children with history of otitis media

Phonological Process	Phonemes Involved	Examples
Stopping of fricatives	/s/, /z/, /ʃ/, /ʒ/, /tʃ/, /dʒ/	"see" → [ti]
	/f/, /v/, /θ/, /ð/	"John" → [dɑn]
		"thumb" → [tʌm]
Initial consonant deletion	Any consonant	"see" → [i]
		"John" → [ɑn]
Glottal fricative replacement	/h/ used for initial consonant	"see" → [hi]
		"John" → [hɑn]
Glottal stop replacement	Any consonant	"see" → [ʔi]
		"John" → [ʔɑn]
Nasal replacement	/m/, /n/, /ŋ/	"my" → [naɪ] or [baɪ]

Source: Bankson, J. E., & Bernthal, N. W. (1998a). Factors Related to Phonologic Disorders. In J. E. Bernthal & N. W. Bankson, *Articulation and Phonological Disorders* (4th ed.). Boston: Allyn and Bacon. Copyright © 1998 by Allyn and Bacon. Reprinted by permission.

Neuromuscular Disorders

The dysarthrias are a group of motor-speech disorders caused by neuromuscular deficits that result in weakness or paralysis and/or poor coordination of the speech musculature. Dysarthrias typically affect respiration, phonation, resonance, and articulation. They are described in more detail in Chapter 12, "Neurogenic Speech Disorders."

About 75% to 85% of children with **cerebral palsy** have impaired speech production skills (Love & Webb, 2001). Cerebral palsy (CP) is a neuromotor disorder caused by brain damage before, during, or soon after birth (Pena-Brooks & Hedge, 2007). The location and severity of brain damage will predict dysarthria type(s) and degree of communication impairment. However, articulatory difficulties are the most prominent deficit for children with CP (Hedge, 2001a, Mecham, 1996).

SPEECH CHARACTERISTICS

The speech characteristics associated with dysarthria depend on the type of cerebral palsy. The most common type is spastic CP, caused by lesions to motor neurons in one or both frontal lobes. If the lesions are bilateral, then the child exhibits spastic dysarthria, which results in a slow speech rate, imprecise articulation of consonants, harsh voice, hypernasality (with possible air escape out of the nose), and prosodic abnormalities (e.g., equal and excess stress patterns). Errors tend to be similar whether reading aloud, speaking to a group, or during one-to-one conversation. Speech training or the use of augmentative or alternative communication may be required.

LIFESPAN ISSUES

In cerebral palsy, the general motor and speech signs are present from early childhood onward. Approximately a third of individuals with CP have normal intelligence; the rest exhibit varying degrees of cognitive deficits. Accompanying deficits may include epilepsy, visual processing deficits, and/or hearing impairment (Cummings, 2008). Although the damage to the brain does not progressively worsen, general motor functioning may deteriorate over time (Long, 1994).

Childhood Apraxia of Speech

Childhood apraxia of speech (CAS) is a neurological speech-sound disorder that affects the ability to plan and/or program the movement sequences necessary for accurate speech production. It is not the result of neuromuscular weakness (ASHA, 2007). Recall from Chapter 3 that before speech is produced, the motor plan/program that specifies all of the necessary parameters for accurate production of that utterance (e.g., positioning and timing of the articulators; amount of muscle activation) is accessed in the brain. This enables speech to be produced rapidly, yet accurately. If we had to think about how each structure needed to move (i.e., lips, tongue, jaw, vocal folds, respiratory muscles), and with how much force every time we spoke, we might need several minutes to produce a sentence versus the several seconds that is typical.

Because children with apraxia of speech have impaired motor planning and/or programming capabilities, they are unable to learn the motor plans/programs necessary for rapid, accurate speech production in the same fashion as unimpaired children. As a result, their connected speech is often highly unintelligible, segmented or choppy, disfluent, and/or lacking in prosodic variation. Children with severe apraxia of speech with normal cognition and receptive language abilities are often aware that speech is difficult and may initially be unwilling to try to talk because they know they will fail. It is therefore important that the SLP build a trusting relationship with the child and assure him or her that we can help. It is essential that children at least attempt to imitate words with the SLP to determine if he or she does in fact have CAS. Specific treatment for children with CAS is discussed later in this chapter.

SPEECH CHARACTERISTICS

Although there are no definitive neurological or behavioral markers of CAS, the following constellation of speech characteristics has been proposed by ASHA to help guide SLPs in properly diagnosing CAS. They include:

- Inconsistent errors on consonants and vowels in repeated productions of syllables or words
- Lengthened and disrupted transitions between sounds and syllables
- Inappropriate prosody, especially in the realization of word or phrasal stress (ASHA, 2007).

In addition, children with CAS often have limited consonant and vowel repertoires, may exhibit groping and/or trial-and-error behaviors, frequently omit sounds or inappropriately add sounds, and produce single words better than running speech (Davis et al., 1998). Although CAS is considered by most to be a motor-speech disorder, because speech is necessary to learn language and linguistic sound representations, children with CAS have concomitant expressive language and phonological impairments as well.

LIFESPAN ISSUES

Children can be diagnosed with CAS as early as 3 or 4 years of age; however, to make this diagnosis correctly, children need to attend and focus on the clinician and attempt multiple repetitions of word stimuli. Standardized assessments are available, such as the Verbal Motor Production Assessment for Children (Hayden & Square, 1999) and the Kaufman Speech Praxis Test for Children (Kaufman, 1995); however, no one test has been shown to be completely reliable or valid with regard to diagnosing CAS (McCauley & Strand, 2008). Children with severe CAS initially may be nonverbal. Therefore, children may need to rely on other means to help them communicate effectively (i.e., augmentative or alternative communication) as they are learning to speak.

Children with normal or near-normal cognition and receptive language abilities have a good prognosis for verbal communication. However, they may continue to have poor intelligibility throughout the school-age years. They will likely also have difficulties with phonological awareness skills, reading, writing, and spelling. Children with CAS continue to exhibit phonological patterned errors well past the age at which these should have resolved. They may continue to have difficulties with certain classes of sounds and/or production of multisyllabic words (e.g., umbrella) into adolescence and young adulthood. The apraxia Web site listed at the end of the chapter provides the latest research in the area of CAS.

The most readily apparent difficulties in individuals who persist with motor planning/programming difficulties are prosodic abnormalities. Even if speech is intelligible, they may continue to have flattened prosodic contours, a segmented speech pattern, and/or incorrect word and sentential stress. Note that CAS is a speech diagnosis that changes with maturation and with treatment. A child may present early on with a primary diagnosis of CAS, but this may change as he or she gets older. Some children present with a primary diagnosis of phonological impairment but may also exhibit some minor motor planning/programming difficulties. It is the job of the SLP to correctly differentially diagnose the child in order to select the appropriate treatment approach and targets (Strand & McCauley, 2008).

Structural Functional Abnormalities

Rapid and accurate movements involving the jaw, lips, tongue, hard and soft palates, and teeth are necessary for normal speech production; however, usually only gross abnormalities of these structures can negatively impact speech intelligibility. Individuals are remarkably adept at compensating for most structural abnormalities, even partial or complete surgical removal of the tongue. Severe deformity of the hard and soft palates as a result of clefting is far more detrimental to speech production as you'll see in Chapter 11, "Cleft Lip and Cleft Palate."

LANGUAGE AND DIALECTAL VARIATIONS

If you are a native speaker of American English and went to another country, such as Greece, to live, you would learn Greek to communicate with those around you. When you spoke in Greek, your speech would reveal your American background. You would speak Greek with an "American accent." This is not a speech disorder.

Similarly, if you are from Georgia and moved to Massachusetts, you would bring your Georgia regionalism with you. Again, this is not a disorder but a dialectal difference to those in your new environment. Many Americans take pride in their regional and linguistic backgrounds and cherish the cultural diversity that characterizes this country.

In assessing phonological skills, an SLP must guard against over- and underdiagnosis, especially with bilingual and minority dialect speakers (Yavas & Goldstein, 1998). The SLP must differentiate between disordered

A person whose speech reflects a regional or foreign language influence may also have a speech disorder. However, the regionalism or foreign dialect in itself is not a disorder.

phonology and that which is simply different due to foreign language or dialect influences. This can be accomplished by doing the following:

1. Recognize cultural differences
2. Evaluate phonological competence in all relevant languages whenever possible
3. Select appropriate assessment tools
4. Use nonstandard assessments often with the help of bilingual assistants
5. Describe phonological patterns
6. Diagnose any phonological disorders that exist (Yavas & Goldstein, 1998)

The SLP then plans and engages in intervention as appropriate. If dialect differences are targeted, the SLP must assess the client's attitude toward his or her dialect and the individual's motivation for accent reduction. Some generalizations can be made regarding the speech of individuals from various linguistic and regional backgrounds. Table 10.6 highlights just a few of these.

TABLE 10.6

Sample phonological characteristics of American English dialects and non-English language influences on spoken English

Rule	Example
African American Vernacular	
Final cluster reduction	"presents" → "presen"
Stopping of interdental initial and medial fricatives	"they" → "dey"
	"nothing" → "noting"
Deletion of "r"	"professor" → "puhfessuh"
Appalachian English	
Addition of "t"	"once" → "oncet"
Addition of initial "h"	"it" → "hit"
Addition of vowel within clusters	"black" → "buhlack"
Portugese, Italian, Spanish	
Final consonant deletion	"but" → "buh"; "house" → "hou"
Cantonese	
Confusion of /i/ and /ɪ/	"heat" → "hit"; "leave" → "live";
	"hit" → "heat"; "live" → "leave"
Spanish	
Confusion of /d/ and /ð/	"they" → "day"
Devoicing of "z"	"lies" → "lice"
Affrication of /ʃ/	"shoe" → "chew"

Sources: Based on Iglesias & Goldstein (1998) and Yavas & Goldstein (1998).

Characteristics of Articulation and Phonology

It is impossible to describe all the variations in articulation and phonology that reflect non-English or dialectal influences. The first language may interfere with languages that are learned later. For example, in Spanish, /d/, and /ð/ are allophones or variations of the same phoneme, whereas in English, these are two separate phonemes, as can be seen in the words "dough" [do] and "though" [ðo]. Native Spanish speakers, however, may confuse the /d/ and /ð/ and pronounce both words the same way (Yavas, 1998). Some first-language interferences are neutral or positive.

Lifespan Issues

Some adults for whom English is a second (or third or fourth) language choose to modify their foreign accent. Often this desire is based on professional considerations. Teachers of English as a second language and speech-language pathologists may contribute to the improvement of English expression and comprehension. However, for adolescents and beyond, the articulatory patterns of a first language are often firmly established and are difficult to entirely eliminate. The goal, then, is not to make a non-native speaker sound like a native, but rather to improve intelligibility and thereby the person's communicative effectiveness.

Assessment

Comprehensive assessment by the SLP is necessary to determine the nature of the speech-sound disorder. In addition to the general procedures described in Chapter 4, "Assessment and Intervention," formal and informal measures specifically designed to assess phonological and articulation impairments are discussed in the following sections. The goals of speech-sound assessment are as follows:

- Describe the individual's speech-sound inventory
- Identify patterns of errors (i.e., phonological processes)
- Determine impact of speech-sound errors or error patterns on communicative effectiveness
- Identify factors that may relate to etiology or maintenance of the speech-sound impairment
- Plan treatment when appropriate
- Make a prognosis
- Monitor change over time (Bernthal et al., 2009).

> Disorders of articulation and phonology sometimes, but not always, occur with other communication impairments.

In addition, the case history, interview, hearing screening, and oral peripheral examination may provide insight into the etiology of the disorder and contribute to predictions of improvement. Collection of baseline data from which to measure change over time with or without intervention is an integral part of the initial assessment. Typical assessment procedures are briefly described and explained in the following sections.

Description of Phonological and Articulatory Status

The SLP should obtain data on several aspects of speech-sound production. Samples of three children with phonological impairments are presented on the book's CD-ROM.

SPEECH-SOUND INVENTORY

A speech-sound inventory and description of word and syllable shapes are highly appropriate for children who are at a very early stage of development and for others whose speech is markedly unintelligible. A recommended system for listing phonemes is by manner of production and syllable and word position (Grunwell, 1987; Klein, 1997). Table 10.7 shows a speech-sound inventory for Pablo, a 4-year-old boy who is receiving speech and language therapy.

> If a client has only one or two speech-sound errors and all other phonemes are correctly produced, a statement to that effect is sufficient. A listing of all the correct phonemes is not needed.

SYLLABLE AND WORD STRUCTURE

A listing of the consonant-vowel (CV) patterns that have been produced in words suggests their complexity. The SLP might list the word and syllable shapes that are most characteristic of the client's speech as well as the reductions or simplifications that have occurred. Figure 10.5 provides a list of the words in Pablo's language sample in both standard orthography and phonetic transcription.

TABLE 10.7
....
Phonemes produced in various word positions by Pablo, age 4 years

Manner of Production	Syllable Initial Word Initial	Syllable Initial Word Within	Syllable Final Word Within	Syllable Final Word Final
Nasals	/m/ /n/ "more," "no"	/n/ "nana"	/m/ "Sam-uel"	/m/ "drum"
Stops	/p/ /b/ /t/ /d/ "put," "ball," "top," "drum"	/p/ /b/ /d/ "happy," "Toby," "lady"		
Fricatives	/h/ /f/ /s/ "house," "face," "see"	/f/ "coffee"		
Glides	/w/ /j/ "wet," "you"	/j/ "yo-yo"		

Note: Words were taken from spontaneous language sample. Words in quotes are exemplars of produced phoneme in given word position. Production accuracy of the entire word is not suggested.

FIGURE 10.5

Words in Pablo's language sample in standard orthography and phonetic transcription.

"more" → [mɔə]	"happy" → [hæpi]	"baseball" → [bebɔ]
"no" → [no]	"Toby" → [tobi]	"ice cream" → [aɪtim]
"banana" → [nænə]	"lady" → [ledi]	"face" → [fe]
"Samuel" → [sæmu]	"house" → [hau]	"wet" → [wɛ]
"put" → [pʊ]	"face" → [fe]	"you" → [ju]
"ball" → [bɔ]	"see" → [si]	"yoyo" → [jojo]
"top" → [tɑ]	"shoe" → [su]	"light" → [jaɪ]
"drum" → [dʌm]	"coffee" → [tɔfi]	"balloon" → [bʌju]

The word shapes produced include CV ([no]), CVCV ([jojo]), CVC ([dʌm]), and VCVC ([aɪtim]).

The word shapes that were reduced are

CVC → CV	("put" → [pʊ])
CVCVCV → CVCV	("banana" → [nænə])
CVCCVC → CVCV	("baseball" → [bebɔ])
VCCCVC → VCVC	("ice cream" → [aɪtim])

SOUND ERROR INVENTORY

In all cases, the SLP needs to identify phonemes that the client misarticulates. This list is typically compiled on the basis of formal testing of sounds in words. The Goldman-Fristoe Test of Articulation-2 (GFTA-2) (Goldman & Fristoe, 2000) and the Structured Photographic Articulation Test II-Featuring Dudsberry (SPAT-DII) (Dawson & Tattersall, 2001) are two commonly used published tests. Sound errors are reported as **substitutions, omissions, distortions,** and **additions** in syllable/word positions. For example, if 8-year-old Amanda pronounced "lemon" as "wemon," the SLP might record

> w/l (I) [meaning "w" was substituted for "l" in the initial position; i.e., at the beginning of a word]

Errors can be compared with norms for the child's age. A sample of an administration of the GFTA-2 is presented on the accompanying CD-ROM.

PHONOLOGICAL PROCESS ANALYSIS

Many research studies have shown that targeting a process rather than an individual phoneme has the advantage of encouraging generalization of learning to similar phonemes and phonological contexts (Gierut, 1998). Therefore, if an individual has numerous errors, it is helpful to identify which phonological processes are apparent. Phonological process information may be analyzed by the SLP on the basis of transcriptions of the child's conversational or single word utterances. Often SLPs will use a published test such as the Khan-Lewis Phonological Analysis-2 (Khan & Lewis, 2002), which analyzes phonological processes on the basis of the findings of the

Goldman-Fristoe Test of Articulation-2 (Goldman & Fristoe, 2000). Other published tests for determining phonological processes include the Hodson Assessment of Phonological Patterns-3 (HAPP-3) (Hodson, 2004) and the Bankson-Bernthal Test of Phonology (Bankson & Bernthal, 1990). One version of the Comprehensive Test of Phonological Processing addresses the needs of older individuals ages 7 through 24 years (Wagner et al., 1999).

Phonological processes also may be analyzed by using a computerized program. These systems often save time and provide more detailed information than hand-scored procedures. Examples of computerized phonological analysis programs include Computerized Articulation and Phonological Evaluation System (Masterson & Bernhardt, 2001) and Macintosh Interactive System for Phonological Analysis (Mac-ISPA; Masterson & Pagan, 1993). The HAPP-3 noted in the previous paragraph is also available in a computerized version called Hodson Computerized Analysis of Phonological Patterns (Hodson, 2003).

In the case of Amanda above, if her only phoneme error was /l/ → /w/ (I), this would not be indicative of a phonological process; it is a *single* sound substitution, an error of articulation. If, however, Amanda produced /l/ → /w/ (I,M) and /r/ → /w/ (I,M), this *pattern* could be described as the phonological process gliding for liquids because /l/ and /r/ are liquids and they were produced as the glide /w/.

> Although computer analysis of phonological processes might save time, once the program is learned, the SLP must still understand the nature of the processes to work effectively with the client.

INTELLIGIBILITY

Speech **intelligibility** refers to how easy it is to understand the individual. Poor intelligibility has a negative impact on communicative effectiveness. Intelligibility depends on such factors as the number, type, and consistency of speech-sound errors. The person's voice, fluency, rate, rhythm, language, and use of gesture also contribute to ease of comprehension, and these should be noted. Other factors beyond the speaker include the listener's hearing acuity, familiarity with the speaker, and experience listening to disordered speech, plus, environmental noise, message complexity, and environmental cues. Figure 10.6 illustrates a commonly used subjective way of reporting intelligibility.

A more objective measure of intelligibility is percentage of intelligible words. If speech is exceedingly poor, intelligibility may be measured in terms of syllables or consonants (Strand & McCauley, 1997). A recorded sample of continuous speech is transcribed, and the percentage of intelligible words is computed as follows:

$$\text{Percentage of Intelligible Words} = \frac{\text{Number of Intelligible Words}}{\text{Total Number of Words}} \times 100$$

1. Readily intelligible even when the context is not known
2. Intelligible with careful listening when the context is not known
3. Intelligible with careful listening when the context is known
4. Unintelligible with careful listening even when the context is known

FIGURE 10.6

Subjective descriptors of intelligibility.

The percentage of intelligible syllables or consonants is computed in a similar fashion. Intelligibility measures are becoming increasingly common in research and clinical use (Shriberg et al., 1997; Wilcox & Morris, 1999). In general, highly unintelligible speech signals a severe disorder, whereas readily intelligible speech suggests that the disorder may be mild.

Prognostic Indicators

Detailed description of the client's speech provide some insight into the prognosis for improvement with and without therapy. The client's age, severity of the disorder, other medical or concomitant problems, and availability of family support also help predict the client's improvement. For adults, the etiology of the speech-sound impairment largely impacts prognosis (i.e., stroke versus neurodegenerative disease). For children, the consistency of speech-sound errors, stimulability for correct production of error sounds, and possibly the ability to discriminate error sounds from target sounds may help determine prognosis.

Consistency

Think about your own speech. If you are reading aloud in front of a class, you are likely to be very careful in how you produce all the sounds of the words. In contrast, when you are speaking casually to a friend, your articulation is probably far less precise. Inconsistency is normal, and it may be a clue to the exact nature of an articulation or phonological error. Let's go back to Amanda. If her misarticulation of /l/ occurs only when she is in conversational speech and then only at the beginning of words, her speech-sound error may be more amenable to change. Lack of consistency is considered a positive prognostic indicator. Ironically, an individual with consistent errors may be easier to understand than someone whose error pattern is inconsistent. Consistency of phoneme errors is achieved by evaluating the client's speech during more than one task and in more than one word position and phonemic context (Bernhardt & Holdgrafer, 2001).

Stimulability

Assessment should always include trial therapy. **Stimulability** is the ability of an individual to produce the target phoneme when given focused auditory and visual cues. Typically, the SLP will say, "Look at me. Listen to me. Now say exactly what I say: _____." The SLP will first prompt correct production of the error phoneme or pattern within the word in which it had been misarticulated. If the client does not correctly imitate the SLP, the prompt is moved to the syllable or phoneme level.

Although stimulability is often a positive prognostic indicator, research studies suggest a more complex relationship. Children who are stimulable may respond more quickly to correction of the target phoneme and may also be more likely to self-correct without therapy than those who are not stimulable. Those sounds for which a child is not stimulable are highly unlikely to change without treatment. However, among children in therapy, those with low stimulability scores often make more progress, especially with untreated sounds, than do those who are more stimulable.

Error sound discrimination is often assessed both externally and internally. External discrimination, or **interpersonal error sound discrimination,** refers to the ability to perceive differences in another person's speech. For example, in external discrimination, the SLP might ask the client, "Are these the same or different: 'wemon'—'lemon'?" Sometimes two words are contrasted, and the client is asked to point to pictures that can be labeled using either the targeted phoneme or the one that was substituted; for example, shown two pictures, the client is told, "Point to awake. Now point to a lake." **Internal error sound discrimination,** sometimes termed **intrapersonal error sound discrimination,** is the ability to judge one's own ongoing speech. The client may be asked to judge the accuracy of her or his phoneme productions.

The relationship of speech-sound discrimination to articulation and phonology remains unclear. Perception of a contrast such as /r/ or /l/ and /w/ usually precedes production in children who are developing typically (Strange & Broen, 1980). In addition, children who are better at internal discrimination have been reported to have more correct articulations (Lapko & Bankson, 1975). From this, we might conclude that error sound discrimination ability signals a more favorable prognosis than the absence of this ability. Two warnings about phoneme discrimination testing are warranted: (1) Only the error phonemes appear to relate to therapeutic prognosis, so only these should be routinely assessed. (2) Many young children do not understand the concept of same versus different; therefore, their error sound discrimination is difficult to judge.

> Improvement in non-targeted phonemes, in addition to those that are taught, is often made when the targets are relatively difficult.

INTERVENTION

If the results of the assessment suggest that treatment is appropriate, the SLP must determine how to proceed. Initial questions to be answered include the following:

- Where will therapy occur? (Clinic, center, school, or home setting?)
- How frequently will the client be seen? (Once or twice a week or three, four, or five times weekly?)
- How long will the sessions be? (Twenty to 60 minutes is the typical range.)
- Will therapy be one to one or in a group setting?

Answers to these questions will be related to the facilities that are available as well as to the needs of the client. In addition to such administrative type decisions, the SLP must determine the following:

- What are the treatment targets?
- What treatment approach appears most suitable?

> Family members may be enlisted to reinforce therapy under the guidance of a speech-language pathologist. Carefully structured homework assignments can provide a client with additional beneficial practice.

Target Selection

The major goal of therapy should be to make the client easier to understand and improve communicative effectiveness. One factor is the frequency of a particular misarticulated phoneme within the language: For example, /ʒ/, as in "treasure" ([trɛʒɚ]), does not occur in many American English words, so it would not normally warrant early attention. However, targets that may generalize to correction of phonological processes would be extremely helpful in improving intelligibility. If a child exhibits the process stopping of fricatives, as in saying "zoo" as [du] and "five" as [paɪb], intervention for correct production of /z/ may generalize to other fricatives, including /f/ and /v/.

A second factor in target selection is likelihood of success. The SLP might initially choose targets that the client will probably master relatively quickly. The best predictors of ease of mastery are stimulability and inconsistency. If the client can produce the target phonemes when prompted to imitate with increased visual and auditory stimulation, this is a favorable sign. In addition, if the client does not misarticulate a particular target in all words or situations, this demonstrates that successful intervention is likely (Miccio et al., 1999).

Some current research studies have demonstrated that greater generalization to nontarget phonemes occurs when the targets are more difficult—that is, not stimulable, later developing, and more phonetically complex (Gierut, 1998). The complexity approach is discussed later in this chapter. It is up to the SLP to determine whether early success on a few targets or more long-term progress on multiple phonemes is best for the individual client.

Intervention Approaches

A variety of therapy approaches and techniques exist. The SLP might target one or two phonemes or multiple phonemes at a time. Therapy might focus on phonological patterns of errors, emphasize motor-speech production, or target the nonsegmental aspects of speech such as rate, rhythm, and stress and intonation. Most SLPs adjust their approach to suit each client and combine procedures to provide individually tailored therapy. Highlights of select therapy approaches are provided in the next few sections (c.f. Kamhi, 2006b, for more details), and the evidence in support of specific approaches of techniques is summarized in Box 10.1 at the end of the chapter.

BOTTOM-UP DRILL APPROACHES

Bottom-up drill approaches focus on discrete skills, with progression from the simplest to the most complex movements. Some begin with auditory discrimination training, oral-motor exercises, or isolated sound productions and work up to correct production of the error sound in connected speech (Kamhi, 2006b). No evidence supports the use of oral-motor exercises, however, so these are not recommended. The utility of auditory discrimination training is also not well established, and more research is needed.

BOX 10.1
Evidence-Based Practices for Individuals with Articulation and Phonological Disorders

General intervention

- Approximately 70% of preschool children who receive intervention for speech-sound disorders exhibit improved intelligibility and communication functioning.
- Approximately 50% of children who are unintelligible to both familiar and unfamiliar listeners progress so that they are intelligible to all listeners.
- More therapy is equated to more improvement.

Specific behavioral treatment approaches or techniques

- The *traditional motor* and *sensory-motor* approaches are highly effective for children who have only one or a few sounds in error (e.g., /l/, /r/) and for whom language skills are within normal limits.
- *Dynamic Temporal and Tactile Cueing (DTTC)* was shown to be effective for a small number of children with severe childhood apraxia of speech. This intensive treatment involves speech production practice sessions two times per day (30 minutes each), 5 days per week for a total of 6 weeks. More research is needed to determine the long-term effectiveness of DTTC.
- The *Lee Silverman Voice Treatment* was shown to be effective in four young children with spastic cerebral palsy. Improvements in loudness and speech intelligibility were maintained at 6 months follow-up.
- The *complexity approach,* based on the work of Judith Gierut and colleagues, has shown that targeting later-acquired sounds and/or consonant clusters leads to increases in treated and in untreated sounds, both within and across sound classes. Also,

using phoneme pairs that are maximally contrasted (i.e., differ by major class distinctions) and compare two new phonemes (versus including the child's error sound) also results in greater systemwide changes.

- The steps of *whole language* used during storybook reading improve phonological performance in some children, but more research is needed. This approach is not suitable for children with severe speech-sound disorders who require direct, structured therapy.
- The *cycles approach* targets multiple phonological processes over an extended period of time and is effective for children who are highly unintelligible. Three to six cycles of phonological intervention involving 30 to 40 hours of instruction are reportedly necessary for the child to become intelligible.
- The *multiple oppositions approach* is best suited for children who substitute one sound for many different sounds. This approach has been shown to be effective for children who are highly unintelligible, particularly during the early stages of treatment.
- The *Metaphon approach* (Howell & Dean, 1994) is aimed at developing the child's metaphonological awareness skills in two phases. Limited evidence is available about the effectiveness of this approach, however.

Source: Based on Fox et al. (2006); Gierut (2009); Gierut et al. (1996); Hodson & Paden (1991); Hoffman et al. (1990); Jarvis (1989); Strand et al. (2006); Williams (2000).

In bottom-up drill approaches, each error sound is targeted one at a time. Speech production practice may involve production of the error sound in isolation, nonsense words, structured phrases, sentences, and conversational speech. Various ways to establish correct production of an error sound may be used, including phonetic placement (e.g., using a tongue blade to push the articulators into position) or sound shaping (i.e., using a sound the child can produce to help produce the new sound).

When the sound is mastered in the therapy setting, speech assignments are provided to allow clients daily practice of their new skills and promote generalization outside of the therapy setting. Instruction on self-monitoring of correct speech-sound production and/or monitoring by others in the child's environment may also be introduced (Pena-Brooks & Hedge, 2007).

The **traditional motor approach** and **sensory-motor approach** are two well-known bottom-up drill approaches. The traditional motor approach begins with auditory discrimination training (i.e., ear training), establishment of the new sound using sound-evoking techniques (e.g., phonetic placement), production practice with the newly established sound in isolation, nonsense syllables, words, phrases, sentences, and conversation, and generalization and maintenance practice (e.g., homework assignments, practice in other communicative settings or situations) (Van Riper & Emerick, 1984). The sensory-motor approach is similar but it does not include auditory discrimination training and begins with production at the syllable level, rather than the sound in isolation (McDonald, 1964; Pena-Brooks & Hedge, 2007).

LANGUAGE-BASED APPROACHES

Language-based approaches integrate the learning of error sounds into meaningful, functional contexts either through play or through the reading and retelling of story books. The focus is actually on increasing language and/or narrative complexity without explicit instruction on speech-sound production. Rather, instruction is implicit, or within the context of language learning. Such an approach is not suitable for children who exhibit severe speech delays and require more direct, structured speech practice. Rather, language-based approaches have proven effective for promoting generalization of newly learned sounds to spontaneous speech following successful drill-type therapy (Williams, 2000).

PHONOLOGICAL-BASED APPROACHES

Children who have multiple speech-sound errors and are highly unintelligible may benefit from phonologically based treatment that focuses on targeting phonological patterned errors (processes) as opposed to individual sounds. By targeting a phonological process, for instance *final consonant deletion*, many sounds can be practiced at any given time, thereby increasing the child's speech-sound inventory and improving speech intelligibility more rapidly.

One of the most well known and widely used phonologically based approaches is the **cycles approach** (Hodson & Paden, 1991). A cycle can be one 60-minute session, two 30-minute sessions, or three 20-minute sessions. Only one phonological process is targeted at a time, and several cycles may be necessary per target process. Therapy begins with the most stimulable phonological process and progresses through multiple cycles until all phonological processes have been addressed (Pena-Brooks & Hedge, 2007).

Cycles training sessions are highly structured. Each session involves review of the previous session, auditory-perceptual training, and production training that incorporates use of **minimal pair** contrasts, or the contrasting of phonemes in pairs of words. This is accomplished by presenting the child with two pictured words that differ by one phoneme; one pictured word contains the child's error sound/error pattern and the other is the correct form (e.g., pig-big). These production exercises involve having the child produce both words in sentences and asking the child if the sentences make sense (e.g., "The *big* lives on the farm").

In addition to minimal pair contrasts that differ by one or a few phoneme features, treatment approaches may use phoneme contrasts that differ by many different features, including place, manner, and voicing (e.g., chop-mop). These phoneme pairs are called **maximal contrasts**. The **multiple oppositions approach** uses maximal contrast word pairs. This approach is effective for children who substitute one sound for multiple sounds, which results in production of the same word for different words (e.g., "dip" is produced for *chip, trip, ship,* and *kip*). Word pairs are created to contrast all error sounds at the same time.

Other phonologically based approaches aim to increase the child's **metaphonological skills,** or the ability to analyze, think about, and manipulate speech sounds (Pena-Brooks & Hedge, 2007). One such approach is the **Metaphon approach,** which is designed to increase the child's active cognitive participation in the remediation of his or her speech-sound disorder. Metaphon theorists believe a child must be aware of his or her speech errors, have a desire to modify them, know the relevant speech targets, and have the neuromotor capability to produce the targets correctly with adequate speed in various speech contexts (Hewlett, 1990).

The Metaphon approach consists of two phases. Phase 1 focuses on expanding the child's knowledge of the sound system of the language, thereby preparing him or her to learn how sounds are produced and how they differ from one another. Phase 2 focuses on transferring this knowledge to communicative situations and teaches the child to self-monitor and correct speech output (Howell & Dean, 1994).

COMPLEXITY APPROACH

It has been argued that *what* is treated in therapy is more important than *how* it is treated (Gierut, 2005). Given that no one treatment approach for articulation or phonological impairments has proven more effective than another, eliminating error sound patterns and increasing the child's speech-sound inventory in a shorter time frame may be a better goal in some cases. The complexity approach involves training more difficult sounds (e.g., teaching a 3-year old to produce /v/, which is not mastered until much later), which then leads to generalization of untreated but less complex sounds (e.g., /f/).

This approach is considered more efficient because only a few complex targets need to be trained to promote change in the child's overall speech-sound system (Gierut, 2001, 2005). The caveat, however, is that it may take longer initially to train children to produce more complex speech targets.

As a result, they may remain unintelligible for longer periods at first, thereby becoming frustrated with their continued lack of communicative effectiveness. Therefore, success of this approach depends on the severity of the child's disorder, his or her frustration level, and the overall goal of therapy (i.e., increase speech intelligibility versus promote significant changes in the child's overall speech-sound system) (Kamhi, 2006b; Pena-Brooks & Hedge, 2007).

Treatment of Neurologically Based Motor-Speech Disorders

Two evidence-based approaches are gaining in popularity for use with children with neurologically based motor-speech disorders. One was specifically designed for children with childhood apraxia of speech, and the other was adapted from the adult version used with patients with Parkinson disease for children with dysarthria. These specific approaches are discussed in the next section.

DYNAMIC TEMPORAL AND TACTILE CUEING

Dynamic temporal and tactile cueing (DTTC) is an intensive motor-based, drill-type treatment designed for children with severe apraxia of speech (Strand et al., 2006). Unlike the bottom-up approach, treatment targets include a small number of functional words and phrases. Speech production practice of each word or phrase involves use of techniques that are effective for adults with apraxia of speech (Rosenbek et al., 1973; Strand & Skinder, 1999). For instance, the clinician says to the client, "Watch me, listen to me, and do what I do" and then provides various levels of cues (e.g., tactile, simultaneous productions) depending on the client's needs.

In DTTC, the target words are practiced slowly and produced simultaneously with the clinician at first. In addition, this approach incorporates principles that promote motor learning (e.g., daily, repetitive practice, systematic feedback). The clinician may use tactile cues (e.g., physically maneuvering the child's jaw into the correct position) to help the child achieve the correct starting position for the desired utterance. As the child's productions improve, direct imitation, delayed imitation, and spontaneous productions of target utterances are elicited.

The eventual goal is to have the child produce the word correctly spontaneously, both in and out of the clinic. Five to 10 minutes of home practice with family members is also recommended. The rationale for only practicing a small set of words is that it will foster neural maturation of motor planning/programming substrates, thus facilitating future speech motor learning (Strand et al., 2006).

LEE SILVERMAN VOICE TREATMENT

The Lee Silverman Voice Treatment (LSVT), discussed briefly in Chapter 9, "The Voice and Voice Disorders," an intensive treatment provided 4 sessions per week, 60 minutes per session, for 4 weeks, was originally designed to increase loudness levels of patients with Parkinson disease. This treatment has since been used successfully with children with CP, with only slight modifications (Fox et al., 2006). Pre-/post-LSVT speech samples of a child with spastic CP can be heard on the book's CD-ROM. Note that SLPs must obtain proper training and certification prior to using this approach with clients. Go to the LSVT Web site listed at the end of the chapter to learn more.

COMPUTER APPLICATIONS

Computer programs and games are available that can be used in conjunction with direct treatment provided by the SLP. These programs provide exercises in both perception and production of speech-sound targets, as well as nonsegmental targets (i.e., pitch, duration, and loudness). Computer applications provide an opportunity for daily practice of treatment targets, which is essential to the learning of new skills. Some computer games are even designed to involve caregivers in the treatment process, which facilitates effective communication between the child and his or her primary communication partner (Patel & Salata, 2006).

Generalization and Maintenance

Once the client has achieved an acceptable level of correct phoneme production, the SLP must ensure that slippage does not occur and that the new speech pattern becomes habitual. Many SLPs introduce self-monitoring exercises from the very beginning of therapy. In this way, clients understand that they are ultimately responsible for their own success. Once the SLP believes that the client is ready for dismissal from therapy, follow-up sessions may be scheduled at progressively longer intervals. If the progress has been maintained over time, the remediation has been effective.

> Success of therapy is determined by the application of what has been learned in a clinical setting to everyday life.

SUMMARY

Producing the sounds of a language during speech is a complex process. It involves an inner conceptualization of phonemes and phonotactic rules so that in our "mind's ear" we know how the language we are speaking should sound. Speech production also requires the neuromotor ability to move our articulators to form the desired sounds in a smooth, rapid, and automatic fashion. As children develop spoken language, they typically employ phonological processes that simplify adult forms. If these persist beyond the expected ages, they may present difficulties. Hearing disorders, neurological impairments, and structural abnormalities may contribute to phonological and articulatory disorders. Foreign language background and regional dialects contribute to variations in speech. Assessment of articulation and phonology includes a detailed description of the individual's phonological output, as well as investigation of etiology and determination of prognosis. Intervention strategies may include perceptual training, contrasted phonemes in word pairs, and speech production drill practice. The general goal is improved intelligibility in spontaneous speech.

THOUGHT QUESTIONS

- How does speech differ for someone who is congenitally deaf versus someone who becomes deaf later in life? Why?
- If you had your own clinic or private practice, which standardized articulation or phonological tests (if any) would you purchase and why?
- How would you determine if a child has a phonological impairment or a motor-speech/articulation disorder (i.e., childhood apraxia of speech, dysarthria)? How would your treatment approach differ depending on the diagnosis?
- How might you explain the difference between a phonological disorder and a motor-speech/articulation disorder to a family member?

SUGGESTED READINGS

Bernthal, J., Bankson, N., & Flipson, P. (2009). *Articulation and phonological disorders: Speech sound disorders in children.* Boston: Pearson Education.

Caruso, A., & Strand, E. (1999). *Clinical management of motor speech disorders in children.* New York: Thieme.

Gildersleeve-Neumann, C. (2007, November 6). Treatment for childhood apraxia of speech: A description of integral stimulation and motor learning. *The ASHA Leader, 12*(15), 10–13, 30.

Kahmi, A. (2006b). Treatment decisions for children with speech-sound disorders. *Language, Speech, and Hearing Services in Schools, 37,* 271–279.

Strand, E., & McCauley, R. (2008, August 12). Differential diagnosis of severe speech impairment in young children. *The ASHA Leader, 13*(10), 10–13.

ONLINE RESOURCES

Childhood Apraxia of Speech Association
www.apraxia-kids.org
The Childhood Apraxia of Speech Association site contains the latest research on CAS and is also a great resource for parents.

Lee Silverman Voice Treatment

www.lsvtglobal.com/

The Lee Silverman Voice Treatment site provides updated information about the LSVT approach for children and adults with neurological speech disorders, as well as upcoming LSVT training and certification workshops.

University of Iowa

www.uiowa.edu/~acadtech/phonetics/about.html

The University of Iowa site has animations and videos of speech-sound production. It can serve as an excellent intervention tool.

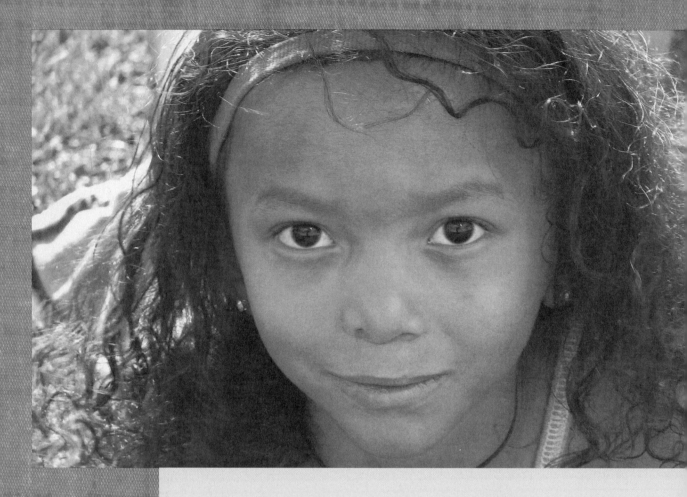

CHAPTER LEARNING GOALS

When you have finished this chapter, you should be able to:

- Describe the embryological development of the face and palate

- Describe how clefts of the lip and palate form

- Describe the clinical features and possible causes of a cleft of the lip

- Describe the clinical features of bilateral and unilateral clefts of the lip and palate

- Describe the team approach and general management procedures used for treating people with clefts, along with the research evidence supporting specific treatment approaches or techniques

11

Cleft Lip and Cleft Palate

In this chapter, we explore **craniofacial anomalies,** or congenital malformations involving the head and face and affecting speech. There are hundreds of different craniofacial anomalies, many of which are accompanied by malformations of the upper lip, hard palate, and soft palate. Malformations of the upper lip and hard and soft palate are called **clefts.** A cleft is an abnormal opening in an anatomical structure (Shprintzen, 1995), representing a failure of structures to fuse or to merge early in embryonic development. This fusion process is discussed later in this chapter.

Clefts may involve an entire anatomical structure, such as the entire hard palate, or only a part of it. Clefts of the lip that may involve the dental arch (**alveolus**) and the anterior aspect of the hard palate (**premaxilla**) develop between the fifth and eighth weeks of gestation. Isolated clefts of the hard and/or soft palate develop between the eighth and twelfth weeks of gestation.

Velopharyngeal inadequacy (VPI) is a term that we use frequently in this chapter. It means that the velopharyngal mechanism is incapable of separating the oral and nasal cavities during swallowing and speech production (Pannabacker, 2004). VPI is a frequent result of palatal clefts and associated with velar soft tissue and muscle tissue deficiencies. We have more to say about VPI later in the chapter.

Clefts of the lip and palate create a condition that interferes with basic biological functions such as breathing and swallowing, and they can inhibit severely a child's development of speech and language. We discuss some of the unique communicative problems associated with palatal clefts and the wide range of medical, dental, and behavioral treatments that children with clefts require. We also discuss the necessity of an interdisciplinary treatment approach for people with clefts.

Clefts of the lip and palate may present challenges well beyond infancy, and these challenges change across the individual's lifespan. We briefly consider some of the major challenges that present themselves across the lifespan of persons with clefts. Case Study 11.1 describes a youngster presenting with residual speech sound production difficulties following cleft lip and palate repair.

CASE STUDY 11.1
Case Study of a Child with Cleft Palate: Colin

Colin is a 6-year-old boy with a repaired bilateral complete cleft of the lip and palate. When Colin was born presenting with the bilateral complete cleft, he was taken to the major medical center in his home town for surgical repair of his lip and palate. In the years following his surgery, Colin was followed carefully by the craniofacial team at the medical center. This team of different specialists ensured that Colin received appropriate dental and orthodontic care, otologic and audiologic management, and speech-language therapy. During his preschool years, Colin had received speech therapy at the medical center. He was dismissed from therapy when he was $4\frac{1}{2}$ years old because his speech and language production was within normal limits.

When Colin enrolled in kindergarten at his local school, he received a standard speech-language screening that was administered to all new students. The SLP who screened Colin noted that he had a mild nasal resonance, particularly on vowels adjacent to nasal consonants, and a small degree of nasal emission noted primarily during production of stop consonants. When the school SLP informed Colin's parents about the problem, they asked her to add Colin to her caseload. The SLP declined their request explaining that Colin should be thoroughly evaluated by

the craniofacial team. The SLP explained that such an evaluation would ensure that Colin's velopharyngeal mechanism was physically capable of closure during speech production. If it was determined that the velopharyngeal mechanism was physically incapable of closure, speech therapy may be contraindicated.

Colin was evaluated by the medical center's craniofacial team. Multidimensional videofluoroscopy revealed that Colin's velopharyngeal mechanism was capable of closure. The hypernasal resonance and nasal emission in his speech was determined to be the result of faulty learning subsequent to Colin's dismissal from speech therapy. The team recommended that Colin resume speech therapy in school. The school SLP agreed to keep the craniofacial team apprised of Colin's progress.

As you read this chapter, think about

- The types of speech problems that result from structural abnormalities of the upper lip, and of the hard and soft palate.
- Why Colin demonstrated nasal emission on stop consonants.
- Why Colin demonstrated hypernasal resonance on vowels that were adjacent to nasal consonants.

PHYSICAL CHALLENGES OF CLEFTS THROUGH THE LIFESPAN

At birth, the infant with a cleft may have obstructive breathing problems and need immediate medical attention. Depending on the severity of the cleft, the child may also have problems with food intake. Typical feeding problems include poor oral suction, lengthy feeding times, nasal regurgitation, gagging, and excessive air intake. Unfortunately, no single feeding method is successful for infants with different types of clefts. The infant's performance during the initial feedings will dictate the feeding method, and individual modifications will need to be made to ensure adequate nutrition. SLPs, occupational therapists, nutritionists, and nurse practitioners will be involved in assisting the mother and infant (Peterson-Falzone et al., 2006).

At 3 months of age, clefts of the lip are surgically closed and the infant is carefully monitored for possible middle ear infection. The SLP is involved very early on to help parents with feeding issues and provide techniques and strategies to facilitate speech and language development. Between 9 and 12 months of age, surgeons close the clefts of the hard and soft palate. Additional surgery, referred to as secondary surgery, may be necessary later to treat continued difficulties with velopharyngeal closure.

When the child is around 2 years of age, dental specialists begin reconstruction of abnormal dentition and dental occlusion. SLPs work closely with dental specialists to ensure normal speech and language development. The adolescent child may require extensive orthodontic treatment in addition to secondary surgeries for VPI and/or cosmetic improvements. Psychological counseling and speech-language therapy may also be required.

From the teenage years through adulthood, a number of potential issues may require attention. These include middle ear disease, potential hearing loss, psychological status, and genetic counseling regarding the risk of having an infant with a cleft. Generally, however, adequate and appropriate health care and specialized services throughout the lifespan will result in an individual who is capable of leading a fulfilling life. We now turn our attention to a more detailed discussion of the information just presented.

DEVELOPMENT OF THE FACE AND PALATE

To begin our discussion of cleft lip and palate, we focus on the normal development of the face and the palate. A brief examination of how the face and palate are formed will shed light on the underlying nature of clefts and how they form. The third through the twelfth week of gestation are when the face and the palate are formed. The formation of cleft lip with or without cleft palate and of isolated cleft palate are well understood.

Facial Development

The face and anterior aspects of the mouth are formed between the fifth and eighth weeks after conception. Normal development of the face and mouth is a result of a complex fusion among five embryonic processes: the right and left **mandibular processes,** the **frontonasal process,** and two **maxillary processes.** These processes are illustrated in Figure 11.1a.

Fusion of the right and left mandibular processes, which forms the mandible and the lower lip, occurs early in the development of the face, during the fourth and fifth weeks of gestation. The right and left mandibular processes grow toward one another and fuse in the midline of the face. This fusion process has been completed in the 6-week-old embryo shown in Figure 11.1a. Mandibular fusion is relatively simple when considered in light of fusion processes that occur above the mandible.

During the fifth week of gestation, the frontonasal processes grow in a downward direction, separating into two distinct tissue masses on both sides of the face called the **nasomedian processes** and the **lateral nasal processes.** Depressions between the nasomedian and lateral nasal processes

During the embryonic and fetal periods of life, humans are at a higher risk of death than at any other period of life except extreme old age. Half of all conceptions are not recognized clinically, and approximately 15% of clincally recognized pregnancies result in miscarriage (Peterson-Falzone & Imagire, 1997).

FIGURE 11.1
....

Embryonic face at 6
weeks of development
(a), embryonic face at
8 weeks of development
(b), adult face illustrating
fusion of embryonic
processes (c).

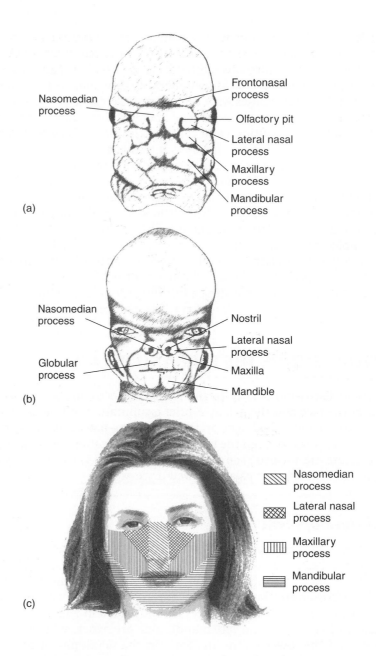

FIGURE 11.1

Embryonic face at 6 weeks of development (a), embryonic face at 8 weeks of development (b), adult face illustrating fusion of embryonic processes (c).

called the **olfactory pits** ultimately become the right and left nasal cavities. The lateral nasal processes fuse with the maxillary processes to form the **nasal alae** (the flared portion of the nostrils) and the anterior aspects of the face just beneath the eyes as shown in Figure 11.1b.

The nasomedian processes also fuse with the paired maxillary processes. Primitive tissue contained in the nasomedian processes become the anterior portion of the upper lip, the anterior aspect of the alveolar process (the portion of the maxilla or upper jaw that holds teeth) containing the upper frontal incisor teeth, and the anterior aspect of the hard palate, called the premaxilla. Facial development is completed during the eighth week of gestation, as shown in Figure 11.1b. Clefts of the lip that may include a cleft of the alveolar process and premaxilla occur when the fusion process between the nasomedian and maxillary processes has been interrupted by some abnormal genetic condition or by environmental agents (e.g., certain drugs, chemicals, nicotine, irradiation) called **teratogens** that adversely affect the developing child.

Development of the Secondary Palate

The secondary palate includes the bony hard palate and the soft palate. Although development of the anterior aspects of the face is complete by the end of the eighth week of gestation, complete separation of the oral and nasal cavities has not yet been achieved. Between the eighth and twelfth weeks of gestation, embryonic processes that give rise to the hard and soft palate fuse, separating the oral and nasal cavities.

Two **palatal shelves,** which are wedge-shaped tissue masses, grow downward from the inner aspects of the maxillary processes. Up to the ninth week of gestation, the tongue projects into the nasal cavity. A rapid growth spurt during the eighth and ninth weeks of gestation increases the length and width of the mandible, pulling the tongue downward and away from its position between the palatal shelves, which then begin fusing with one another in an anterior to posterior fashion. Figure 11.2 shows the general aspects of this anterior to posterior fusion process. As the palatal shelves are fusing, the nasal septum grows downward to meet the palatal shelves in the midline, separating the left and right nasal cavities.

Muscles of the soft palate also evolve from the palatal shelves. The soft palate begins forming during the tenth week of gestation, and fusion of the secondary palate is completed by the end of the twelfth week. Aberrations that prevent fusion of the palatal shelves will result in an isolated cleft of the hard and/or soft palate. As with cleft lip, genetic and nongenetic factors have been identified as causing an isolated cleft of the secondary palate. These factors are discussed later in this chapter.

CLEFT LIP AND PALATE CLASSIFICATION SYSTEMS

Clefts vary in size and severity, and it is important clinically and for clinical research to classify clefts accurately. At present, no universally accepted classification system exists, but there are some classification systems that are useful for clinical reference (Bzoch, 1997).

A cleft lip and palate classification scheme that was developed originally in the 1930s is still in use today. The **Veau system** is useful for a quick general reference regarding the nature and extent of clefts (Bzoch, 1997). Four classes of clefts, identified by Roman numerals, comprise the

Contemporary cleft palate classification systems are based on the embryological development of the face and palatal structures.

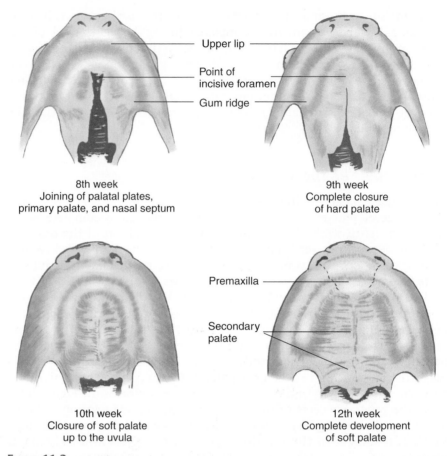

Upper lip

Point of
incisive foramen

Gum ridge

8th week
Joining of palatal plates,
primary palate, and nasal septum

9th week
Complete closure
of hard palate

Premaxilla

Secondary
palate

10th week
Closure of soft palate
up to the uvula

12th week
Complete development
of soft palate

FIGURE 11.2

Fusion of the palatal shelves, forming the hard and soft palates.

Veau system and are listed in Table 11.1. More modern clinical classification systems include **Kernahan's Striped Y,** a visual identification system based on location, and one developed by the American Cleft Palate-Craniofacial Association (ACPA) that focuses on the primary and secondary palates.

CLINICAL FEATURES OF CLEFTS

Clefts vary greatly in type and severity, ranging from a small V-shaped notch of the lip to a complete separation of the upper lip, dental arch, and the right and left sides of the hard and soft palate. Clefts are classified commonly as (1) unilateral or bilateral cleft of the lip, (2) unilateral cleft of the lip and palate, (3) bilateral cleft of the lip and palate, (4) submucous cleft, or (5) bifid uvula. Some of the clinical features of these clefts are discussed here.

TABLE 11.1
The Veau cleft lip and palate classification system

Class	Descriptor
I	Cleft of the soft palate only
II	Cleft of the hard and soft palate to the incisive foramen
III	Complete unilateral cleft of the soft and hard palate and of the lip and alveolar ridge on one side
IV	Complete bilateral cleft of the soft and hard palate and/or the lip and alveolar ridge on both sides

Cleft of the Lip

A cleft of the lip involves the reddish (**vermilion**) portion of the upper lip and may extend through the lip toward the nostril. For example, an **incomplete cleft** of the lip may be a minor V-shaped notch in the vermilion portion of the lip, whereas **complete cleft** of the lip continues through the upper lip into the floor of the nostril. A cleft of the lip has an adverse affect on the shape of the nose characterized by a flattening of the nose and a flaring of the nostril on the side of the cleft. Additionally, the **columella,** the strip of tissue connecting the base and tip of the nose, is short and misaligned. Clefts of the lip may be unilateral or bilateral. When the cleft lip is unilateral (see Figure 11.3),

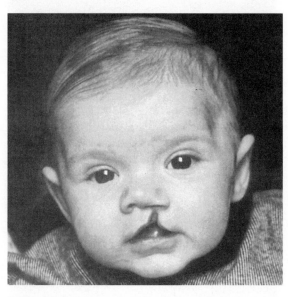
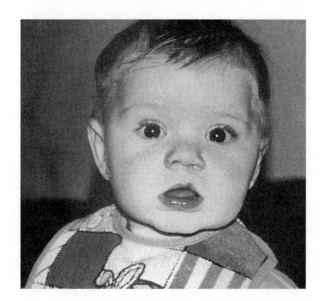

FIGURE 11.3

Unilateral cleft of the lip presurgery (a) and postsurgery (b). Note the "V" shaped notch in the vermilion border of the lip extending toward the left nostril and the flattening of nose and flaring of nose and flaring of the nostril on the side of the cleft. (Photographs courtesy of Donald Warren, D.D.S., Ph.D., University of North Carolina, Chapel Hill) it most commonly occurs on the left side. If the cleft lip is bilateral, it is generally accompanied by a cleft of the palate as well.

An isolated cleft of the lip is rare, accounting for less than 5% of all cleft cases (Shprintzen, 1995). Usually, clefts of the lip extend posteriorly through the alveolar process. Such clefts may be minor notches in the alveolar process, or they may extend completely through the alveolar process and involve the premaxilla.

Unilateral Cleft of the Lip and Palate

A unilateral complete cleft of the lip and palate extends from the external portion of the upper lip, through the alveolus, and through the hard and soft palate (see Figure 11.4). The nasal septum attaches to the larger of the two palatal segments.

As discussed earlier, a cleft of the secondary palate alone without a cleft lip is sometimes observed. Clefts of the secondary palate alone vary in severity, involving all of the hard and soft palate or only a small portion of the hard or soft palate.

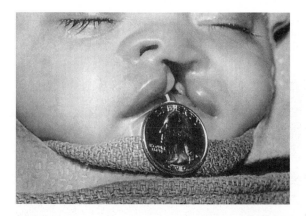

(a)

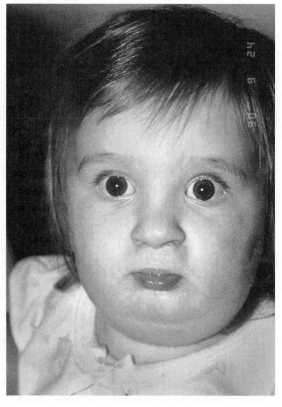

(b)

FIGURE 11.4

Unilateral cleft of the lip and palate presurgery (a) and postsurgery (b). Observe that this cleft extends completely through the lip into the left nostril and the alveolus is also cleft. The cleft of the hard and soft palates cannot be seen in this photograph. (Photographs courtesy of Donald Warren, D.D.S., Ph.D., University of North Carolina, Chapel Hill)

Bilateral Cleft of the Lip and Palate

A bilateral complete cleft of the lip and palate (see Figure 11.5) is the most severe type of cleft due primarily to a severe tissue deficiency. The lip and the alveolus are cleft under both nostrils and the central portion of the lip (**prolabium**), alveolar process, and the premaxilla is positioned abnormally at the tip of the nasal septum as a protruding mass of tissue that is sometimes called the free-floating premaxilla (Seagle, 1997; Shprintzen, 1995). In bilateral complete clefts, the columella is usually absent, resulting in the tip of the nose attaching directly to the lip. The nasal septum is not attached to either of the palatal shelves in bilateral clefts.

Submucous Cleft

A submucous cleft is a muscular cleft in the region of the soft palate (see Figure 11.6). The cleft is covered by a thin layer of mucosal tissue that can conceal the underlying lack of muscular fusion. Unlike the clefts just discussed, the submucous cleft may not be discovered until late in childhood. Physical characteristics such as a **bifid uvula** (the uvula appears to be split in half) may indicate the presence of a submucous cleft. However, a bifid uvula may be present in the absence of a submucous cleft. In fact, about 1 in 80 people has a bifid uvula (Bradley, 1997).

Another symptom of a submucous cleft is a bluish coloration in the middle of the soft palate where the muscles failed to fuse termed "zona

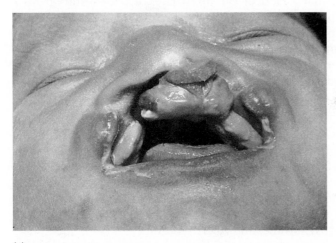

(a)

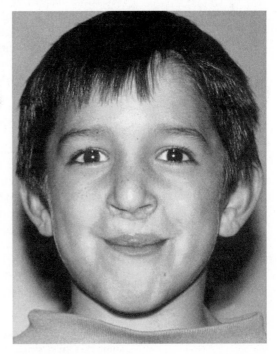

(b)

FIGURE 11.5

Bilateral cleft of the lip and palate presurgery (a) and post-surgery (b). Note the clefts on both sides of the face and the protruding tissue mass in the central position of the upper lip. (Photographs courtesy of Donald Warren, D.D.S., Ph.D., University of North Carolina, Chapel Hill)

FIGURE 11.6

Submucous cleft. (Photograph courtesy of Donald Warren, D.D.S., Ph.D., University of North Carolina, Chapel Hill)

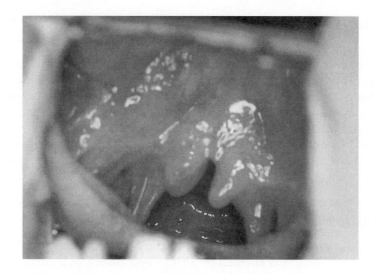

pellucida." This may be accompanied by a notch on the posterior border of the hard palate that can be felt. Submucous clefts may lead to velopharyngeal incompetence.

ETIOLOGIES OF CLEFTS

We have already seen that a cleft of the lip, palate, or both results from a fusion failure among primitive embryonic structures. But what causes such a fusion failure? It is generally accepted that four different categories of etiologies can produce cleft lip, cleft palate, or both cleft lip and cleft palate (Shprintzen & Goldberg, 1995): genetic disorders, chromosomal aberrations, teratogenically induced disorders, and mechanically induced abnormalities.

Genetic Disorders

Genetic disorders account for a substantial percentage of clefting. Clefting is associated with over 400 multiple anomaly **syndromes,** or combinations of symptoms, that occur together in predictable and consistent combinations of traits.[1] Some of the major syndromes that SLPs are likely to encounter include Pierre Robin syndrome (Robin sequence), Treacher Collins syndrome, velocardiofacial syndrome, and Apert syndrome.

The primary symptoms of Pierre Robin syndrome, or, more properly, Robin sequence, include **micrognathia** or an underdeveloped mandible, a retracted and elevated tongue into the pharyngeal airway, an isolated cleft of the hard and soft palate, congenital heart problems, digital anomalies,

[1]Another definition for syndromes is "A syndrome may be defined as the presence of multiple anomalies in a single individual with all those anomalies having one primary cause" (Shprintzen, 1995).

conductive hearing loss, and developmental deficits. Communication deficits are related to cognitive and learning deficits, and severely delayed language development is common (McWilliams et al., 1990). The small mandible is believed to interfere with the descent of the tongue around the eighth or ninth week of gestation. Position of the tongue between the palatal shelves prevents palatal fusion. The isolated palatal cleft is a result of the tongue's failure to descend.

Treacher Collins syndrome is characterized by **malar hypoplasia,** or an underdevelopment of the cheekbones, underdevelopment of the mandible, malformation of the external ear and the ear canal, conductive hearing loss, cleft palate, and a projection of scalp hair onto the cheek. Brain dysfunction is rare with these individuals, and the major communication problems result from conductive hearing loss and VPI.

Of special interest to the SLP is Velocardiofacial syndrome because of the universality of language deficits and learning disabilities in conjunction with a palatal cleft. Individuals with this syndrome are usually of small stature with a broad, flattened nose and have underdeveloped cheekbones and heart problems. A delayed onset of expressive language and persistent language difficulties are primary communication problems among these individuals. The cognitive behavior of individuals with velocardiofacial syndrome is concrete, and they sometimes demonstrate perseverative behaviors (Peterson-Falzone, et al., 2010).

Apert syndrome has an invariable feature called **craniosynostosis,** or a premature closing of the sutures of the skull that greatly disfigures the forehead, and **syndactyly,** or webbing of the fingers and toes with bone fusion. The palate is very high and narrow, giving the appearance of a cleft, but actual clefts occur in only 30% of people with Apert syndrome. Conductive hearing loss is frequent, and language development is commensurate with mental ability. Expressive language development is typically delayed.

Before turning our attention to chromosomal aberrations, some mention of general familial inheritance patterns associated with clefting should be made. Table 11.2 summarizes the risk factors for having a child with a cleft.

Chromosomal Aberrations

Within the nucleus of human cells are 46 chromosomes arranged in 23 pairs. A chromosomal aberration known as trisomy 13 results in a cleft lip with or without cleft palate in 60% to 70% of cases. Trisomy 13 is a rare condition resulting from the appearance of a third #13 chromosome. This condition occurs about once in 6,000 births. Like syndromes, disorders associated with chromosomal aberrations are characterized by multiple congenital abnormalities (Peterson-Falzone et al., 2010).

Teratogenically Induced Disorders

Environmental teratogens are agents that interfere with or interrupt normal development of a fetus and create congenital malformations. Recognized

Thalidomide caused thousands of birth defects, including clefting, in the 1960s when the drug was administered to pregnant women. As a result, the drug was outlawed for over 30 years. In 1998, the Food and Drug Administration approved its use for the treatment of certain serious conditions such as leprosy and some cancers associated with AIDS.

TABLE 11.2
....
Risks for cleft lip with or without cleft palate (CL [+/2] CP) and cleft palate (CP)

Situation	(CL [+/–] CP)	(CP)
Frequency of defect in the general population	0.1%	0.04%
My spouse and I are unaffected. We have an affected child. What is the probability that our next baby will have the same condition if:		
We have no affected relatives?	4%	2%
We have an affected relative?	4%	7%
We have two affected children.		
What is the probability that our next child will have the same condition?	9%	1%
I am affected or my spouse is. We have no affected children.		
What is the probability that our next child will be affected?	4%	6%
We have an affected child.		
What is the probability that our next child will be affected?	17%	15%

Source: Adapted from Grabb et al., (1971).

teratogens associated with clefting include drugs such as dilantin, an anti-convulsant; thalidomide, a drug that was formerly used as a sedative; excessive use of aspirin, and retinoids, nontopical acne medication. In excessive amounts, ingestion of alcohol, nicotine, and caffeine are also considered to be teratogens responsible for clefting. In addition, X-rays, certain viruses, and some naturally occurring environmental substances have teratogenic properties. The effects of teratogens vary with an individual's unique genetic makeup, the time during pregnancy when the agent was encountered, the amount, and the mother's metabolism (Kummer, 2001; Shprintzen & Goldberg, 1995).

Mechanically Induced Abnormalities

Mechanical factors that cause clefts are those that impinge directly on the embryo. With such clefts, the embryo is developing in a normal fashion, and the cleft is induced by something external to the embryo (Shprintzen & Goldberg, 1995). The most frequent cause of mechanically induced clefts is amniotic rupture (loss of amniotic fluid). Intrauterine crowding as when there is a twin, a uterine tumor, or an irregularly shaped uterus can also result in clefts.

INCIDENCE OF CLEFTS

Clefts occur in approximately 1 in every 750 live births. Clefts of the lip with or without cleft palate occur more frequently than clefts of the palate alone. Submucous clefts occur in approximately 1 in every 1,200 births (Peterson-Falzone et al., 2010). There are some indications that the incidence rate for clefts may be increasing because improved prenatal treatment is resulting in the birth of more high-risk fetuses. Additionally, improved postnatal treatment results in adults with clefts who look, speak, and function in a typical manner, making it more likely than it once was that they will have children of their own. Both factors could serve to increase the size of the genetic pool that carries the cleft trait, resulting in more children being born with clefts (McWilliams et al., 1990; Peterson-Falzone et al., 2010).

SEX AND RACIAL DIFFERENCES

Clefts of the lip with or without clefts of the palate occur about twice as frequently in males and tend to be more severe. Clefts of the palate alone, however, occur more frequently in females than males. Submucous clefts occur at approximately the same frequency in males and females. In the United States, Native Americans have the highest incidence rates, followed by people of Asian descent, whites, and people of African descent. These incidence differences have been attributed to genetic and environmental factors (McWilliams et al., 1990). Regardless of sex and race, individuals with clefts present many different interrelated problems that require the cooperation of a wide variety of specialists for effective management (Peterson-Falzone et al., 2006).

THE CLEFT PALATE TEAM AND GENERAL MANAGEMENT ISSUES THROUGH THE LIFESPAN

The group of specialists working together providing care for individuals with cleft palate is referred to as a **cleft palate team.** The concept of a cleft palate team, sometimes called the craniofacial team, was developed originally at the Lancaster Cleft Palate Clinic in Lancaster, Pennsylvania, in the 1930s. Cleft and craniofacial teams listed by state can be found on the American Cleft Palate-Craniofacial Association web site. Figure 11.7 lists the professions that constitute a typical cleft palate team.

Effective clinical management of people with clefts requires the efficient integration of information among professionals. For example, a surgeon might require information about speech production ability from the SLP when deciding whether to perform a particular operation. Advantages of a team approach include the following:

- The family can see several specialists during one appointment.
- The family associates all aspects of care with one setting.

FIGURE 11.7

Composition of a cleft palate team.

Anesthesiologist	Nurse practitioner	Plastic surgeon
Audiologist	Oral surgeon	Prosthodontist
Coordinator	Orthodontist	Psychiatrist
Educator	Otolaryngologist	Psychologist
Endodontist	Parents	Radiologist
Geneticist	Pediatrician	Social worker
Genetic counselor	Periodontist	Speech-language pathologist

- Only one contact is required if an emergency arises.
- Follow-up is managed in a controlled manner (McWilliams et al., 1990).

The needs of a person with a cleft and his or her family change during the lifespan, requiring team member compositions and roles to change accordingly.

SLPs, surgeons, dental specialists, and audiologists work closely together on the team. Therefore, the SLP needs to have some familiarity with the specific roles and concerns of the other team members. In the next four sections of this chapter, we discuss surgical, dental, audiological, and psychosocial concerns regarding clefts. This discussion is followed by a detailed account of the communicative problems faced by persons with clefts and the SLP's role as a member of a cleft palate team.

Surgical Management of Clefts

Although the recorded history of clefts dates back to the Ching dynasty (390 B.C.), surgical repair of clefts did not occur until the 19th century. Surgical repair of clefts, or **palatoplasty,** is divided into two stages: primary surgical correction followed by secondary procedures to correct velopharyngeal inadequacy.

PRIMARY SURGICAL CORRECTION

The first stage of primary surgical correction is lip surgery if the child has a cleft of the lip and palate. Lip surgery is performed generally before 3 months of age (Kuehn & Henne, 2003). Surgical correction of a cleft palate is designed to create a velopharyngeal valving mechanism that is capable of separating the oral cavity from the nasal cavity during speech production. Early surgical closure of the palate also improves swallowing function and reduces the number of middle ear and upper respiratory infections. Recent surgical trends advocate closure of the palatal cleft between 9 and 12 months of age. Early closure has a positive influence on velopharyngeal function, midfacial symmetry, and overall appearance (Kuehn & Henne, 2003).

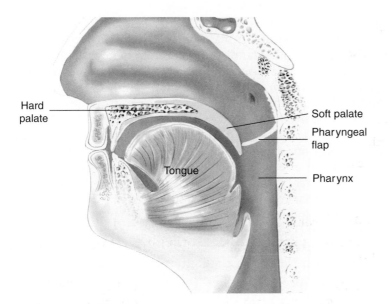

FIGURE 11.8
....
Stylized drawing of a
pharyngeal flap.

Hard
palate

Soft palate

Pharyngeal
flap

Tongue

Pharynx

SECONDARY SURGICAL CORRECTION

The efficacy of primary palatal surgery is assessed by the adequacy of the velopharyngeal mechanism for speech production. Approximately 1 in 4 individuals who have primary palatal surgery fail to achieve adequate velopharyngeal closure for speech production, requiring additional surgical management to correct the velopharyngeal incompetence (Riski, 1995).

A commonly used secondary surgical procedure designed to correct VPI is called a **pharyngeal flap** operation. A pharyngeal flap is created by cutting a flap of soft tissue from the posterior pharyngeal wall, as shown in Figure 11.8. One end of the flap remains attached to the posterior pharyngeal wall, and the other is sutured to the velum. To permit nasal breathing and the production of nasal speech sounds, small openings are maintained between the flap and the lateral walls of the pharynx. Closure of these openings during swallowing and the production of nonnasal speech sounds is accomplished by active movement of the lateral walls of the pharynx (toward the midline) (Riski, 1995; Sloan, 2000). Pharyngeal flap procedures are performed generally between the ages of 6 and 12, and it has been reported that "normal" speech is realized following most of these operations (Peterson-Falzone et al., 2010).

Dental Management of Clefts

People with cleft lip and palate have significant dental problems that can interfere with chewing, swallowing, and in some cases, speech production. During the lifespan, various dental specialists will be involved in care ranging from developing devices to assist the infant's swallowing to treatment focusing on improving the positions of teeth and maxillary bone segments (Peterson-Falzone et al., 2010). **Orthodontists** are crucial members of cleft palate teams who are concerned primarily with the alignment of teeth and dental **malocclusions.** A malocclusion is the improper alignment of the maxillary and mandibular dental arches. Pressure is applied to the teeth and/or the dental arches with metal bands and various dental appliances.

Abnormal **dentition** based on the kind, number, and arrangement of teeth and malocclusions can have adverse effects on speech production, particularly if present during early speech-language learning. Nearly 90% of all English consonants are made in the anterior portion of the mouth, the area of the mouth most affected by clefts. Missing or misaligned teeth and malocclusions can affect adversely the production of sounds that require accurate tongue placement on the teeth or dental arch, such as /t/, /d/, and /l/. Sounds that require a constriction between the tongue and teeth, such as /s/, /th/, and /sh/, will be adversely affected by the absence or misalignment of teeth (Le Blanc & Cisneros, 1995).

A **prosthodontist,** a dental specialist, is frequently involved in the care of individuals with clefts. Prosthodontics is a dental specialty concerned with the replacement of missing teeth and other oral structures with various appliances. For some individuals with clefts, palatoplasty is not recommended because of other complicating medical conditions, religious beliefs, or simply personal choice. In such circumstances, closure of the cleft can be achieved by a prosthodontic *obturator.* An obturator is a special kind of dental prosthesis designed to occlude or fill the cleft and partition the oral cavity from the nasal cavity. Obturators may be used as primary management of a cleft or as a secondary procedure after unsuccessful palatoplasty (Peterson-Falzone et al., 2010).

Obturators are made of acrylic material and custom built to conform to the general configuration of an individual's oral cavity. The obturator is held in place by clasps that anchor it to the teeth. The palatal portion of the obturator covers the cleft, and the posterior portion extends into the pharynx and terminates in a bulblike structure, called a **speech bulb,** that fills the velopharyngeal space. Velopharyngeal closure is achieved by movement of the lateral pharyngeal walls making contact with the bulb.

Audiological Management of Clefts

People with clefts exhibit a higher incidence of hearing disorders and middle ear disease than the general population. Middle ear disease is universal during a cleft palate child's infancy, resulting in a conductive hearing loss that may persist into adulthood (Peterson-Falzone et al., 2010). It has been estimated that 58% of the cleft palate population has some degree of hearing loss (Kemker, 1995). Later in this section, we discuss the potential impact of hearing loss on speech and language development, but first we consider how middle ear disease leads to conductive hearing loss in the cleft palate population.

The middle ear is an air-filled cavity in the temporal bone of the skull bounded on the outside by the tympanic membrane (eardrum) and on the inside by the cochlea, a spiral-shaped structure that contains the nerve endings for hearing. A tube runs from the middle ear down into the nasopharynx (the portion of the pharynx above the velum). This tube, called the auditory or eustacian tube, permits drainage from the middle ear into the pharynx and serves to equalize air pressure in the middle ear with atmospheric pressure.

The eustachian tube is normally closed, opening only when one swallows or yawns widely. The tube is opened by contraction of the **tensor veli palatini** muscle of the soft palate. When a cleft of the soft palate occurs, the muscle does not function properly and will not open the tube. Dysfunction of the eustachian tube results in poor middle ear ventilation, which, in turn, leads to inflammation and abnormal fluid accumulation. This fluid accumulation is a disease called *otitis media,* which causes mild to moderate conductive hearing loss. Otitis media frequently needs to be treated with a **myringotomy,** which is a surgical puncture of the tympanic membrane and insertion of a ventilating tube for pressure equalization.

You can develop some appreciation of how a mild conductive loss affects your hearing sensitivity by plugging your ears gently with your fingers. Note that you still hear some sounds but not others. In general, loud sounds can be heard, but soft sounds cannot. Try this little experiment with a friend: Have your friend stand behind you and produce a vowel sound such as /a/ for three seconds and then produce /s/ for 3 seconds. If you have normal hearing, you will hear both these sounds clearly. With your friend still standing behind you, plug your ears gently and have him or her produce those sounds again in the same manner. With your ears plugged, you probably heard the /a/ but not the /s/. If you did hear the /s/, it was very muffled and distorted.

Your little experiment demonstrates that even a mild conductive loss can prevent a listener from hearing many of the sounds of spoken English. Longstanding conductive hearing loss associated with otitis media can have a devastating effect on speech and language development, compounding the already adverse conditions created by the cleft.

The audiologist is a vital member of the cleft palate team who provides critical information to the SLP about an individual's hearing status. For people with clefts, hearing testing should be done routinely every 3 to 6 months. During episodes of active otitis media, hearing should be checked more frequently.

Psychosocial Management of Clefts

No strong evidence indicates that children with repaired clefts are more maladapted psychosocially than their noncleft peers, and they have no documented personality deviations. Frequently, however, these children suffer from social isolation owing to discrimination by peers and teachers who overemphasize the residual evidence of the cleft condition and underestimate the child's real capabilities. Such social isolation may lead to low self-esteem, decreased participation in group activities, inhibited behavior, and lowered expectations on the part of parents, teachers, and peers (McWilliams et al., 1990).

Children with clefts encounter unusual social pressures, and there is a continuing need to ensure their psychological well-being. The SLP needs to be keenly aware of the child's psychological and social needs and "provide treatment or referral as required in individual cases" (McWilliams et al., 1990, p. 144).

TABLE 11.3
Psychosocial concerns during the lifespan of a person with a cleft palate

Developmental Stage	Areas of Concern
Prenatal/Perinatal Period	Parental adjustments to impending birth/birth of a child with cleft palate
Toddler Years	Parental attempts to protect the child from negative reactions of extended family and community members; stress of medical intervention
Preschool Years	Self-concept, peer relationships
Early School and Teen Years	Self-concept, peer relationships, school adjustment, negative judgments by teachers
Adults	Social interactions, life partners, and employment

Source: Based on Peterson-Falzone et al., (2010).

Table 11.3 highlights some of the psychosocial concerns as they change during the lifespan of individuals with cleft palate. More information can be found on the Web site listed at the end of the chapter.

COMMUNICATION PROBLEMS ASSOCIATED WITH CLEFTS

Approximately 80% of people born with clefts that are not associated with a syndrome and receiving palatal repair by 12 months can be expected to develop reasonably good speech without therapeutic intervention. For the other 20% born with clefts and for children with associated syndromes, "the road to normal speech often seems long and arduous" (Golding-Kushner, 1995, p. 327). The child with a cleft palate may have voice disorders, resonance disorders associated with VPI, articulation disorders associated with VPI, dental malocclusions, and possible hearing loss. In addition, children with clefts may exhibit language disorders. In this section, we discuss the presumed causes, assessment, and treatment of these communicative problems.

An SLP who specializes in craniofacial disorders probably has fewer adolescents and adult patients with cleft palate than once was the case. Persons with cleft palate now receive effective treatments earlier in their life and generally speak normally by the time they are adolescents (Peterson-Falzone et al., 2010). Thus this section of the text focuses on communicative problems that are likely to be diagnosed and treated during childhood.

Voice Disorders

Clinical research indicates that phonatory disorders are far more common in people with clefts then in those without clefts, possible involving over 80% of the cleft population. The most common vocal fold pathology is bilateral vocal nodules, which produce a hoarse, breathy vocal quality. The high incidence of individuals with vocal nodules among the cleft palate population is likely related to vocal hyperfunction (Peterson-Falzone et al., 2006). Vocal hyperfunction is also the presumed cause of vocal nodules in noncleft children, usually associated with excessive yelling and screaming.

Vocal hyperfunction among children with cleft palate appears to be a compensatory behavior related to VPI. Children with VPI are unable to increase their vocal loudness in a normal fashion owing to the loss of energy into the nasal cavity. To compensate for this inability, these children position their larynx high in the neck during speaking, and this behavior exerts unusually high tension on the vocal folds, causing the vocal nodules.

Another voice disorder that occurs in children with cleft palate is called **soft-voice syndrome.** Soft-voice syndrome is also a compensatory behavior by which the child purposely reduces vocal loudness to prevent air escape through the nose and reduce hypernasality. Soft-voice syndrome is frequently accompanied by a monotone voice characterized by little variation in pitch.

ASSESSMENT OF VOICE DISORDERS

Four general steps have been recommended for the assessment of suspected voice disorders associated with clefts (McWilliams et al., 1990). First, a case history should be taken to determine whether the vocal symptoms are of recent origin or longstanding. If the symptoms have been present for a long time, patterns of potential vocal misuse need to be explored in detail.

The second step should explore the individual's personality. Vocal hyperfunction is commonly associated with people who are tense, loud, and/or aggressive. These personality characteristics are not typical of individuals with clefts, but the possibility of such a personality factor contributing to vocal hyperfunction needs to be explored.

A detailed phonation examination to determine the nature of the voice disorder is the third general step. Of interest is the appropriateness of the vocal pitch range, loudness, and voice quality. Specific techniques and instruments for such assessments have been discussed in numerous texts on voice disorders and in Chapter 9.

The fourth step is to determine whether the person can modify his or her voice. A straightforward procedure to determine an individual's ability to change the voice is to have him or her "sigh" or produce an "um-hum." People who exhibit vocal hyperfunction during connected speech may demonstrate unconsciously the ability to change vocal quality when producing these easy, natural phonations.

As with any suspected disorder of voice, the individual needs to be examined by a physician before commencing therapy. When a hoarse voice quality accompanies a cleft, there is a strong possibility that bilateral vocal nodules exist. Voice therapy is usually the initial treatment of choice with the goal of reducing vocal hyperfunction.

TREATMENT OF VOICE DISORDERS

The treatment techniques and approaches described in Chapter 9 to reduce or eliminate vocal hyperfunction are applicable here as well.

An additional goal of voice therapy is elimination of **hard glottal attacks.** A hard glottal attack occurs when a client initiates speech using hypertensive vocal fold adduction.

To eliminate hard glottal attacks, the individual is trained to initiate words beginning with vowels using a gentle onset of voice. This strategy is taught by having the individual begin by producing a prolonged /h/ and then gradually moving into the initial vowel in the word. This breathy, relaxed voicing onset can be felt and heard, and the individual is taught to sense the relaxed phonation. Initiating words with the /h/ is gradually phased out, and therapy progresses into two-word combinations, sentences, and finally conversational speech.

Habituating the new voice is divided into two phases: limited habituation and overall habituation (McWilliams et al., 1990). Limited habituation involves having the individual use his or her new voice only in the presence of the SLP and then in highly controlled situations outside the clinic. Overall habituation involves using the new voice during the entire therapy session, then in specific classes in school, and during certain hours at home. The times and situations are gradually extended. Therapy is terminated when the individual and his or her caregivers or significant others report a consistent use of the new voice.

Resonance Disorders

People with VPI are said to have a hypernasal voice quality. Hypernasality is not a problem associated with phonation; rather, it is the result of not partitioning the oral and nasal cavities by actions of the velopharyngeal mechanism. Hypernasality is a resonance problem created by the nasal cavity acting inappropriately as a second "filter" coupled to the oral cavity. Addition of this second filter alters the vocal tract's output in such a way that it sounds as though the individual is talking through the nose.

Several different instruments are commercially available that will obtain nasalance scores. The computation and interpretation of these scores varies according to the instrument.

Some nasal resonance is normal. To illustrate this point, say the sentence "Where were you last year?" aloud. Now pinch your nostrils shut and listen to the difference in your voice quality. Pinching your nostrils shut while speaking reduces normal nasal resonance, and as a result your voice sounds unnatural. This lack of nasal resonance is called **hyponasality.** Your voice may have a hyponasal quality when you experience a bad head cold.

Individuals with VPI exhibit increased nasal resonance and decreased oral resonance, and the voice quality is abnormally nasal sounding, or hypernasal. Hypernasality is associated mainly with vowels. High vowels such as /i/ tend to be perceived as more nasal than low vowels such as /a/, and perceived hypernasality may be greater in connected speech than during the production of isolated words.

ASSESSMENT OF RESONANCE DISORDERS

There are a number of standardized rating scales for assessing vocal resonance. Rating scales permit the assignment of numbers to express increasing

(a)

		Hypernasality				
Normal		Mild		Moderate		Severe
1	2	3	4	5	6	7

(b)

		Hypernasality					
Hypo-nasality	Normal		Mild		Moderate		Severe
−1	0	1	2	3	4	5	6

Source: Based on McWilliams et al., (1990).

FIGURE 11.9

Two examples of scales used to rate the degree of resonance disorders: (a) a 7-point scale emphasizing hypernasality, and (b) an 8-point scale for rating nasal resonance.

severity of the disorder. In general, such rating scales are reliable and valid. Two such rating scales are presented in Figure 11.9.

Noninstrumental procedures to assess velopharyngeal functioning are the mirror test and the nostril-pinching test. To determine the presence of nasal airflow during speech production, a small dental mirror can be is placed under the nose while the client produces words or sentences containing high-pressure consonants (e.g., Buy Bobby a puppy). If the mirror fogs during this task, then air may be escaping from the nose. It is important to place the mirror under the nose at the right time because normal air leakage can occur just before the start of the utterance, and again right at the end (Kuehn & Henne, 2003).

To assess abnormal nasal flow during speech using the nostril-pinching test, have the client produce nonnasal words first while pinching the nostrils and then again with the nostrils open. The perceived resonance and quality should sound the same; if there is a perceptual difference, it may suggest the velopharyngeal port is open (Kuehn & Henne, 2003).

Specially designed instruments are also available to assess resonance disorders. One such instrument, manufactured by Kay Elemetrics, is called a **nasometer.** The nasometer measures simultaneously the relative amplitude of acoustic energy being emitted through the nose and mouth during phonation. A numerical value, the **nasalance score,** is computed that reflects the magnitude of hypernasality. Nasalance scores correlate well with rating scales and with the actual degree of velopharyngeal opening (Dalston, 1995, 2004; Dalston & Seaver, 1990). Nasometry can also be used as an effective therapeutic feedback technique. Examples of nasometry can be seen on the book's CD-ROM.

The definitive procedure for assessing velopharyngeal function is **multiview videofluoroscopy.** Videofluoroscopy is motion picture X-rays recorded on videotape. Multiview videofluoroscopy permits the imaging of velopharyngeal function from three different perspectives: from the front, from the side, and from beneath. These images provide a complete picture of velopharyngeal closure or the lack thereof.

TREATMENT OF RESONANCE DISORDERS

Behavioral treatments designed to improve velopharyngeal functioning and reduce hypernasality have a 50-year history in the United States. Although for some individuals velopharyngeal closure may be improved without additional surgery (Tomes et al., 1997), those who have anatomical limitations such as a velum that is too short to contact the posterior pharyngeal wall or a velum that is completely immobile will not benefit from behavioral treatments alone. Such individuals will require further surgery or a prosthesis to achieve velopharyngeal competence. The decision to try behavioral treatments to improve velopharyngeal function must be made through careful collaboration with the cleft palate team. If the cleft palate team determines that behavioral management is appropriate, the SLP may want to try a resistance exercise approach such as continuous positive airway pressure (CPAP).

CPAP treatment is an 8-week muscle resistance home-training program designed to strengthen the muscles of the soft palate. The CPAP device, like the one used for patients with obstructive sleep apnea, generates continuous positive air pressure delivered through a nose mask. Treatment involves production of 50 specified words and 6 sentences while pressure is delivered through the nose. The amount of pressure delivered and the amount of practice time progressively increases each week (Kuehn, 1991; Peterson-Falzone et al., 2010).

CPAP therapy is based on the exercise physiology principle of progressive resistance training. Progressive resistance training asserts that when muscles are subjected systematically to weights greater than those to which they are accustomed, they adapt by adding muscle tissue and strength is increased. To continue building muscle tissue, weights are increased systematically until the desired muscle strength is achieved.

The CPAP procedure attempts to strengthen the muscles of the velopharyngeal mechanism by having the velar musculature work against systematic increases of weight. Because it would be quite impractical and probably impossible to use miniature free weights, CPAP uses air pressure in the nasal cavity as a substitute. Heightened air pressure in the nasal cavity is the "weight" that the velopharyngeal mechanism works against (Tomes et al., 1997).

During therapy, the velum works against the increased air pressure in the nasal cavity while producing syllables that contain nasal consonants /n/or/m/, vowels, and nonnasal consonants. The velum is lowered during production of the nasal consonant and elevated during vowel and nonnasal consonant productions. Nasal air pressure is increased systematically during velar elevation associated with production of the nonnasal consonant.

Articulation Disorders

Individuals with clefts are at high risk for disordered articulation. Disordered articulation can be the result of VPI, structural deviations in the oral cavity, misaligned or missing teeth, faulty learning, or combinations of these factors. Sounds that tend to be produced incorrectly more than 60% of the time in the cleft population include /s/, /z/, /θ/, /tʃ/, and /ts/ (McWilliams et al., 1990). Vowels and some consonants are produced with a hypernasal quality, as discussed previously.

Production of consonants that require an air pressure buildup in the oral cavity, such as the stop consonants /p/, /t/, and /k/, is frequently accompanied by air escaping inappropriately through the nose. Air escaping through the nose during speech production is called **nasal emission.** Nasal emission is not the same as hypernasal speech quality. Rather, nasal emission is an audible or inaudible leakage of air into the nasal cavity.

People with clefts may also exhibit **compensatory articulation errors** apart from the articulation errors discussed here. A compensatory articulation error is a gross sound substitution error that is an attempt to compensate for the physical inability to produce a given sound correctly. A common compensatory articulation error is a **glottal stop** similar to /h/. Other examples are provided in Table 11.4.

Individuals with VPI are unable to build the requisite oral air pressure to produce stops such as /p/, /t/, and /k/ because of air escaping into the nasal cavity, as discussed above. Stop sounds require a brief stoppage of air flow and a buildup of oral air pressure followed by a sudden release of that pressure. The normal production of a /p/ sound, for example, requires a buildup of oral pressure that is accomplished by holding the upper and lower lips together briefly (the stop) followed by a sudden release of that built-up air pressure. The person with VPI is incapable of producing the /p/ in this fashion and compensates by stopping the air at the glottis, approximating the vocal folds. Air is stopped, and pressure is built up beneath the vocal folds instead of behind the lips.

Compensatory behaviors may become strongly habituated and still be present after the structural deficit that caused them has been corrected. The SLP needs to make a careful inventory of such behaviors during the articulation assessment of people with clefts.

TABLE 11.4

Compensatory articulations often present among individuals born with a cleft palate

Target	Phonemes Involved	Compensatory Articulation
Stop	/p/, /b/, /t/, /d/, /k/, /g/	Glottal stop /ʔ/, stop produced at the glottis
		Pharyngeal stop, stop produced near pharynx
		Middorsum stop, stop produced in middle of tongue
Fricative	/s/, /z/, /ʃ/, /ʒ/	Pharyngeal fricative, closure occurs near pharynx
		Velar fricative, posterior nasal fricative
Affricate	/tʃ/, /dʒ/	Pharyngeal fricative, velar fricative, posterior nasal fricative

The overall effect is speech that is hypernasal and contains nasal emission and weak and distorted consonants.

Source: Based on text material in Air et al., (1989).

ASSESSMENT OF ARTICULATION DISORDERS

A number of widely used articulation tests can be used to assess the sound production skills of people with clefts. Some of these are the *Templin-Darley Test of Articulation*, the *Goldman-Fristoe Test of Articulation*, and the *Fisher-Logemann Test of Articulation Competence*. The *Fisher-Logemann Test* is particularly useful for assessing individuals with clefts because it allows for an analysis of patterns of articulation errors regarding the place, manner, and voicing characteristics of sounds (McWilliams et al., 1990).

Specialized tests of articulation have been developed for use with people who are suspected of having VPI. The *Iowa Pressure Articulation Test* is a subtest embedded in the *Templin-Darley Test of Articulation*. This test is composed of 43 sounds that have been identified as likely to be misarticulated by people with VPI. The test emphasizes sounds that require the buildup of oral pressure. Individuals who score poorly on this test because of VPI will produce a unique pattern of errors characterized by nasal emission, a lack of oral pressure, and gross compensatory substitutions (McWilliams et al., 1990).

The *Bzoch Error Pattern Diagnostic Articulation Test* is another specialized instrument designed for people with clefts and/or suspected VPI. The test is constructed to facilitate identification of error patterns in speech that are related more to VPI than to functional learning problems.

Phonological process analysis can also be used to assess the sound production skills of people with clefts. Because sound formation difficulties caused by structural anomaly may lead to persistent phonological process simplifications, phonological process analysis should accompany more articulation-based assessment (Witzel, 1995).

TREATMENT OF ARTICULATION DISORDERS

Direct intervention for speech-sound development should begin prior to the first palatal surgery, and as early as 5 to 6 months of age, just before the onset of babbling (Peterson-Falzone et al., 2006). Early speech-language intervention should focus on increasing the child's consonant inventory, especially pressure consonants and increased oral airflow (Hardin-Jones et al., 2006). The behavioral treatment approaches and techniques described in Chapter 10 for children with articulation and phonological disorders also apply to the treatment of the cleft population. The procedures and techniques used in bottom-up drill approaches may be particularly useful for treating habituated, compensatory misarticulations.

In addition, teaching the difference between nasal and oral sounds, as well as how to direct the air stream through the mouth, might also be useful. This can be accomplished using swimmer's nose clips to prevent nasal air escape, and help the child learn how airflow feels when it is directed through the mouth during speech production (Peterson-Falzone et al., 2006).

For children who continue to substitute glottal stops (i.e., production of a grunt-like sound in the glottis or throat) for high-pressure consonants such as stops, fricatives, or affricates even after surgical correction of the cleft, direct speech treatment should begin as soon as possible. Glottal stops are far easier to eliminate early on, and specific treatment procedures are available (c.f. Kuehn & Henne, 2003; Peterson-Falzone et al., 2006).

A promising technique for speech sound production training is **electropalatography (EPG).** This technique uses an artificial palatal plate containing electrodes connected to a computer. The palatal plate is fitted in the client's mouth and when the tongue contacts these electrodes during speech production, the articulatory patterns can be seen on the computer screen. Children with cleft palate can learn correct placement of the articulators for speech sound production using EPG.

Language Disorders

Research studies have found evidence of language delays or less well-developed language skills in children with cleft palate. A number of factors have been suggested as possible contributors to language delay in this population, including lengthy hospital stays, hearing loss, and poor speech production skills. A study by Broen and colleagues (1998) found significant differences (not delays) in the language skills of children with and without cleft palate, and determined that these differences were likely related to very early hearing loss and poor speech production skills due to velopharyngeal inadequacy. More research is needed, however, to determine the relation of these factors, and the specific syndromes and language differences or delays in the cleft palate population.

ASSESSMENT OF LANGUAGE DISORDERS

Children born with clefts should be routinely examined for potential delays in language development and specific language impairments. Language evaluations should include information about environmental factors, motor and mental development, and hearing acuity. Language assessment of children with clefts is the same as language assessment of other children (McWilliams et al., 1990). Standardized tests of receptive and expressive language like those discussed in Chapter 5 can be used effectively with the cleft palate population.

TREATMENT OF LANGUAGE DISORDERS

As with language assessment, treating language disorders for children with clefts does not differ substantively from treating language disorders in the noncleft population. In fact, it has been shown that delayed language development can in large part be prevented in this population. Early and repeated family counseling regarding receptive and expressive language development, aggressive treatment of middle ear disease, and language enrichment programs have been shown to prevent language difficulties (Bzoch, 1997). See Box 11.1 for a brief review of evidence-based treatment of resonance, articulation, and language disorders in children with cleft palate.

One last issue regarding language development in children with clefts should be noted. Mothers of cleft children may engage in significantly less verbal play with their child than mothers of noncleft children. The SLP should be mindful of this possibility and counsel new parents about how

BOX 11.1
Evidence-Based Practices for Individuals with Cleft Palate

Surgical intervention

- Although about 90% of children with non-syndromic clefts are expected to have good velopharyngeal function after the first surgery, speech therapy may still be needed. As structures of the head and face grow, velopharyngeal function may deteriorate.
- The type of secondary surgical procedure used in some children (i.e., secondary palatal surgery and/or pharyngeal flap surgery) depends on the severity of velopharyngeal inadequacy. Following secondary surgery, speech therapy is often needed to eliminate habituated compensatory misarticulations and nasal air emission during production of pressure consonants.

Specific behavioral treatment approaches or techniques

- *Continuous positive airway pressure (CPAP)* treatment is best suited for individuals with a small velopharyngeal gap (less than 2 mm) and a moveable velum, and it has been found to be effective in some patients with mild to moderate hypernasality.
- *Electropalatography (EPG)* provides visual feedback on the location and timing of tongue–palate contacts and continues to show promise for remediation of speech-sound disorders in the cleft palate population. EPG is effective in teaching correct

production of /s/ in preschool children with cleft palate.
- Bottom-up articulation drill procedures that focus on phonetic placement and sound shaping are recommended for children with repaired clefts, and they may be effective for sounds that are often difficult for this population. For instance, to teach the production of /s/ without nasal emission, have the child produce /t/ with the teeth closed. Then have the child prolong this sound, which should result in the correct production of /s/. The technique can be applied to other fricative or affricate sounds. For remediation of vowels produced with an abnormally high tongue position, have the child yawn while producing the vowel sound. Yawning causes the tongue to go down and the velum to go up.
- *Focused stimulation* and *enhanced milieu training (EMT)* models are naturalistic methods of stimulating speech and language development in young children that parents can do at home. Success of these approaches has been documented, particularly for children living in rural areas.

Based on Hardin-Jones et al., (2006); Kuehn et al., (2002); Kuehn & Henne (2003); Kummer (2006); Michi et al., (1993); Peterson-Falzone et al., (2006).

important early verbal play is to good language development. As the child matures, parents should be encouraged to read to the child and talk about daily events and experiences. Perhaps most important, parents should provide a good language model for their child. The SLP can be invaluable in helping parents to achieve this goal.

SUMMARY

Children with cleft palate face a myriad of problems from early infancy through adulthood. These problems can be treated effectively only when a team of professionals works cooperatively toward their resolution. The speech-language pathologist is an integral member of the cleft palate team who works in conjunction with surgeons, orthodontists, and other professionals to facilitate the development of normal speech and language for the child with a cleft. Surgical correction of the cleft by reconstruction of the palate and velopharyngeal mechanism must in many cases be followed by long-term therapy to remediate voice, resonance, and articulation disorders.

THOUGHT QUESTIONS

- Given the timeline of embryological development of the face and palate, why might it be important for couples planning to have a child to be as drug free as possible?
- Can you think of some environmental teratogens that you might be exposed to regularly?
- What impact might a cleft palate have on family–infant bonding?
- What are your impressions of the postsurgical results of the clefts you have seen (if any)? How do you think they differ in less well-developed countries? How do you think repaired clefts will function during speaking and eating?

SUGGESTED READINGS

Peterson-Falzone, S., Hardin-Jones, M., & Karnell, M. (2010). *Cleft palate speech* (4th ed.). St. Louis, MO: Mosby.

Peterson-Falzone, S., Trost-Cardamone, J., Karnell, M., & Hardin-Jones, M. (2006). *The clinician's guide to treating cleft palate speech*. St. Louis, MO: Mosby.

Shprintzen, R. (2000). *Syndrome identification for speech-language pathology: An illustrated pocket guide*. San Diego, CA: Singular.

ONLINE RESOURCES

American Cleft Palate-Craniofacial Association
www.acpa-cpf.org
The American Cleft Palate-Craniofacial Association site lists local organizations and has information for parents and professionals.
www.cleft.org/
Web site includes stories by families with children born with cleft lip and/or cleft palate, with links to related information.

National Craniofacial Association
www.faces-cranio.org/
National Craniofacial Association site has links to enable you to explore disorders associated with craniofacial anomalies.

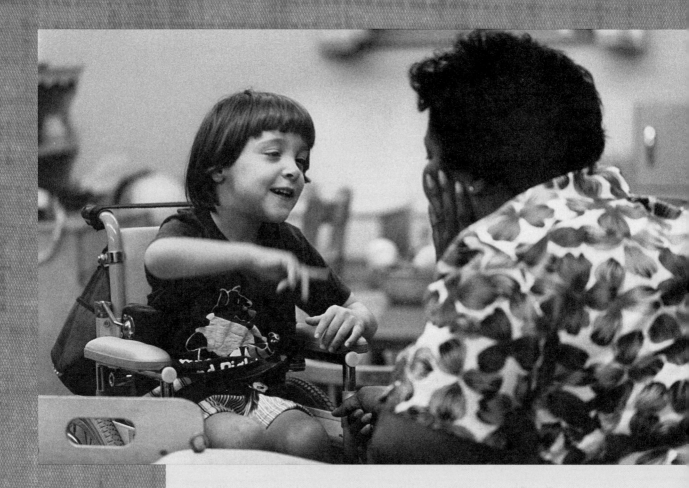

CHAPTER LEARNING GOALS

When you have finished this chapter, you should be able to:

- Describe the major differences between cerebral palsy, dysarthria, and apraxia of speech

- Explain the causes of neurogenic speech disorders

- Name the types of cerebral palsy and dysarthria

- Explain the general assessment and intervention techniques that are used with neurogenic motor-speech disorders and research-based findings on efficacy

Neurogenic Speech Disorders

12

Neurogenic speech disorders are difficulties related to problems of movement as a result of some neurological disorder or injury. They are sometimes referred to as motor-speech disorders. The term "motor" refers to movement.

Neurogenic speech disorders are a heterogeneous group of neurological impairments that affect the planning, coordination, timing, and execution of the movement patterns that are used to produce speech in both children and adults. Any or all of the processes of respiration, phonation, resonation, and articulation, described in previous chapters, may be affected. Although voice and fluency may also be involved, these are addressed in other chapters. In addition, language disorders often co-occur with neurogenic speech disorders. These are described in Chapter 7, "Adult Language Impairments."

That brief explanation does not begin to hint at the complexity of the disorders that fall within the boundaries of neurogenic speech disorders. So finite and particular are the movements needed for speech that more area in the brain is devoted to control of your vocal folds, tongue, lips, and other articulators than to any other bodily movement, even walking. Given this complexity, it is amazing that the process of producing speech becomes almost automatic for you and that you give little thought to it when speaking. In fact, we rarely consider the process unless something is wrong.

As with language, there does not seem to be a speech production area. Even those areas of the frontal lobe that are important for speech are not solely devoted to speech-specific tasks. They also participate in nonspeech tasks. Remember that accurate motor movements also depend on feedback so that muscles know when to moderate or extend movement.

In this chapter, we limit our discussion to the production of speech. We discuss three types of neurogenic speech impairments: cerebral palsy, dysarthria, and apraxia of speech. There may be overlap. For example, many individuals with cerebral palsy also exhibit dysarthria and apraxia of speech. Several very informative Web sites listed at the end of the chapter will further your exploration of these disorders.

CASE STUDY 12.1
Case Study of a Teen with a Neurogenic Speech Disorder: Caitlin

Caitlin, a cheerleader and member of the high school theater group, began experiencing slight speech problems in 11th grade. Her speech became slurred and difficult to understand. Even when she repeated herself to correct her speech, she often made the same errors. Both her parents and teachers noted the difference but assumed that Caitlin was talking too fast. Her parents became worried, however, when their daughter began complaining of severe headaches. After a neurological evaluation including a brain imaging scan, it was determined that she had a tumor that was putting pressure on the left frontal lobe of her brain.

Although surgery was successful, Caitlin still experienced speech difficulties and was referred to a speech-language pathologist who did a complete evaluation of Caitlin's motor speech abilities. The speech-language pathologist coordinated intervention services with a second speech-language pathologist in Caitlin's school district who agreed to provide similar services in the school. Several of Caitlin's friends and teachers were approached by the school SLP and enlisted to talk with Caitlin to ensure that she had to speak in school. Her parents were also part of the intervention team. After 8 months, Caitlin's speech has returned to the pretrauma level of performance.

As you read the chapter, think about

- Possible explanations for Caitlin's difficulties.
- Possible measures of Caitlin's speech that might have been used by her speech-language pathologist.
- Possible reasons for enlisting the help of so many individuals in Caitlin's intervention plan.

It might help you to remember these disorders if we make a somewhat artificial distinction. Because cerebral palsy occurs before, at, or shortly after birth, it is considered a *developmental* neuromotor deficit. In contrast, most but not all cases of dysarthria and apraxia occur after the neuromotor system is fully mature and therefore are considered to be *acquired* disorders.

CAUSES OF NEUROGENIC SPEECH DISORDERS

The major causes of neurogenic language and neurogenic speech disorders are similar.

Many conditions can result in disturbances in brain function. Stroke or cerebrovascular accident, discussed in Chapter 7, is the leading cause of neurogenic speech disorders. Certain racial/ethnic and gender differences exist in the incidence of strokes. In the United States, African Americans are more susceptible to strokes and hypertension than are individuals from other ethnic backgrounds (Singh et al., 1996). Although men of all backgrounds have more strokes than women, women seem particularly vulnerable to aneurysms (Leblanc, 1996). Cerebral hemorrhaging is also one of the leading causes of cerebral palsy in infants.

Traumatic brain injury (TBI), also discussed in Chapter 7, is another leading cause of neurogenic speech disorders. Males who experience TBI far outnumber females, and nearly 70% of injuries resulting in TBI occur in the under-35 age group.

Brain injury also may result from deprivation of oxygen as in a drowning accident. Greatly reduced oxygen, or **anoxia,** is a more common cause of parenatal, natal, and neonatal brain injury than of adult injury.

Brain tumors, or neoplasms, can also lead to neurogenic speech disorders, destroying healthy brain tissue by taking nutrition, impinging on healthy cells, or increasing the pressure within the brain cavity. At any given time, over 60,000 individuals in the United States have tumors of the nervous system. Not all of these affect speech. Some individuals may experience a slow degeneration of their cognitive abilities; others have a steep decline. Shortly before her death from a brain tumor, a friend was reduced to eye blinks and finger squeezes to communicate. Six months earlier, she had little impaired functioning. Some, but not all, tumors are operable or treatable with either chemotherapy or radiation.

Infections and toxins may also cause trauma to the central nervous system (CNS), although the incidence of these causes is changing. Infections such as meningitis and viral and fungal inflammations that once threatened healthy brains are now usually treatable by antibiotics if intervention begins in the early stages. The developing embryo is especially susceptible to infections. Some neural infections, such as those associated with new drugresistant microbes and the human immunodeficiency virus (HIV), the virus that causes AIDS, offer a challenge to our pharmacological methods of treatment.

The list of brain-injuring toxins is lengthy, and new products are being introduced daily. Obvious neurotoxins are lead, mercury, certain pesticides, and pollution, but the most prevalent culprits are alcohol and drug use by pregnant women. Some toxins can pass the placental barrier between the mother and the fetus.

Diseases, either inherited or acquired, can also affect the CNS. Many are slow, degenerative diseases that gradually rob their victims of muscular control. A "Who's Who" of this rogues's gallery includes, but is not limited to, multiple sclerosis, amyotrophic lateral sclerosis (ALS), Parkinson disease, Huntington's disease, and myasthenia gravis. Muhammed Ali, former world heavyweight champion boxer; Janet Reno, former attorney general of the United States in the Clinton administration; and actor Michael J. Fox all have Parkinsons disease. Each of the authors of this text has been touched in some way by a friend or relative with a neurological disease. Maybe you have too.

Whatever the cause, the speech of affected individuals may vary widely. Even individuals with the same etiology may have very different speech problems, depending on the severity of the disorder, the age of the client, the time since the incident, and the extent of the affected area. To the untrained ear, two very different clients may sound the same and both be classified as having speech that is slurred, sloppy, thick, or unclear. Such descriptors do little to differentiate between the various etiologies, and an SLP must describe these behaviors much more thoroughly.

CEREBRAL PALSY

The term *cerebral palsy* (CP) describes a heterogeneous group of neurological difficulties resulting from brain injury that occurs very early in fetal or infant development. The disorder is nonprogressive, meaning the condition does not worsen over time. Affected areas include motor movement, communication, growth and development, locomotion, learning, and sensation. Physical manifestations may range from extreme rigidity and immobility to being ambulatory, or capable of moving about relatively freely. Cerebral palsy may affect one or more limbs and might or might not be accompanied by speech difficulties. The cognitive abilities of people with cerebral palsy range from mental retardation through superior intelligence. One of the authors of this text, Dr. Owens, has a grandson with CP.

Movement patterns are learned from many, many repetitions. Therefore, faulty movement results in faulty patterns being learned. If you have typical motor patterns, you can probably pick up an object without looking at it.

Although the reported incidence of CP is low—1.5 to 4 per 1,000 births—the data may reflect poor reporting, misdiagnosis, or assignment of other labels, such as mental retardation, because the person has greater disorders in these areas. At present, more than 500,000 individuals in the United States have CP; most are under 21 years of age. Anywhere from 30% to 90% also have some dysarthria (Yorkston et al., 1988).

Three characteristics distinguish CP from some of the other neurogenic speech disorders that are discussed in this chapter. First, it is a developmental neurogenic disorder. Most neurogenic speech disorders are considered to be acquired; that is, typical speech patterns were established before the disorder occurred. The insult to the neurological system with cerebral palsy occurs before the neuromotor system has matured. As a result, the child must learn motor movements for which no patterns have been established.

Second, cerebral palsy is not a disease. It is a nonprogressive, noninfectious injury occurring before, at, or shortly after birth. Some children may improve with maturity, especially in the first few years of life as the brain matures rapidly.

Finally, the motor patterns in cerebral palsy are much more predictable than those in acquired neurogenic impairments. Although a person who has suffered a stroke may have severe impairment in an arm and a mild impairment in a leg on the same side, a person with CP is more likely to have similar severity in all affected limbs. These may include involvement of the legs (*paraplegia*), all four extremities (*quadriplegia*), one side (*hemiplegia*), or one limb (*monoplegia*).

Types of Cerebral Palsy

Not everyone with CP is alike. Clients vary in age, culture, education, and type and severity. The type of CP varies with the areas of the CNS that are affected. Injury may occur in the motor cortex, the pyramidal or extrapyramidal tracts, and the cerebellum as shown in Figure 12.1.

Most types of CP can be classified in one of three ways: spastic, athetoid, or ataxic. Although some infants with CP exhibit poor muscle tone and

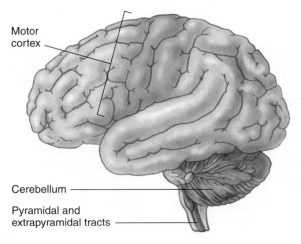

Motor cortex

Cerebellum

Pyramidal and extrapyramidal tracts

FIGURE 12.1

Areas of the brain important for motor function.

Signals to the muscles originate in the motor cortex and are sent deep into the brain to begin their descent. The cerebellum sets the overall tone and posture that gives the motor cortex the ability to execute intentional movements. In addition, although the motor cortex determines where to move, the cerebellum implements the proper timing and force. Motor nerve impulses continue through the pyramidal tract that relays intentional movement and the extrapyramidal tract that relays automatic, involuntary movement.

weakness, a condition called **hypotonia,** muscle movement and control almost always evolve during infancy into one of the three predominant types discussed here. *Spasticity,* or **hypertonia,** is a condition in which there is too much muscle tone, especially in the muscles that oppose the bending of joints and that help us to stand erect. Tone increases as muscles are stretched. *Athetosis,* or **dyskinesia,** is a slow, involuntary movement of the body. With a change in an individual's emotional state, such as being under stress, excited, angry, or amused, there may be an accompanying increase in muscle tone. **Ataxia** is uncoordinated movement.

It may be difficult to keep the types of cerebral palsy clear in your mind. The major features of each are presented on Table 12.1.

SPASTIC CEREBRAL PALSY

For approximately 60% of individuals with CP, the prominent characteristic is spasticity or increased muscle tone. When a muscle of someone with **spastic cerebral palsy** contracts, the opposing muscle may react abnormally to stretch by increasing muscle tone too much. Rigid opposing muscle groups make movement extremely difficult. Described as "exaggerated stretch reflex," movement is characterized by increased muscle tone in the muscles opposing the movement that is attempted. Because tone increases as these muscles are stretched, muscle movement is described as jerky, labored, and slow. Individuals with spastic CP may also exhibit infantile reflex patterns that in nonaffected children typically disappear within a few months of birth.

> Individuals with CP are a very heterogeneous group, varying in severity, type, and portion of the body affected. Like all individuals, they also differ in personality, interests, and maturity.

TABLE 12.1
Characteristics of cerebral palsy

Type of Cerebral Palsy	Characteristics	Area of Brain Affected
Spastic	Spasticity, increased muscle tone in opposing muscle groups	Motor cortex and/or pyramidal tract
	Rigidity and exaggerated stretch reflex	
	Jerky, labored, and slow movements	
	Infantile reflex patterns	
Athetoid	Slow, involuntary writhing	Extrapyramidal tract, basal ganglia
	Disorganized and uncoordinated volitional movement	
	Movements occur accompanying volitional movement	
Ataxic	Uncoordinated movement	Cerebellum
	Poor balance	
	Movements lack direction, force, and control	

Spasticity results from damage to the motor cortex of the brain and/or lower brain areas. Unable to direct and control lower structures, higher centers of functioning cannot block signals to increase muscle tone or rigidity; the result is hypertonicity.

In severe cases, the limbs may be rotated inward with the arms drawn upward and the head drawn to one side. Walking or even standing may be extremely difficult. Figure 12.2a shows the posture of an individual with severe spastic cerebral palsy.

ATHETOID CEREBRAL PALSY

Accounting for approximately 30% of individuals with CP athetoid CP is characterized by a slow, involuntary writhing, most pronounced when the individual attempts volitional movement. The resultant behavior may be

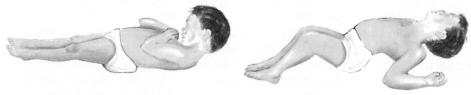

(a) Spastic cerebral palsy   (b) Athetoid cerebral palsy

FIGURE 12.2
Characteristic posture of severe spastic and athetoid cerebral palsy.

disorganized and uncoordinated. Individuals with athetoid CP may also exhibit infantile reflex patterns throughout their lives. In nonaffected children, these typically disappear within a few months of birth.

Athetosis is caused by injury to lower brain areas that help to plan motor patterns and modify motor cortex impulses. When damage occurs, cortical impulses cannot be moderated. Inhibitor mechanisms cannot appropriately monitor the excitation mechanisms of the motor cortex. The result is too much muscle activity.

In its most severe form, athetosis causes the individual's feet to turn inward, the back and neck to arch, and the arms and hands to be overextended above the head. The mouth may be open, resulting in drooling. Breathing may also be affected. Figure 12.2b shows the posture of an individual with severe athetoid CP.

The severity of athetoid CP varies between individuals. In a given person, the moment-to-moment strength of the athetosis varies with the situation. When the individual is quiet or at rest, athetosis might not be evident. Athetoid movements occur or are exaggerated when purposeful movement is attempted and when the individual is excited or emotionally upset.

ATAXIC CEREBRAL PALSY

Ataxic CP, accounting for approximately 10% of the population with CP, is characterized by uncoordinated movement and disturbed balance. The individual with ataxia seems clumsy and awkward. Movements lack direction, and hypotonic muscles lack adequate force and rate and have poor direction control. Walking is particularly difficult for the individual with ataxia and, in the most extreme cases, may be characterized by a wide stance with the head pushed forward and the arms back in an almost birdlike appearance. Even those who are less affected may have a gait resembling that of someone who is intoxicated.

Ataxia results from injury to the cerebellum. Injury to this part of the brain impairs the monitoring of balance information from the inner ears and of proprioceptive information from the muscles regarding the rate, force, and direction of movements. Coordination of muscle movement is difficult without accurate feedback. It is easy to see why walking would be especially problematic.

Motor-Speech Problems Associated with Cerebral Palsy

Not everyone with CP has motor-speech difficulties. For example, individuals might have spastic CP that involves primarily their legs (paraplegia). Nearly all people with athetoid CP exhibit an accompanying motor-speech disorder that affects all aspects of production. Ataxic speech difficulties may be related to cognitive impairment and phonological processing problems (Love, 1992).

Although adults with acquired motor-speech disorders once had typical speech, the developing child did not and consequently may develop atypical

The different types of CP result in differing speech characteristics.

motor patterns of production in the process of learning speech using a faulty motor system. In working with individuals with CP, the SLP considers both the control dysfunction and the overlaid learning problem.

All aspects of speech production—respiration, phonation, resonation, and articulation, plus prosody—may be affected. Speech may be slow and labored. In severe cases, it may be unintelligible. Swallowing may also be affected, and individuals may exhibit dysphagia (see Chapter 13).

Many individuals with CP have breathing difficulties, which, in turn, may affect speech. Breathing may be rapid and shallow. Vital capacity or the total amount of air expelled after a deep inhalation may be decreased, making it difficult for an individual to exhale sufficiently to produce speech. A client's speech may be limited to a word or short phrase.

Inconsistent or inadequate airflow and involvement of the laryngeal muscles will affect phonation. Voice quality may demonstrate hypertonia in several ways, from a breathy voice with puffs of air to a strained voice with hard glottal attack. A breathy voice may indicate a compensatory movement to force air from the lungs.

Resonance difficulties may be characterized by hypernasality resulting from dysfunction of the velopharyngeal mechanism. Inability to seal off the nasal cavity results in loss of air pressure, a critical component for good consonant production.

Articulation may be extremely difficult if there is involvement of the tongue, lips, and/or jaw. The tongue of an individual with CP may move as one unit with limited ability to differentiate its parts. Consequently, consonants, especially those made with the aid of the tip of the tongue—/s/, /z/, /l/, and /r/—will offer a particular challenge. Lip movement may be slow and restricted. Jaw and tongue movements may be unspecified, and they may move together. Articulation problems in athetoid CP seem to result from excessive jaw movement, limited tongue mobility, and velopharyngeal insufficiency.

> In the absence of established motor speech patterns, the child with cerebral palsy may develop abnormal movement patterns, further complicating intervention.

The prosodic aspects of speech—pitch, loudness, and duration—may be very monotonous. The client may be unable to perform the subtle oral movements that are necessary to convey shades of meaning or mark grammatical structures or morphological changes. Poor muscle control can make it difficult to initiate phonation and sustain it. The resultant speech may be choppy with short phrases or words and frequent interruptions. Speech may be characterized as nonrhythmic or nonfluent.

Other factors may also complicate the production of meaningful speech. These include intellectual, auditory, information-processing, and language impairments. Although many individuals with CP have average or above average intelligence, approximately half have some significant cognitive deficits (Bottenberg & Hanks, 1986). Hearing and speech sound discrimination may also be problematic, especially for individuals with athetoid CP. Attentional disorders may also be exhibited.

All of these factors plus injury to adjacent areas of the brain account for the language impairment that is found in many individuals with CP. This impairment may include delayed language development and immature linguistic structures and use.

Etiology

It would be impossible to catalog all the possible prenatal, natal, and neonatal conditions that could result in brain damage for an embryo, fetus, or infant. In general, the younger the developing being, the more rapidly the brain is maturing, and the more susceptible his or her brain is to damage. The incidence of CP is higher for extremely high-birthweight and extremely low-birthweight infants, nonwhite babies in the United States, children born to older mothers, in multiple births, and among males.

Premature infants account for only 2% of all live births but represent a substantially larger percentage of the population of individuals with disability. In some cases, the premature birth is related to prenatal difficulties, including malformation of the CNS. Premature infants are also more susceptible to neonatal complications, including respiratory dysfunction, that can lead to anoxia.

The two most common causes of CP are anoxia and hemorrhages in the brain. Anoxia, especially to the neuromotor areas of the brain, which are high oxygen users, can kill neurons in the CNS. Any interruption in the blood supply, as occurs in a hemorrhage in the vascular system, a not uncommon event in utero, can cause damage to a developing brain.

Infections and toxins may also disrupt brain development. Bacterial and viral infections, such as HIV, may infiltrate the brain from other bodily organs or be transported within the blood supply. During the first few months of pregnancy, before the development of a placental barrier, the embryo is especially susceptible to infections of the mother, such as influenza, rubella, and mumps, that can damage the developing brain. Toxic agents, such as heavy metals, mercury, and lead, may lodge in the brain and disrupt development. The use of alcohol and illicit drugs by pregnant women can also result in children born with brain dysfunction.

Finally, accidents during pregnancy and in the neonatal period also can result in fetal brain injury. The incidence of fetal injury due to automobile accidents has risen in recent years. Sadly, some infants are also physically abused.

Lifespan Issues

Early symptoms of CP may include irritability, weak crying and sucking, excessive sleeping, little interest in surroundings, and persistence of primitive reflexes beyond the newborn stage. Initial parental reactions on learning that their infant has CP vary and may include guilt, grief, anger, and denial. Typically, parents adjust well to their child but may exhibit *chronic grief,* or the continuing desire for their child to be "normal." The parent-child bonding process may be strained as the child fails to respond in predictable ways. In addition, the care of a child with CP may tax the family and introduce stress into the familial relationship.

It may take up to 2 years to confirm a diagnosis of CP among infants with mild involvement. The type of CP may change within the first few years, and it is important for the child and family to be in contact with medical and educational professionals. Motor delays associated with CP are often the first sign.

Children with CP usually begin school or receive intervention services early in life. Training emphasis is on physical movement and communication. Communication training may focus on both speech and language, and augmentative/alternative communication (AAC) methods, discussed in Chapter 15, may be introduced.

Variables such as severity, associated disorders, parental involvement, and school system flexibility are important in determining the appropriate educational environment. In general, children with average or better intelligence and mild CP are more likely to have a more typical educational experience. It is extremely important to assess the cognitive abilities of people with severe motor disabilities appropriately because a physical handicap may obscure intellectual functioning.

Many individuals, especially those with mild physical and cognitive difficulties, obtain higher education and/or go into competitive employment. Often, physical adaptations are made to improve performance. Other individuals may work and learn in centers run by agencies or the state. Workshops and day treatment programs also provide training in daily living and vocational skills for individuals with severe involvment and/or cognitive impairment. Case Study 12.2 presents the story of a young man with cerebral palsy.

Assessment

Intervention team membership changes in response to the changing lifespan challenges of the individual with CP.

As with many other disorders discussed in this text, assessment and rehabilitation for people with CP is a team effort. The team usually includes a pediatrician who often first identifies a disorder; a neurologist who confirms the diagnosis and describes the child's disability; a physical therapist who, along with an orthopedic surgeon, identifies motor patterns and implements muscle training and exercise to increase muscle tone, strength, and timing, and movement accuracy; an otolaryngologist who investigates and makes recommendations about the ear, nose, and throat; and a speech-language pathologist. Over the individual's lifespan, other professionals, including an occupational therapist, special education teacher, clinical psychologist, audiologist, ophthalmologist, rehabilitation engineer, and/or social worker, may also be involved. It is essential that professionals and parents become involved in the intervention process together as soon as possible.

Speech and language problems differ with the type and severity of cerebral palsy and with the age and functioning level of the individual. In addition to the procedures outlined in Chapter 4, the SLP will want to make a more thorough evaluation of the oral mechanism and, in many cases, to assess potential client success with an augmentative/alternative form of communication. Within the oral peripheral examination, the SLP will note the following with particular interest:

Symmetry, configuration, color, and general appearance of the tongue, palate, lips, teeth, and jaw

CASE STUDY 12.2
Personal Story of a Boy with Cerebral Palsy

Tony was born 3 months prematurely in a small rural hospital. The delivering obstetrician was concerned about possible oxygen deprivation at the time of birth, although Tony was placed in an incubator shortly after he was born.

Because of their son's prematurity, Tony's parents were counseled to expect developmental delays. They reported that he was irritable and seemed to have difficulty ingesting milk. At 4 months, his pediatrician expressed concern because of the continued presence of some reflexive behaviors, such as the whole-body response to startle, and the lack of motor responding, such as eye-hand coordination. She referred Tony to a developmental team in a large urban hospital.

The interdisciplinary team consisted of a pediatrician, neurologist, physical therapist, occupational therapist, developmental specialist, and speech-language pathologist. They determined that Tony had cognitive and motor delays and moderate dyskinesia or athetoid cerebral palsy.

As a result of the evaluation, it was recommended that Tony participate in a home-based interdisciplinary program with periodic reevaluation at the hospital. During the evaluation and subsequent consultation, Tony's parents heard the term "cerebral palsy" used to describe their child for the first time. The team recommended that the parents receive counseling and participate in a parents' group as a portion of their son's intervention plan.

By age 3, Tony was able to self-feed handheld food with some difficulty. Dressing was limited to completing tasks, such as pulling down a shirt that had been fitted over his arms and head. He could walk with great difficulty and usually needed support to steady himself. His speech consisted of a few words and phrases that were often unintelligible to people other than family. When unsure of his meaning, the family often used the immediate situation for interpretation.

At this time, Tony was enrolled in a special preschool for children with disabilities. On the advice of the school's speech-language pathologist, he began training with AAC. At first, this involved pointing to pictures on a communication board. Although his pointing response was somewhat imprecise, he continued to use the communication board until he entered elementary school. In first grade, Tony began to use a direct selection method of communicating using a computer and a joystick interface. Pictures evolved into words, then to individual letters. Now in third grade, Tony is communicating using a combination of his own speech and selection of pictures, words, and simple spelling on a computer, which he accesses by using the joystick control. He has a computer at home and in school for his use.

Movement of the tongue, soft palate, lips, and jaw

Swallowing (see Chapter 13 for details)

Valving

    Lung capacity and control

    Phonatory initiation, maintenance, and cessation

    Pitch and volitional pitch variations

    Loudness and volitional loudness variations

    Volitional pitch-loudness variations

Velopharyngeal adequacy

Range, velocity, and direction of tongue, lip, and jaw movement

The specific tasks are modified for young children, who may be unable to follow directions.

One form of instrumentation used in assessment of speech production is the electropalatograph (EPG) (Gibbon & Wood, 2003). The EPG consists of an artificial palate embedded with electrodes that record tongue contact with the palate during speech production. The artificial palate is connected to a computer display for analysis of tongue-palate contact patterns.

Oral motor abilities are very important in determining the appropriateness of augmentative/alternative communication (AAC). As the individual matures and develops, the AAC system must be continually reevaluated to determine whether it still maximizes the client's potential for communication (see Chapter 15).

The long-term nature of CP necessitates the establishment of realistic long-term goals. Limits to motor function improvement exist and must be considered. Once set, goals must be continually reevaluated. Team members can often help each other to set achievable goals.

> It is extremely important that the AAC systems evolve with the client's abilities and needs.

Intervention

Speech and language training is essential for many individuals with CP to correct or compensate for faulty motor speech patterns. Efficient motor patterns are strengthened, and inefficient ones are modified.

Because one motor pattern, such as breathing, may affect another, such as phonation, most SLPs now believe that it is best to use a systems approach, one that targets efficient use of the entire speech production system, rather than one that focuses exclusively on one organ or structure. For example, a systems approach might consider poor lung capacity to be adequate for speech if the client can be taught to use shorter units of production, thus negating the need to strain the breathing system by increasing the demand. In other words, speech production may be possible within the physiological limitations of the individual. In contrast, a focused approach might target lung capacity and efficient breathing alone. In a second example, an SLP using a systems approach might train rate control or the slowing of speech rate to increase overall speech intelligibility. A focused approach might target speech sound production exclusively.

Prosthetic devices and/or intraoral surgery may help to decrease hypernasality. These procedures alone will be insufficient, and the client must be trained with the new or repaired structure (see Chapter 10).

Exercises to improve oral nonspeech movement are usually minimal. Little carryover exists from nonspeech to speech movement patterns (Love, 1992). Likewise, exercising specific muscle groups, such as those for respiration or articulation, does little to improve speech.

Specific sounds are targeted on the basis of the ease of production. For the child with accompanying language deficits, these sounds and the child's interests will be important in the selection of initial words to be trained. Likewise, the child's interests and the demands of the environment will also be important in content selection with AAC.

The electropalatograph (EPG), mentioned in the assessment section, has application for intervention as well and can be used to train tongue movement by offering visual feedback of motor movement. EPG technology has wide application for a variety of motor-speech problems. Although the device may be awkward at first, wearing an EPG palate for as little as 2 hours results in speech that sounds typical for a client (McLeod & Searl, 2006). Through a combination of EPG computer display, speech monitoring, and biofeedback, some clients can learn better tongue control. EPG use is not limited to CP and has been used successfully with clients having all the neurogenic disorders presented in this chapter.

Speech perception and comprehension by others may be increased with additional linguistic knowledge in the form of alphabet cues and semantic predictability (Hustad, 2007). Alphabet cues are supplied via an alphabet board on which speakers indicate the first letter of each word while simultaneously speaking. Semantic predictability is the use of predictable sentences in specific contexts.

> To be maximally effective, AAC must be integrated into the user's everyday routine, and conversational partners must be trained in its use.

For many individuals with severe CP, unaided AAC systems, such as sign, are inappropriate. For these individuals, aided electronic AAC can greatly enhance communication abilities. Individual assessment is needed to determine the optimal system, including the client-device interface or input mode (Angelo, 1992; Light & Lindsay, 1991; Silverman, 1995; Yorkston et al., 1990). See examples on the accompanying CD-ROM.

Much research needs to be done on the effects of AAC on language acquisition in children with CP. Research findings suggest that making the process more typical facilitates acquisition (Rhea, 1997). Emphasis on the communication environment of these children is particularly important (Calculator, 1997; Light, 1997). Successful use of AAC requires operational, linguistic, social, and strategic competence (Light, 1989). Operational competence enables a client to make maximal use of the device. Linguistic and social competence is needed for the give and take of conversation. Finally, strategic competence includes individual strategies that each client uses to maximize the communication process and make it as typical as possible. These topics are discussed in more detail in Chapter 15.

The SLP often works closely with the physical therapist to maximize and facilitate movement patterns. Some employ the *Bobath method,* a procedure using head, body, and limb postures that inhibit reflexive and uncontrolled movements. The child is placed in positions that prohibit certain reflexive movements. For example, the child with athetoid CP may be seated with her or his legs bent or flexed and feet firmly supported to inhibit extensor motor patterns. Once the child can perform desired movements within a reflex-inhibiting posture, the posture is gradually changed to a more functional one while attempting to maintain the desired movement. Even SLPs who do not subscribe to this method of intervention generally accept the notion of using either postural supports or seating systems to improve movement.

> Motor performance of individuals with CP can often be improved by consideration of positioning and placement of the trunk, neck, and head for maximum facilitation.

Parents must be consulted by the SLP and other professionals regarding their expectations for their child. Parents must learn to be realistic about their child's functioning level and the prognosis for change. SLPs must be careful not to mislead parents who have a natural desire for their child to improve. Attempts to reach unattainable goals result in the placing of unrealistic demands on children. Interaction between the family, child, and professionals is essential, and the family should be involved as a fully participating member of the intervention team.

THE DYSARTHRIAS

It might seem strange that movement would be altered but the pattern remain. Have you ever broken a bone? Although movement is altered, you still remember how to make that movement.

As we mentioned previously, dysarthria is a group of neuromuscular impairments that may affect the speed, range, direction, strength, and timing of motor movement as the result of paralysis, weakness, or discoordination of the muscles. Motor movements that were previously established may have been lost or modified in some way, though the pattern for that movement still exists. The processes of respiration, phonation, resonation, and articulation all may be affected. Motor function may be excessively slow or rapid, decreased in range or strength, and have poor directionality and coordination. It may be more appropriate to speak of *the dysarthrias,* given the wide variety of impairments included under this name.

As you read, keep in mind that we are describing specific types of dysarthria that may only rarely be seen in their pure form in real individuals. It is not uncommon for dysarthrias to occur with other disorders. One study found that all of the subjects identified as having apraxia of speech (AOS) and motor neuron disease (MND), a degenerative disorder, also had spastic or mixed spastic-flaccid dysarthria (Duffy et al., 2006).

Speech may be slowed or, in some disorders, be excessively fast or contain involuntary movements. The range of movements may decrease until only tiny, barely discernible ones are possible. Direction of movement may become imprecise and nonrepeatable. Strength may decrease, and timing may become either erratic—fluctuating wildly—or monotonous. Unlike apraxia, a problem of motor planning and coordination, which we discuss later in this chapter, the dysarthrias represent difficulties in motor-speech control.

Speech intelligibility is most affected by motoric impairment of the tongue, lips, jaw, and soft palate. A variety of speech features may be affected. Problems of articulation, voicing, prosody, and respiration may be intertwined. Accurate description requires the SLP to

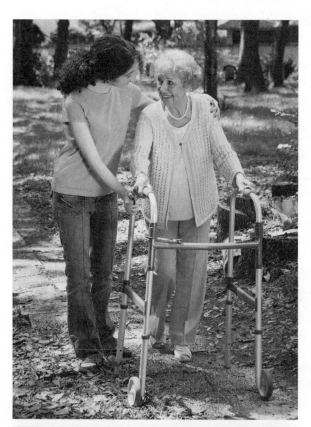

Dysarthrias can occur with or be a symptom of other cognitive or neuromuscular disorders.

Figure 12.3

Possible speech dimensions of dysarthria.

Source: Based on Darley et al. (1975).

Respiration

Forced expirations and/or inspirations

Grunt at end of expiration

Audible inspiration

Voice

Pitch

Inappropriate pitch level

Monopitch

Pitch breaks

Voice tremor

Loudness

Inappropriate loudness level

Alternating loudness

Excess loudness variation

Monoloudness

Loudness decay

Quality

Harsh, strained/strangled, or continuous or transient breathy voice

Hyponasality or hypernasality

Nasal emissions

Voice stoppages

Prosody

Inappropriate rate

Increased overall or in segments or variable

Prolonged intervals

Short rushes of speech

Short pauses

Inappropriate silences

Stress

Reduced or excess and equal

Articulation

Imprecise consonants

Phonemes repeated or prolonged

Vowels distorted

unweave each speech parameter. The speech pattern presented by a client depends on the location and extent of the neural damage as well as on the etiology. Figure 12.3 presents speech dimensions that may be observed in clients with dysarthria. Note that several parameters of voice, mentioned in Chapter 9, are present.

Dysarthria is not a language disorder. The individual with dysarthria but no other complications exhibits good language structure and vocabulary, has good reading comprehension, can participate in the give and take of conversation as well as her or his physical limitations permit, and is able to convey by other means, such as a computer, sentences that she or he seems unable to produce freely through speech. Audio and video speech samples of persons with dysarthia are presented on the accompanying CD-ROM.

Types of Dysarthria and Associated Etiologies

The muscular disorders found in dysarthria represent a variety of neurological diseases. Although individuals with dysarthria share some common symptoms, distinct clusters of neurological and speech characteristics exist that describe particular variations of the disorder.

Different types of dysarthria are the result of lesions to different parts of the CNS and PNS as presented in Figure 12.4. Certain commonalities exist, as noted in Table 12.2. These include inadequate breath supply; voice deviations, such as pitch variations and breaks and voice quality anomalies; prosodic problems of slow, rapid, or varying speed; nasality; and articulation errors.

Five distinct types of dysarthria can be identified by their speech characteristics and the impaired neuromuscular processes (Bloom & Ferrand, 1997; Darley et al., 1975; Rosenbek & LaPointe, 1985). These include **flaccid, spastic, ataxic, hyperkinetic,** and **hypokinetic dysarthria.** Disorders affecting multiple motor systems may yield a mixed dysarthria, as is found in amyotrophic lateral sclerosis (ALS); multiple sclerosis, and Wilson's disease, to name a few. Each type of dysarthria and etiology is discussed briefly here.

> Dysarthria is a group of related motor disorders with a variety of etiologies and sites of lesion.

Flaccid Dysarthrias

Flaccid muscles possess a weak, soft, flabby tone, called *hypotonia,* resulting in weakness or paralysis of the affected muscle. Dysarthria of this type usually results from lesions in the cranial and spinal nerves or in the muscle unit itself. Weak muscles tire quickly. Affected muscles may cause reduced vital capacity and shallow breathing, breathy voice and aphonia, reduced pitch and loudness levels, monotone, hypernasality, and imprecise articulation. Bell's

Figure 12.4

....

Central and peripheral nervous systems.

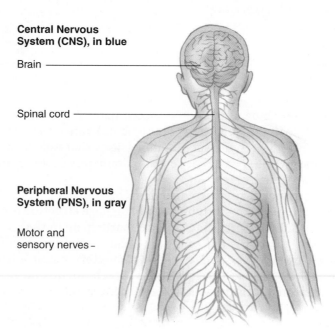

Central Nervous System (CNS), in blue

Brain

Spinal cord

Peripheral Nervous System (PNS), in gray

Motor and sensory nerves

TABLE 12.2
....
Characteristics of the dysarthrias

Type of Dysarthria	Voice Quality	Speech Rate	Articulation
Flaccid dysarthria			
Weak, soft, flabby muscle tone; lesions in the lower motor neurons (cranial and spinal nerves) or in the muscle unit itself	Breathy voice, monopitch/tone, hypernasality, reduced pitch/loudness	Short phrases	Imprecise consonants
Spastic dysarthria			
Stiff and rigid muscles; lesions in the upper motor neurons and the pyramidal tract	Monopitch/loudness, reduced stress, harsh voice, hypernasality, strained/strangled voice	Slow	Imprecise consonants
Ataxic dysarthria			
Damage to the cerebellum; muscle weakness and coordination problems involving accuracy, timing, and direction	Excessive and equal stress, harsh voice	Prolonged pauses and rate	Imprecise consonants, irregular articulatory breakdown
Hyperkinetic dysarthria			
Increased movement from lesions of the extrapyramidal tract and basal nuclei	Monopitch, harsh voice, excess loudness	Variable rate, silences, prolonged intervals	Imprecise consonants, distorted vowels
Hypokinetic dysarthria			
Decrease or lack of appropriate movement from lesions of the extra pyramidal tract and basal nuclei; muscles rigid and stiff	Monopitch/loudness, reduced stress, harsh/breathy voice	Variable rate, silences, prolonged intervals	Imprecise consonants
Mixed dysarthrias			
Severe muscle weakness from diffuse brain damage	Hypernasality, harsh voice, low pitch, monopitch/loudness, excess and equal stress	Slow rate, prolonged intervals	Imprecise consonants, distorted vowels

Source: Based on Darley et al. (1975).

palsy, a facial nerve disorder; bulbar palsy; myasthenia gravis; and muscular dystrophy are characterized by flaccid paralysis.

Bulbar Palsy   A flaccid dysarthria, **bulbar palsy** results from involvement either at the neuron (nerve cell) level or in the synapse (space between neurons). Most likely, the neurons or synapses fail or are slow in chemically resetting after nerve firing. In addition, bulbar palsy is characterized by muscle atrophy and by random and irregular contractions (**vasiculation**) of nerve bundles. These rapid, minute contractions have been described by individuals with bulbar palsy as feeling like a bubbling under the skin. Tremors may be obvious in the tongue when it is extended. In general, the speech of these individuals is weak, hypernasal, and monopitched with articulation difficulties. A sample of the speech of a person with bulbar palsy is presented on the accompanying CD-ROM.

Myasthenia Gravis   A common disorder, **myasthenia gravis** affects the neuromuscular juncture. The disorder is characterized by a rapid weakening of the muscle due to the inadequate transmission of the nerve impulse. Muscles tire quickly but regain their strength after a short interval of rest. Velar and laryngeal muscles are often affected.

Muscular Dystrophy   In **muscular dystrophy,** the muscles themselves are affected. Muscles may be unable either to contract or to relax. A progressive degenerative disease, muscular dystrophy may eventually affect all aspects of speech.

SPASTIC DYSARTHRIAS

Spastic paralysis—stiff and rigid muscles—is the result of lesions in the lower brain. The most common cause is stroke, and the results may be temporary or permanent. Lesions in the left hemisphere may be accompanied by aphasia and result in mild spasticity (see Chapter 7). More severe spastic dysarthria is bilateral, with the site of lesion in areas such as the brain stem where left and right innervation are in close proximity. Hypertonia makes movement difficult, and speech is characterized as slow with jerky, imprecise articulation and reduction of the rapidly alternating movements of speech.

Pseudobulbar Palsy   *Pseudobulbar palsy* is an example of spastic paralysis. Although individuals with pseudobulbar palsy exhibit the muscle weakness and loss of movement that are found in bulbar palsy, muscle atrophy and vasiculation do not seem to be present. Movement is characterized by hyperflexia, a combination of overreaction and overreach. The voice of individuals with pseudobulbar palsy is strained and strangled-sounding, resulting from intermittent spasticity. The rate is slow, and articulation is imprecise.

ATAXIC DYSARTHRIA

Damage to the cerebellum can result in a combination of muscle weakness or reduced tone or hypotonia and problems with muscle coordination, called *ataxia* (Kent, et al., 2001). Ataxic dysarthria is the result of breakdown in motor organization and control (Duffy, 1995). Little or no paralysis exists, and the problem is one involving the accuracy, timing, and direction of movement. Movements overshoot. The signal to start a movement is received, and the accompanying inhibition is impaired. As a result, movements are jerky and imprecise. Congenital ataxia is a form of cerebral palsy that is seen in children.

Speech is characterized by a shift in fundamental frequency and variability in the slow rate of moving between different speech sounds (diadochokinesis) (Kent et al., 2000). Energy varies across repeated syllables, respiration is poorly coordinated, and voicing and articulation are inadequate and imprecise.

HYPERKINETIC DYSARTHRIAS

Hyperkinesia, or increased movement, called tremors and tics, results from lesions of the mid and lower brain. *Tremors* are involuntary, nonpurposeful, rhythmic movements caused by contractions of antagonistic muscles. Several types of tremors exist. **Tics** are involuntary, rapid and repetitive, stereotypic movements. Unlike tremors, tics can be suppressed for short periods of time. One characteristic of hyperkinetic dysarthria is inaccurate articulation. Two disorders, dystonia and chorea, are forms of hyperkinetic dysarthria.

Dystonia   **Dystonia** is characterized by a slow increase and decrease of hyperkinesia involving either the entire body or localized sets of muscles. Excessive movement is slow and sustained, often writhing in nature. Like chorea, dystonia may involve either the entire motor system or be localized. As a result, there are excessive pitch and loudness variations, irregular articulation breakdown, and vowel distortions.

Chorea   Unlike dystonia, **chorea** is characterized by rapid or continual hyperkinesia. Chorea movements are characterized as random, irregular, and/or abrupt, usually lasting less than one second (Roseneldt, 1991). Movement may involve the entire body or a particular segment. Hyperkinesia impairs control and reduces coordination, especially in rapid successive movements such as speech. Speech, when affected, may be characterized by inappropriate silences caused by voice stoppage; intermittent breathiness, strained harsh voice, and hypernasality; imprecise articulation with prolonged pauses; and forced inspiration and expiration resulting in excessive loudness variations (Duffy, 1995).

Huntington's Chorea   An inherited progressive disease, also known as Huntington's disease, Huntington's chorea results from a genetic defect on chromosome 4 (American Psychiatric Association, 1994). Initial symptoms include involuntary movements and behavior change. As the disease progresses, movements become rigid with reduced speed and difficulty with coordination. Jerky, irregular movements affect the diaphragm, laryngeal muscles, tongue, and lips. In addition to the speech difficulties, language may be affected as a result of cognitive and memory changes. In general, individuals with Huntington's chorea have the same verbal output as their non-Huntington peers, but they are less informative with their language (Murray, 2000). Their language is characterized by a smaller proportion of grammatical utterances and a larger proportion of simple sentences than both non-Huntington individuals and those with Parkinson disease.

Accompanying personality changes may include depression, paranoia, delusional thoughts, and intellectual decline (Greenamyre & Shoulson, 1994).

HYPOKINETIC DYSARTHRIAS

Like hyperkinetic dysarthria, hypokinetic dysarthria is caused by lesions of the mid and lower brain, though the result is just the opposite: a decrease or lack of appropriate movement. Muscles become rigid and stiff, resulting in restricted motor movement. One form of hypokinetic dysarthria is found in many people with Parkinson disease.

Parkinson Disease   In Parkinson disease (PD), the individual's muscles become rigid as opposing pairs of muscles contract simultaneously. Motor movements become increasingly reduced, a condition called **hypokinesia.** Other characteristics include involuntary shaking or tremors when at rest, slowness of movement, and difficulty initiating voluntary movements. Symptoms reflect the reduced supply of dopamine, a neurotransmitter, a result of loss of dopaminergic neurons. Tremors may be controlled by different neural systems rather than one central tremor generator (Gurd et al., 1998). Comments by a professional with Parkinson disease are presented in Case Study 12.3.

CASE STUDY 12.3
The Story of Carlos, a Man with Parkinson Disease

Carlos is 64 and retired. He had to retire because the effects of PD would no longer allow him to work as a foreign language professor. His wife, 3 years younger, has also retired in order to take care of her husband. About 15 years ago, Carlos noticed small nerve twitches, usually when he was at rest. At first, they were intermittent and he thought they were the result of nervousness, stress, or muscle fatigue. As they became more frequent, Carlos found it harder and harder to ignore the symptoms.

Carlos's disease has progressed to the point where he walks by shuffling his feet and he can only climb stairs with assistance and support. In danger of falling when he walks, Carlos has found that even getting over the upturned edge of a carpet can offer a genuine challenge. For this reason, he and his wife rarely go out, although they daily walk the lightly traveled road in front of their house because it is flat and easy for him to manage. Carlos calls it his "workout routine."

Carlos finds meals less satisfying than before because the consistency of some foods makes them difficult for him to chew. Although Carlos eats independently, his food must be cut beforehand into small pieces. If he uses a knife at all, it is for spreading, not cutting.

Although his speech is affected and comes in short quiet bursts, Carlos has maintained his sense of humor and his sarcastic wit. If anything, he's modified his speech so these short barbs are even more pointed. He still loves to tell stories of growing up in New York City.

Along with the tremors and decreased range of movement, Carlos has experienced other physiological changes related to PD. He tires easily, quickly becomes short of breath, and has difficulty concentrating. At other times, he seems to become lost in seemingly repetitive tasks, such as picking up lint. Medication, which raises his level of dopamine, gives him smoother movement but is only temporary at best. He is sometimes frustrated by his response to the medication and his inability to time its effect on his movement for special times, such as a visit by his grandchildren.

PD may result from different pathogenetic mechanisms, including genetic or environmental factors or an interaction of both (Liss et al., 2006). For example, pallido-ponto-nigral degeneration (PPND), a neurodegenerative syndrome, is a familial disorder linked to chromosome 17q21–22. The characteristics include dementia and rapidly progressing parkinsonism usually occurring in middle age or later.

Almost all individuals with PD develop voice and speech problems (Ho et al., 1998). These include reduced loudness; breathy, harsh, or hoarse voice quality; reduced pitch inflection; imprecise and reduced range of articulatory movements; short bursts of speech; voice tremor; dysfluencies; and overall reduction in speech intelligibility (Ramig et al., 2004; Sapir et al., 2006). Although speakers with PD are able to produce higher variation or contrastivity levels in sentence repetition tasks, they are limited in their ability to do so (Rosen et al., 2006). Contrastivity includes the acoustic characteristics of sound frequency, intensity, and shape and contributes to the ability to produce distinguishable speech sounds.

These deficits are usually accompanied by orofacial abnormalities such as disturbed swallowing, reduced facial expression, and tremor (Perez et al., 1996; Sharkawi et al., 2002; Spielman et al., 2003). All orofacial muscles are involved, but tongue movement is affected more than jaw and lip movement (Yunusova et al., 2008).

Although speech rate increases, it may be perceived to be even faster than it actually is (Tjaden, 2000). Voice changes may occur early in the course of the disease, although articulation deficits typically do not. Dysarthria is a symptom in the more advanced stages of PD. Speech may become extremely rapid, accompanied by imprecise consonant formation as a result of weak tongue strength and endurance (Solomon et al., 2000). Speech deficits may be accompanied by a decrease in nonlinguistic communication, such as gestures and facial expression.

Although individuals with PD have a similar verbal output to their non-PD peers, they are less informative with their language (Murray, 2000). Individuals with PD also have a smaller proportion of grammatical sentences.

The most common form of Parkinson disease occurs in 1% of the population over age 60. (www.michaeljfox.org/living_aboutParkinsons_parkinsons101.cfm#q1, 2006). In real numbers, approximately half a million individuals have PD in the United States, and about 50,000 new cases occur annually (www.ninds.nih.gov/disorders/parkinsons_disease/parkinsons_research.htm, 2009). A sample of the speech of a person with PD is presented on the accompanying CD-ROM.

Mixed Dysarthrias

Some dysarthrias are not easily classified within the system just described. Called **mixed dysarthrias,** these disorders are characterized by symptoms or areas of brain injury that cross several dysarthrias. Diffuse brain damage may result from degenerative disorders, toxins, metabolic disorders, stroke, trauma, tumors, and infectious diseases. Amyotrophic lateral sclerosis is one example of this category.

Amyotrophic Lateral Sclerosis Commonly called Lou Gehrig's disease for the baseball player who was afflicted with it in the early 20th century, **amyotrophic lateral sclerosis (ALS)** is a rapidly progressive degenerative disease that involves both the upper and lower motor neurons and spinal cord.

Mental capacity is not affected, but the individual gradually loses control of her or his musculature. ALS is characterized by fatigue, muscle atrophy (loss of bulk), involuntary contractions, and reduced muscle tone. Speech deficits are common in the later stages of the disorder (Yorkston et al., 1993). These include a labored, slow rate; short phrasing, long pauses, hypernasality, and severely impaired articulation (Duffy, 1995). The slow rate influences the timing of elements within each sound, distorting its production (Tjaden & Turner, 2000). Vowel production differs across speakers and vowels, and with the surrounding sounds in a speech (Yunusova et al., 2008).

ALS combines both flaccid and spastic dysarthria. Dysarthria increases as the disease progresses, and approximately 75% of affected people are unable to speak at the time of death. Age of onset is usually in the mid-50s. Incidence figures vary but may be as high as 2 per 100,000 individuals. Males are affected more frequently than females. Death usually occurs within 5 years after the initial diagnosis. A sample of the speech of a person with ALS is presented on the accompanying CD-ROM.

Lifespan Issues

Most acquired dysarthria occurs in adults. Even the individual with mild dysarthria may be reluctant to speak, leading to assumptions by others that the person is frightened, tense, shy, or unfriendly. For some individuals, even a slight speech imperfection can be cause for embarrassment or depression. In the more advanced dysarthrias, individuals may be frustrated as loved ones and acquaintances attempt to communicate for them by finishing sentences or ordering for them in restaurants. In turn, the individual may communicate and socialize less. Difficulty communicating may limit the opportunities to participate in social, occupational, and educational activities, leading to feelings of isolation.

Some individuals with dysarthria are unable to live independently and may need daily living assistance or institutional care. The social, physical, psychological, and familial adjustments in this situation can be enormous.

In the later stages of progressive degenerative disorders, the individual may be unable to care for herself or himself. Movement may be very difficult, and the person may be unable to speak. AAC devices may be helpful even for the most severely affected individuals.

Neuromotor problems are not limited to speech production and may have a profound effect on many aspects of an individual's life.

Assessment

The SLP is an important member of the diagnostic team. By identifying differing speech patterns characteristic of specific neurological conditions, the SLP provides valuable information on localized neurological conditions to other team members.

The purposes of evaluation for dysarthria are many and include the following:

To determine whether a significant long-term problem exists

To describe the nature of impaired functions, specifically, the types of problems, their extent/severity, and the effect of these impairments on everyday, functional communication

To identify functions that are not impaired

To establish appropriate goals and decide where to begin intervention

To form a well-reasoned prognosis based on the nature of the disorder, the client's age, the age or stage of injury or disease, the presence of other accompanying conditions, client motivation, and family support

As described in Chapter 4, the speech-language pathologist thoroughly evaluates oral peripheral function, conversational speech, and speech in special tasks. The oral-motor mechanism is evaluated as outlined in the section on CP. Of particular importance in assessment of dysarthria are the range, speed, and direction of oral movement.

Although very few commercial test procedures are available, most SLPs working in hospitals or outpatient clinics have a standard assessment protocol that they use for motor-speech evaluations. These procedures might or might not rely on the use of instrumental approaches and computerized analysis.

Given the difficulty of precise assessment of motor-speech disorders in adults with acquired neurological impairment, one promising technique is the use of online real-time videoconferencing among several SLPs during an evaluation (Hill et al., 2006). Although pilot studies have been conducted, additional refinement of the technology and of assessment procedures will determine if such technology is feasible in the future.

Intervention

Some basic principles underlie intervention for acquired motor-speech disorders (Darley et al., 1975):

Compensatory strategies: Maximize individual strengths while working to bypass physical limitations.

Automatic to volitional shift: Foster more purposeful control over automatic and overlearned behaviors.

Just as the AAC system of the child with CP must change as the child matures, so that of the individual with a degenerative disorder must change as the disorder progresses.

Behavior change monitoring: Maintain precise records and foster self-monitoring by the client.

An early start: Early intervention forestalls formation of bad habits.

Motivation: Provide information and support.

The SLP begins with this basic foundation.

The type of intervention, its course, and the prognosis vary with the underlying cause of the dysarthria. Some diseases, such as PD or Wilson's, are *progressive,* the client's condition degenerating gradually over time. As severity increases or a client becomes less motivated, the prognosis becomes less optimistic. In cases of irreversible disease, therapy goals become holding actions in which the client and the SLP attempt to hold the client's performance at a certain plateau, maintaining the client's speech abilities even as the client's overall function decreases (Yorkston et al., 1995). Other goals might include teaching compensatory skills, such as the use of an augmentative/alternative form of communication. One young man we know used a keyboard to communicate through his computer. When this became too difficult, he used a joystick to navigate the keyboard. Spelling became too arduous, and electronic picture communication using the joystick was substituted. After several modifications, he now communicates with a combination of eye gazes and hand squeezes.

Because dysarthria affects all aspects of speech production, intervention must address the client's difficulties in respiration, phonation, resonance, and articulation, as well as prosody. Of concern within each area are muscle timing, strength, and tone. Therapy might focus on sustaining phonation, production of nasal and nonnasal words (*met-pet, neat-beat, king-kid*), and speech-sound production in meaningful words.

Intelligibility of words improves with repeated training, although the mode of presentation of words—audiovisual versus audio only—does not seem to affect production accuracy (Hustad & Cahill, 2003).

Speech supplementation strategies that provide additional information to a listener can also significantly increase speech intelligibility (Hustad & Beukelman, 2001; Yorkston & Beukelman, 2004). The most effective strategies seem to be alphabet cues or combined cues and slower speech (Hustad et al., 2003). With alphabet cues, speakers point to the first letter of each word as they say the word. Combined cues include both alphabet cues and topic cues in which the listener is supplied with the topic prior to the speaker's beginning to talk.

Traditionally, intervention has included nonspeech oral motor treatments (NSOMTs), including exercise, massage, blowing, positioning, icing, sucking, swallowing, cheek puffing, and other nonspeech activities. Data on the value of this methodology were mostly weak and anecdotal. Despite the popularity of NSOMTs, evidence-based practice suggests that sufficient evidence does not exist to support their effectiveness in improving speech (Lass & Pannbacker, 2008). See Box 12.1.

Intervention is best when it occurs within a meaningful speech context but may include drill, progressively more complex tasks, and feedback. The SLP works with the physical and occupational therapists to coordinate

BOX 12.1
Evidence-Based Practice with Motor Impairments

Repetition of movement

- Repetition is important for maintaining changes in the brain and their related functional benefits. In general, maintenance of intervention gains requires long-term, consistent use of a skill.

Intensity of intervention

- Following a stroke, early overuse of a weak limb can result in greater deficits, but complete disuse can also slow recovery. Therefore, intervention should be less intense at first and then become more intense over time.
- There are more beneficial results from practice distributed over time than from intensive mass practice.

Techniques

- Electropalatograph (EPG) technology offers modest gains in speech production.

- Evidence does not support the use of nonspeech oral motor treatments (NSOMTs) as a standard treatment. These methods should not be used as a speech production intervention.

Parkinson disease

- Pharmacological, surgical, and traditional speech therapy methods for PD yield little in long-term intervention effects.
- The Lee Silverman Voice Treatment (LSVT) produces marked and long-term improvement in voice and speech functions in individuals with PD.
- Intense intervention for phonation shows positive results.
- Intervention improves speech intelligibility for two thirds of clients.

Source: Based on Lass & Pannbacker (2008); Raymer et al. (2008); Sapir et al; (2006, 2007), Yorkston (2008).

exercises to increase muscle functioning or to decrease hypertonia through relaxation techniques.

Respiratory exercises emphasize efficient breath control and sustained exhalation. These exercises inevitably lead into sustained phonation. Either vocal fold exercises or relaxation techniques accompanied by easy phonation may also be a part of the intervention regime. Intervention for voice disorders is discussed in Chapter 9. Likewise hypernasality, the primary disorder of resonance, is treated through exercise. In addition, prosthetic devices similar to those discussed with cleft palate (see Chapter 11) may be fitted; the client is then trained to use them properly to achieve either velopharyngeal closure or approximation. Although progress in all these areas will improve articulation, such improvement does not preclude working directly with the client's articulation abilities. Exercises focus on auditory and proprioceptive feedback and placement of the articulators.

One technique that holds some promise for those with PD is the Lee Silverman Voice Treatment (LSVT). The LSVT, an intensive, 1-month speech therapy regimen, has been shown to produce marked and long-term improvement in voice and speech functions (Farley et al., 2008; Sapir et al., 2007; Trail et al., 2005). In general, the LSVT trains speakers to use a louder voice while using self-monitoring.

New evidence about nonspeech motor recovery and brain plasticity or the ability of the brain to adapt to injury may offer new avenues of intervention for neurogenic speech disorders (Maas et al., 2008). Because speech is a motor skill, motor-learning research may provide important insights into how to enhance relearning and/or reorganization of the speech-motor system. At present, it is unknown whether speech-motor control will respond to the same types of intervention.

Many individuals with severe dysarthria never regain enough intelligible speech to communicate even simple conversational messages. These clients may benefit from the use of AAC (see Chapter 15) as a substitution for or a complement to oral forms of communication to increase the intelligibility for severely dysarthric speech (Hustad & Beukelman, 2001). Most of the considerations mentioned in the discussion of CP are also applicable.

As long as there is no accompanying cognitive or language impairment, adults may find spelling of words on an AAC device to be an acceptable substitute for, or accompaniment to, speech.

Unaided AAC systems such as sign may be taught if the client does not have accompanying severe aphasia or severe motor involvement, such as those found in PD, that may interfere with communication (Garcia et al., 2000). People who have a language disorder in addition to a speech disorder still may have some difficulty forming messages.

Aided systems, such as communication boards or electronic devices, have been used successfully, although the most common AAC devices for speakers with dysarthria are speech amplifiers that increase loudness. Only very careful evaluation can help the SLP to determine the appropriate device and symbol system for a client.

Neurosurgical, genetic, and pharmacological interventions hold great promise for individuals with some forms of neurological impairment, although speech and nonspeech movements respond differently to these interventions (Camicioli et al., 1998). For example, surgical placement of an electronic stimulator on the globus pallidus of the brain of individuals with PD modifies some abnormal neural activity (Solomon et al., 2000). As a result, oral tremors decrease and the amount of voluntary responding increases.

APRAXIA OF SPEECH

Apraxia is a disorder in volitional or voluntary motor placement and sequencing that is unrelated to muscle weakness, slowness, or paralysis. It is the result of an acquired neurological impairment of the ability to program—organize and plan—and execute movement of the muscles for speech production. Because apraxia can involve any muscle group, apraxia that affects the initiation and execution of the movement patterns for speech is called **apraxia of speech (AOS).** Apraxia of the mouth area is termed **oral apraxia** and is often, but not always, associated with apraxia of speech.

Apraxia of speech is a problem of speech-sound articulation and prosody or rhythm caused by a neurologically based movement disorder

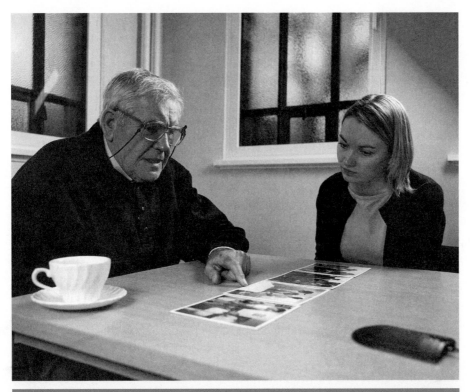

The individual with apraxia of speech may say the name of common objects differently on repeat attempts, reflecting programming difficulties.

(Darley et al., 1975; Duffy, 2005; Kearns & Simmons, 1988; Yorkston et al., 1988). Difficulties are not the result of muscle or linguistic processing deficits, although these disorders may co-occur with apraxia of speech. Individuals with apraxia have difficulty planning and executing the movements to position the articulators for correct sound production.

The speech of individuals with apraxia is characterized by groping attempts to find the correct articulatory position, with great variability on repeated attempts. There are frequent speech-sound substitutions and omissions with sound-sequencing difficulties. Distortions and additions also occur. Unlike the person with dysarthria, who makes predominantly distortions and related substitutions, the person with apraxia makes unrelated substitutions, repetitions, and additions.

Recognizing errors, the individual with apraxia of speech will make repeated attempts to correct them. As she or he tries to produce the correct sound, there are inordinately frequent pauses and reinitiations of words and sentences (Wertz et al., 1991). Unlike the person with dysarthria, who repeats the same error, the individual with apraxia of speech often produces widely varying productions on repeated attempts. A sample of speech from a person with apraxia follows:

> O-o-on . . . on . . . on our cavation, cavation, cacation . . . oh darn . . . vavation, oh, you know, to Ca-ca-caciporenia . . . no, Lacifacnia, vafacnia to Lacifacnion . . . On our vacation to Vacafornia, no darn it . . . to Ca-caliborneo . . . not bornia . . . fornia, Bornifornia . . . no, Balliforneo, Ballifornee, Balifornee, Californee, California. Phew, it was hard to say Cacaforneo. Oh darn.

Consonants and consonant clusters and blends offer a particular challenge, although more frequently used phonemes and words are produced with more accuracy. As you might expect, complex, long, or unfamiliar words are more difficult to produce.

Individuals with apraxia of speech may have no difficulty producing words on one occasion that they struggle to produce on another. In fact, clients may exhibit periods of error-free speech during automatic or emotional utterances. It is not uncommon to have a client struggle with volitional production of a word such as "vacation" only to hear the client easily say later, "Boy, I sure had a lot of trouble with *vacation!*" A sample of the speech of a person with apraxia of speech is presented on the accompanying CD-ROM.

The speaker with apraxia is typically aware of errors and may even anticipate them but be unable to correct them. Monitoring of speech in anticipation of these errors results in a slowed, almost cautious rate of speech with even stress and spacing. Clients frequently report that they know what they want to say but can't initiate the sequence or keep it going. Faced with a naming task, these individuals frequently respond, "I know it, but I can't say it."

Although apraxia and aphasia often co-occur in an individual, the two are not the same. Aphasia is a language disorder; apraxia is a motor-speech problem. The individual with aphasia has difficulty with word recall in all modalities, whereas the person with apraxia of speech can recall the word easily when writing but may be unable to say it accurately. In addition, the individual with apraxia of speech has no difficulties with the structure of language. Case Study 12.4 presents the story of a woman with apraxia.

At this point, no doubt, your head is swimming with seemingly overlapping characteristics of the dysarthrias and apraxia of speech. Table 12.3 presents the major differences between the two disorders although there will be many individual variations.

Although we have defined apraxia as a disorder of the mature nervous system, children can also exhibit apraxia of speech, termed *developmental apraxia of speech* (Hall et al., 1993) (see Chapter 10). Data are complicated by causal factors such as TBI. Most frequently, children who are diagnosed as having developmental apraxia of speech exhibit multiple articulation errors, including addition of speech sounds, sound and syllable repetitions, and sound prolongations.

CASE STUDY 12.4
Personal Story of a Woman with Dysarthria and Apraxia of Speech

Ruth is a 75-year-old woman who suffered a stroke in the frontal lobe of the left cerebral hemisphere after surgery. On release from the hospital following her stroke, Ruth began receiving services twice weekly at a rehabilitation center for her speech and for other motor difficulties.

Six months after the incident, her speech is characterized by moderate dysarthria, which is evidenced in poor breath control, decreased loudness, and decreased articulatory precision. In addition, she exhibits apraxia in her ability to initiate and complete functional communication. Her speech is characterized by cluster reduction and inconsistent omission, substitution, and distortion of speech sound and consists primarily of single words. In reading samples, intelligibility decreases with increasingly complex material. Ruth has difficulty beginning speech initiation and with sound and syllable sequencing. Her speech seems to improve with preformulation of the message, word-by-word attack, and gesturing.

Auditory comprehension of both conversation and directions and silent reading comprehension of directions are good. Although she reads the newspaper, she seems uninterested in the more substantial pleasure reading that occupied much of her time previously. Ruth's memory and attention seem unaffected.

A retired schoolteacher and widow, Ruth lives alone. She has six children. Her two oldest daughters are attempting to supplement the home health care she receives. Ruth's diet consists primarily of soft foods and semiliquids, which require more time for ingestion than was previously allotted for meals.

TABLE 12.3
....
Differences between dysarthria and apraxia

Dysarthria	Apraxia of Speech
Speech-sound distortions	Speech-sound substitutions
Substitution errors related to target phoneme	Substitution errors often not related to target phoneme
Highly consistent speech-sound errors	Inconsistent speech-sound substitution
Consonant clusters simplified	Schwa (/ə/) often inserted between consonants in a cluster
Little audible or silent groping for a target speech sound	Audible or silent groping for a target speech sound
Rapid or slow rate	Slow rate characterized by repetitions, prolongations, and additions
No periods of unaffected speech	Islands of fluency
Little difference between reactive or automatic speech and volitional speech; both affected	Often very fluent reactive or automatic speech, nonfluent volitional speech

Etiology

In most clients, apraxia of speech is the result of a lesion in the central programming area for speech: Broca's area in the left frontal lobe of the brain (Kent, et al., 2001). Broca's area details and plans the coordination of sequenced motor movements for speech, much as an assembly line computer would organized the various aspects of car production. Breakdown in Broca's area makes speech difficult, just as a glitch in an automobile factory computer might cause a chassis to arrive after the component parts to be installed have already moved on. Without a plan, the person with apraxia of speech has difficulty placing the articulators and sequencing his or her movement. Chewing, sucking, and swallowing may be possible, but speech is inconsistent. The language message is sent from the left temporal lobe, but production through speech is difficult. The most common causes of AOS in adults are stroke, degenerative disease, and trauma.

> In apraxia of speech, it is not the nerves or muscles that are defective but the part of the brain that coordinates and activates them.

Assessment

Because of the nature of apraxia of speech, the SLP must pay special attention to additional aspects of assessments. These include the following:

Imitation of single words of varying lengths

Sentence imitation

Reading aloud

Spontaneous speech

Rapid repetition of "puh," "tuh," "kuh," and "puh-tuh-kuh"

Note that a number of the tasks are repetitive or imitative. Recall that in apraxia, performance may vary with repeated performance. Modes of stimulus presentation are also important because the person with apraxia responds better to auditory-visual stimuli than to either auditory or visual stimuli alone.

Intervention

In conjunction with other health professionals, the SLP attempts to increase muscle tone and strength, especially those of the speech mechanism. The sequenced production of speech sounds and motor planning that are needed to accomplish this may begin with practice of nonspeech movements

Intervention often begins with sensory bombardment, in which the client hears the correct sound or word repeatedly and sees it in print. Gradually, the client moves to imitation, followed by simultaneous production and finally spontaneous speech. The SLP and the client discuss how the sound or word felt when the articulators were moved. More difficult sounds, consonant clusters, and words are gradually introduced. For clients with severe apraxia of speech, AAC may be introduced (see Chapter 15).

Some individuals need additional input to be successful. The SLP may provide visual and physical cues and/or aid with physical manipulation. Electromagnetic articulography (EMA), which tracks oral movement, can remediate some articulatory deficits by providing visually guided biofeedback for tongue tip position improvement (Katz et al., 1999).

A decreased rate of production may also improve production. Some clients benefit from the use of carrier phrases that are repeated with each word, such as "I like _____" or "I want _____." Frequently used phrases such as "How are you?" are also practiced and incorporated into the client's verbal repertoire to help the client's speech to sound more normal.

SUMMARY

The major types of neurogenic motor speech disorders are cerebral palsy (CP), dysarthria, and apraxia of speech. CP is characterized as a group of developmental, nonprogressive neurological difficulties resulting from brain injury that occurs very early in fetal or infant development and affects motor movement, communication, growth and development, locomotion, learning, and sensation. The three main types of CP—spastic, athetoid, and ataxic—result in very different motor patterns and speech difficulties.

Dysarthria is a group of acquired impairments that affect the speed, range, direction, strength, and timing of motor movement as the result of paralysis, weakness, or discoordination of the speech muscles. Unlike apraxia of speech, the dysarthrias represent difficulties in motor speech control. Five distinct types include flaccid, spastic, ataxic, hyperkinetic, and hypokinetic dysarthria. Disorders affecting multiple motor systems may yield a mixed dysarthria.

In contrast, apraxia is an acquired disorder in voluntary motor placement and sequencing that is unrelated to muscle weakness, slowness, or paralysis and results from a lesion in the central programming area for speech in the left frontal lobe that details and plans the coordination of sequenced motor movements for speech.

Neurogenic motor speech disorders, both developmental and acquired, offer a special challenge to the affected individual, family, friends, and the speech-language pathologist. Many clients are in the very frustrating position of being able to formulate the message but unable to produce it intelligibly.

Intervention methods differ greatly. The child with CP may be learning to communicate and to acquire language using an AAC. Meanwhile, the older adult with a motor-speech problem may be relearning or retrieving older speech patterns. Finally, the individual with a progressive degenerative disease, such as Parkinson disease or ALS, may be attempting to cling to the level of effective communication that was previously possible or exploring additional methods of communication. Changing intervention techniques and promising new surgical procedures and drugs will continue to offer hope to individuals with neurogenic speech disorders.

THOUGHT QUESTIONS

- What are the major differences between CP, dysarthria, and apraxia?
- Name some of the causes of neurogenic speech disorders.
- Describe the main types of cerebral palsy.
- Describe the major types of dysarthria.
- What are the differences between dysarthria and apraxia of speech?
- How do the assessment and intervention techniques used with each neurogenic motor speech disorder differ? How are they similar?

SUGGESTED RESOURCES

Brookshire, R. H. (2007). *Introduction to neurogenic communication disorders* (7th ed.). St. Louis, MO: Mosby.

My Left Foot. (1989). Miramax Pictures.

ONLINE RESOURCES

4Mychild
www.cerebralpalsy.org/
4mychild Web site has useful information on CP for parents and families.

American Speech-Language-Hearing Association
www.asha.org/public/speech/disorders/dysarthria.htm
ASHA site addresses multiple topics related to dysarthria.

National Institute on Deafness and Other Communication Disorders
www.nidcd.nih.gov/health/voice/apraxia.htm
National Institute on Deafness and Other Communication Disorders describes apraxia of speech and has links to other sites.

National Institutes of Health Medline Plus
www.nlm.nih.gov/medlineplus/brainandnerves.html
National Institutes of Health's Medline Plus Web site contains information and links to other sites.

National Institute of Neurological Disorders and Stroke
www.ninds.nih.gov/disorders/disorder_index.htm#C
Index for the National Institute of Neurological Disorders and Stroke Web site contains in-depth discussion of neurogenic disorders and links to other organizations and sites.

New York Online Health
www.noah-health.org/en/bns/
New York Online Health (NOAH) site Brain and Nervous System page has multiple links for all the neurogenic topics discussed in this chapter.

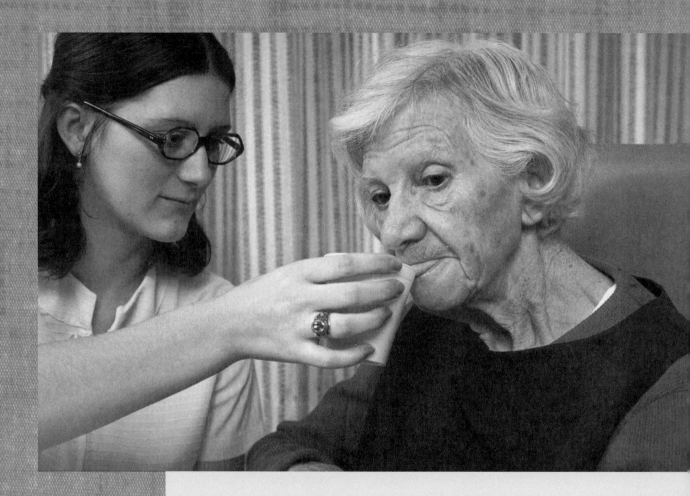

CHAPTER LEARNING GOALS

When you have finished this chapter, you should be able to:

- Explain why speech-language pathologists are concerned with swallowing

- Describe the basic process of human swallowing

- Identify some causes of swallowing disorders in children and adults

- Describe basic clinical and instrumental assessment techniques

- Discuss evidence-based practices in swallowing treatment

13

Disorders of Swallowing

Speech-language pathologists play a major role in the evaluation and management of dysphagia, or swallowing disorders. ASHA's 2005 *Health Care Survey in Speech-Language Pathology* found that 87% of respondents reported they were the primary providers of dysphagia management in their work settings. In this same survey, 16% of SLPs working in medical settings reported that they provide feeding and swallowing services to infants and children. Furthermore, SLPs may be required to manage dysphagia in children in their school-based setting (ASHA, 2005).

The SLP is responsible for identifying, evaluating, and treating individuals with feeding and swallowing disorders. With the continually growing number of adult and pediatric patients identified every year with feeding and swallowing disorders, specific knowledge about normal and abnormal swallowing patterns is essential for effective evaluation and management of this clinical population. Case Study 13.1 describes an elderly woman with swallowing difficulties similar to those that the speech-language pathologist will frequently encounter in the aging population.

As with much of the work that speech-language pathologists do, they do not function alone. SLPs who treat patients with swallowing problems are generally part of a team consisting of a physician, nurse, nutritionist, radiologist, gastroenterologist, dentist, otolaryngologist, neurologist, occupational therapist, physical therapist, respiratory therapist, and family members. The role of each of these specialists will become clear when we discuss evaluation and treatment later in this chapter.

Swallowing and the efficient intake of food have both medical and psychosocial implications. Eating is essential to physical health. Without proper nourishment, one cannot grow, develop, or survive. Swallowing disorders increase the risk of choking and may lead to *aspiration* of food into the lungs and respiratory illnesses such as pneumonia (Langmore et al., 1998). Inadequate swallowing may result in **gastroesophageal reflux (GER),** the movement of food or acid from the stomach back into the esophagus. Eating is also one of our major social activities. Feeding difficulties in children may stress the parent-child relationship. Among older

CASE STUDY 13.1
Case Study of a Women with Dysphagia: Rhea

Rhea is an 80-year-old woman who lives alone. Her son was concerned about a rapid and noticeable weight loss and approached Rhea's primary care physician with his concerns. A routine physical examination did not reveal anything that could be contributing to the loss of weight. During the doctor-patient interview following the physical examination, Rhea mentioned that she felt a frequent tightness in her throat and would sometimes gag when she was eating. Her son also told the physician that Rhea's normally robust appetite has recently become significantly diminished and that she seemed unduly anxious during mealtime. Based on the negative results of the physical examination regarding the cause of Rhea's weight loss and the information presented in the follow-up interview, her physician referred Rhea to the hospital for an evaluation for a potential swallowing disorder.

The staff SLP in charge of swallowing disorders performed the initial portion of Rhea's swallowing examination. Following a review of the case information, the SLP conducted an interview with Rhea and her son. The SLP noted that Rhea was alert during the interview and cognitively intact. During the oral-motor examination, the SLP evaluated head and body posture, the anatomy and general health of Rhea's mouth, and her ability to produce a strong cough. No problems were found in any of these areas. A modified barium swallow study (videofluoroscopy) showed an efficient swallow. Further testing with variegated textures of liquids and foods revealed that foods that were thick or sticky and hard to chew such as peanut butter or tough cuts of meat increased Rhea's anxiety, often causing her to gag.

Upon reviewing the swallow examination results, the swallowing team agreed that Rhea's difficulty with swallowing was related to life circumstances. The team recommended that Rhea be provided with more opportunities to eat with others rather than alone. Additionally, they recommended modifications to her dietary intake, reducing thick, tough, and chewy foods. By following the recommendations of the swallowing team, Rhea has begun to gain weight and her family reports that she experiences less anxiety when eating.

As you read this chapter think about

- How the consistency of a food might affect the person's ability to swallow.
- How a swallowing disorder might affect a person's daily life.
- Conditions other than old age that might adversely affect a person's ability to swallow.

The term "dysphagia" comes from the Greek and literally means difficulty with eating.

people, dysphagia may lead to isolation, depression, frustration, and diminished quality of life.

In this chapter, we describe the basics of swallowing, characteristics and correlates of disordered swallowing, evaluation, and treatment.

LIFESPAN PERSPECTIVES

Feeding and swallowing problems exist in both children and adults. They may occur at any point in the lifespan. Newborns may be unable to suckle and/or ingest nutriment. As they age, they may refuse food and develop unhealthy food preferences. Neuromotor problems and structural anomalies that are congenital or acquired at any age can interfere with feeding, as can a host of psychosocial factors. Dysphagia may be related to many diverse conditions; therefore, we describe only some of the more common ones. The correlates

TABLE 13.1

Correlates of swallowing problems in children and adults

Congenital Difficulties	Acquired Conditions
Cerebral palsy	Stroke
Spina bifida	Mouth, throat, laryngeal, or esophageal cancer
Mental retardation/developmental delay	
	HIV/AIDS
Pervasive developmental disability/ autism	Multiple sclerosis
	Amyotrophic lateral sclerosis
HIV/AIDS	Parkinson disease
Cleft lip or palate	Spinal cord injury
Pierre Robin syndrome	Medications and drugs
Treacher Collins syndrome	Dementia
Pyloric stenosis	Depression and social isolation

of swallowing disorders are not mutually exclusive; for example, an individual may be impaired in swallowing because of mental retardation as well as laryngeal cancer. Whatever the etiology, the outcomes of a swallowing disorder at any age include malnutrition, ill health, weight loss, fatigue, frustration, respiratory infection, aspiration, and even death. Table 13.1 lists common correlates of swallowing disorders in children and adults.

THE SWALLOWING PROCESS

Most of us don't typically think about how we swallow food. We know very generally that we put something edible in our mouth, chew for a while, and then swallow. Sometimes, however, we experience difficulty that calls attention to the process. For example, we might eat and cough or feel that the food has "gone down the wrong pipe." Occasionally while drinking, we might laugh and find that fluid comes out of our nose. Once in a while, we feel "all choked up" for an emotional reason and feel unable to eat and swallow. Before we can understand disorders of swallowing, we need to examine the basics of nonproblematic swallowing. Normal swallowing can be described in four phases: anticipatory, oral, pharyngeal, and esophageal. Normal swallowing is presented on the accompanying CD-ROM.

Anticipatory Phase

Do you occasionally salivate as you pass a candy shop? How about when you're selecting ice cream at your local grocery store? When you do, you are preparing your mouth to take in food. You probably position yourself to eat by sitting down. A pleasant aroma and an attractive presentation stimulate your hunger, and you become physiologically ready to take in food. Many individuals have a ritual that they perform before a meal, such as hand washing, silent or spoken grace, or a sip of water or other beverage that helps to set the stage for eating. Without this premeal interlude, eating might feel rushed and less satisfying.

Oral Phase

The oral phase is sometimes considered in two stages: oral preparatory and oral transport.

ORAL PREPARATORY

When you are ready to eat, you put food or beverage into your mouth and close your lips. In the oral preparatory stage of drinking, the tongue forms a cupped position and holds the fluid in a liquid **bolus,** the substance that is to be ingested, against the front portion of the hard palate. In preparation for swallowing solid foods, the tongue and cheeks move the food to the teeth for chewing and mixing with saliva to form a solid bolus. The prepared liquid or solid bolus is held in the mouth by the soft palate, which moves forward and down to touch the back of the tongue and close the passage to the pharynx or throat.

ORAL TRANSPORT

Once the bolus is formed, oral transport begins. This stage consists of the movement of the bolus from the front to the back of the mouth. When the substance reaches the anterior faucial arch at the rear of the mouth, the pharyngeal swallow reflex is triggered. Oral transport typically takes about 1 second.

Pharyngeal Phase

The oral and pharyngeal phases of swallowing involve much of the same anatomy that is used in speaking. There is wisdom to the traditional advice "Don't eat and talk at the same time."

The velum now moves up to meet the rear wall of the pharynx and to prevent the bolus from going into the nasal cavity. The base of the tongue and the pharyngeal wall move toward one another to create the pressure that is needed to project the bolus into the pharynx. The pharynx contracts and squeezes the bolus down. While this is occurring, the hyoid bone rises, bringing the larynx up and forward. The larynx prevents the bolus from entering the trachea, or windpipe, by closing the true and false vocal folds and lowering the epiglottis covering the airway. The pharyngeal phase is complete when the cricopharyngeal sphincter opens and the food or liquid moves into the esophagus. The pharyngeal phase occurs very quickly and is usually complete in less than 1 second.

Esophageal Phase

The last stage of the swallowing process occurs when the muscles of the esophagus move the bolus in peristaltic or rhythmic, wavelike contractions from the top of the esophagus into the stomach. This typically takes 8 to 10 seconds in an unimpaired individual.

DISORDERED SWALLOWING

Problems in swallowing can occur in any or all phases of the process. A person may lack appetite or be unable to form a bolus and transport it to the rear of the mouth. In addition, difficulties may arise later if the bolus moves inadequately or is blocked as it passes through the pharynx and esophagus to the stomach.

Anticipatory Phase

Lack of interest in food may be the result of depression or limited alertness. Sensory impairments involving vision and scent may interfere with a person's readiness to accept food. Some individuals, because of neuromuscular difficulties, cannot position themselves appropriately to take in food or liquid. Infants might not be guided to breastfeed adequately, and their lack of success may lead to a downward spiral culminating in termination of attempts to nurse.

Oral Phase

If the lips do not seal properly, drooling can occur. Chewing may be impaired because of poor muscle tone or paralysis involving the mouth or because of missing teeth. Insufficient saliva will impede adequate bolus formation. The muscles of the tongue might not function purposefully or efficiently enough to move the food to the teeth for chewing and to transport the bolus from the front to the rear of the mouth to prepare for the pharyngeal phase.

Pharyngeal Phase

Several serious problems are associated with limitations during the pharyngeal phase. If the swallow is not triggered or is delayed, material may be *aspirated,* or fall into the airway, eventually ending in the lungs. Failure to close the velopharyngeal port, the passageway to the nose, can lead to substances going into and out of the nose. Poor tongue mobility may result in insufficient pressure in the pharynx, which is needed to drive the bolus into the esophagus. Aspiration is presented on the accompanying CD-ROM.

Esophageal Phase

If peristalsis is slow or absent, the complete bolus might not be transported from the pharynx to the stomach. Residue might be left on the esophageal walls, resulting in infection and nutritional problems.

Pediatric Dysphagia

Infants and children with swallowing disorders may experience inadequate growth, ill health, fatigue, difficulty learning, and poor parent-child relationships. Children with central nervous system or peripheral nervous system deficits, and/or neuromuscular disease, are vulnerable to feeding and swallowing disorders (Arvedson, 2000). Dysphagia may occur at any phase and may range from mild to severe. Some of the more prevalent correlates of pediatric dysphagia are described next.

CEREBRAL PALSY

As you'll recall, CP is a nonprogressive neuromotor disorder that occurs as a result of brain damage prior to or during birth, or soon thereafter. It is the most common cause of neuorgenic pediatric dysphagia (Arvedson & Brodsky, 2002). An infant with spastic cerebral palsy exhibits excessive muscle tone, abnormal postures and movements, and possibly a hyperactive gag reflex. The child may be difficult to hold because of his or her increased tone, causing excessive flexion of the arms, an arched posture, and abnormal posturing of the legs. The infant may also gag during breastfeeding and/or be unable to move the tongue rhythmically to suckle. The unpleasantness of the feeding situation will undoubtedly have adverse affects on the quality of the child-mother interaction.

Gastroesophageal reflux is common in infants and children with CP, and ingestion of food may become painful. Uncoordinated swallowing is also a problem for individuals with CP, thereby increasing their risk of aspriation (Sullivan, 2008). In severe cases of dsyphagia, children with CP require gastrostomy tube feedings.

SPINA BIFIDA

Approximately 1 in 1,000 infants is born with **spina bifida,** a congenital malformation of the spinal column typically involving associated neural damage, resulting in limited sensation and motor control difficulties. A child with spina bifida may experience feeding difficulties in all phases of the process. Sucking and intake of food are often disturbed, owing to sensory impairments and frequently exhibited dyspraxia (difficulty coordinating movement). The pharyngeal and esophageal stages of swallowing may be affected by cranial nerve damage due to the disorder (Prontnicki, 1995).

MENTAL RETARDATION AND DEVELOPMENTAL DELAY

About 2 to 3 of every 100 individuals are considered to have intellectual functioning that is enough below average to be labeled as mental retardation. Children with mental retardation are also delayed in mastering motor coordination, and the delay may interfere with development of eating skills and the oral phase of swallowing. Communication disorders are common in this population, and children may be limited in their ability to express food desires and preferences, thereby causing disturbances in the anticipatory phase of swallowing.

AUTISM SPECTRUM DISORDERS

Although children with autism spectrum disorders (ASD) do not usually exhibit swallowing disorders, they may have significant feeding problems. Recall that children with ASD may be socially withdrawn, have impaired communication, and/or may exhibit repetitive or stereotypic behaviors. They may also be hypersensitive to sound, light, pain, smell, and touch. This pattern of symptoms often contributes to feeding difficulties. For instance, social withdrawal and communication deficits may impede the child's ability to indicate hunger or thirst to an adult or caregiver. Further, repetitive patterns of behavior and/or sensory issues may restrict the types of food that are consumed, possibly leading to poor nutrition (Lukens & Linscheid, 2008).

HIV/AIDS

HIV (human immunodeficiency virus) causes the illness known as **AIDS (acquired immunodeficiency syndrome)**. It infects white blood cells, the brain, skin, and other tissues of the body. Children infected with HIV often acquire the disease from their mothers either in utero, during the delivery process, and/or through the mother's breast milk. The number of HIV-positive children increases daily in the United States, and feeding and swallowing disorders are quite prevalent in this population (McNeilly, 2005). One study found that 20.8% of 150 children were determined to have feeding or swallowing problems (Pressman, 1992). These may be due to lowered immunity to infections like oral herpes that can cause pain during eating.

In the final stages of the disease, HIV-positive children have difficulty managing oral secretions and exhibit **odynophagia,** or painful swallowing. Because HIV is a progressive disease, HIV-positive children often exhibit developmental delays, mental retardation, language deficits, and poor attention skills (McNeilly, 2005). Such deficits can interfere with the anticipatory stage of swallowing.

STRUCTURAL AND PHYSIOLOGICAL ABNORMALITIES

Children born with cleft lip or palate are impaired in the oral phase of swallowing. Congenital abnormalities of the jaw, as in **Pierre Robin syndrome,** or of the face, as in **Treacher Collins syndrome,** also negatively affect the ability to use the mouth for intake of food and swallowing. **Esophageal atresia,** which occurs when the esophagus does not have an open connection to the stomach, prevents normal esophageal swallowing and results in choking. This is a life-threatening condition for newborns and must be surgically treated immediately (Prontnicki, 1995).

Similarly life threatening is **pyloric stenosis,** in which the pyloric sphincter at the outlet of the stomach narrows and prevents food from passing to the small intestine. When this is a congenital condition, the infant vomits and cannot ingest milk or water. Prompt surgical intervention usually successfully corrects this difficulty. Pyloric stenosis may also be acquired later in life; it is caused by peptic ulceration or carcinoma.

Infants who are born today do not spend much time in a hospital. Rapid diagnosis of and attention to congenital defects are essential for the welfare of the child.

Dysphagia in Adults

Approximately 6,228,000 Americans older than age 60 have dysphagia, and about 300,000 to 600,000 Americans with neurological disease are identified with swallowing disorders each year (AHCPR, 1999). As such, there is an increased demand for qualified speech-language pathologists who can provide feeding and swallowing services to adult patients in various clinical settings.

Common neurological etiologies of dysphagia include stroke, head trauma, and progressive neurological disease. Swallowing problems can be seen in patients treated for head and neck cancer who require surgical resection of their tumors. Many other conditions can also cause feeding and swallowing problems in the adult population. These are addressed in the following sections.

STROKE

Persistent dysphagia is a serious problem for 5% to 10% of stroke survivors, and about twice that number may experience swallowing problems during the first 6 months after the stroke. Facial paresis (muscle weakness) appears to be the primary factor associated with dysphagia due to stroke. All phases of ingestion are likely to be slowed and impaired. Swallowing and breathing are poorly coordinated, putting the patient at risk for aspiration pneumonia (Nilsson et al., 1998). Pneumonia is the cause for about a third of deaths following stroke (Odderson et al., 1995).

CANCER OF THE MOUTH, THROAT, OR LARYNX

Surgery, radiation, and chemotherapy are used to treat tumors of the mouth, throat, and larynx. Swallowing problems are likely after any type or combination of treatments. Surgery requires removal of the tumor and closing of the wound. For larger lesions, tissue from another area may be excised and used to help patch the deficit. The degree of swallowing impairment is closely related to the size and location of the original tumor and the surgical procedure used to close or reconstruct the area. For example, if a relatively small area of the tongue has been removed, a short-term swallowing problem is likely owing to the swelling following surgery. In more radical surgical procedures in which the tongue is sewn into the mandible to close the floor of the mouth, oral swallow is severely affected (Logemann, 1998).

A visit to the dentist often makes the oral phase of swallowing difficult. Imagine how much more impaired a person is after oral surgery or radiation.

Radiation therapy may result in diminished salivation, swelling, and sometimes mouth sores. The swallowing reflex may be reduced. These interferences with normal swallowing may occur during, soon after, or even a year or two after oral radiation therapy. Chemotherapy may cause nausea, vomiting, and loss of appetite, which interfere with the eating process (Tierney, 1993).

HIV/AIDS

Individuals with AIDS are susceptible to numerous opportunistic infections because of the immune deficiency nature of the disease. A situation was reported in which a 61-year-old man with AIDS complained of swallowing difficulties. The results of the clinical evaluation revealed perforations and growths in the esophagus, which were attributable to Hodgkin's disease, a form of cancer (Gelb et al., 1997). Esophageal ulcers and esophagitis, or inflammation of the esophagus, were reported in about 16% of a group of heterosexual men with AIDS (Yang et al., 1996).

MULTIPLE SCLEROSIS

Multiple sclerosis (MS), a central nervous system disorder, may affect one or several cranial nerves. Multiple sclerosis is of unknown cause and is typically characterized by periods of both relapse and remission. The major general symptoms are poor coordination, muscle weakness, and often speech and visual disturbances. Delayed swallowing reflex and reduced pharyngeal peristaltic action are the primary forms of dysphagia associated with multiple sclerosis (Logemann, 1998).

Numbness or a "pins-and-needles" sensation in the extremities or on one side of the face may be an early sign of MS.

AMYOTROPHIC LATERAL SCLEROSIS (LOU GEHRIG'S DISEASE)

Amyotrophic lateral sclerosis (ALS), discussed in Chapter 12, is a progressive disease that may begin in middle age. It is characterized by muscle atrophy due to degeneration of motor neurons. Poor tongue movement is sometimes an early sign. ALS may interfere with swallowing in several ways. Reduced tongue mobility may result in spillage into the airway before the pharyngeal swallow has been triggered. The larynx might not elevate and close adequately during the pharyngeal phase. Pharyngeal peristalsis is frequently reduced, causing material to remain in the pharynx. Any of these difficulties could result in aspiration of food or liquid (Hardy & Robinson, 1993; Logemann, 1998).

PARKINSON DISEASE

Parkinson disease (PD), also discussed in Chapter 12, is a progressive disorder, typically of midlife, and is characterized by slowness of movement, muscle rigidity, and tremor. About 30% of individuals with PD have been reported to exhibit dysphagia; however, this does not seem to be related to the severity or duration of the disease (Castell, et al., 2001).

Tremors and rigidity that are visible in a person's extremities may also occur within the body, resulting in swallowing and other difficulties.

Any or all phases of the swallowing process may be impaired, although in a recent study, only 10% percent of people with PD were found to need dietary aid (Clarke et al., 1998). When dysphagia occurs, the bolus is usually formed normally in the oral preparatory stage. However, oral transport may be impaired by a front-to-back rolling pattern until the back of the tongue finally lowers sufficiently to permit the bolus to pass to the pharynx. Pharyngeal swallow may be delayed and laryngeal closure may be impaired in advanced cases of PD. Aspiration sometimes occurs when the patient inhales after a swallow, and material remaining in the pharynx falls into the airway (Logemann, 1998). Esophageal motor abnormalities that impede swallowing may occur in PD even in early stages of the disease (Bassotti, et al., 1998; Johnston et al., 2001).

SPINAL CORD INJURY

Individuals who have injured their spinal cords because of accidents have a higher incidence of esophageal dysphagia than noninjured people do.

Among the problems that they experience are heartburn, chest pain while swallowing, and slow, abnormal peristaltic contractions of the esophagus (Stinneford et al., 1993).

Surgery to the front portion of the upper (anterior cervical) spine may result in dysphagia. These swallowing problems may affect any phase of swallowing. Oral preparatory and transport stages are impaired in some postsurgical patients; others experience weakness in the pharyngeal phase or suffer upper esophageal sphincter malfunctioning (Martin et al., 1997).

MEDICATIONS AND NONFOOD SUBSTANCES

Although medications are used to cure and manage disease, they may also have negative side effects. Some medications, including decongestants, cough suppressants, and muscle relaxants, might make the patient feel drowsy and/or confused. This condition can interfere with anticipation and the oral phase of swallowing. A dry mouth, or insufficient saliva, has been reported to be a side effect of more than 300 medications (Toner, 1997). High doses of steroids may impede pharyngeal swallowing. Antipsychotic drugs may result in **tardive dyskinesia** (involuntary, repetitive facial, tongue, or limb movements) after a year or more of use. At the extreme, tardive dyskinesia may result in the inability to chew and swallow (Feinberg, 1997).

Behaviors such as smoking and ingesting excessive amounts of caffeine and alcohol may also interfere with normal swallowing. Appetite may be depressed and sensations dulled, resulting in anticipatory phase impairment. Alcohol abuse has been implicated in pharyngeal phase dysphagia (Feinberg, 1997).

DEMENTIA

Unlike mental retardation, dementia is an acquired disorder. Although found in some older people, diminution of intellectual function is not an imperative of aging. We all know people in their 80s and 90s whose minds are sharp and capable. As we learned in Chapter 7, dementia is associated with Alzheimer's disease, several small strokes, Parkinson disease, multiple sclerosis, and other ailments that may occur among older people. The cognitive deficits of dementia may impede attention and orientation to food. Oral preparatory tongue and jaw movements may be lacking in purpose, resulting in poor bolus formation and

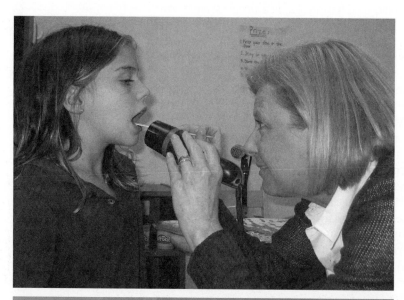

The clinician evaluates the oral mechanism for health, structure, and function.

drooling. Transport of the bolus may be prolonged. Pharyngeal swallow may be delayed and laryngeal elevation reduced, resulting in possible aspiration (Cherney, 1994; Hardy & Robinson, 1993).

DEPRESSION AND SOCIAL ISOLATION

Life circumstances among the elderly may interfere with several phases of swallowing. Taking a meal is traditionally a social event. We eat with family and friends. As people enter old age, they may find themselves alone and lonely. Spouses and friends have died. Children have moved away. Some may have no experience preparing food and so do not have adequate meals. Others are not motivated to cook just for themselves. Communal meals in retirement homes or long-term care facilities may feature unfamiliar foods and be served in a noisy, hurried environment. For example, mealtime difficulties in one home for the aged were documented in 87% percent of the residents (Steele et al., 1997).

Feelings of depression among elderly people are common. Depression is associated with diminished interest in food, restlessness, and fatigue. The throat may feel tight, making swallowing uncomfortable. Some individuals may feel too tired to eat and then are exhausted after they do eat. This may prompt a cycle of inadequate food intake, weight loss, and malnutrition (Toner, 1997).

EVALUATION FOR SWALLOWING

Not everyone with the correlates described in the previous sections has a swallowing disorder. Furthermore, swallowing problems are not always readily apparent. Patients may not report difficulties, and some may experience **silent aspiration** (lack of cough when food or liquid enters the airway) (Logemann, 1996). Therefore, the first step in evaluation is to identify the individuals who are at risk for dysphagia. Following this screening (refer to Chapter 4, "Assessment and Intervention," for a discussion of screening), the speech-language pathologist will serve on a team to obtain background information and to use clinical and instrumental techniques to assess swallowing. A determination is made about appropriate intervention, and treatment strategies are developed and implemented in coordination with other professionals. Speech-language pathologists are advocates for their clients and help to provide education and counseling to them, their families, and related others (ASHA, 2001e).

> Some birthing centers have lactation consultants who encourage and assist mothers and infants in the nursing process.

Screening for Dysphagia in Newborns and the Elderly

A primary indication of dysphagia in infants is **failure to thrive.** Infants in a neonatal intensive care unit are carefully monitored for weight gain and development. Full-term infants who are not accepting breast or bottle are signaling feeding problems. The *Non-Instrumental Clinical Evaluation (NICE)* is a systematic way of obtaining clinical and family history and

FIGURE 13.1
·················

Three-ounce water swallow test.

Source: Based on DePippo et al., (1992).

Task: Patient drinks three ounces of water from a cup without interruption.

Outcome:

1. No problems.

2. Coughing during swallow.

3. Coughing after swallow.

4. Wet-hoarse voice quality after swallow.

Pass: Outcome 1 *Fail:* Outcome 2, 3, or 4.

observing the child being fed by a caregiver (Scott, 1998). The child's breathing and physical coordination are evaluated. The child's ability to form a seal and suck are assessed by direct observation and by techniques that enable quantification of nutritive and nonnutritive sucking skill (Lau & Kusnierczyk, 2001). Caregivers can be counseled and instrumental evaluation recommended when warranted.

Checklists to screen for dysphagia in older individuals are also available. The *Burke Dysphagia Screening Test* is a relatively quick way to screen patients who have had a stroke (DePippo, 1992). The 3-ounce water swallow test used in the *Burke* has been found to identify between 80 to 98% of patients who were aspirating as later confirmed by more elaborate tests (DePippo et al., 1992; Suiter & Leder, 2008). Figure 13.1 outlines this procedure.

Additional screening instruments include the *Examine Ability to Swallow (EATS)* (Wood & Emick-Herring, 1997) and the *Repetitive Oral Suction Swallow (ROSS),* which screens swallowing function as individuals sip water through a straw (Nilsson et al., 1998). Stroke patients who, at bedside, exhibit a delay in moving food from the front to the rear of the mouth and incomplete oral clearance signal the likelihood of dysphagic complications (Mann & Hankey, 2001).

For mentally retarded adults and others, inappropriate weight for the person's size may be an indication of nutritional problems that could be due to dysphagia (Sheppard, 1991). All of these measures and indicators have been reported to be useful in identifying serious swallowing difficulties and the need for more complete clinical and instrumental assessment.

Case History and Background Information Regarding Dysphagia

A parent, caregiver, physician, nurse, or professional from an early intervention program or adult day treatment center may make a referral to a dysphagia team, typically based on three general areas of concern:

- Difficulties have been observed related to feeding and ingestion of food or liquid.
- The client appears to be at risk for aspirating food or liquid into the lungs.

Does the infant accept breast or bottle?	When was the problem first observed?
Does the individual refuse certain foods? Which ones?	Did it worsen slowly or rapidly?
Does the individual appear to chew food?	What exactly happens when the person tries to swallow?
Has drooling been observed?	Does material seem to stop somewhere? Where?
Does the child or adult eat excessively slowly?	What medical diagnoses or conditions may affect the swallow?
Does the child or adult eat excessively rapidly?	Has the person had surgery that may relate to swallowing?
Does coughing or choking occur at mealtimes?	Is the individual using any medications?
Is food or liquid expelled from the nose?	How is the client's respiratory health?
Is food or liquid regurgitated?	How attentive is the client?
Is the child gaining weight?	Is the client able to follow directions?
Is the adult maintaining weight?	

FIGURE 13.2

Important questions pertaining to swallowing.

Source: Based on Hardy & Robinson (1993).

- The client appears not to be receiving adequate nourishment (Rosenthal et al., 1995).

The SLP will then seek answers to questions such as those presented in Figure 13.2. The answers to these questions provide preliminary information about the location of the swallowing problem (oral, pharyngeal, or both), the kinds of food substances that are easiest and hardest to swallow, and the nature and severity of the disorder (Logemann, 1998).

Clinical Assessment

CAREGIVER AND ENVIRONMENTAL FACTORS

The treating clinician will want to observe feeding as it occurs normally between caregiver and client. The therapist will pay special attention to the following:

- Is the caregiver patient and attentive?
- Does feeding take place in a reasonably quiet environment that is free from distractions?
- What position is the individual in when eating or drinking?
- How does the client express feeding preferences?

The parent or caregiver is an important part of the swallowing team. Careful observation and communication will help the speech-language

CASE STUDY 13.2
The Personal Story of a Man with Dysphagia

Mr. M. was 51 years of age when he was referred as an outpatient by the director of Neurology and Rehabilitative Medicine at Municipal Hospital to Ms. R., the staff SLP in charge of swallowing disorders. The referral note read "myotonic dystrophy, dysarthria, dysphagia for solids." Ms. R. recognized her role in ensuring the patient's safety. Difficulty in swallowing foods could result in choking and/or aspiration pneumonia. Ms. R. was also concerned about the dysarthria and wondered to what degree this affected Mr. M.'s communication.

At their first meeting, Ms. R. learned that Mr. M., a recent immigrant from Colombia, had limited English proficiency. Once again, Ms. R. was grateful for her own Spanish language skills; the summer she had spent in Spain after her third year of college had been worthwhile in a multitude of ways. Many of the patients and staff at this inner-city hospital had Spanish as their primary language. Although Mr. M. was mildly dysarthric, his speech was readily intelligible. His responses during the interview were appropriate in form (Spanish) and content. Mr. M. reported that he choked on rice, a staple of his diet. Other foods and liquids did not appear to be a problem. Mr. M. reported that he smoked "a little, just at the Saturday evening dances." A cursory

evaluation of the oral mechanism revealed adequate strength and motion of the lips, tongue, velum, and mandible. Although coughing, choking, and gurgling were not observed during trial feeding, an apparent delay in the pharyngeal swallow reflex was noted with both liquids and solids. Ms. R. recommended a modified barium swallow study to confirm and document dysphagia.

Several types of foods were mixed with barium in preparation for the X-ray procedure. Mr. M. ate a spoonful of applesauce and then pudding as the radiologist and Ms. R. watched the X-ray monitor. No difficulties were noted in the oral phase. However, they observed food lingering in the esophagus and building up with each successive swallow. Although the larynx elevated for swallowing, the bolus did not clear, and residue remained on the right **aryepiglottic fold.** Mr. M. was instructed to produce an abdominal cough, but he was unsuccessful, and the food remained on the fold.

Ms. R. made the following recommendations: Mr. M. should not eat alone. He should avoid clear liquids and take only a small amount of food before swallowing. He should try to cough deeply when he feels food stuck in his mouth. At the next appointment, in 2 weeks, Mr. M. would be instructed in the supraglottic and hard swallow techniques. Because myotonic dystrophy is a progressive disease, Mr. M. requires regular monitoring.

pathologist to assess how best to improve this person's contributions. This is also the opportunity for the SLP to learn about the client's position within the family and cultural and individual factors that may influence therapy. For example, certain foods and spices may be preferred to others. When possible, personal and cultural desires should be respected and accommodated (Logemann, 1998). Case Study 13.2 describes portions of the assessment of a 51-year-old man who was referred for a swallowing evaluation.

Cognitive and Communicative Functioning

Is the client alert and awake during feeding? Can he or she follow directions? What is the client's general level of functioning? Answers to these questions will influence the type of intervention that is most suitable for the client.

HEAD AND BODY POSTURE

It is important to note whether the patient can hold his or her head erect. Does it lean to one side or the other? Does it tend to tilt forward or back? Can the client position the head when asked to do so? The SLP will also note general body posture and tone. Swallowing and ingestion of food and drink involve more than the head, so a complete picture of the individual is important.

ORAL MECHANISM

The integrity of the anatomy and health of the mouth needs to be determined. Abnormalities of structure of the lips, teeth, tongue, palate, and velum are noted. The SLP looks for facial symmetry and will note sagging and imbalances. Motor difficulties such as tremor, flaccidity, excessive muscle tone, and poor coordination are observed. Oral reflexes are examined. Certain reflexes such as sucking and rooting (turning in the direction of a stroke to the cheek) are expected in infants but should disappear as the child matures. The SLP observes any drooling, which may signal neuromuscular deficits, gum and tooth infections, or upper airway obstruction (Sheppard, 1995). The SLP also notes the client's response to sensation. Does the client accept touch such as face washing? If the client is an older child or adult, is she or he aware of food residue or saliva on the face? (Cherney, 1994).

> Myotonic dystrophy is a rare, slowly progressive hereditary disease. It is characterized initially by poor muscle relaxation following contraction and later by muscle atrophy especially of the face and neck.

LARYNGEAL FUNCTION

The SLP cannot directly observe the larynx in the way that he or she can look at the oral mechanism. So the SLP looks for indirect signs of difficulty. In older children and adults, a hoarse, gurgly, or breathy voice quality before, during, or after a swallow may signal laryngeal dysfunction. Other indications of laryngeal problems include the following:

- Inability to rapidly repeat the syllable /ha/ with a clear voiced vowel sound
- Inability to produce vocal tones up and down the musical scale
- An s/z ratio greater than 1.3 (See Chapter 9, "The Voice and Voice Disorders")
- Inability to produce a strong cough (Hardy & Robinson, 1993; Logemann, 1998)

If any difficulties are observed, the SLP should refer the client to an otolaryngologist for a thorough laryngeal evaluation.

BEDSIDE SWALLOWING EXAMINATION

If the client is alert and does not have a history of aspiration, a bedside swallow evaluation can be completed. Usually, food or beverage is used, although some SLPs prefer to conduct this assessment with a piece of gauze that has been soaked in water to reduce the risk of aspiration. If real food substances are used, anticipatory and the oral phases swallowing can be assessed. Pharyngeal phase swallowing efficiency can be judged in part by noting specific behaviors during food or drink intake.

The SLP evaluates the client's reaction to the appearance of food or drink and the associated utensils, observing whether the client's activity level changes and the person appears eager to receive food. A small amount (a quarter of a teaspoon) of thin or thick liquid may be placed in the mouth, and the client is then encouraged to swallow. Oral mechanism function is observed throughout the swallow.

The SLP examines the client's lips to see whether they are together before the taking in of food. The SLP is interested in answering questions such as the following:

> The SLP should observe swallowing on more than one occasion. The nature of the food presented and the client's comfort level and hunger will influence the acceptance of foods.

- Do the lips open and then close around the nipple, cup, or spoon?
- Is there sucking activity on the nipple?
- Is food successfully removed from the spoon?
- Is liquid or food dribbled out of the sides of the mouth?

The SLP also observes tongue movement. Again, answers to certain questions are vital:

- When the mouth opens to take in food, does the tongue cup in anticipation?
- Does the client move the tongue to one side of the mouth if food is presented laterally?
- Does the client move the tongue adequately to form a bolus?
- Is the bolus transported efficiently from the front to the back of the mouth?
- Is the tongue used to remove food substances from the lips?

In addition, the SLP notes movements of the jaw and chewing patterns when solid foods are presented:

- Does the client bite food efficiently?
- Does the client isolate tongue and jaw movement?
- Does chewing continue for an adequate period of time?
- Is the jaw clenched?

Several observations pertaining to the adequacy of pharyngeal swallow are performed. If the client is unable to cough, this may suggest difficulty closing the larynx to protect the airway. Nasal regurgitation points to possibly inadequate velopharyngeal closure. The SLP observes the movement of the hyoid bone and thyroid cartilage in the neck by watching and possibly placing a finger gently on this area. These should move up during pharyngeal swallow. The SLP records the number of times the client swallows while ingesting each amount of food or drink. Multiple swallows may suggest inadequate pharyngeal contraction. If vocal quality changes after swallowing this may indicate pooling of liquid (Cherney, 1994).

Of importance to the SLP are which food consistencies appear to cause difficulties and which seem to be swallowed efficiently. Similarly, the SLP notices whether there is a preferential placement in the mouth for food or liquid.

Managing a Tracheostomy Tube

Some clients will have a **tracheostomy tube** in place to facilitate breathing. A swallowing evaluation can still be conducted in most of these cases with the physician's approval. The SLP or nurse deflates the cuff of the tube before assessment and suctions secretions from the mouth and above the cuff. The swallowing evaluation is similar to the one just outlined; however, the patient is instructed to cover the tube with a gauze pad or gloved finger before each swallow to normalize tracheal pressure (Logemann, 1998). See the online resource *Aaron's Tracheostomy Page*.

Instrumentation

Although the bedside swallowing evaluation is useful in identifying the presence or absence of a swallowing problem, it cannot adequately determine the nature or severity of the dysphagia (Coyle et al., 2009). Complete, accurate assessment of swallowing function requires the use of instrumentation. The SLP collaborates with other team members such as the physician, radiologist, and X-ray technician in the use of diagnostic technology. Some of the more commonly used instrumental procedures are described in the following paragraphs.

Modified Barium Swallow Study

The **modified barium swallow study,** also referred to as **videofluoroscopy,** is an X-ray procedure that has been considered "the gold standard" in dysphagia diagnosis in children or adults (Sonies & Frattalli, 1997). This procedure is used when clinical evaluation or screening suggests dysphagia and/or aspiration. Barium, a substance that can be seen on X-rays, is coated onto or mixed into the food or beverage to be ingested. The SLP typically determines the size, texture, and consistency of the food or beverage to be presented and the head and body position of the patient during the study. A radiologist and an X-ray technician use fluoroscopic (X-ray) equipment to observe the movement of the barium throughout the swallow. These views are videorecorded for later analysis by the physician and SLP. The study provides real-time visualization of the swallowing process and is highly useful in determining whether the client should be fed orally or nonorally, what food textures are safest, and what types of therapy are appropriate (Hardy & Robinson, 1993; Rogers et al., 1994).

Solid knowledge of anatomy and physiology is essential in order to interpret videofluoroscopic swallowing studies accurately (Wooi et al., 2001).

Fiberoptic Endoscopic Evaluation of Swallowing

Fiberoptic endoscopic evaluation of swallowing (FEES) may be used with adult patients who are too ill to be brought to a radiology department for the modified barium swallow study. FEES is not an X-ray procedure. Instead, following topical or localized anesthesia, an otolaryngologist inserts

The FEES procedure is increasingly used because of its convenience and portability.

a flexible fiberoptic laryngoscope through the patient's nose and down into the pharynx. A specially trained SLP can also perform this procedure in consultation with a physician. When the scope is in place, the patient may be asked to cough, hold his or her breath, and swallow foods of different textures and thickness that have been dyed for better visualization. The views may be videotaped. FEES may reveal bolus spilling into the pharynx before swallowing and closing of the airway during swallow. Oral and esophageal phases of swallowing are not visible with FEES. Nevertheless, observations with FEES can be performed at the bedside and provide valuable information about desirable body and head posture during feeding, preferred food types, and aspiration. FEES may also be more cost effective than videofluoroscopy, particularly for patients with head and neck cancer (ASHA, 1992; Aviv et al., 2001; Leder et al., 1998; Sonies, 1997).

SCINTIGRAPHY

Scintigraphy is a computerized technique sometimes used with adults for measuring the amount of aspiration during or after a swallow. A specialized physician such as a radiologist, gastroenterologist, or otolaryngologist performs scintigraphy; however, the SLP plays a role in positioning the patient, suggesting swallowing procedures, and interpreting test results. A radioactive tracer is mixed with the food or liquid to be ingested. Radioactive markers may be placed externally on the chin, lip, thyroid notch, and other anatomical landmarks to facilitate measurement. A specialized gamma scintillation camera is used. When scintigraphy is used, it is generally to supplement information obtained from other tests. Scintigraphy provides insight regarding esophageal function and may help in the determination of the safety of oral feedings (ASHA, 1992; Sonies, 1997).

ULTRASOUND

Ultrasound, or **ultrasonography,** is an imaging technique that uses sound waves at a frequency that is inaudible to human ears, over 20,000 Hz. It is a noninvasive procedure that is safe to use with infants and children as well as adults. A transducer that generates and receives sound waves is placed below the chin for views of the oral cavity and on the thyroid notch for visualizing the laryngeal area. The acoustic images are videotaped. Ultrasonographic real-time measures are particularly helpful in assessing the duration of the oral phases of swallowing as well the structure and movement of the tongue and hyoid bone. One drawback is that ultrasound does not permit visualization of the pharyngeal stage of swallow (ASHA, 1992; Logemann, 1998; Sonies, 1997).

DYSPHAGIA INTERVENTION AND TREATMENT

Disorders of swallowing present medical, nutritional, psychological, social, and communicative problems, so many individuals are involved in working toward their resolution. As was mentioned earlier, the speech-language pathologist is usually the coordinator of services and the professional who is most likely to implement dysphagia therapy. Nevertheless, input from other team members is essential to a satisfactory outcome.

Feeding Environment

Whether the patient is an infant, a young child, or an adult, the environment for feeding sets the stage for a satisfactory experience. It is especially important for people with swallowing problems to have their meals in an environment that is conducive to success. Visual and auditory distractions should be minimized. This means that the eating area should not contain nonrelevant objects. Lighting should be comfortable, neither too bright nor too dark. Noise should be reduced and replaced with pleasant familiar music.

The caregiver should have a relaxed, unhurried manner. He or she must be tuned in to the patient's signals regarding feeding speed, food choices, and quantity. When necessary, these communication strategies may be developed and trained. The caregiver should indicate an interest in the person being fed and reinforce his or her healthy, effective eating behaviors. When possible, the goal is the development of self-feeding skills.

Utensils for feeding need to be appropriate to the patient's functioning. For infants, a slow-flow nipple may be helpful in controlling the amount of liquid taken at a time. A Teflon- or latex-covered spoon may be used for children with infantile tonic bite reflex, who will bite hard on any object that is placed on the teeth or gums. Children and adults with motor coordination difficulties may benefit from the use of a shallow-bowled spoon. Special cutout cups may help to improve tongue positioning in drinking (Hall, 2001; Jelm, 1994; Sheppard, 1995).

Whereas children who have excess muscle tone (hypertonia) benefit from low lighting, soft music, and minimal stimulation, children with insufficient muscle tone (hypotonia) often respond better to bright lights, peppy music, and physical stimulation.

Body and Head Positioning

Body posture and stability have a strong influence on oral-pharyngeal movements. The basic premise is that controlled mobility stems from a solid base (Woods, 1995). An upright, 90° hip angle, symmetrical position with sufficient postural support to provide stability is generally needed. The individual's head and neck must be positioned and prevented from making extraneous movement.

Occasionally, a child or adult may benefit from a hip angle other than 90°. For example, some infants with severe respiratory and swallowing problems may feed better when placed on their stomach. Some older individuals who have a considerable amount of pharyngeal residue may eat more safely at a bent-over 45° angle to prevent regurgitation of food from the esophagus into the airway (Martin, 1994; Woods, 1995).

The SLP works closely with the physical therapist and occupational therapist in obtaining optimum positioning for feeding. The **chin tuck** posture is often recommended for patients with delayed pharyngeal swallow. This position helps prevent food and liquid from entering the airway. The chin tuck posture is presented on the accompanying CD-ROM. The **head-back position** is useful for patients with poor tongue mobility if they have excellent airway closure. **Head tilt** and **head rotation** postures are used when an individual has impairment on one side. In these positions, the head may be moved in the direction of (rotation) or away from (tilt) the impairment. Clients who have been found to have residue in the pharynx during videofluoroscopy may be advised to lie on one side while eating (Hall, 2001; Logemann, 1998; Martin, 1994).

Modification of Foods and Beverages

TEXTURES, QUANTITIES, AND TEMPERATURES

During the assessment, liquids and foods of varying consistencies, amounts, and possibly temperatures will have been presented to the patient. On the basis of the findings of these tests, appropriate recommendations will be made.

Certain foods that are hard to chew, are small or slick when wet, or are thick and sticky are not recommended for children under age 5 who exhibit neuromotor difficulties. Specific foods for these infants and young children to avoid are listed in Figure 13.3.

Clients may exhibit a range of food consistency requirements. They might not tolerate any food by mouth, accept only thin or thick liquids, require a pureed consistency, or be able to ingest the range of normal foods. Figure 13.4 lists possible food consistencies.

The amount of food that clients can manage in their mouth at a time may be determined by the modified barium swallow study. In general, the goal is to reduce the amount that is presented. Drinking through a straw typically causes too much fluid to enter the mouth, so straws are usually not advised. Spoons with a shallow bowl are helpful in limiting food amounts. Caregivers and patients must avoid placing food in the mouth until the previous bolus has been swallowed. Finally, patients may be encouraged to swallow twice per bite or sip.

Providing foods of varying temperatures may increase the client's sensory awareness of the food and improve swallowing. Cold food or drink sometimes improves tongue movement during the oral transport phase and helps to stimulate pharyngeal swallow, although some patients with respiratory problems prefer all substances to be ingested at room temperature (Martin, 1994).

PLACEMENT

Food or drink should be placed in the mouth where the patient has intact sensation and adequate muscle strength. For example, an individual who

FIGURE 13.3

Specific foods that should be avoided for children under age 5 with neuromotor problems.

Source: Based on Lotze (1995).

Hot dogs	Nuts	Chewing gum
Grapes	Seeds	Raw carrots
Popcorn	Hard candy	

NPO	From the Latin, *non per os,* meaning nothing by mouth. If an individual aspirates more than 10% of all foods or is unable to swallow one bolus of food within 10 seconds, alternative means of feeding must be used.
No Liquid by Mouth	Liquids will need to be provided via a nasogastric tube or intravenously for patients who can tolerate pureed or more solid food but are at risk for aspiration of liquids.
Thin Liquid Consistency	This includes foods such as gelatin desserts, which are tolerated by some patients better than thicker consistencies.
Thick Liquid Consistency	Beverages are thickened to the consistency of fruit nectar or tomato juice. A variety of commercial thickeners are available.
Pureed Consistency	Foods are blended to the consistency of mashed potatoes or pudding. This may be recommended for individuals with oral preparatory or oral transport stage difficulties.
Crushed Medication	Pills and capsules are often difficult to swallow, and crushing may facilitate the process. Some medications are time-released, however, and lose effectiveness when crushed. The physician must be consulted before using this approach.
Mechanical Soft Consistency	This consistency is sometimes referred to as *dental soft.* It includes soft foods such as cooked vegetables, fruits, and pasta and may be easier than firmer foods for patients with oral or pharyngeal phase dysphagia to tolerate.
Regular Dietary Consistency	A patient with mild dysphagia may tolerate regular food textures but may need to adjust body or head posture, amount per mouthful, rate of eating, and so on.

FIGURE 13.4

Dietary consistencies.

Source: Adapted from *Swallowing Disorders Treatment Manual,* 2nd ed. (pp. 97–103), by E. Hardy and N. M. Robinson, 1999, Austin, TX: PRO-ED. Copyright 1999 by PRO-ED, Inc. Adapted with permission.

has had oral cancer has diminished sensation in the region where surgery occurred. Similarly, the ability to feel may be reduced after radiation therapy. Neurological disease and damage may also impair a person's full awareness of foods that are placed in the mouth. Surgery and neurological problems may also compromise muscle tone and make the person less able to move parts of the tongue, lips, or cheeks. Appropriate placement along with the adjustments in texture, quantity, and temperature is critical to successful dysphagia intervention (Martin, 1994).

Behavioral Swallowing Treatments

Each of the procedures described here is used only after clinical and instrumental assessment has demonstrated its safety and appropriateness. Clients will also need to be able to follow instructions. All of the techniques may be practiced without food. However, the swallowing techniques are specific to improving the actual swallowing process and are described with the use of food or drink. The evidence bases for these treatments are presented at the end of the chapter.

STRENGTHENING EXERCISES

The swallowing physiology may be improved through exercise. Clients with impaired swallowing may have restricted mouth opening, tongue or lip movement, and laryngeal elevation. **Range of motion** may be improved by practicing specific exercises. Bite blocks of differing sizes may be used to encourage lowering the mandible. Flavored gauze or a toothette may be placed in various places around the mouth to stimulate tongue and lip movement. A licorice stick or a candy LifeSaver on a string may also be used to improve tongue movement. The client may be instructed in moving her or his lips from pucker to smile and back again. Exercises to facilitate awareness of laryngeal movement may involve placement of the hand on the neck at the level of the hyoid bone. A mirror is often used to provide visual feedback to the patient.

Lip strength and seal may be improved by having the client attempt to hold a tongue depressor with the lips. Pushing the tongue against a tongue depressor is a technique for strengthening that muscle. Improved coordination is taught by asking the client to follow instruction such as moving the tongue to explore the outside, then inside of the upper and lower front teeth. Pharyngeal muscle-strengthening exercises involve head-lift exercises, where the patient lies flat on his or her back, then raises the head and holds this position for 1 minute. After three sustained head raisings, the patient rests for 1 minute. The patient then performs 30 additional head-raisings (Shaker et al., 2002). Clark (2004) provides an excellent tutorial regarding neuromuscular treatment of swallowing disorders.

EFFORTFUL AND DOUBLE SWALLOWS

A hard or effortful swallow may be helpful for patients whose tongues do not retract enough to trigger pharyngeal swallow. In these cases, the client is instructed to swallow forcefully and try to feel the tongue moving backward. This technique is helpful as swallowing practice with or without food or drink (Logemann, 1997; Martin, 1994).

Double or multiple **swallows** are advised for individuals who, for whatever reason, retain some food in the oral cavity after a single swallow. Very simply, the client is instructed to swallow two or more times for each bolus (Martin, 1994).

SUPRAGLOTTIC SWALLOW

In the normal swallow, the vocal folds are closed to prevent food from entering the airway. The supraglottic swallow may be used for individuals who do not fully close the glottis during swallowing or close the glottis late. This technique teaches voluntary closure of the glottal area and reduces the depth of misdirected swallows (Bulow et al., 2001). The client is instructed to do the following:

1. Breathe in and hold your breath.
2. Put a small amount of food or liquid in your mouth.
3. Swallow.
4. Cough or clear your throat while exhaling.
5. Swallow again (Hardy & Robinson, 1993; Martin, 1994).

Results of physiological studies reveal that the supraglottic swallow technique does in fact close the vocal folds earlier in the swallow, and it keeps them together longer (Wheeler-Hegland et al., 2009).

MENDELSOHN MANEUVER

The Mendelsohn maneuver is useful for clients who do not have adequate laryngeal elevation during swallowing. The patient is taught to hold the larynx manually at its highest point during the swallow (see Figure 13.5). The instructions are as follows (Hardy & Robinson, 1993; Martin, 1994):

1. Place a small amount of food or liquid in your mouth.
2. Chew if necessary.
3. Swallow while placing your thumb and forefinger on either side of your larynx.
4. Manually hold the larynx for 3 to 5 seconds during and after swallowing in the highest position it reached during swallowing.
5. Let go of your larynx and let it drop.

During the assessment process, the SLP determines which of these exercises and techniques are appropriate for a particular client. Evaluation continues, however, and modifications in treatment approaches are often made as therapy proceeds.

Medical and Pharmacological Approaches

DRUG TREATMENTS

Neurological patients, such as those with Parkinson disease and multiple sclerosis who are taking medications to improve their condition, benefit from being medicated with these drugs before eating. In addition, the medication atropine has been reported to control drooling (Logemann, 1998), and nifedipine may be useful in managing dysphagia

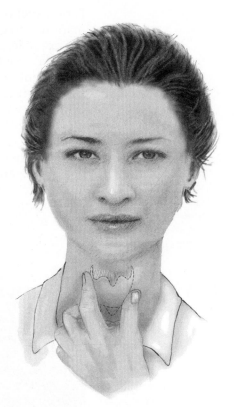

FIGURE 13.5
....

In the Mendelsohn maneuver, the client manually holds the larynx at its highest position to facilitate swallowing.

Source: From *Swallowing Disorders Treatment Manual,* 2nd ed. (p. 121), by E. Hardy and N. M. Robinson, 1999, Austin, TX: PRO-ED. Copyright 1999 by PRO-ED, Inc. Reprinted with permission.

in individuals who have had a stroke (Perez et al., 1998). Injections of botulinum toxin have been shown to improve swallowing in individuals with spasticity and hypertonicity of the cricopharyngeal muscle (Shaw & Searl, 2001). As we discussed earlier in this chapter, some medications actually cause or contribute to swallowing disorders. In these cases, the SLP needs to work with the physician to determine whether alternatives can be used (Feinberg, 1997).

PROSTHESES AND SURGICAL PROCEDURES

Patients who lack an intact swallowing mechanism because of malformation, surgery, or another cause may benefit from a prosthetic device. For example, individuals who had oral cancer and have had a significant portion of the soft palate excised may have a **palatal obturator,** a permanent or removable plate, that helps to close this area during speaking or eating (Logemann, 1998). In addition, children with CP who exhibit dysphagia have been shown to improve their feeding skills and growth significantly when using an appropriately designed intraoral appliance (Haberfellner et al., 2001).

    If less invasive approaches have been unsuccessful, surgery to improve swallowing and prevent aspiration is sometimes needed. Some techniques attempt to correct organic defects. For example, if the patient has bony growths on the cervical vertebrae that displace the rear pharyngeal wall, these may be reduced surgically. Other surgical procedures are used to increase the dimensions of the vocal folds or elevate the larynx. In severe cases of aspiration, the true or false vocal folds may be sutured closed, and

A current reference book describing prescription drugs is an essential part of the personal library of the well-informed SLP.

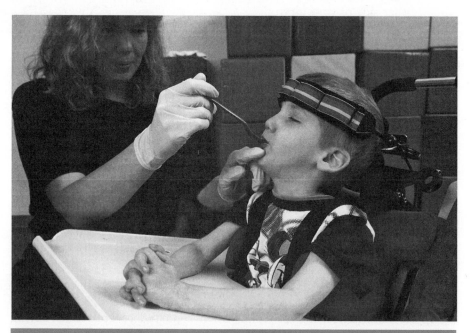

Swallowing disorders may accompany a variety of neuromotor impairments.

breathing will have to occur through a tracheostomy (Logemann, 1998). For patients with esophageal dysphagia, injection of botulinum toxin is sometimes effective (Sonies, 1997).

NONORAL FEEDING

Clients who require more than 10 seconds to swallow a liquid or food bolus or who aspirate more than 10% of either will likely require at least some nonoral feeding (Logemann, 1998). Several approaches are used.

Nasogastric tube (NG tube) feeding requires that a tube be placed from the nose to the pharynx, the esophagus, and finally the stomach. Liquefied food and water are inserted through this opening. Unlike the more long-term procedures described later, NG tubes are typically not used for periods of more than 5 or 6 months.

In **pharyngostomy,** a feeding tube is inserted into a **stoma,** or hole in the external neck region skin, which extends into the pharynx. **Esophagostomy** is a similar procedure; however, a hole is made into the esophagus from the chest area, and a food tube is inserted through it.

In gastrostomy, a hole is surgically made from the abdomen to the stomach. A soft tube is placed through this, and blended regular food can be inserted into the tube. This procedure is used in cases of severe dysphagia.

PROGNOSES AND OUTCOMES FOR SWALLOWING DISORDERS

The overriding objectives of swallowing therapy are to improve the intake of food and drink and to prevent aspiration of these materials into the lungs. The potential for success of swallowing therapy is determined largely by the cause of the disorder, the severity of aspiration, and the onset of treatment (Denk et al., 1997). In young children with developmental disabilities, treatment based on a careful diagnosis of the feeding disorder results in improved nutrition and generally better health (Schwarz et al., 2001). Early identification and successful intervention for swallowing disorders reduces the risk of aspiration and death following stroke, shortens the length of time patients need to stay in the hospital, and improves quality of life (Odderson et al., 1995). Although the original causes of swallowing problems may not be remediable, treatment for dysphagia has been reported to be beneficial in at least 80% of cases (Johns Hopkins, 2000). Box 13.1 provides a brief overview of the research evidence supporting the use of various treatment approaches and techniques for patients with dysphagia.

Speech-language pathologists have sometimes been successful in preventing dysphagia. Caregivers of youngsters who are at risk are instructed in feeding techniques soon after the child's birth. Information for the older population is also valuable. Among the elderly, swallowing disorders are sometimes related to poor dentition, which might be corrected by appropriate dental care. Advice to avoid alcohol, caffeine, spicy products, and foods that are extremely hot or cold may improve swallowing and prevent dysphagia (Toner, 1997).

BOX 13.1
Evidence-Based Practices for Individuals with Dysphagia

General Intervention

- Both clinical and instrumental methods of assessment effectively evaluate dysphagia and guide selection of intervention goals.
- Development of nonnutritive sucking significantly decreases the length of hospitalization for preterm infants.
- Intraoral appliance therapy can result in jaw stability and significantly improved feeding for some children with moderate dysphagia.
- Intervention with adults improves nutrition and hydration and reduces morbidity due to pneumonia and pulmonary problems, thus reducing hospitalization expense and length of stay.
- Compensatory and direct intervention techniques with adults result in improvements in nutrition, feeding efficiency, and swallowing safety, such as less aspiration.
- As a result of SLP intervention, approximately 60% of clients no longer require alternative methods of feeding.

Specific behavioral treatment approaches or techniques

- Diet modifications, particularly modification of thin liquids, is highly effective, at least in the short term, in patients with dysphagia associated with dementia and/or PD. Honey-thickened liquids were most effective for both patient populations, followed by nectar-thickened liquids plus use of the chin tuck technique.
- Postural techniques are effective in eliminating aspiration on thin liquids, although more systematic research is needed in specific patient populations. In neurological patient populations, the chin tuck technique is about 50% effective. The head rotation technique has limited evidence but shows promise for patients with dysphagia of neurological origin (Logemann et al., 1989). The supraglottic swallow technique is difficult for many patients but is successful for some patients with dysphagia associated with neurological disease.
- Muscle-strengthening exercises are effective for patients with pharyngeal phase dysphagia. Patients who participated in a 6-week exercise program involving head-raising exercises three times per day showed significant increases in swallowing functioning following the program.
- Case study research has shown that individualized swallowing programs that use principles that promote motor learning (e.g., maximized practice trials, random practice, systematic feedback) are effective for young children with dysphagia.
- Studies examining the effects of neuromuscular electrical stimulation (NMES) applied to the neck via surface electrodes on functional swallowing outcomes in adults with dysphagia are promising. Well-controlled experimental trials are needed to establish the treatment efficacy of NMES procedures, however.

Sources: Based on Arvedson (2009); Ashford et al. (2009a, 2009b); Clark et al. (2009); Logemann et al. (2008); Nagaya et al. (2004); Shaker et al. (2002); Sheppard (2008). www.asha.org/members/ebp/EBSRS.htm

SUMMARY

Speech-language pathologists who want to focus their careers in the area of dysphagia become specially trained to assess and treat swallowing disorders in the pediatric and adult populations. They work with infants who are unable to nurse adequately, children with feeding problems, and older people who have dysphagia. The anticipatory, oral, pharyngeal, and/or esophageal phases of swallowing may be impaired. Causes include congenital or acquired neurological problems, stroke, cancer, developmental disability, dementia, and accident. Swallowing affects not only nutrition and health, but also social and personal aspects of life. A team approach is used for both assessment and intervention. Evaluation includes a careful history and direct observation of the client while he or she is feeding. The modified barium swallow study uses videofluoroscopic equipment and is considered the "gold standard" in dysphagia evaluation. Treatment procedures address the feeding environment, the client's body and facial posture, food textures and temperatures, oral-motor mobility, and specific swallowing techniques. Medical, prosthetic, and surgical approaches are used when necessary. Nonoral feeding may be required in severe cases.

THOUGHT QUESTIONS

- What connections can you think of between swallowing and speech?
- What special skills and knowledge does the SLP bring to swallowing therapy?
- Can you think of ways that aspiration can be prevented in individuals at risk for dysphagia?
- Do you think patient adherence to certain diet modifications (e.g., honey-thickened liquids, pureed food) is problematic? Why or why not?

SUGGESTED READINGS

Clark, H. M. (2004). Neuromuscular treatment for speech and swallowing: A tutorial. *American Journal of Speech-Language Pathology, 12,* 400–415.

Hall, K. (2001). *Pediatric dysphagia resource guide.* San Diego, CA: Singular.

Logemann, J. A. (1998). *Evaluation and treatment of swallowing disorders* (2nd ed.). Austin, TX: Pro-Ed.

The 2009 issue of the *Journal of Rehabilitation Research and Development, 46(2),* 175–222, provides a systematic review of evidence-based practice in dysphagia treatment.

ONLINE RESOURCES

Aaron's Tracheostomy Page
www.tracheostomy.com
An online resource with information on home care and resources for family members.

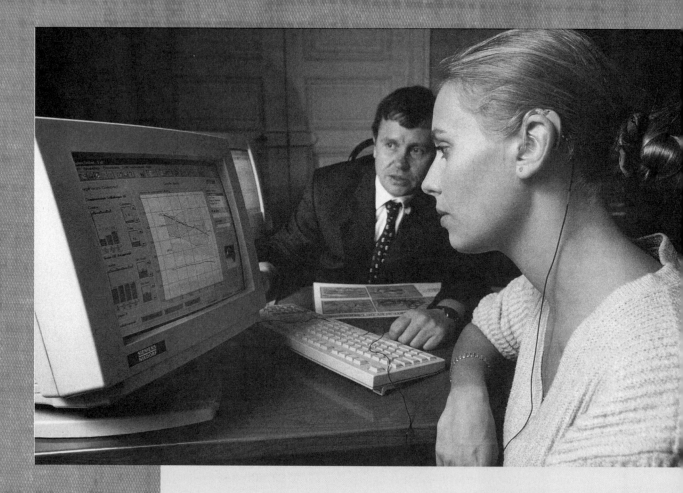

CHAPTER LEARNING GOALS

When you have finished this chapter, you should be able to:

- Describe the psychosocial consequences of hearing loss

- Define *audiology* and describe the role of the audiologist in various employment settings

- Describe the mechanics of sound production and propagation, and demonstrate a basic understanding of the anatomy and physiology of the auditory system

- Identify the general types of hearing loss and potential causes of each

- Identify the components of the audiological test battery and explain the general purpose of and method used in each test

- Define *aural (audiologic) habilitation/rehabilitation* and describe the basic techniques that are used to mitigate the effects of hearing loss on communication

14

Audiology and Hearing Loss

Douglas J. MacKenzie, AuD

Those who are unfamiliar with the topic of hearing loss often have the misconception that it is primarily a disorder specific to the elderly population, occurring simply as a natural consequence of the aging process. Stereotypical images of the elderly being poked fun at, ridiculed, or ignored because they have difficulty hearing abound on television and in movies. In reality, hearing loss is prevalent in people of all ages. From newborns to school-aged children, from teenagers and young adults to seniors, no individual is immune from incurring a hearing problem at some point during their lifetime. Another common misconception is that hearing loss is a disorder that simply impedes one's ability to hear soft to average-level sounds. Although this perception has validity and the consequences should not be downplayed, it is much too simplistic. The impact of hearing loss can be far reaching in terms of overall quality of life. It can have a profound negative impact on speech and language development, reading skills, educational achievement, vocational performance, social interactions, and psychological well-being. It can also have a significant negative impact on family members and close friends. In this chapter, we take a closer look at how hearing loss occurs, the many ways it impacts people's lives, how it is diagnosed, and how it is treated. Case Study 14.1 presents a college student who faced many challenges after experiencing a sudden hearing loss.

INCIDENCE AND PREVALENCE OF HEARING LOSS

Invariably, one of the first questions that comes to mind is "How many people are we talking about?" Although this question is difficult to answer precisely, a general estimate is that approximately 10% of the population in the United States, or 31.5 million people, have some degree of hearing loss (Kochkin, 2005). This number has doubled since the mid-1980s and is

CASE STUDY 14.1
Case Study of David, an Adult with Sudden Sensorineural Hearing Loss

At the age of 22, David was halfway through his senior year at a prominent university, majoring in political science/pre law. He had planned to attend law school the following fall with aspirations of becoming a trial attorney. While attending a party one evening, David suffered a skull fracture when the chair he was sitting in gave way as he leaned back. In a matter of hours, David's world was turned upside down as he went from being able to hear normally to being totally deaf in both ears. David's career goals were suddenly in jeopardy, and he began to experience personal isolation due to problems he had communicating with family and friends. "I feel lost," David confided to his audiologist, "because I can't interact with people around me the way I used to."

David's audiologist recommended that he be fit with hearing aids, but they provided minimal benefit. Ten months after his accident, David underwent surgery to obtain a cochlear implant. He worked closely with his audiologist to develop an individualized aural (audiological) rehabilitation program designed to help him relearn how to make use of sound heard through his cochlear implant. Following intensive auditory training and communication strategy practice, David was now ready to get on with his life and transferred to a college that provided educational support services to deaf and hard-of-hearing students. Unfortunately, David had difficulty developing new relationships. He no longer felt that he fit into the "hearing world," but at the same time he was unable to assimilate into the Deaf Community. He joined a cochlear implant support group and participated in one-on-one auditory therapy with his audiologist to work on specific listening skills. David benefited from these activities and eventually graduated with a degree in computer science. Although David's future is once again bright, this case demonstrates the impact hearing loss can have on all facets of an individual's life.

Not only did David have to cope with the emotional consequences of his sudden deafness, he also had to learn how to hear again through his cochlear implant and deal with the various communication, social, academic, and career challenges stemming from the hearing loss.

As you read this chapter think about

- Possible explanations for David's communication difficulties.
- The psychological and emotional impact of David's hearing loss
- Possible evaluation procedures that could be used to measure David's auditory abilities
- Possible types of intervention that might be considered to help David communicate more effectively

expected to reach 40 million by 2025. Approximately 3 in every 1,000 births results in a child with hearing loss, making it the most frequently occurring birth defect (NCHAM, 2006). Additionally, approximately 1 in every 1,000 births results in a child with a severe to profound degree of hearing loss, or in other words, a child who is considered audiometrically "deaf." Approximately 83 in every 1,000 children in the United States exhibit what is termed an "educationally significant" hearing loss that can have lifelong consequences (National Dissemination Center for Children with Disabilities, 2003).

Over the past two decades, there has been a proliferation of Early Hearing Detection and Intervention (EHDI) programs designed to identify significant congenital hearing loss in newborn babies systematically and follow up with prompt and appropriate audiological habilitation services. Currently in the United States, more than 95% of babies are being screened for hearing loss within the first month after birth (National Center for Hearing Assessment and Management, 2009). The Joint Committee on Infant Hearing (2007) has recommended that babies who fail their newborn hearing screening, and any subsequent rescreening, undergo a comprehensive audiological and medical evaluation before the age of 3 months to confirm or rule out the presence of hearing loss. Although diagnosis of congenital hearing loss is occurring at an earlier age in recent years due to state-mandated and voluntary Universal Newborn Hearing Screening programs, this is only the first step, albeit an essential one, in the audiological habilitation process. It is equally important that appropriate early intervention services be prescribed and treatment promptly initiated once a hearing disorder has been identified. Failure to identify hearing loss and provide appropriate early intervention services can lead to significant difficulties relative to speech-language, social-emotional, and cognitive development, which may ultimately have a negative impact on academic achievement and vocational options (Moeller, 2001; Yoshinaga-Itano et al., 1998). For up to date information on the status of Early Hearing Detection and Intervention programs in the United States, visit the National Center for Hearing Assessment and Management Web site listed at the end of this chapter.

HEARING LOSS THROUGH THE LIFESPAN
••

Psychosocial Aspects of Hearing Loss

The process of adjusting to and coping with hearing loss can be difficult for those who are afflicted, as well as their families. This period of adjustment can also be frustrating for professionals because clients are often slow to follow through on recommendations for treatment when they have not fully accepted the permanency of their condition. People with hearing impairment experience a wide range of psychological, social, and emotional consequences (English, 2002). With children who are hearing impaired, delays in speech and language may present problems with self-awareness and self-expression. Ultimately, this may lead to difficulties in the development of social skills. Children with hearing loss, even if only mild in degree, frequently exhibit lower self-esteem and reduced self-worth that may ultimately impact interpersonal relationships with their peers and family members (Bess et al., 1998).

The psychosocial consequences of hearing loss may not only manifest themselves in children who are afflicted, but also their parents. A somewhat staggering statistic is that approximately 95% of hearing-impaired children are born to parents with normal hearing (Mitchell & Karchmer, 2004). Most parents have little knowledge, let alone experience, pertaining to hearing loss and the challenges it presents when raising a child. The birth of a child is one of the most joyous moments in the life of a parent. It is a time filled with hope and optimism. Feelings of euphoria, however, can quickly turn to feelings of despair and helplessness upon receiving word that one's newborn baby has been identified with a significant hearing loss. Parents may feel as if their lives are suddenly spiraling out of control as they face the reality of raising a child who has a disorder for which they are unprepared to handle. Tanner (1980) has described how the Kübler-Ross grief cycle, associated with the dying process, is applicable to those dealing with hearing loss. Parents of children with hearing loss often go through the various stages of grief, experiencing shock, denial, anger, and depression before they are finally able to accept the reality of the situation.

Adults who have acquired hearing loss over the course of their lifetime, whether suddenly or gradually, are equally susceptible to psychosocial problems. Many go through the same stages of grief as parents of hearing-impaired children. The reality of no longer being able to enjoy social activities to the same degree as in the past, or not being able to understand conversations on the phone, at meetings, or during family gatherings may cause an adult with hearing loss to experience a variety of emotions including anger and frustration that may ultimately lead to depression (Mullins, 2004). Having to rely on others to answer the phone or clarify messages that were misunderstood can lead to feelings of inadequacy, guilt, decreased self-sufficiency, and reduced self-worth. Family relationships may become strained as a hearing-impaired member is increasingly excluded from conversations due to frustration brought on by numerous requests for repetition. The spouse of a hearing-impaired person may become particularly vulnerable to stress imposed by having to assume greater responsibility for assisting with their partner's daily communication requirements. They may also face the likelihood of reduced social interactions with friends and acquaintances as their hearing-impaired partner withdraws from activities that were once routinely engaged in as a couple. It is imperative that professionals identify and explore these psychosocial issues to determine the full impact of a hearing problem on the individual client and his or her significant other.

Classification of Impairment, Disability, and Handicap

When it comes to describing the affects of hearing loss, terminology can be confusing, especially for those who are new to the subject. Terms such as "impaired," "disabled," and "handicapped" are tossed about freely. In 1980, the World Health Organization (WHO) adopted an international classification system in an effort to delineate these terms clearly (WHO, 1980). It has since been revised (WHO, 2000) and used extensively in the disciplines of education, sociology, anthropology, speech-language pathology, and audiology. The WHO defines **impairment** as a loss of structure or function. Relative to the auditory system, impairment can occur due to trauma to the eardrum or the tiny bones of the middle ear, a loss of sensory cells in the inner ear, or compression of the auditory nerve due to a tumor. Simply because an impairment exists does not necessarily mean it will have a significant impact on a person's ability to communicate. The functional consequences associated with a particular impairment are referred to as *activity limitation* or **disability.** For those with hearing loss the resulting disability may be an inability to understand speech in the presence of background noise, difficulty understanding conversations on the phone, or difficulty hearing low-intensity speech sounds. It is important to determine one's degree of disability in order to prescribe an appropriate course of treatment.

Impairment and disability may lead to *participation restriction* or **handicap,** which is defined as the psychosocial consequence of the hearing loss. As we have already seen, hearing loss can have a profound negative effect on one's ability to cope. It may lead to reduced self-concept and self-worth, social isolation, and strained family relationships. Simply put, all people with hearing loss experience impairment. Many of these individuals experience disability. Not all who experience disability, however, necessarily experience handicap. Despite problems hearing on the phone or understanding conversations in noisy settings, many hearing-impaired people are well adjusted, independent, fully participating members of society. In contrast, others are completely debilitated by the same degree, or in some cases, lesser degrees of hearing loss. Professionals need to be cognizant of the full spectrum of psychosocial consequences that can result while at the same time never losing sight of the fact that not all people with hearing loss are impacted to the same degree in terms of communication handicap. As we will see later, counseling plays a critical role in helping clients realize and understand the psychosocial implications of their hearing problem.

Deafness, the Deaf Community, and Deaf Culture

If you've had little or no contact with individuals with significant hearing loss, it may be difficult to conceive of how anyone would resist seeking treatment for their condition or would feel a sense of relief or even elation upon receiving word that their newborn baby is deaf. Such is the case, however, for many hearing-impaired individuals who view deafness not as a disability or handicap but as a cultural trait. These individuals make up what is referred to as the **Deaf Community,** a group who views deafness with a sense of pride that serves to unite its members and positively shape their sense of self-identity and self-concept.

An important distinction needs to be made between the labels "deaf" with a lowercase "d" and "Deaf" with an uppercase "D". Individuals who are "deaf" share a common physiological condition, that being hearing loss that is severe to profound in degree. In contrast, "Deaf" refers to individuals who are members of the Deaf Community. Simply having a severe to profound hearing loss, however, does not automatically indoctrinate one into the Deaf Community. There must be a concomitant identification with what is known as **Deaf Culture.**

A culture is created when a group of people share in a common background of language, traditions, mores, and values. Those who identify with Deaf Culture share a common language, **American Sign Language** (ASL), which is considered the natural language of the Deaf that serves to foster group cohesion and identity. Deaf Culture is further characterized by its rich history, traditions, folklore, and various contributions to the arts including poetry, dance, and theater. Those who embrace Deaf Culture share common beliefs and customs that have been passed on from one generation to the next. The continued existence of any culture depends on the perpetuation of its native language and traditions. Within the Deaf Community this is usually accomplished through education and marriage. Schools for the deaf provide a means for children to interact freely using ASL. Through the socialization process, pride in one's identity as a Deaf person is fostered. Upon reaching adulthood, members of the Deaf Community often marry others who share these same cultural ideals. For many there is a desire to have children who are deaf to whom they can pass on their traditions and values. Needless to say, growing up within the Deaf Community is not without its challenges. Children brought up using ASL as their primary mode of communication encounter many of the same challenges as other nonnative speakers of English in terms of literacy and writing skills. Because most hearing people have no knowledge of sign language, the limited English and spoken language skills of many who are deaf inhibits their ability to communicate effectively with the vast majority of nonsigning people with whom they come in contact.

Living and working in today's culturally diverse society, it is important for professionals in the fields of speech-language pathology and audiology to develop an awareness and understanding of Deaf Culture. Academic training programs have traditionally addressed hearing impairment from a pathological perspective, an approach referred to as the medical model. With this approach, hearing that is audiometrically within normal limits is the standard by which everything else is compared. Therefore, anyone with any degree of hearing loss deviates from the norm. Those who are considering a career in speech-language pathology or audiology should be aware that some members of the Deaf Community view professionals in these disciplines in a negative light due to their affiliation with the medical model. Speech-language pathologists and audiologists are viewed by some as "Audists" who practice under the assumption that it is desirable for those who are deaf to develop spoken language and auditory skills rather than rely on sign language. Professionals have been accused of profiting from deafness through the sale of hearing aids and other assistive devices and supporting efforts to eradicate or "fix" deafness through cochlear implants and gene therapy. Some have even gone so far as to label these efforts as "cultural genocide."

Professionals have also been criticized for focusing on how people who are deaf deviate from the norm, prescribing various treatments to overcome what they perceive to be a disabling or handicapping condition rather than a personal trait. Speech-language pathologists and audiologists must be cognizant of these issues. Having a firm understanding of Deaf Culture and the unique perspective of the Deaf Community will serve to positively shape the direction and quality of services provided to those who are severely to profoundly hearing impaired.

WHAT IS AUDIOLOGY?

We have already alluded to the fact that some speech and language disorders are the direct result of significant hearing loss. A child who is profoundly hearing impaired will experience significant delays in speech and language development if prompt and appropriate intervention services are not provided. Although speech-language pathologists, under their scope of practice, are able to conduct basic hearing screenings, the detailed information provided by a comprehensive audiological evaluation is critical to the development and implementation of an appropriate early intervention plan. Additionally, the complementary nature of habilitative/rehabilitative services provided by their respective disciplines requires speech-language pathologists and audiologists to work closely together. It is appropriate, therefore, that we consider the discipline of audiology in the overall scope of communicative disorders.

The American Speech-Language-Hearing Association (ASHA) defines audiology as the discipline involved in "the prevention of and assessment of auditory, vestibular, and related impairments as well as the habilitation/rehabilitation and maintenance of persons with these impairments." (ASHA, 2004, p. 2). A key point contained within this definition is that audiology consists of professional efforts related to assessment *and* habilitation/rehabilitation. All too often, students new to the area of communicative disorders perceive audiology as a discipline that deals strictly with the diagnosis of hearing loss. Although assessment is a critical component, what is subsequently done in terms of treatment and management of a client diagnosed with a hearing problem is equally important. Audiologists are not simply technicians. They must be adept at providing habilitative/rehabilitative services including counseling, prescribing and fitting **amplification,** and various therapeutic services designed to facilitate communication and improve one's overall quality of life.

Obviously, hearing loss is not a new phenomenon so you might naturally assume that the discipline of audiology has been around for quite some time. Surprisingly, however, audiology is a fairly new field of study, with its roots dating back only to the mid-1940s. Audiology is the product of two disciplines: speech pathology, which by now you are quite familiar with, and otology, a medically based discipline concerned with the diagnosis and treatment of disorders of the auditory system. At the end of World War II, service personnel returning home were in need of rehabilitative services to overcome communication difficulties associated with battle-related hearing loss. Rehabilitation centers were established by medical departments within the military to provide medical and aural rehabilitation services. Eventually these services were extended to the general civilian population through community-based clinics, and audiology began to distinguish itself from speech pathology and otology as a unique and separate discipline.

Today, audiology continues to be an exciting, ever-changing profession with employment opportunities in a wide range of settings. A recent survey of ASHA-certified audiologists revealed that more than half work in nonresidential health care settings (e.g., private practices, community speech and hearing centers, physician's offices), with 26% employed in hospital settings, 11% in schools, and a smaller percentage in universities and residential health care facilities (ASHA, 2003). There is a tendency for audiologists to specialize depending on the setting where they work and the population(s) they serve. For example, audiologists in private practice typically specialize in the fitting and dispensing of hearing aids; educational audiologists specialize in the fitting of personal and classroom amplification systems and the diagnosis, treatment, and management of (central) auditory processing disorders. Some audiologists in medical settings even participate as members of surgical teams by conducting interoperative monitoring of auditory nerve function during surgery.

FUNDAMENTALS OF SOUND

It is unlikely that you've spent much time pondering the question "What is sound?" Perhaps you've taken a course where the professor has asked you to contemplate the classic question *"If a tree falls in the forest and there is no one there to hear it, does it still make a sound?"* To fully appreciate the process of hearing, let's start with a brief overview of the fundamentals of how sound is generated.

Several conditions must exist in order for sound to occur and be perceived. For the purpose of this discussion, let's focus specifically on the speech signal. As described in Chapter 3, there must be an available energy source such as exhalation of air from the lungs, an object capable of vibrating, such as the vocal folds of the larynx for the energy source to act on, and an available medium, such as air, that is capable of conducting the resulting vibrations. Finally, there needs to be a receptor in place to receive, decode, and interpret the resulting sound. The remainder of this chapter focuses exclusively on the human auditory system as the receptor of sound.

How is it that sound is able to travel great distances through the air to reach our ears? Let's take a step back and first consider how an object, such as a simple guitar string, vibrates. Vibration can be thought of as a series of rhythmic back-and-forth movements. As the guitar sting is plucked, it vibrates to and fro. As it moves in one direction, an increase in pressure occurs as air molecules lying in close proximity are displaced and subsequently compressed or packed together tightly in relation to one another. As the guitar string reverses and moves in the opposite direction, the air molecules that were initially compressed begin to rebound or spread apart, creating a subsequent decrease in pressure referred to as a rarefaction. In simplified form, sound is a series of compressions and rarefactions that move outward from a vibrating source. It is important to realize that the individual air molecules themselves do not travel from their original position near the sound source to the listener's ear. Rather, it is the sound wave resulting from changes in pressure that propagates to the ear. For example, imagine a group of people standing single file in a long line. If the person at the end of the line accidentally bumps the individual directly in front of him, that person will make contact with the next person in line and so forth. Although energy is transmitted far away down the line, each individual moves only a short distance before rebounding to his or her original position.

Because a vibrating object moves back and forth relative to its normal resting position, it takes on special qualities. First, the vibrating object travels a measurable distance in either direction. This is referred to as the amplitude of the vibration. The amplitude of a sound determines its **intensity,** which is measured in **decibels** (dB). Secondly, this back-and-forth movement regularly repeats itself, resulting in a certain number of complete cycles during a specified period of time. This is referred to as the **frequency** of the vibration and is expressed in cycles per second, or **Hertz** (Hz). The intensity of a sound is generally associated with the perception of loudness, whereas the frequency is associated with the perception of pitch. Every sound, therefore, can be described in terms of its characteristic intensity and frequency. This information is decoded by the auditory system, enabling one to differentiate the infinitesimal number of sounds exposed to throughout the course of a day.

Audibility Versus Intelligibility

When discussing hearing and hearing loss, it is important to differentiate the concepts of **audibility** and **intelligibility.** Audibility is the ability to detect the presence of sound through one's sense of hearing. As we will later see, many audiological tests evaluate an individual's ability to detect sound to determine how much energy is needed for it to be just barely perceptible. This type of task, however, does not provide any information as to whether the listener actually understands or can make use of what they hear, only that they are able to detect the presence of a given sound. In contrast, intelligibility refers to one's ability to recognize and understand what they hear. Not only can the listener detect a stimulus such as speech, they are able to identify the individual phonemes that make up words and sentences.

As we shall see, hearing loss affects intelligibility as well as audibility. Sounds are softer than usual or may be inaudible altogether. Obviously, this will impede one's ability to understand speech unless audibility can be improved through the use of amplification. One complaint, however, that is common among hearing-impaired persons is that they are often able to hear people talking but can't figure out what they are saying. In other words, speech is audible but not intelligible. You may have found yourself in a situation where you were able to hear a TV or radio playing in a neighboring room. The sound was audible but too muffled to make out more than a few isolated words. This is similar to what is experienced by many hearing-impaired individuals during daily conversations. Unfortunately for some individuals, even if audibility of the speech signal can be increased though amplification, intelligibility may not improve significantly due to distortion imposed by permanent damage to the auditory system.

ANATOMY AND PHYSIOLOGY OF THE AUDITORY SYSTEM

Before we can delve into a discussion of the various types and causes of hearing loss, a general understanding of the anatomy and physiology of the auditory system is essential. Anatomically, the auditory system can be divided into several general areas. They include the outer ear, the middle ear, the inner ear, the vesibulocochlear nerve, the auditory brainstem, and the auditory cortex of the brain. The first four areas (Figure 14.1) are commonly referred to as the peripheral auditory system; the later two comprise the central auditory system. In general, damage to structures within the peripheral system results in a loss of sensitivity, whereas damage to the central auditory system results in deficits related to the processing of sound. We begin our discussion at the point where sound enters the auditory system: the area referred to as the outer ear.

The Outer Ear

The **outer ear** is comprised of the **pinna,** or auricle, and the **external auditory meatus,** or external auditory canal. The pinna is the most outwardly visible structure of the auditory system and composed of flexible cartilage covered with skin. Although somewhat simple in appearance, the various ridges and depressions associated with the pinna serve to enhance sound naturally. The pinna collects and funnels sound into the ear canal while also serving as a natural resonator. In addition, the pinna facilitates in determining where sound originates in space, a process called **localization.**

The external auditory meatus is an elliptical tube lined with skin that extends from the primary bowl-like depression associated with the pinna, known as the **concha,** to the **tympanic membrane** or **eardrum.**

FIGURE 14.1

The peripheral auditory system.

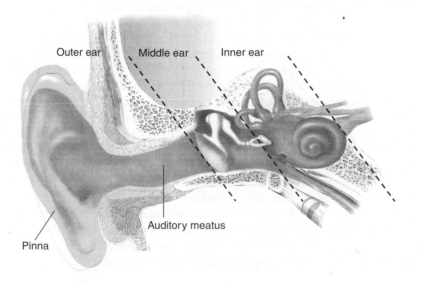

Approximately 1 inch in length in adults, the canal has a slight "S-shaped" contour and narrows slightly as it progresses toward the eardrum. The outer region is marked by a proliferation of fine hair follicles and glands that produce a substance called **cerumen,** more commonly known as ear wax. Because the external auditory meatus is essentially a tube, it functions as a resonator, much like a musical instrument, naturally amplifying sound in the 2,700 Hz to 3,400 Hz region.

The Middle Ear

The external auditory canal leads to the tympanic membrane, which marks the boundary between the outer ear and the **middle ear.** The tympanic membrane is a thin concave-shaped structure that is highly elastic and responds much like a stereo speaker, vibrating in response to sound waves that travel down the canal. Most of the surface area of the tympanic membrane is composed of three distinct layers of tissue. The outer layer is a continuation of the skin that lines the external canal; the inner layer is continuous with the mucous membrane that lines the cavity directly behind the eardrum. Sandwiched between the two is a layer of fibrous tissue that provides strength and accounts for the eardrum's elastic properties. A healthy eardrum is often described as appearing "pearl gray" in color. It is highly vascular, and due to its semitransparent nature it is possible to observe some of the structures of the middle ear when conducting a visual examination.

Located behind the tympanic membrane is the **middle ear space,** or **tympanic cavity.** This air-filled cavity housed within the temporal bone of the skull is roughly cube shaped and lined with mucous membrane. Located near the bottom of the anterior wall is the opening to the **eustachian tube,** which connects the middle ear with the **nasopharynx,** the space located behind the nose and above the roof of the mouth. The eustachian tube is normally closed but opens periodically, providing a passageway for air to ventilate the middle ear space and equalize air pressure on each side of the eardrum.

Spanning the length of the middle ear cavity, much like a suspension bridge, is a chain formed by three small bones. These bones, called the **malleus, incus,** and **stapes,** are collectively referred to as the **ossicles** or **ossicular chain** (see Figure 14.2). The first bone in the chain, the malleus, is the largest of the three. Its primary structure is embedded in the fibrous layer of the eardrum. The upper portion articulates with the second bone in the chain, the incus, which in turn, articulates with the stapes, the smallest bone in the human body. Resembling a stirrup, the stapes contains two curved arms that terminate in a flat, bony disk called the footplate. The footplate rests against the **oval window,** a thin membrane that marks the entrance to the inner ear. Attached to the neck of the stapes is the tendon of the **stapedius muscle.** In a normal ear, intense sounds cause the stapedius muscle to contract, which pulls the stapes posteriorly and dampens the transmission of energy through the middle ear. At one time it was

FIGURE 14.2

Structures of the middle ear.

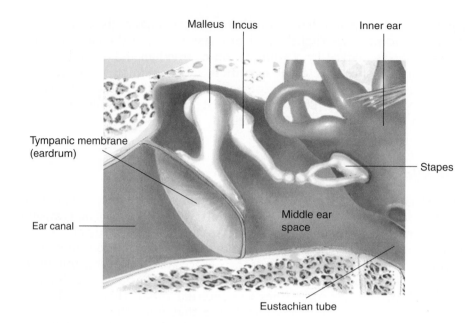

thought that contraction served to protect the delicate structures of the inner ear from high-intensity sound. It has since been shown that the stapedius muscle reflex provides limited attenuation of sound and is insufficient in protecting one's hearing.

The Inner Ear

The **inner ear** is a complex structure that serves two important roles. One major component, the **cochlea,** is responsible for providing auditory input to the central auditory system. The other major component, the **vestibular system,** is responsible for supplying information regarding balance and spatial orientation. Deficits in the vestibular system often result in problems related to **vertigo** (the sensation of spinning), dizziness, and imbalance.

Let's turn our attention first to the cochlea, a coiled structure the size of a pea that resembles a snail's shell. The cochlea spirals 2.5 times around a central core of bone and is the portion of the inner ear that contains the auditory sensory receptor cells. The cochlea is comprised of two concentric labyrinths. The outer labyrinth is composed of bone and filled with a fluid called **perilymph;** the inner labyrinth is composed of membranous material and contains a fluid called **endolymph.**

Running along the center of the membranous labyrinth is an intricate structure called the **organ of Corti** (see Figure 14.3). The floor of the organ of Corti is formed by the basilar membrane. The **basilar membrane** is unique in that it is not of uniform width, thickness, or stiffness throughout the cochlea. Rather, it is narrower, thinner, and stiffer at the base and wider, thicker, and more flaccid at the apex, enabling it to respond differently to sounds that vary in terms of their component frequencies. It is said

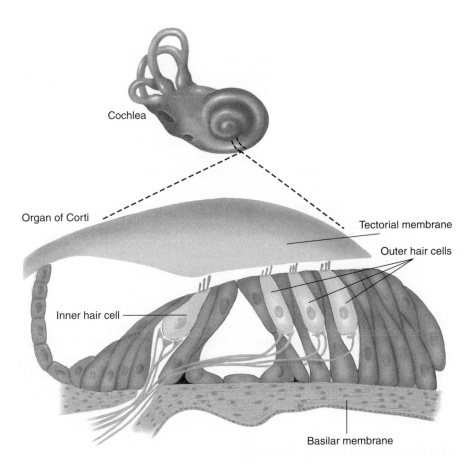

FIGURE 14.3

The organ of Corti.

Cochlea

Organ of Corti

Tectorial membrane

Outer hair cells

Inner hair cell

Basilar membrane

to be **tonotopically** organized. That is, the portion of the basilar membrane closest to the stapes responds best to high-frequency sounds, and the portion nearest the tip or apex of the cochlea responds best to low-frequency sounds. Forming the roof of the organ of Corti is a gelatinous, tongue-shaped structure called the **tectorial membrane.** The tectorial membrane is fixed at one end while the opposite end is free to move up and down in response to displacement of the surrounding fluid.

Situated on the basilar membrane are thousands of tiny **hair cells,** which are considered to be the sensory receptor cells of the auditory system. Located on the top of each cell are small hairlike projections called **stereocilia.** Due to differences in their structure and orientation, the hair cells are separated into two groups: the outer and inner hair cells. As the stereocilia are bent and sheared through the movement of the tectorial and basilar membranes, chemical transmitters are released at the base of the hair cells and neuroelectrical energy is subsequently generated. Innervating the hair cells are auditory nerve fibers that collectively form the acoustic branch of the **vestibulocochlear,** or **VIIIth nerve.**

Before we end our discussion of the inner ear, a brief mention of the vestibular system is in order. The vestibular system is also comprised of bony and membranous sections and contains two important features: the **semicircular canals** and the **otolith system.** A total of three semicircular canals are positioned at right angles to one another. Sensory receptor cells located within the enlarged ends of each canal sense angular acceleration such as up-and-down and side-to-side head movement. The otolith system consists of two membranous sacs that contain additional sensory cells. These cells sense linear acceleration such as that which occurs when riding in a car or elevator. Nerve fibers innervating the sensory cells of the vestibular system collectively form the vestibular branch of the VIIIth nerve. Given the interrelationship between the auditory and vestibular systems, it is considered within the audiologist's scope of practice to conduct vestibular testing and provide nonmedical intervention of balance disorders (ASHA, 2004).

The Vestibulocochlear Nerve

As its name implies, the vesibulocochlear nerve is made up of neural fibers that originate in the vestibular and cochlear portions of the inner ear. This highly organized bundle of nerve fibers traverses through a bony canal called the **internal auditory meatus.** Upon exiting the canal the fibers of the vestibulocochlear nerve join the brainstem at the angle formed by the cerebellum, medulla oblongata, and the pons: a region referred to as the **cerebellopontine angle.** This region marks the juncture of the peripheral and central auditory systems.

The Central Auditory System

The central auditory system is highly complex. It consists of ascending and descending pathways comprised of nuclei, nerve fibers, nerve tracts, and their associated connections. Only a grossly simplified overview of the ascending auditory pathways is presented in this section. Although it may appear that the anatomical structures leading to the brain serve merely as relay centers for the transmission of neural impulses, they actually play a key role in the extraction, enhancement, and processing of auditory signals (Bellis, 2003a).

Nerve fibers from the cochlear branch of VIIIth nerve enter the brainstem and synapse at the cochlear nucleus complex. Beyond this point, nerve fibers from each ear divide into two distinct branches: the ipsilateral and contralateral ascending pathways. Some nerve fibers ascend to the brain on the same, or ipsilateral, side of the brainstem; the majority cross over and ascend on the opposite, or contralateral, side. From the cochlear nucleus, the majority of fibers ascend to the superior olivary complex located in the pons. The superior olivary complex plays a significant role in localization and activation of the stapedius muscle reflex. From there, nerve fibers generally progress subcortically to the lateral lemniscus in the pons, the inferior colliculus in the midbrain, and the medial geniculate body in the thalamus. Additional crossover occurs at some of these sites. Beyond this level, the auditory nerve fibers fan out and proceed as auditory radiations to the **primary auditory cortex,** known as Heschl's gyrus, located in the temporal lobes. In most individuals, the left hemisphere is the primary area where linguistic information is processed, and the right hemisphere is responsible for processing nonlinguistic auditory cues such as rhythm and stress.

Now that we have a general understanding of the anatomical structures of the auditory system, let's briefly review the process of how sound is transmitted from the environment to the brain. Sound waves generated by a vibrating object go through a series of energy transformations as they pass through the auditory system. As acoustic energy travels down the external auditory meatus it is transformed into mechanical energy by the movement of the tympanic membrane and ossicular chain. The resulting mechanical energy, in turn, is converted to hydraulic energy through the motion of the stapes footplate in and out of the oval window. Displacement of the cochlear fluids results in movement of the tectorial and basilar membranes, which in turn leads to the bending and shearing action of the stereocilia located on the tips of the hair cells in the organ of Corti. This process converts the hydraulic energy into neuroelectrical impulses that are transmitted to the auditory cortex of the brain via the auditory branch of the vestibulocochlear nerve and ascending auditory pathways. Amazingly, this complex process takes place within a matter of milliseconds, making it a truly remarkable system.

TYPES OF HEARING LOSS

The previous section described the ear from an anatomical and physiological standpoint. Functionally, the outer and the middle ear serve to collect, amplify, and conduct sound to the cochlea. The outer and middle ear, therefore, are referred to as the conductive system. The cochlea is the actual sensory organ of hearing, and the auditory branch of the VIIIth nerve is responsible for transmitting the resulting neural signal to the brainstem and ultimately to the auditory cortex for processing. The cochlea and auditory nerve, therefore, make up the sensorineural system. In describing peripheral hearing loss, it is most common to describe the loss from a functional perspective, that is, conductive versus sensorineural. Deficits relative to the central auditory system can be functionally described as well in terms of their impact on auditory processing abilities. As we see in the next section, each of these general types of hearing loss can present unique challenges for people of all ages.

Conductive Hearing Loss

A **conductive hearing loss** occurs as a result of a deformation, malfunction, or obstruction of the outer or middle ear. Not all disorders of the outer and middle ear result in a loss of hearing sensitivity. In many cases, however, problems in these areas reduce or eliminate the ear's natural conduction and resonance properties, impeding sound reaching the cochlea. The result is that the intensity of sound arriving at the inner ear is reduced. This usually prevents low to moderate intensity sounds from being audible, with higher intensity sounds perceived as being much softer than normal. It is important to remember that the primary consequence of conductive hearing loss is a loss of loudness or audibility. As long as the sensorineural system remains intact, sound can be heard without difficulty if it is made loud enough for the individual, such as by turning up the volume of a radio or TV, or by raising the level of one's voice.

Although conductive hearing loss can have a significant impact on audibility, it does not result in a total loss of hearing. In other words, a person who is considered "deaf" would not have lost hearing solely as a result of a conductive deficit. Fortunately, most conductive losses are not permanent. Some resolve spontaneously, and most others are medically treatable. In those rare instances, however, where treatment of the underlying disease does not completely resolve a conductive hearing loss, use of amplification may be warranted.

Disorders of the Outer Ear

Starting with the outer ear, several conditions can occur owing to the malformation of structures during embryonic development. The first, **microtia,** refers to a small malformed pinna. By itself, microtia does not result in a loss of hearing sensitivity. When observed, however, the audiologist is alerted to the possibility of other congenital conditions such as **atresia,** a disorder in which there is complete closure of the external auditory meatus. Because sound cannot travel through the ear canal in the usual manner, significant hearing loss is inevitable. Stenosis, a severe narrowing of the external canal, may occur in some individuals. Unlike atresia, however, stenois does not result in significant hearing loss unless debris or earwax becomes trapped in the narrow opening. These conditions most frequently occur in conjunction with other craniofacial disorders (see Chapter 11) as in the case of Down syndrome or Treacher Collins syndrome. Because the structures of the external ear develop from embryological tissue that lies in close proximity to that which gives rise to the cochlea during roughly the same gestational period, whenever a congenital malformation of the pinna or external ear canal is observed, a full hearing evaluation should be conducted to determine if impairment to the cochlea coexists.

A much more common cause of conductive hearing loss in the outer ear is due to impacted cerumen or a foreign object. It may be hard to believe, but cerumen actually serves several useful purposes. Cerumen protects the ear, at least to some degree, from insects and other foreign bodies entering the canal. It also traps dirt and debris, naturally cleansing the external canal as it migrates outward. Cerumen acts as a lubricant to prevent the skin that lines the canal from drying out and serves as a chemical barrier to bacterial and fungal infection. Given these positive attributes and the potential for injury to the lining of the canal and the eardrum, the use of cotton swabs or other implements to remove cerumen should be avoided. Some populations, such as young children and the elderly, are more prone to problems resulting from excessive cerumen production or entrapment in the canal. This can create a slight/mild to moderate degree of hearing loss, necessitating medical intervention to remove the cerumen plug. Interestingly, in many states cerumen management (removal) is within the audiologist's scope of practice, although it should be conducted with extreme caution and only after proper training.

DISORDERS OF THE MIDDLE EAR

Several causes of conductive hearing loss can be traced to the middle ear. The tympanic membrane may be perforated as a result of disease, trauma, or sudden change in pressure, or it may become thickened as a result of calcium plaque formation. Likewise, the bones of the ossicular chain may become disarticulated due to a blow to the head, or their movement may be impeded by fluid or a tumor in the middle ear cavity.

Cholesteatoma is a tumorlike mass composed of epithelial (skin) cells, keratin, and fat that migrates into the middle ear cavity, often through a perforated eardrum. The resulting mass can grow in size and has a propensity to erode bone, including the ossicles and bony walls of the middle ear space. Left untreated, this can lead to irreversible damage to the inner ear, facial nerve, and structures of the cranial cavity. Due to its destructive nature and the potential for serious complications, prompt surgical removal is required.

Otosclerosis is a disorder that afflicts primarily young adults, particularly females, and in the majority of cases is linked to genetic factors. It is characterized by the resorption of healthy bone and subsequent formation of spongy bone in the vicinity of the stapes footplate. This bone often hardens, resulting in partial or complete fixation of the stapes. Because normal movement of the stapes footplate in and out of the oval window is impeded, hearing loss is a likely consequence. Treatment of otosclerosis usually consists of surgical removal of part or all of the fixated footplate and insertion of a prosthetic device that acts as an artificial stapes.

One of the most common causes of conductive hearing loss, particularly in children, is **otitis media,** an inflammation of the mucous membrane lining the middle ear cavity. In fact, otitis media is the most frequently diagnosed disorder in the United States in children younger than 15 years. More than 90% of children experience at least one episode by the age of 7 years, with peak incidence generally occurring during the period from 6 months to 2 years of age (Jung & Hanson, 1999). Children who experience longstanding or frequently reoccurring episodes are of particular concern because the timing tends to coincide with the period that is most crucial for speech, language, and cognitive development (Gravel & Wallace, 1999). Given the potential to negatively affect academic achievement, it is imperative that speech-language pathologists and audiologists educate parents regarding the symptoms and consequences of otitis media to facilitate early identification and prompt intervention.

A number of factors place certain children at risk for otitis media. They include the presence of craniofacial anomalies such as cleft palate and those associated with Down syndrome, day-care placement, and exposure to secondhand smoke. Heredity, race, and gender are also contributing factors. Although it is significantly more prevalent in children, adults are not immune to otitis media. Despite its prevalence, a great deal of confusion and controversy surround the disorder, particularly when it comes to terminology and treatment.

Otitis media generally results from eustachian dysfunction, often following an upper respiratory infection, which prevents proper ventilation of the middle ear cavity. A normal functioning eustachian tube opens periodically as one chews, yawns, or swallows, allowing for the equalization of air pressure between the middle ear and the external environment. In children, the eustachian tube is shorter, wider, oriented more in the horizontal plane, and more pliable than in adults, making it less efficient in ventilating the middle ear. If adequate ventilation cannot be provided by the eustachian tube due to enlarged adenoids or swelling of the tissue lining the nasopharynx, oxygen within the middle ear cavity is absorbed into the mucous membrane lining, forming a partial vacuum. This, in turn, results in a reduction in air pressure within the middle ear compared to the pressure in the ear canal. This pressure imbalance, a condition known as negative middle ear pressure, causes the eardrum to retract into the middle ear cavity, diminishing its ability to vibrate freely. If normal ventilation of the middle ear is not restored, further retraction of the eardrum into the middle ear cavity will continue. At this point, the person may experience a sensation of their ear feeling plugged or slight discomfort.

The vacuum within the middle ear can lead to the secretion of fluid, a condition referred to as **otitis media with effusion** (OME). As fluid fills the cavity, further stiffening the eardrum and the ossicular chain, the medium through which sound normally travels is altered. That is, sound must now be conducted through a less efficient fluid-filled medium instead of the usual air-filled environment. If the fluid is sterile, the condition is classified as **serous otitis media.** However, when pathogens are present and make their way from the nasopharynx through the eustachian tube, infection of the middle ear cavity is likely. Pus forms within the middle ear cavity as a direct result of the infection of the mucous membrane. This condition is referred to as **purulent** or **suppurative otitis media.** Symptoms associated with an active infection include restlessness, irritability, ear pain, fever, and vomiting. During this process the tympanic membrane may appear reddish in color or bulging. Spontaneous rupturing of the tympanic membrane may occur along with concomitant fluid discharge.

Otitis media can be further classified based on the general time course of the disease process. **Acute otitis media** is characterized by rapid onset, with resolution within approximately 3 weeks. When the condition persists for longer than 8 weeks, it is referred to as **chronic otitis media.** Episodes lasting between 3 weeks and 8 weeks are referred to as **subacute otitis media.**

Treatment of otitis media is a complex process because an active infection may or may not be involved. In some cases the recommended course of treatment is simply to monitor the situation to see whether it will resolve spontaneously. Decongestants and antihistamines may be prescribed to resolve the underlying problem of inadequate eustachian tube function. Antibiotics such as amoxicillin are frequently used in cases of acute otitis media to prevent the development of chronic disease and reduce the risk of complications such as damage to the structures of the middle and inner ear, and meningitis. There has been strong concern expressed in recent years regarding the increased resistance of certain pathogens to antibiotics that in the past were successful in treating acute otitis media (Rosenfeld et al., 1994). Surgical treatment is sometimes warranted and involves a relatively simple procedure called a **myringotomy** whereby an incision is made in the tympanic membrane and fluid within the middle ear cavity is drained. This is frequently followed by insertion of a **pressure equalization** (PE) or **tympanostomy tube** into the tympanic membrane. These tubes or grommets are very small in diameter and serve the same purpose as the eustachian tube, allowing air to pass into the middle ear space. However, instead of passing from the nasopharynx in the usual manner, air enters the middle ear from the external auditory canal via the open PE tube situated in the eardrum. Images of various outer and middle ear disorders are available on Roy Sullivan's video otoscopy Web site listed at the end of this chapter.

Sensorineural Hearing Loss

A second general type of hearing loss, **sensorineural hearing loss,** results from the absence or malformation of, or damage to the structures of the inner ear, most notably the hair cells within the cochlea. Sensorineural hearing loss may be present at birth or develop over the course of one's life. It may be sudden in onset, occurring over a matter of hours, or gradual, manifesting over a period of years. Some forms of sensorineural hearing loss have a genetic basis; other forms are acquired, resulting from factors exogenous to the individual. Hearing may remain stable, become worse, or fluctuate. It is in many ways the direct opposite of conductive hearing loss because sensorineural losses are usually permanent. Recent advances in auditory hair cell regeneration in animals through gene therapy hold promise because they may one day become a viable means of restoring hearing in humans who have experienced significant hair cell damage (Izumikawa et al., 2005).

Although sensorineural hearing loss may affect sensitivity for any range of frequencies, most cases are characterized by hearing loss predominantly in the higher frequency range; sensitivity in the lower frequencies often remains unaffected. Unlike conductive hearing loss where the problem stems from sound not being loud enough, sensorineural hearing loss presents an additional problem, the lack of clarity. Not only are certain sounds inaudible or difficult to hear, but sounds that are audible are often perceived as being distorted. To illustrate this point, let's consider a standard AM/FM radio. When a radio is tuned to a particular station but is set at a very low volume level, it simulates a conductive hearing loss. That is, sound is softer than normal, making it difficult to perceive. If, however, the volume is increased (i.e., the conductive disorder is overcome), the radio signal not only becomes easier to hear, but its clarity remains true and easy to understand. If we now take the same radio but this time adjust the tuner slightly so that it is no longer centered directly on the desired station, the signal remains audible but is distorted and harder to understand. Increasing the volume does little to improve the signal's clarity. This simple demonstration reveals how sensorineural hearing loss is not simply a problem of reduced audibility, but reduced clarity as well that may negatively impact intelligibility.

Because of its permanency and corrupting effect on the quality of the auditory signal, sensorineural hearing loss can be expected to have a negative impact on speech, language, and cognitive development. To what degree this will happen depends on several factors including the cause of the hearing loss, the person's age when the hearing loss occurred (age of onset), when it was discovered, and the type and quality of intervention received.

Age of onset is usually described as **congenital** (present at birth) or acquired (occurring sometime after birth). Another way of looking at this is to consider whether the hearing loss occurred **prelingually,** that is, before speech and language skills have developed, or **postlingually,** after the person has acquired spoken language skills. There is no precise age that delineates the two, although generally hearing loss that occurs prior to the age of 2 years is considered prelingual in onset, whereas hearing loss that occurs after the age of 5 years is considered postlingual. If a congenital hearing loss goes undetected until a child is 4 or 5 years of age, it will have a far more adverse effect on speech and language development than if it is discovered as a newborn and appropriate early intervention services are provided. In the later case, the prognosis for development of age-appropriate speech and language skills is much more encouraging.

DISORDERS OF THE INNER EAR

Now that we have a general understanding of sensorineural hearing loss, let's take a look at some of the causes starting with those that are congenital and hereditary. When a hearing loss is due to the absence or malformation of inner ear structures during embryonic development, it is referred to as **aplasia** or **dysplasia.** There are several types of aplasia depending on which part of the inner ear (i.e., the hair cells, the organ of Corti, or the entire cochlea itself) is affected. Very often, congenital hereditary sensorineural hearing loss is one component of a group of disorders associated with a syndrome. For example, **Usher's syndrome** is a genetic disorder characterized by sensorineural hearing loss ranging from severe to profound in degree and retinitis pigmentosa, a degenerative visual impairment that results in night blindness and reduced peripheral vision. **Waardenburg's syndrome** is another genetic disorder characterized by mild to severe sensorineural hearing loss, pigmentary discoloration of the irises and hair, and craniofacial malformation of the nasal area. **Alport's syndrome** is marked by sensorineural hearing loss and kidney disease. Case Study 14.2 presents

CASE STUDY 14.2
Story of a Woman with Usher's Syndrome

Although Marie was born with a hearing loss in both ears, it was not identified until age 6. At that time she was fit with hearing aids. At 15, Marie began to experience periodic episodes of dizziness and feelings of being "off balance." She also noticed a steady decline in her ability to hear. While attending college, Marie began to experience problems with her vision. Initially she noticed difficulty only at night and simply attributed it to being "clumsy." Over time, however, Marie began to experience difficulty with greater frequency. A follow-up medical evaluation revealed that Marie was suffering from Usher's syndrome, a progressive genetic disorder of the auditory and visual systems.

From the time Marie graduated from college until she reached her early 30s, she continued to experience a steady decline in her ability to hear and understand speech. In addition to her night blindness, she began to experience "tunnel vision." Although her primary mode of communication up to this point had been spoken language, a continued decline in hearing prompted her to learn sign language to supplement auditory and visual speech cues.

Marie currently works as a guidance counselor at a residential school for the deaf. She continues to use hearing aids to help her hear important environmental sounds, identify talkers, and facilitate lipreading but finds them to be bothersome in noisy environments.

At age 50, Marie has begun mobility training to learn how to use a cane to help her navigate her home and work environments in preparation for the day when she will lose her vision completely. For assistance in identifying important sounds around the home, she recently acquired a trained "hearing dog." As her ability to hear continues to decline, Marie's next step in the rehabilitative process is to investigate getting a cochlear implant to facilitate listening.

an adult woman with Usher's Syndrome, a progressive genetic disorder affecting both the auditory and visual systems.

Although sensorineural hearing loss may be present at birth, it is not always the result of genetic factors. Instead, an illness or toxic agent experienced by the mother during pregnancy may be the cause. One of the most notorious examples is hearing loss resulting from **maternal rubella** (German measles), which resulted in approximately 10,000 to 20,000 children born in the early to mid-1960s. Although a rubella vaccine is now available, other viruses such as the human immunodeficiency virus (HIV) and cytomegalovirus (CMV) continue to be major causes of congenital sensorineural hearing loss when contracted by the mother during pregnancy. Sexually transmitted bacterial diseases such as syphilis can seriously damage the central nervous system of a developing fetus, leading to intellectual and developmental disabilities, and hearing loss. Aside from infections, complications during pregnancy such as Rh incompatibility and anoxia (oxygen deprivation) can also result in sensorineural hearing loss.

Sensorineural hearing loss can occur as a result of circumstances encountered at any point during one's lifetime. Acquired hearing loss may be due to viral infections such as mumps, rubeola, and herpes zoster oticus, or due to bacterial infection such as **meningitis.** Meningitis is an inflammation of the fluids and layers of tissue covering the brain, and it frequently leads to a severe or profound hearing loss in young children and adults. The structures of the inner ear are particularly susceptible to damage either from the bacteria that cause the disease or from the high fever that often accompanies the illness. Moreover, because bacterial meningitis is potentially life threatening, it requires treatment with high doses of potent antibiotics that can be **ototoxic.** Sadly, in this case it may be the treatment rather than the disease that causes the hearing loss. Specific drugs known to be ototoxic include aminoglycocides, particularly those belonging to the -mycin family, cisplatin and carboplatin used to treat cancer, loop diuretics, aspirin taken in large doses, and drugs used to treat HIV and AIDS. Hearing loss resulting from ototoxicity may be permanent or reversible. Frequent monitoring of hearing is often recommended for individuals being treated with these medications so that drug type and dosage can be adjusted as needed.

Although the majority of sensorineural hearing losses are gradual in terms of their onset and progression, sudden hearing loss is possible, occurring in approximately 10 to 20 per 100,000 individuals (Wilson, 1994). This can be a particularly tenuous situation for those afflicted, most of whom are adults between the ages of 30 and 60 years because they go from being able to hear normally to experiencing a significant hearing loss in a matter of hours or days. In the vast majority of cases only one ear is affected. Some can be traced to a specific incident involving trauma to the head. In many cases, however, sudden hearing loss occurs seemingly without cause or advanced warning. It is thought that the majority of these cases are due to either viral infection or vascular insult. Individuals who experience sudden hearing loss frequently complain of vertigo, **tinnitus** (ringing in the ears), or fullness in the ear. These individuals must be referred for prompt treatment because this condition constitutes a medical emergency. Surprisingly, hearing often recovers spontaneously in most cases (Byl, 1984). When it fails to do so, however, various treatments are employed including the administration of steroids, vasodilators, anticoagulants, and histamines. Inhalation of carbogen, a combination of carbon dioxide and oxygen, is also recommended in some cases.

Meniere's disease is another disorder that can produce hearing loss that is rather sudden in onset. First described by Prosper Meniere in 1861, Meniere's disease is caused by pressure resulting from the build-up of endolymph within the membranous labyrinth of the inner ear: a condition called endolymphatic hydrops. Both the cochlear and vestibular portions of the inner ear may be involved or the disorder may be specific to only one region. The classic symptoms associated with Meniere's disease are fluctuating and progressive sensorineural hearing loss, roaring or low-pitched tinnitus, vertigo, and a feeling of fullness in the ear. It should be noted, however, that not all of these symptoms are experienced by all who are afflicted. In addition, the disorder is episodic, whereby symptoms intensify and abate over a matter of hours or days. This can be particularly disconcerting to those afflicted because they may have little or no warning of an impending attack of vertigo that may leave them incapacitated. Treatment may include drug therapy, surgical intervention, or regulation of one's diet to alleviate symptoms.

Although quite rare, an **acoustic neuroma** or auditory nerve tumor may develop in some individuals. These tumors, found mostly in adults, are typically benign and slow growing, and they tend to form on only one side. Most tumors originate from cells that form the outer covering of the vestibular branch of the VIIIth nerve, in the area of the cerebellotine angle. Pressure exerted by the tumor can disrupt blood flow that may ultimately affect the function of the vestibulocochlear and facial nerve. Symptoms of an acoustic neuroma include dizziness, tinnitus, and hearing loss marked by significant difficulty understanding speech. Treatment usually involves surgical removal of the tumor because it can grow to a size where it can compromise other structures and possibly result in death. Unfortunately, surgical removal often necessitates excising part of or all of the auditory nerve, resulting in permanent hearing loss. Radiation treatment is an option for those who cannot undergo surgery.

Another type of inner ear disorder, referred to as **auditory neuropathy/ auditory dyssynchrony** (AN/AD), has received considerable attention in recent years as more information has become available about its origin. In general, AN/AD is characterized by a lack of synchrony in the firing of auditory nerve fibers in response to sound in conjunction with normal outer hair cell function. The degree of hearing loss can vary greatly, but most who suffer from this disorder demonstrate poor receptive speech skills, particularly when listening in background noise.

Let's now turn our attention to a cause of sensorineural hearing loss that in most cases is avoidable, that is, hearing loss resulting from excessive exposure to high levels of sound (noise). We live in an age where we are inundated with ever-increasing amounts of noise. From machines at factories and construction sites to common everyday items such as power tools, motorcycles, and musical instruments, it is almost impossible to escape the constant bombardment of noise associated with occupational and recreational activities. It should come as no surprise then that **noise-induced hearing loss** is one of the leading causes of acquired sensorineural hearing loss in young and middle-aged adults. Even children are not immune to the potential negative effects of noise exposure because many of today's popular toys, electronic games, and personal stereos emit sound levels that are potentially hazardous. Exposure to high-intensity sound subjects the delicate structures housed within the cochlea to considerable stress that may inevitably lead to irreversible damage.

Hearing loss that occurs from exposure to high levels of noise can be temporary or permanent. **Temporary threshold shift** (TTS) is a term used to describe hearing loss that results from short-term exposure but recovers spontaneously. Most people are familiar with this effect. After attending a loud party or concert it is not uncommon to experience a slight reduction in hearing accompanied by tinnitus. After several hours of rest the ringing ceases and hearing returns to normal. Of course, if short-term exposure involves sound that is sufficiently intense, such from an explosion, immediate and irreversible hearing loss can occur from just a single episode.

Frequent exposure to high levels of noise over time may eventually lead to **permanent threshold shift** (PTS). A PTS is typically characterized by a loss of sensitivity in the high frequency range (between 3000 and 6000 Hz), with better hearing for frequencies on either side. As damage resulting from long-term exposure increases, the range of frequencies affected widens. Increased difficulty understanding speech, particularly in the presence of background noise, is often associated with noise-induced sensorineural hearing loss.

What is particularly disconcerting about PTS is that in most cases it is preventable. The risk of experiencing PTS is a function of how long a person is exposed relative to the intensity of the sound: a time-intensity tradeoff. The Occupational Safety and Health Administration (OSHA) has established regulations for industrial settings that limit daily exposure to no more than 90 dBA for an 8-hour period (OSHA, 1983). For every 5 dBA increase in the noise level, the maximum allowable exposure time is cut in half, so that at 95 dBA a worker can only be exposed for 4 hours, and at 100 dBA exposure must be limited to 2 hours, and so forth. Workers exposed to these levels daily must wear hearing protection. Additionally, all workers with daily noise exposure at or exceeding 85 dBA must have their hearing tested annually to monitor any changes. Not all persons are equally susceptible to the potential risks of noise exposure. Factors such as age, genetics, medication use, and exposure to certain chemicals can all influence one's susceptibility. If you are a musician or music lover, learn more about how you can protect yourself against noise-induced hearing loss by visiting the Hearing Education and Awareness for Rockers Web site listed at the end of this chapter.

Finally, the reality is that most of us will eventually experience some degree of sensorineural hearing loss in our lifetime, and sadly we have little control over it. Hearing loss that occurs through the aging process is referred to as **presbycusis** (Willot, 1996). Although included in our discussion of sensorineural hearing loss, note that the aging process may not only result in dysfunction of the structures of the inner ear, such as hair cells and acoustic nerve fibers, but other structures of the peripheral auditory system such as the tympanic membrane and ossicular chain. As we see later, the aging process can also affect the central auditory system. As a result, the consequences of presbycusis may involve not only reduced hearing sensitivity, particularly for high-frequency sounds, but deficits in auditory perception as well. Some individuals with presbycusis experience difficulty understanding speech that is far greater than one would predict based on their degree of hearing loss. This condition is referred to as **phonemic regression** and may be attributed to deficits beyond the inner ear (Gaeth, 1948). What makes these cases particularly challenging is that the use of amplification, although helpful in improving the audibility of speech, may not significantly improve intelligibility. Cruickshanks et al., (1998) estimate that approximately 45% of adults between the ages of 48 and 92 years have some degree of hearing loss, with men demonstrating a higher prevalence than women. Given that the elderly population continues to be one of the fastest growing segments within the United States, it is imperative that speech-language pathologists and audiologists have a good understanding of presbycusis and its associated consequences, including those related to psychosocial adjustment.

Mixed Hearing Loss

The third general type of hearing loss, **mixed hearing loss,** is the simultaneous presence of conductive and sensorineural hearing loss. For example, a person with a sensorineural hearing loss resulting from noise exposure may develop otitis media or impacted cerumen, which further decreases their hearing sensitivity. In most cases the conductive component can be medically treated, leading to some improvement in overall hearing sensitivity. However, because the sensorineural component remains, the person's hearing cannot be restored to normal levels. Audio simulations of different degrees of hearing loss are available on Scott Bradley's Web site listed at the end of this chapter.

(Central) Auditory Processing Disorders

The three types of hearing loss described in the preceding section refer to impairment of the peripheral auditory system or the structures of the ear spanning from the pinna to the auditory nerve. The function of the peripheral auditory system is what is routinely assessed during the course of a comprehensive audiological evaluation. Because we hear with our brains, audiologists must consider the *entire* auditory system including problems that affect the central auditory system. This can generally be thought of as the auditory structures, pathways, and neural synapses that span from the level of the brainstem to the cortex of the brain (see Figure 14.4). Problems associated with the central auditory system do not typically result in a loss of hearing sensitivity. Instead, they are characterized by an inability to efficiently and effectively use and interpret acoustic information. This is often reflected in problems associated with sound localization and lateralization, auditory discrimination and temporal (timing and order) processing of speech, and understanding speech in background noise or other acoustic conditions that significantly degrade the quality of the speech signal. Such deficits are collectively referred to as **(central) auditory processing disorders,** or (C)APD.

Despite a significant rise in awareness among professionals in recent years, establishing a consensus in terms of how to define and diagnose (C)APD has been difficult and at times controversial. Deficits associated with the central auditory system manifest themselves in a variety of ways, with the associated signs and symptoms often similar to those exhibited by individuals with higher-order language impairments, learning disabilities, attention deficit hyperactivity disorder (ADHD), and autism, to name a few. Although (C)APD can coexist with these other disorders, it is not an outcome. These disorders frequently present problems in the ability to understand or retain auditory information. However, in their purest form, the underlying neural structures responsible for processing auditory information remain intact. The ASHA Working Group on Auditory Processing Disorders has defined (C)APD as "difficulties in the perceptual processing of auditory information by the central nervous system" (ASHA, 2005, p. 2). As we see later, differentiating (C)APD from problems related to other higher-order processes poses a significant challenge to professionals. (Central) Auditory processing disorders are prevalent in children and adults

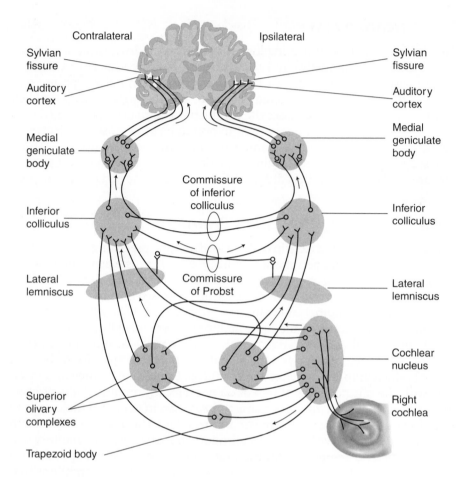

and may be the result of delayed neuromaturation of the central auditory system, neurologic disorders, diseases, or insults such as a stroke, tumor, head trauma, complications resulting from surgery, or neurologic changes associated with the aging process (Chermak & Musiek, 1997). Some forms of (C)APD may have a genetic link (Bellis, 2003b) or develop as a result of auditory deprivation suffered as a consequence of chronic otitis media (Hall & Grose, 1993). It has been estimated that (C)APD occurs in 2% to 3% of children, with males outnumbering females by a ratio of 2 to 1. In older adults, prevalence estimates range anywhere from 10% to 20% to as high as 70% (Chermak & Musiek, 1997; Stach et al., 1990). With children, we are usually concerned with how APD impacts language development and learning, which naturally has significant implications for academic achievement. With adults, (C)APD may have greater implications for communication in social situations or in the workplace.

A variety of behavioral characteristics have been identified that raise suspicion concerning the possible presence of (C)APD. For example, individuals with (C)APD may be easily distracted and demonstrate difficulty comprehending rapid speech or understanding speech in poor acoustic environments such as settings with competing noise or **reverberation** (echo caused by reflected sound). Difficulty localizing sounds in space, following complex auditory directions, or differentiating speech sounds that are acoustically similar are also common characteristics. Individuals with (C)APD may demonstrate difficulty paying attention or frequently request repetition when they misunderstand spoken information. Other characteristics include responding slowly or inconsistently to verbal messages, increased dependency on visual cues, or a tendency to watch the speaker's face intently when engaged in spoken communication. Note that individuals with (C)APD do not necessarily demonstrate all of these characteristics. Also remember that these characteristics are often associated with other disorders. It is critical, therefore, that one does not automatically jump to the conclusion that a person has a (C)APD if he or she exhibits one or more of these tendencies. Only by administering a comprehensive battery of appropriate tests, and not solely through the use of checklists and behavioral observation, can an audiologist diagnose the presence of a (C)APD.

DEGREES OF HEARING LOSS

When describing a person's hearing loss, audiologists use terminology such as *conductive, sensorineural, mixed,* and so forth, to specify the "site of lesion" or region of the auditory system affected. Although this is a critical part of the diagnostic process, it is equally important to quantify the degree of hearing loss. Quantitatively, the degree of hearing loss is expressed in units called decibels (dB). A decibel is a mathematically derived unit based on the pressure exerted by a particular sound. The lowest decibel level at which a given sound is barely audible represents a person's auditory threshold. The greater the decibel value required to reach a person's threshold relative to what is considered "normal," the greater the degree of hearing loss. As we see later, this type of measurement is often conducted using tones that vary as a function of frequency. Remember that an individual's degree of hearing loss may not be the same at all frequencies. In other words, there may be a greater degree of hearing loss for high-frequency sounds, for example, compared to sounds in the low- or mid-frequency range. This can have significance in terms of which speech sounds are audible and which need to be amplified.

Audiologists have adopted the terms presented in Table 14.1 to apply descriptive labels corresponding to the degree of hearing loss (HL). Notice that the range considered "normal" is different for children and adults. Specifically, whereas adult thresholds up to 25 dB HL are considered within normal limits, the cutoff for children is set more conservatively at 15 dB HL. Children who are in the process of developing speech and language may miss some of the subtle intricacies specific to the acoustic speech signal when auditory thresholds are in the 16 to 25 dB range (Bess et al., 1998). Adults, in contrast, typically experience no difficulty despite having thresholds in this same range because of their mature language system and their ability to fill in the missing pieces, a process referred to as auditory closure. In very

TABLE 14.1

Degrees of hearing loss

	Degree of Hearing Loss		
Threshold	Children	Adults	Description
−10 to 15 dB HL	Normal	Normal	
16–25 dB HL	Slight	Normal	Children who are in the process of developing speech and language may miss some of the subtle nuances of speech.
26–40 dB HL	Mild	Mild	Difficulty with faint or distant speech.
41–55 dB HL	Moderate	Moderate	Difficulty following conversational-level speech.
56–70 dB HL	Moderately severe	Moderately severe	Can hear only loud speech.
71–90 dB HL	Severe	Severe	Difficulty understanding even loud speech without amplification.
>90 dB HL	Profound	Profound	Usually considered "deaf"; without amplification cannot depend on auditory system alone to obtain information.

general terms, individuals whose degree of hearing loss falls within the slight/mild to moderately severe range are classified as hard of hearing. These individuals depend extensively on their residual hearing for receptive communication for the learning of new concepts. For people whose auditory thresholds fall in the severe to profound range, however, the auditory system provides limited or no access to speech without the use of amplification. As previously mentioned, these individuals are often referred to as "deaf" and present significant challenges compared to those with normal hearing.

AUDIOLOGICAL ASSESSMENT PROCEDURES

Having described the basic principles of sound, the anatomy and physiology of the auditory system, and the various types and causes of hearing loss, we are now ready to take a look at how this knowledge is applied clinically in the assessment of hearing. It is important to stress that no single test can accurately represent the full extent of a person's hearing loss or the effect it has in terms of overall communication function or psychosocial well-being. Instead, the audiologist must rely on a battery of tests and other measures to obtain an accurate picture of an individual's hearing problem. A battery approach also enables the audiologist to cross-check the results of individual tests to identify any trends or inconsistencies.

Before continuing, now is a good time to differentiate "assessment," as we discuss in this section, from "screening," referred to earlier in this chapter.

Screening is the process used to determine which individuals, whether children or adults, are *likely* to have a hearing loss. If you ever had your hearing tested as part of a school-based program, it is likely you participated in a screening. As previously mentioned, newborn hearing screening programs have been implemented across the country to identify those infants born with a significant hearing impairment. For each screening program, specific tools and protocols are selected and appropriate pass/fail criterion are established. Those who pass the screening in all likelihood have normal hearing, although periodic monitoring is advised because hearing loss can occur at any point afterward. However, it cannot be definitively concluded that those who fail a screening are indeed hearing impaired. Failure of a hearing screening simply indicates that additional in-depth assessment is warranted to determine if a hearing loss truly exists, and if so, to quantify the type and degree. The remainder of this section focuses on the types of tests available for inclusion in a comprehensive audiological assessment battery.

Assessing Infants and Children Versus Adults

The special skills of the pediatric audiologist are called into play when assessing infants and young children because obtaining reliable information from this population can be challenging to say the least. As with speech and language, auditory behavior is developmental, and as long as the audiologist is familiar with the different stages of auditory development, in most cases age-appropriate response can be elicited. In addition to information gained from behavioral, electroacoustic, and electrophysiological tests, a number of commercially available instruments can be used with younger children to assess progress relative to functional auditory development (Anderson 2002; Stredler-Brown & Johnson, 2003).

Assessing adult clients can also present challenges to the audiologist. Adults with developmental, neurogenic, language, or cognitive disorders frequently require modifications to the test battery, test materials, and administration procedures. Cases of nonorganic hearing loss are particularly challenging and at times frustrating. **Nonorganic hearing loss** is a term used to describe the condition in which an individual portrays having a hearing loss when one does not exist or exaggerates the degree of a true organic impairment (Martin & Clark, 2003). The audiologist must be skilled in identifying these individuals and obtaining an accurate measure of their true auditory function. Finally, geriatric clients often present challenges during testing due to fatigue and slower reaction time. Fortunately, modifications to test procedures can be made to address these issues.

Counseling

Although not a test per se, counseling is an essential component of any audiological service. Counseling is usually thought of as the process of imparting information. In this somewhat narrow view, the audiologist provides information while the client listens, occasionally interjecting a pertinent comment or question. For example, the audiologist might explain the results of individual tests, provide technical information on the anatomy of the ear, or explain how hearing loss occurs so the client can better understand the nature of his or her problem. The audiologist might also present possible courses of treatment including amplification and rehabilitation options designed to facilitate spoken communication. This type of counseling, referred to as **informational counseling,** is critical and requires great skill on the part of the clinician so that information is communicated in a manner that is easily understood and remembered. It has been reported that only 50% of the information conveyed by health care providers is actually retained by clients, and that approximately half of this information is remembered inaccurately (Kessels, 2003; Margolis, 2004). Although important, informational counseling is only one facet of the counseling process. Counseling should be thought of as a process that is much broader in scope than simply providing information.

As discussed earlier in this chapter, hearing loss can have a profound impact on a person's psychological, social, and emotional well-being. Clients may struggle as they try to come to terms with feelings of anger, anxiety, fear, frustration, and despair that are a direct result of their hearing loss. These feelings are not limited to the hearing-impaired client. They often transcend to others who are in close contact with the individual such as parents or a spouse. Unless these individuals receive support from an empathetic clinician, they cannot proceed with efforts to remediate the problem. The process of assisting the client and family in dealing with the emotional consequences of hearing loss is referred to as **personal adjustment counseling.** As part of this process, the audiologist must pay close attention to a client's affective statements and questions to uncover any underlying personal adjustment issues. This involves listening intently and encouraging the client to "tell their story" of what it's like to live with a hearing loss. Clients need to accept and assume ownership of their hearing loss before any efforts to remediate the condition can proceed. Simply telling a client what they should do will not lead to compliance if they do not first acknowledge and accept the fact that a problem exists. The audiologists must be adept at determining when a client is asking for "information" as opposed to seeking acknowledgment of an affective or emotional concern that conveys personal feelings about their hearing problem (English, 2007).

Several key points regarding the counseling process must be stressed. First, clinicians must be cognizant of the client's/family's cultural background and linguistic needs to ensure appropriate communication (Scott, 2000). Secondly, audiologists should seize the moment by providing counseling whenever the opportunity presents itself, not only at the conclusion of the clinical session. Additionally, clinicians need to remember that clients and family members process information at different rates. Some want as much information as possible at the time of the diagnosis; others need time to deal with the initial shock before they can move on and consider various treatment options. Finally, clinicians should always be aware of their professional boundaries. When potential psychological or mental health issues arise, clinicians should not hesitate to refer clients to a qualified professional counselor.

Referral and Case History

Referral for audiological testing may originate from a variety of sources, including physicians, school nurses, speech-language pathologists, psychologists, teachers, and family members, to name a few. Self-referral is also common. The referring source may be able to provide important background information that is helpful in gaining a better understanding of the client's specific problem.

Before conducting any tests, the audiologist spends time interviewing the client and collecting case history information. This process provides an opportunity to obtain background information from the client's perspective and helps the audiologist map out an appropriate assessment plan. It is important to know why the client has come in for the evaluation, whether there is a family history of hearing loss, whether the client has sustained a recent head injury or is taking medication, whether he or she has been exposed to noise, and so forth. The audiologist will ask the client to describe the situations in which he or she is having difficulty or any symptoms that may be present such as tinnitus, ear pain, or dizziness. A complete case history can often provide the audiologist with a strong indication of what the problem is even before any tests are administered. An audiological interview can be seen on the book's CD-ROM.

Formal self-assessment questionnaires are available to assist the audiologist in obtaining the client's perspective on the types of communication problems he or she is experiencing, including measures of hearing disability (activity limitation) and handicap (participation restriction). For example, a particular item might ask the client to rate the degree of difficulty experienced when listening in a noisy restaurant. Several of these questionnaires contain a companion version that can be completed by the client's significant other. Obtaining input from someone the client is close to can shed additional light on the particular problems encountered as a result of the hearing loss. As an added benefit, these self-assessment instruments facilitate the counseling process by providing a vehicle for promoting self-reflection, self-disclosure, and discussion of one's attitudes and feelings about their hearing problem.

Otoscopic Examination

One of the first procedures performed during an evaluation is a visual or otoscopic examination. The examination is conducted using a small hand-held device called an otoscope that illuminates the external auditory meatus and allows the audiologist to visually inspect the canal and tympanic membrane. The audiologist will also visually inspect the external surface of the pinna for any signs of abnormality. This is a critical first step in the assessment process because it promptly calls attention to any conditions that may impede sound during testing such as excessive cerumen, or warrant immediate medical referral such as drainage from the ear. A more elaborate version of this device, called a video-otoscope, projects the image of the ear onto a television or computer monitor, allowing the client and family members to observe simultaneously. In addition to enhancing the counseling process, this technology enables the audiologist to print and store images to facilitate communication with medical personnel. A demonstration of an otoscopic examination can be seen on the book's CD-ROM.

Electroacoustic and Electrophysiological Testing

Over the past 40 years, advances in technology and in our understanding of the hearing process have led to the development of specialized electroacoustic and electrophysiological tests of the auditory system. These tests evaluate the integrity of the peripheral and central auditory systems without the need for an overt behavioral response on the part of the client. Although they are not true "hearing" tests because hearing requires the person to be able to recognize and use sound, they represent a major step forward in the early diagnosis and comprehensive evaluation of the auditory system.

Electroacoustic measures record acoustic signals from within the client's external auditory canal using specialized equipment. Two types of electroacoustic measures commonly performed on children and adults are tests of acoustic immittance and otoacoustic emissions.

Acoustic immittance measures are useful in the diagnosis of conductive pathology and can be completed in a relatively short period of time. No behavioral response is required, making it an excellent tool for children, including infants, as well as adults. All that is necessary is for the client to remain relatively still and refrain from vocalizing. Acoustic immittance testing is performed using an electronic device that consists of a small probe containing a microphone, air-pressure pump, and sound generator connected to a recording instrument. The probe is inserted into the external auditory meatus, creating an airtight seal. During testing, a continuous tone is emitted into the canal as air pressure is systematically increased and decreased. This change in air pressure sets the eardrum into motion. The microphone measures any changes in the intensity of the tone as it flows through the canal and is subsequently reflected by the tympanic membrane. This process results in a graph called a **tympanogram** that plots the compliance of the middle ear as a function of changes in air pressure within the ear canal (see Figure 14.5). Quantitative data obtained as part of this process, as well as the overall shape of the tympanogram, can assist in identifying the presence of conductive pathology and differentiating whether it is likely due to otosclerosis, a break in the ossicular chain, otitis media with effusion, or a perforation of the eardrum.

Frequently included as a part of the acoustic immittance battery is a test involving the acoustic reflex. As previously discussed, the stapedius muscle contracts in response to high-intensity sounds causing the ossicular chain and tympanic membrane to stiffen. The same device used to generate a tympanogram is capable of measuring the contraction of the stapedius muscle in response to different stimuli. By analyzing whether or not the reflex is present, and if so, at what intensity level, the audiologist is able to make important inferences as to the possible site of the disorder. A demonstration of acoustic immittance testing can be seen on the book's CD-ROM.

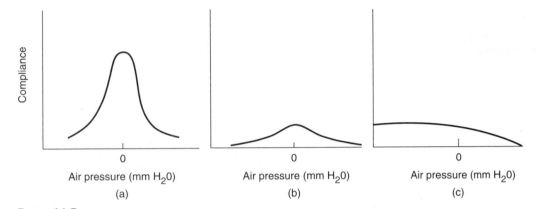

FIGURE 14.5

Schematic of three common tympanogram patterns: (a) normal middle ear function, (b) somewhat reduced compliance due to otosclerosis, (c) minimal compliance due to olitis media with effusion.

Otoacoustic emissions (OAEs) are a second type of elecroacoustic measure that has received considerable attention during the past two decades. Discovered by David Kemp (1978), otoacoustic emissions are low-intensity sounds, commonly referred to as "echoes," that are generated within the cochlea as a result of movement of the outer hair cells. These tiny emissions propagate outward from the cochlea, through the middle ear, to the external auditory canal where they can be recorded. Otoacoustic emissions occur spontaneously in some individuals, but for clinical purposes they are evoked by presenting a moderate-intensity acoustic stimulus by way of a small probe placed in the ear canal. The stimulus used to generate these emissions consists of a series of clicks or pairs of tones that are closely spaced in terms of their frequency. The same probe that generates these stimuli contains a miniature microphone capable of recording the low-level emissions returning from the cochlea. Specialized equipment is used to extract the emissions from extraneous noise in the ear canal. Results are interpreted by analyzing the absolute amplitude of the resultant waveform relative to the frequency of the stimulus as in Figure 14.6, by analyzing the amplitude relative to the noise level measured in the ear canal, and by analyzing how reproducible or consistent the responses are over repeated trials.

Generally, when OAEs are present, hearing sensitivity is presumed to be normal or no worse than a mild loss (Glattke & Robinette, 2007). In contrast, reduced or absent OAEs are indicative of outer hair cell dysfunction. Caution, however, must be exercised when interpreting "absent" results because conductive pathology can impede the return path of the emission in the same manner that it attenuates sound that naturally enters the auditory system.

OAE testing has several important clinical applications. Because OAEs measure the integrity of the outer hair cells, they are a powerful tool in differentiating disorders that are cochlear in origin from those that occur beyond the cochlea, as well as differentiating disorders of the outer hair cells from those of the inner hair cells. OAEs are also useful in monitoring outer hair cell function for clients being treated with potentially ototoxic

FIGURE 14.6
················

Example of a transient-evoked otoacoustic emission generated by a click stimulus to a normal ear.

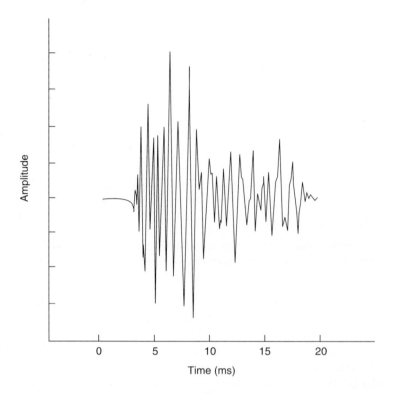

Time (ms)

drugs such as those used in chemotherapy. Frequently, early signs of cochlear damage are revealed during OAE testing before they show up on more traditional behavioral hearing tests. This may also be the case for those who demonstrate early signs of outer hair cell damage due to excessive noise exposure (Lonsbury-Martin, 2005). Finally, because the measurement of OAEs is noninvasive and can be accomplished while a child sleeps, this powerful tool is used extensively in newborn hearing screening programs.

In addition to electroacoustic tests, several electrophysiological tests are available to the audiologist. Electrophysiological tests record neuroelectric responses (nerve impulses) generated by the auditory system in response to acoustic stimulation. These responses are collectively referred to as **auditory evoked potentials,** or AEPs, and can be further classified based on when they occur (measured in milliseconds) following presentation of a stimulus and the anatomical site(s) where they are generated.

Neuroelectric responses are recorded by small electrodes placed at strategic points on the surface of the head while a stimulus is delivered to the ear. These tiny responses are extracted from the greater ongoing electrical brain activity using specialized computer equipment. Once the resulting waveform is recorded and displayed, analysis can occur by measuring the amplitude or height of specific peaks associated with the response, and the latency or number of milliseconds it takes to generate the various peaks of the waveform following presentation of a stimulus.

Several unique types of AEPs can be recorded and evaluated by the audiologist. The first type, called **electrocochleography** (ECochG), measures the electrical responses arising from the hair cells within the cochlea and the

VIIIth nerve within the first 1.5 to 2 ms after stimulation. Recordings are made using a tiny electrode that is either surgically placed on or near the cochlea, or positioned in the external auditory meatus. Electrocochleography has many useful applications, including the monitoring of cochlear and VIIIth nerve function during surgery and the evaluation of those suspected of having Meniere's disease.

A second type of auditory evoked potential, the **auditory brainstem response** (ABR), measures the neuroelectric activity of the auditory nerve and structures in the lower brainstem. In normal ears this response is characterized by five to seven distinct peaks in the waveform that occur within the first 5 to 6 ms following stimulation. Although varying somewhat from person to person, these waves have a typical form with regard to their amplitude and latency that allows them to be used for diagnostic purposes (see Figure 14.7). It is thought that the first two waves reflect neuroelectric activity generated by the cochlea and VIIIth nerve, whereas the remaining waves are generated by sites within the brainstem (Jewett et al., 1970). ABR testing is most useful in the estimation of auditory threshold in those who are unable or unwilling to be evaluated using conventional behavioral techniques, such as infants and young children. Testing can be conducted while the child sleeps, or in some cases mildly sedated, making this an ideal tool for early identification of hearing loss. Other applications of the ABR include neurological assessment of the central auditory system including suspected cases of auditory neuropathy/auditory dys-synchrony, acoustic neuroma, and multiple sclerosis. A new approach to ABR testing, referred to as the **stacked ABR,** has demonstrated promise in the identification of small acoustic nerve tumors that may be missed by conventional ABR.

Other types of AEPs include the auditory middle latency response (AMLR) and the auditory late response (ALR). The auditory middle latency response consists of a series of waves that occur approximately 12 to 50 ms after stimulation, whereas waves associated with the auditory late response occur anywhere from 50 to 500 ms (Hall, 2007). The AMLR evaluates anatomical sites

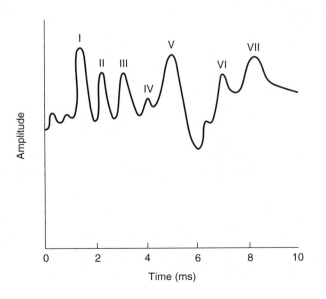

FIGURE 14.7

Schematic drawing of a typical auditory brainstem response (ABR) waveform for a normal ear.

spanning from the brainstem to the cortex and is more effective than the ABR in estimating auditory sensitivity for low- and mid-frequency signals. Unlike the ABR, however, the AMLR is more affected by the individual's sleep state, particularly in children. Measurement of the auditory late response can be performed using a variety of signals including tones and speech. Responses are highly affected by the client's attention and are more effective in evaluating higher-level auditory processing functions than other types of AEPs.

Behavioral Testing

A fundamental limitation of electroacoustic and electrophysiological measures is that although they yield information about the integrity of the auditory system, they do not provide information on how the individual perceives or responds to sound. Therefore, behavioral measures are necessary to fully define a person's ability to hear and process sound.

Most behavioral tests are administered using a specialized piece of electronic equipment called an **audiometer,** which contains numerous controls that allow for the selection, manipulation, and presentation of various stimuli used to assess hearing. Testing is usually carried out in a specially treated sound booth that limits the penetration of extraneous noise that can interfere with hearing and thus confound the results of behavioral measures.

The most basic form of behavioral assessment used with infants is a process referred to as **behavioral observation audiometry** (BOA). As the term implies, the audiologist presents a stimulus such as speech or tones through a loudspeaker and observes the child's reaction. Basic responses the audiologist looks for in response to sound are gross body movements such as startling, widening of the eyes, and facial grimacing. Cessation of movement may also indicate a response to loud sounds.

Although fairly simple to administer, BOA has been criticized for its poor reliability and validity (Hicks et al., 2000). Making judgments as to whether a child's bodily movement was in direct response to the stimulus or simply occurred spontaneously can be a difficult task, and because there are no formal means of reinforcement used during this procedure, the child may quickly habituate to the task, ceasing to respond after only a few presentations. Recently Madell (2008) described a more reliable technique for conducting BOA that analyzes changes in sucking by an infant in response to sound. Generally, however, electroacoustic and electrophysiological measures are preferred over BOA when assessing children younger than 5 months of age. As a child reaches the age of 5 to 6 months, the natural ability to localize, or turn toward a sound, emerges and the audiologist can begin to employ a technique called **visual reinforcement audiometry** (VRA) to assess behavioral responses to speech and frequency-specific tones. With VRA, the child is rewarded for a head-turn response toward the stimulus by way of an appealing visual display such as an animated or lighted toy. VRA is more reliable and less prone to problems related to habituation than BOA and has been shown to be an effective tool for accurately assessing hearing sensitivity in young children (Diefendorf, 1988).

By $2\frac{1}{2}$ years of age, a child should be able to engage in testing procedures that approximate those used with adults. The child should be able to wear earphones and taught to respond to pure tones using various techniques. A popular technique, referred to as **conditioned play audiometry** (CPA), involves the use of toys such as blocks, puzzle pieces, or stacking rings to engage the child in a listening game. The child is conditioned to put a block in the bucket, a ring on the post, or the like, each time the test signal is heard. After a few demonstrations most children are able to comply with the task, allowing the audiologist to obtain frequency-specific results for each ear. Conditioned play audiometry can be used until a child is able to be tested via conventional pure tone audiometry, which usually occurs somewhere around the age of 5 to 8 years.

PURE TONE AUDIOMETRY

A great deal of information can be obtained about a person's hearing through **pure tone audiometry.** In fact, the pure tone test is considered to be one of, if not *the* most fundamental behavioral tests in the standard audiometric assessment battery. **Pure tones** are sounds that contain energy only at a single frequency. Those that are routinely used in evaluating hearing sensitivity are octave frequencies ranging from 250 Hz to 8000 Hz. By following this progression from low frequency to high frequency, the integrity of the cochlea spanning a broad range from apex to base is evaluated.

The purpose of pure tone testing is to determine a person's threshold at each test frequency for the right and left ears. **Threshold** is defined as the lowest (quietest) intensity level, measured in decibels, at which a person can just barely detect a given stimulus approximately 50% of the time. The audiologist measures a client's threshold by presenting a single pure tone (e.g., 1000 Hz) for approximately 1 to 2 seconds and looking for a response from the client indicating whether or not it was heard. Adult clients are typically instructed to raise their hand or finger, or press a button to signal when they have heard the tone. Each time the tone is detected, the intensity level is reduced by 10 dB and presented again. This process continues until the tone becomes inaudible as it reaches a level below the client's auditory threshold. Once the tone can no longer be heard, the audiologist reverses the process by increasing the intensity in 5-dB increments until once again it becomes audible. This process of raising and lowering the intensity continues until

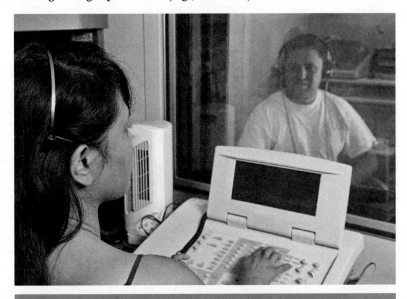

Within schools, audiologists may provide both screening and diagnostic testing

the audiologist finds the lowest presentation level at which the person is just barely able to detect the tone approximately 50% of the time for a specific number of trials (e.g., 2 of 4, 3 of 6). Once the threshold is established for a 1000-Hz tone, the audiologist repeats the procedure at 2000 Hz, then 4000 Hz, and so forth, until all of the octave frequencies ranging from 250 Hz to 8000 Hz have been tested. In some cases, additional frequencies such as 125 Hz, 750 Hz, 1500 Hz, 3000 Hz, and 6000 Hz are also evaluated. Pure tone threshold results are recorded by placing symbols on a graph called an audiogram. An example of an audiogram is shown in Figure 14.8. The presence or absence of hearing loss is determined by comparing the client's thresholds to normative values for each frequency.

Auditory thresholds are established by delivering pure tones in two different ways; through **air conduction** and **bone conduction.** Air conduction

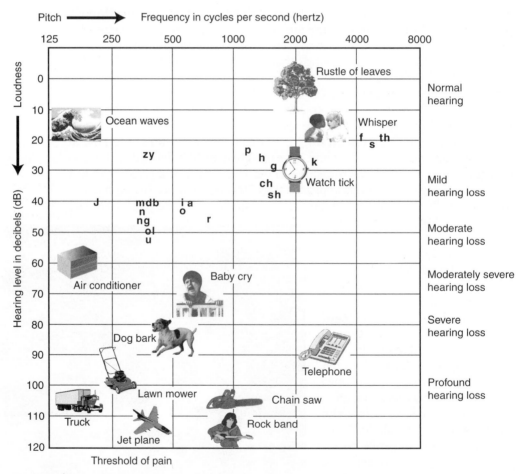

FIGURE 14.8

Audiogram showing typical frequency range and intensity of common environmental and speech sounds.

Source: Based on information from *Hearing in Children* (2nd ed.), by J. Northern and M. Downs, 1976, Baltimore, MD: Williams and Wilkins.

testing is administered while the client wears either insert phones or supra-aural earphones. Insert phones contain pliable, foam-like receivers that are placed within the external auditory meatus; supra-aural earphones are mounted on a more traditional headset and placed over each pinna. Presentation by air conduction results in transmission of sound to the cochlea via the outer and middle ear. Hence hearing loss resulting from disorders occurring within any of the three major (outer, middle, inner) sections of the peripheral auditory system is identified in this manner. Once air conduction testing is completed, the process is repeated using a bone oscillator, a small vibrating device that is positioned against the skull, either on the forehead or the mastoid process located directly behind the pinna. When a stimulus is presented through the oscillator, the bones of the skull are set into vibration at the same frequency. This vibration directly stimulates the cochlea by displacing the fluids encased within its two concentric labyrinths, which, in turn, leads to the bending and shearing action of the hair cells. Consequently, the person is able to hear the stimulus even though it has not passed through the outer or middle ear.

By comparing the results of air conduction testing to those obtained from bone conduction testing, it is possible to identify the type of hearing loss. Consider the audiograms in Figures 14.9 and 14.10. In Figure 14.9, the right ear air conduction thresholds (represented by the circles) fall within the moderate hearing loss range. However, the bone conduction thresholds

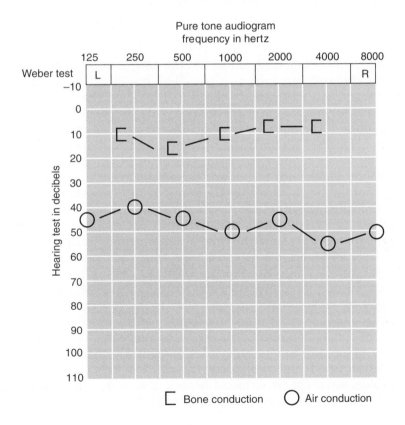

FIGURE 14.9

Audiogram representing a moderate conductive hearing loss in the right ear. (Note: The symbol used to denote bone conduction thresholds depends on the method used to assess it.)

FIGURE **14.10**
....

**Audiogram representing
a severe sensorineural
hearing loss in the
right ear.**

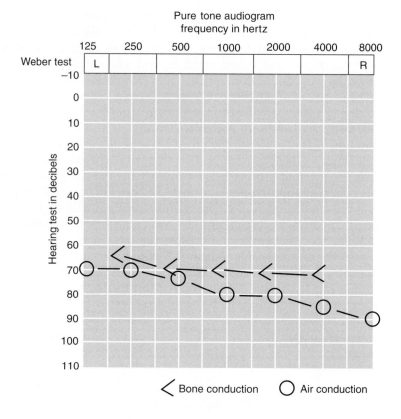

(represented by the brackets) fall within the normal range of hearing. From this the audiologist can infer that the client has difficulty hearing sound when it is introduced in the conventional manner, that is, through the external auditory meatus. Notice, however, that the client has no difficulty hearing sound if the outer and middle ear are bypassed and the cochlea is stimulated directly. Therefore, the conclusion can be drawn that the client is suffering from a conductive hearing loss occurring in the outer or middle ear. In Figure 14.10, both the air and bone conduction thresholds fall outside the normal limits to within the severe range. Because the results are unchanged when the inner ear is stimulated directly via bone conduction, the audiologist can conclude that the inner ear itself must be affected. Therefore, this client is suffering from a sensorineural hearing loss.

In Figure 14.11, again both the air and bone conduction thresholds fall outside the normal range. However, the degree of hearing loss represented by the air conduction thresholds is greater than the degree of hearing loss represented by the bone conduction thresholds. In this case the audiologist concludes that although there is obvious damage to the inner ear as evidenced by the bone conduction results, the person has the potential to hear better if the outer and middle ear are bypassed. Consequently, there is evidence that both a sensorineural and a conductive hearing loss exist simultaneously. In other words, the client has a mixed hearing loss. A demonstration of pure tone audiometry can be seen on the book's CD-ROM.

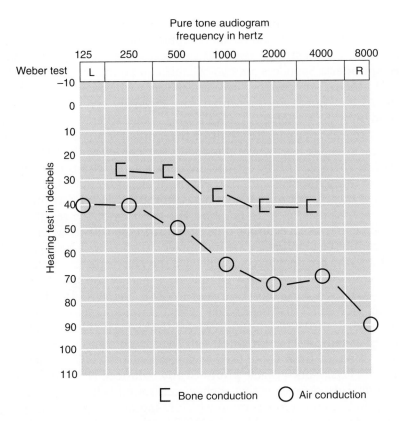

Pure tone audiogram
frequency in hertz

FIGURE 14.11

Audiogram representing a moderate to severe mixed hearing loss in the right ear.

☐ Bone conduction　　○ Air conduction

SPEECH AUDIOMETRY

Although pure tone audiometry is often considered to be the most fundamental component of an audiological evaluation, we must keep in mind that people typically seek the services of an audiologist because they are having difficulty understanding speech, not pure tones. It is only natural, then, that we evaluate a client's ability to hear and understand speech as part of the assessment battery.

Numerous tools are available to assess a client's auditory skills for speech. Most are commercially available on compact disc and can easily be routed through the audiometer. Use of recorded materials ensures consistency of the signal from one administration to the next, which is essential when making comparisons of an individual's performance over time or from one clinical facility to another. In some cases, such as when testing young children, the audiologist may opt to use his or her own voice rather than recorded speech to administer a test. This process is referred to as monitored live voice testing and requires the audiologist to speak into a microphone connected to the audiometer. As with any type of assessment, it is critical to select tests and materials that are age appropriate, reliable, have normative data, and tap the specific auditory skills necessary to diagnose the problem and make appropriate recommendations for treatment and management.

Two measures typically included in the speech audiometry battery are the Speech Recognition Threshold and the Word Recognition Test. The

Speech Recognition Threshold (SRT) is a measure of the lowest (softest) intensity where a person can recognize approximately 50% of the words presented. The speech stimuli used for this test are a special group of words called **spondees.** Spondees are two-syllable compound words, such as "hotdog," "birthday," or "cowboy," that are spoken with equal stress on both syllables. As the words are presented, the intensity level is systematically adjusted until the audiologist finds the lowest level where the client is able to correctly repeat approximately half of the words for a specified number of trials. The intensity level where this occurs is recorded as the SRT for a given ear. The decibel value of the SRT should closely agree with the average of the pure tone threshold values for 500 Hz, 1000 Hz, and 2000 Hz for the same ear. When there is poor agreement between the pure tone data and the SRT, the audiologist may begin to question the accuracy of the results. The SRT may also be used as an estimate of overall hearing sensitivity when pure tone results cannot be obtained or are incomplete, such as with younger children and adults who are unable to comply with the pure tone test protocol.

A second measure routinely conducted as part of the speech audiometry battery is the **word recognition test** (WRT). The WRT is different from the other procedures discussed so far in that it is not a measure of sensitivity per se. Instead, the WRT assesses how well the client is able to identify words presented at some level above threshold. The speech stimuli used in the WRT are also different from those used to assess a client's SRT in that they are taken from lists of one-syllable **phonetically balanced** (PB) words. The term *phonetically balanced* means that each speech sound is incorporated into the word list in the same proportion in which it appears in everyday language.

The intensity level at which the WRT is administered varies depending on the type of information of interest. If the goal is to make inferences as to how well an individual understands speech (words) when presented at a typical or average level of conversational speech, then the test is usually administered at an intensity level of 45 to 50 dB HL. Many individuals with hearing loss demonstrate significant difficulty at this level because the signal is not loud enough. Therefore, it is desirable to increase the intensity of the stimulus to determine maximal word recognition performance because this may be helpful in determining the potential for improvement if the client is ultimately fit with hearing aids that amplify the speech signal. Additionally, in some cases it may be useful to present word lists at multiple intensity levels to assist in determining the type of hearing loss, most notably those that involve auditory nerve tumors. A demonstration of word recognition testing can be viewed on the book's CD-ROM.

In recent years there has been much debate as to whether traditional word recognition testing is truly reflective of real-world performance. Obviously, most conversational exchanges consist of connected discourse rather than single-syllable words that are unrelated to one another. Talkers engaged in conversation also make use of linguistic and contextual cues to decipher the message. In addition, real-world conversations do not typically occur in sound-treated environments where there is little or no background noise, and except for telephone communication, additional information can be gained through speech reading (lipreading). To address these limitations, a variety of speech tests have been developed that incorporate sentence-length stimuli. Several have been recorded with competing background noise to evaluate those who complain of difficulty hearing in noisy situations, or they contain sentence lists recorded with and without visual cues to determine how much a client benefits when listening and speech reading are combined compared to listening alone. These types of tests hold considerable promise in presenting an overall picture of how an individual functions under conditions that are more representative of "typical" real-world settings.

AUDITORY PROCESSING ASSESSMENT

The audiologist is the professional responsible for the diagnosis of (central) auditory processing disorders. However, because other types of disorders may present similar symptoms, the process of assessing an individual for a possible (C)APD requires a multidisciplinary approach. Typically, personnel involved in the assessment process include the audiologist who administers specific auditory tests of the peripheral and central auditory pathways, the speech-language pathologist who assesses the individual's expressive and receptive oral language skills, the psychologist who assesses cognitive function, and when dealing with children, parents and school personnel who can provide input on academic performance and the functional impact of the problem.

Numerous auditory tests, both behavioral and electrophysiological, are available to evaluate a variety of auditory processes. The overall goal is not just simply to determine whether an auditory processing disorder exists, but to analyze the nature of the disorder in order to recommend appropriate strategies for treatment and management. In each case, therefore, it is critical to design an individualized assessment plan that taps the specific characteristics or deficits demonstrated by the individual. No single test can adequately assess all levels of the central auditory system or all aspects of auditory processing. Instead, a battery approach is necessary. Unfortunately, because of the high degree of variability associated with the maturation of the central auditory system in younger children, most behavioral tests for (C)APD are generally not appropriate for those younger than 7 years. In addition, impairment of the peripheral auditory system may affect the results obtained on some auditory processing tests. Therefore, assessment of the peripheral system is a prerequisite to any type of auditory processing evaluation.

Although it is beyond the scope of this chapter to present all of the tests available for inclusion in an individualized assessment battery, it is helpful to discuss some of the general types of measures frequently administered in the evaluation of the central auditory system. One general category consists of what are called **dichotic** measures. Dichotic tests involve the simultaneous presentation of different stimuli to each ear. Depending on the specific test, stimuli may consist of digits (numbers), consonant-vowel pairs, words, or sentences. The individual may be asked to direct their attention to only one ear and identify what is heard, or attend to and identify what is heard in both ears. These types of tasks assess the person's ability to separate or integrate competing signals.

A second general category includes tests of temporal processing. These tests are used to evaluate a client's ability to process timing cues associated with speech such as ordering and sequencing. Specific tests may require the individual to identify differences in the duration pattern (e.g., long-long-short or long-short-long) for a series of three tones or clicks, differences in the frequency pattern (e.g., high-high-low or high-low-high) for a series of three tones, or the presence of short gaps separating pairs of tones or clicks.

A third general category of auditory processing measure involves what is referred to as monaural low-redundancy speech. These tests are termed *monaural* because the stimulus is directed to only one ear at a time. Low redundancy means that the stimulus has been altered in some way so as to reduce the speech signal's inherent redundancy and tax the auditory system because those with (C)APD often demonstrate increased difficulty with auditory closure when the signal is compromised. This can be accomplished by having the individual identify words where acoustic energy above a specific frequency has been filtered out. It can also be accomplished by altering the rate of speech or by presenting speech in various levels of competing background noise or reverberation.

The final general category includes tests that assess **binaural integration,** which is the process of assimilating different information presented to each ear into a single unit. For example, a portion of a word may be presented to the left ear while another portion is presented to the right ear. The individual must combine the two components to identify the target word.

Although behavioral tests such as those just mentioned are the most popular means of assessing auditory processing function, the incorporation of electrophysiological measures such as the auditory brainstem response and the auditory middle and late responses into the assessment battery can be extremely useful. Due to neuromaturation of the central auditory system and the contributions of learning, it is critical that any test administered be scored according to age-appropriate norms. Also, all data collected must be interpreted in conjunction with the findings obtained by other specialists on the multidisciplinary team.

AURAL (AUDIOLOGICAL) HABILITATION/REHABILITATION

After the audiological assessment has been completed and the various tests analyzed, it is time to recommend and implement an appropriate course of treatment. This may entail referral to a physician for a medical evaluation. It may also involve various therapeutic services referred to as **aural (or audiological) habilitation/rehabilitation,** which can be defined as "intervention aimed at minimizing and alleviating the communication difficulties associated with hearing loss" (Tye-Murray, 2009, p.2). Before discussing the specific intervention options available, it is important to differentiate the terms *aural habilitation* and *aural rehabilitation. Aural habilitation* refers to intervention conducted with individuals whose hearing loss occurred at an early age and therefore prevented normal development of auditory and spoken language skills. In general, this refers to services and therapies used primarily with children who are prelingually hearing impaired. Because these individuals essentially have had little or no time to develop spoken language, the focus of aural habilitation is to teach those skills that are missing. In contrast, *aural rehabilitation* refers to services and therapies provided to individuals who have lost their hearing later in life, after spoken language skills have fully developed. In this case, the focus is on preservation and restoration of communication skills that have been negatively impacted by a loss of hearing. Despite these differences, professionals frequently use the term *aural rehabilitation* to refer to both habilitative and rehabilitative aspects of intervention, and for the sake of convenience, we use it in the remainder of this section.

An important first step in the aural rehabilitation process is to identify, describe, and clarify the individual's communication problems resulting from their hearing loss. This can usually be accomplished by synthesizing information obtained from the case history interview, self-assessment questionnaires, and results of the audiometric test battery. By identifying the specific needs of the individual and selecting treatment methods using principles of evidence based practice, both the client and the clinician can feel confident that the rehabilitation process will proceed based on the best available information (see Box 14.1).

Audiologists may find themselves working closely with professionals from other areas in the development of a comprehensive aural rehabilitation program. Depending on the specific needs of the individual, this may include medical personnel, speech-language pathologists, special education teachers, teachers of the deaf and hard of hearing, psychologists, and vocational rehabilitation counselors.

BOX 14.1
Evidence-Based Practice in Audiology

Universal newborn hearing screening

- By the time they reach school age, infants screened for hearing loss demonstrate higher language outcomes compared to those who are not screened.
- Infants who are identified with permanent hearing loss through newborn screening programs are referred, diagnosed, and treated earlier than those who are identified using other methods.

Early intervention for children with permanent hearing loss

- Outcomes are influenced by age of onset, age of identification, duration of hearing loss, age of (cochlear) implantation, and type of educational placement.

Cochlear implants in children

- Children implanted before the age of 2 years demonstrate improved communication skills compared to those implanted later.

Hearing aids

- Hearing aids improve quality of life among users.

Source: Based on Ali and O'Connell (2007), Chisolm et al., (2007); Nelson et al., (2008); Queensland Health (2008).

The overall goal of most aural rehabilitation programs is to improve functional communication. Typically, key areas considered when designing an individualized program include amplification, hearing assistive technology, auditory training, communication strategy training, and communication methodology, to name a few. Depending on the degree to which the hearing loss affects communication, goals are developed relative to one or more of these areas. We address each of these separately, but it should be emphasized that many of these areas are routinely attended to at the same time because work in one area will have implications for performance in others.

Amplification

Amplification is often considered the core of most aural rehabilitation plans. The success of other treatment strategies incorporated into the plan is often predicated on the use of appropriate amplification. Therefore, one of the first steps in the aural rehabilitation process is the selection, fitting, and evaluation of amplification. In most cases amplification consists of **personal hearing aids,** although as we will later see, other amplification options are available.

HEARING AIDS

Hearing aids come in a variety of styles and sizes ranging from tiny custom models that fit entirely within the external auditory canal, to custom in-the-ear models that fit into the concha region of the pinna, to slightly larger instruments that are worn behind the ear (see Figure 14.12). Even "disposable" models intended for short-term use are available. Regardless of the style, every hearing aid contains three basic components: a microphone, an amplifier, and a receiver. The microphone picks up acoustic energy from the environment, converts it to an electrical signal, and sends it to the amplifier. The amplifier increases the voltage of the electrical

FIGURE 14.12
....
Styles of hearing aids.
(Photos courtesy
of Siemens Hearing
Instruments)

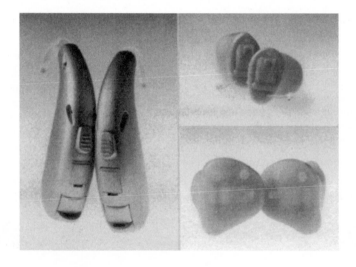

signal and sends it to the receiver, which, in turn, converts it back into acoustic energy and routes it to the user's ear canal.

There have been numerous advances in hearing aid technology in recent years. The vast majority of hearing aids dispensed today incorporate sophisticated digital signal processing. Sound entering the hearing aid is converted into a digital code that can be uniquely processed by applying a series of mathematical formulas. These formulas allow the signal to be manipulated in various ways to improve audibility while maintaining comfort, reducing unwanted background noise, and eliminating acoustic feedback (the annoying "whistle" that occurs when amplified sound leaks out of the ear canal is picked up by the microphone and reamplified by the hearing aid).

Most modern hearing aids are programmed by the audiologist using a computer and sophisticated fitting software. Many hearing aid models contain directional microphone technology that automatically suppresses background noise originating from in back of, or to the side of, the user. Some hearing aids even incorporate a handheld remote control that allows the user to adjust the volume or turn the hearing aid on and off.

The primary goal in most hearing aid fittings is to make speech audible to the user to improve intelligibility. This is not a simple task because people often have greater hearing loss at some frequencies compared to others. In addition, some frequencies, such as those in the higher range, are more critical in making speech intelligible and may require greater amplification. These factors must be taken into account when determining how much amplification to provide. Additionally, although the overall goal is to make speech audible, it is essential that the amplified signal never becomes uncomfortably loud for the user or cause additional trauma to the auditory system.

Unlike eyeglasses, which can restore a person's sight to 20/20, a hearing aid will not return hearing to normal. Although audibility for speech should improve, amplification of the speech signal may not necessarily restore its clarity. When a person is considering amplification, he or she must be counseled on this point so as not to develop unrealistic expectations. It usually takes time, training, and practice before a person makes maximal use of their new hearing aids. As part of the counseling process, the audiologist also instructs the client on hearing aid care and maintenance, and how to adjust the controls properly for different listening situations. Specific strategies designed to facilitate listening are also reviewed. If the audiologist does not take the time to cover this information, more than likely the hearing aids will end up in the drawer. A demonstration of hearing aid counseling can be seen on the book's CD-ROM.

Those with conductive hearing losses that are not medically treatable, such as atresia, may benefit from a bone conduction hearing aid. This device consists of a headband and bone vibrator coupled to a conventional hearing aid. With the bone vibrator placed firmly against the skull, sound is converted to mechanical vibration that stimulates the inner ear, bypassing the impaired outer or middle ear. A newer version of this device, called a **bone-anchored hearing aid,** functions in the same manner. However, unlike a traditional bone conduction hearing aid that can be cumbersome to wear, the bone-anchored version consists of a small titanium screw that is surgically implanted into the skull directly behind the pinna. A small external device containing a microphone and other electronic components attaches to the screw and converts sound to mechanical vibration, which stimulates the cochlea via bone conduction.

COCHLEAR IMPLANTS

Some people with severe-to-profound hearing losses receive little or no benefit from traditional hearing aids because they fail to provide enough amplification to make sound audible and facilitate speech perception. For this select group, a **cochlear implant** (Figure 14.13) may be an option. A cochlear implant is a neural prosthesis designed to bypass the damaged hair cells of the cochlea and directly stimulate the surviving auditory nerve fibers with electrical energy.

A cochlear implant consists of externally worn and internally implanted components. The external components consist of the microphone, speech processor, and external transmitter. The internal components include the receiver-stimulator that is surgically coupled to the skull and the electrode array inserted approximately 22 to 30 mm into the cochlea. In the past, only one ear was selected for implantation even when there was significant hearing loss in both ears. Today, bilateral implantation has become more routine in children and adults.

Let's take a closer look at how a cochlear implant works. The microphone is typically positioned on the head, at or near the pinna. It picks up sound, converts it to electrical energy, and transmits it to the speech

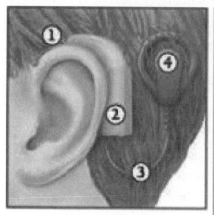
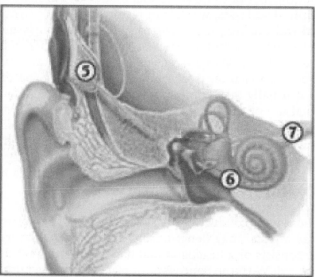

FIGURE 14.13

Schematic depicting the components of an ear-level cochlear implant (1) microphone, (2) speech processor, (3) transmitting cable, (4) transmitting coil, (5) receiver-stimulator, (6) electrode array, (7) VIIIth nerve.

(Courtesy of Cochlear Corporation, Inc.)

processor. The speech processor is a sophisticated microcomputer that is custom programmed for each user to maximize reception of the speech signal. Only certain aspects of the input signal are sent to the cochlea. These are defined by the processing scheme, or coding strategy, incorporated into the device. The intent is to send the impaired ear those features of the speech signal that are critical to intelligibility. Most modern speech processors are worn behind the ear. The coded signal is sent through a cable to the external transmitting coil that is magnetically secured to the head. Using FM radio waves, the signal is transmitted across the skin to the internal receiver-stimulator and finally to the individual electrodes implanted in the cochlea. Modern cochlear implants contain multiple electrodes that provide electrical stimulation to many sites along the basilar membrane, taking advantage of the way the cochlea naturally codes frequency information. The resulting neural impulses are transmitted to the brain in the usual manner via the ascending auditory pathways.

When cochlear implants were originally introduced, only adults who were postlingually deafened were candidates. Today, cochlear implant surgery is routinely conducted on severely to profoundly hearing impaired children as young as 12 months, and even younger in certain cases, and adults of all ages including those with prelingual and postlingual onset. Postlingually deafened adults tend to benefit extensively because they have acquired spoken language skills before losing their hearing and can more readily make use of the auditory cues provided by the device. Children who are implanted at an early age and receive intensive auditory therapy also demonstrate significant gains relative to speech perception, language acquisition, speech production, and literacy development (Papsin et al., 2000; Waltzman & Roland, 2005).

It is important to understand that a cochlear implant does not restore a person's hearing to normal and that performance varies widely among those who use the device. Some rely on a cochlear implant strictly to provide greater awareness of environmental sounds. Others find that an implant provides sufficient auditory cues to enhance their ability to speech-read or improve speech production. Some individuals are able to understand connected speech without visual cues including over the phone. The degree of benefit obtained from a cochlear implant depends on many factors, including when the person became deaf (prelingually or postlingually), the amount of time between when they became deaf and received an implant, the number of surviving auditory nerve fibers available for stimulation, and the scope and quality of aural rehabilitation services received following implantation, to name just a few. Given the impressive results demonstrated by many recipients, particularly young children who are identified and implanted early on and receive appropriate early intervention services to stimulate the auditory pathways leading to the brain, the number of individuals who will receive and benefit from cochlear implants will no doubt continue to grow. Speech-language pathologists and audiologists must be prepared to provide aural rehabilitation services to these individuals to maximize their perceptual and spoken language skills.

Hearing Assistive Technology

Hearing assistive technology (HAT) is another category of devices routinely incorporated into the aural rehabilitation plan. Although hearing aids and cochlear implants provide benefit in many situations, it is not uncommon for users to experience difficulty in environments where there are high levels of background noise and reverberation, or environments where they are situated at a significant distance from the person they want to hear. Use of various assistive devices can be helpful in overcoming these problems in settings such as classrooms, restaurants, meeting rooms, and auditoriums.

The principle behind most devices is to position the microphone of the device in close proximity to the desired sound source. For example, the microphone can be clipped to the talker's lapel or placed at the center of a conference table, increasing the intensity of the desired signal compared to unwanted noise in the background. Using various types of wired or wireless technology, the signal is delivered directly to the listener via headphones or to their hearing aid or cochlear implant. In many cases, use of HAT allows the listener to be seated at a significant distance yet still be able to hear as if they were positioned right next to the talker.

One type of device that is very popular, particularly in educational settings, is the personal **FM system.** This device operates on the same principle as conventional FM radio. The talker speaks into a lapel or headset microphone attached to a small body-worn transmitter that "broadcasts" on a designated frequency or channel. The hearing-impaired listener accesses the FM signal through a body-worn receiver tuned to the same FM radio frequency or "channel" as the transmitter. The signal picked up by the receiver is directed to the listener's ear(s) by way of headphones or ear buds. In cases where the person uses a hearing aid or cochlear implant, a small FM "boot" can be plugged directly into the hearing instrument, eliminating the need for cumbersome cords and conspicuous bodyworn devices.

Another type of technology also widely used in schools is **sound field amplification.** Similar to personal FM, sound field amplification consists of a lapel or boom microphone worn by the talker (teacher) and a wireless transmitter. The main difference, however, is that instead of broadcasting the signal to individual receivers, the signal is sent to loudspeakers that are strategically placed around the room. Small portable desktop speakers are also available. The primary advantage of sound field amplification over other types of systems is that all students in the room can benefit from the device, including those with transient hearing loss due to otitis media.

A variety of devices are available for specialized applications such as TV and telephone listening. For those who have losses so severe that they do not benefit from amplification, specialized devices are available that alert the user, usually by way of a flashing (strobe) light, of important sounds in the environment. For example, devices are available that visually alert the person of a ringing phone, alarm clock, smoke detector, or baby cry. For phone communication, deaf callers often rely on a portable keyboard called a **teletypewriter** (TTY) that allows text conversations to be conducted over regular phone lines. In recent years the Internet and various forms of wireless technology have played a significant role in expanding communication options for those who are deaf by enabling them to converse through e-mail, text messaging, synchronous chat, and videoconferencing. Last but not least, many deaf people look to the assistance and companionship of a "hearing dog" to facilitate receptive communication. Similar to guide dogs for the visually impaired, a hearing dog is trained to alert its client to important sounds in the environment such as the doorbell, microwave, or smoke alarm. Further information on hearing dogs is available on the Dogs for the Deaf Web site listed at the end of this chapter.

Auditory Training

Once a client has been fit with an appropriate amplification device, he or she may need to learn (or relearn) how to make sense of what is being heard through some type of formal or structured listening practice. This process is referred to as **auditory training.** The goal of auditory training is to maximize a person's use of their **residual hearing** to enhance the perception of speech and nonspeech cues (Schow & Nerbonne, 2007). Improvements in auditory perceptual skills should lead to progress in other areas including speech and language development, cognition, reading, and learning.

The principle of **neural plasticity** is paramount to the process of auditory training. Neural plasticity, as it relates to the auditory system, refers to physiological and functional changes within the central nervous system in response to auditory stimulation (Greenough, 1975). The underlying principle of auditory training is to promote neural plasticity through auditory stimulation to overcome the negative consequences of auditory deprivation brought on by the hearing loss. Neural plasticity is greater in children than adults, further supporting the importance of early identification and early intervention. With adults, neural plasticity involves relearning how to recognize and make use of critical speech cues as new neural patterns develop through the use of amplification.

When developing an individualized auditory training plan, it is important to consider the individual's degree of hearing loss and whether they are prelingually or postlingually hearing impaired. In most cases, intensive and enriched auditory training activities are conducted with children, particularly those who have recently received hearing aids or cochlear implants. Prelingual hearing-impaired adults, particularly those with severe to profound losses who have begun using amplification for the first time or are resuming amplification after many years of nonuse, may also benefit from structured listening practice.

Development of an individualized training program usually begins with a thorough assessment of the person's auditory perceptual skills. This type of assessment goes beyond what is routinely conducted as part of the basic audiological evaluation previously described. Several commercially available tools are available that assess a wide variety of perceptual skills ranging from simple phoneme awareness to comprehension of connected discourse. Tests are available for children and adults, most of which contain normative data relative to the individual's age and degree of hearing loss. In some cases it is helpful to administer speech perception tests that evaluate how a person makes use of both visual and auditory cues to determine how well they are able integrate the two modalities to facilitate receptive communication.

Many of the instruments that assess auditory perceptual skills are components of larger, comprehensive auditory training curricula. Some of these programs have been designed specifically for hearing-impaired children, including infants with severe to profound losses. These curricula are developmentally based and designed to be integrated into the child's overall speech and language intervention plan. Many of these programs are designed specifically for the home with the child's family assuming an active role in the training process.

Although there is no universally recommended approach to auditory training, one of the most widely used models is that advocated by Erber (1982). This model is appropriate for children and adults and can be used for visual as well as auditory perceptual training. The general framework of this model is a matrix comprised of two distinct variables: the complexity of the training stimulus and the complexity of the perceptual task. Stimulus complexity is arranged in hierarchical order from environmental sounds and suprasegmental aspects of speech, to consonants and vowels, syllables, words, phrases, sentences, and ultimately more complex forms of connected discourse. The most basic perceptual task is detection or awareness, that is, being able to determine the presence or absence of a stimulus. The basic premise is that a stimulus cannot be processed unless it can first be detected. Therefore, at this level the task is to determine which environmental (e.g., telephone ring, smoke alarm) or speech sounds are audible to the individual.

Auditory awareness is followed by the next level, "auditory discrimination," whereby a person makes judgments as to whether pairs of stimuli are the same or different. For example, when presented with the syllable pair /pa/ - /sa/, the client must determine whether or not they sound the same. This can be done for environmental sounds, words, phrases, and sentences as well. At the next level, training focuses on "identification" whereby the client must label what he or she hears, such as by repeating or pointing to a picture representing the target. The final level, "comprehension," focuses on the person's ability to understand the meaning of the spoken message.

This model is highly flexible in that it can be adapted for use in a variety of settings, and training activities can be infused into many facets of an individual's daily routine such as listening in the classroom or on the phone. In addition, it can accommodate a variety of materials that are geared specifically toward the individual, making the process both interesting and relevant. Although some levels of this model are characterized by significant drill and practice, it is flexible enough to allow clinicians to incorporate listening activities that are less formal.

Communication Strategy Training

Most adults with hearing loss can improve their conversational interactions through the use of specific strategies designed to facilitate communication or repair breakdowns that occur during the course of a conversation

(Tye-Murray, 2009). Demonstrating and practicing how to implement these strategies is a major component of most adult aural rehabilitation programs. The ultimate goal is for clients to manage communication problems efficiently and effectively that arise during their daily activities.

As part of the training process, clients must first increase their awareness of the various environmental barriers that may preclude successful communication, including background noise, poor lighting, and distance. Clients are taught to recognize these obstacles and assertively, yet tactfully, request appropriate modifications such as turning off a radio in the background, adjusting the lighting, or moving to another location. In addition, the hearing-impaired listener may need to instruct talkers to modify their speaking behavior by asking them to slow down, speak louder, or face them to facilitate speech reading. Simply revealing one's hearing loss to the talker can facilitate communication because it raises awareness that accommodations may be necessary.

Another critical component of communication strategy training is to teach clients to anticipate or predict what is likely to be said during a conversation. Walking into your favorite fast-food restaurant, you can probably guess the types of questions, statements, and vocabulary the person behind the counter will use. For example, the first thing they will likely ask is "Can I take your order?" rather than a question about your political views or thoughts on the latest Hollywood scandal. By anticipating what is likely to be said based on the context of the conversation and the environment, clients can eliminate vocabulary that is unlikely to be spoken, allowing them to better predict the message and fill in any missing pieces. Having a good handle on the English language is also extremely helpful because it allows the hearing-impaired person to predict a missed word by analyzing the grammatical structure of the utterance. For example, if the talker says "Let's go to the movies" but the hearing-impaired person misses the final word, knowing the grammatical rules of English enables the listener to realize that the missed word must be a noun, limiting the number of possible choices to some degree. Having a good understanding of semantics further limits the number of choices.

For most of us, when we miss what someone has said, we usually respond with "what?" or "pardon?" to indicate that we would like the talker to repeat the message. Although not very instructive, this type of response is quick to implement and fairly effective for those with normal hearing. Asking for repetition, however, is usually not as effective for a hearing-impaired person because it tends to elicit a rote response that provides no additional information and, as a result, is likely to be missed again. Used excessively, the "repeat" strategy also has a tendency to increase the frustration level during a conversation. A more effective strategy is for the hearing-impaired individual to ask for the message to be rephrased, which may provide enough additional information to facilitate comprehension. Other effective repair strategies include asking the talker to provide a key word, identify the topic of the conversation, provide additional information, or restate the message using less complex syntax and terminology. Gestures and writing may also be helpful in repairing a breakdown. The end result is likely to be a more fluent conversational exchange between the hearing-impaired person and those with whom he or she interacts regularly.

Treatment and Management of (Central) Auditory Processing Disorders

Recall from our earlier discussion that a (central) auditory processing disorder refers to deficits of the central auditory system that affects one's ability to efficiently and effectively use and interpret auditory information. The treatment and management of (C)APD must be based on the findings obtained as part of a comprehensive evaluation. No single form of treatment is appropriate for all cases. Treatment generally encompasses three general areas: environmental accommodations, compensatory strategies, and direct therapy to remediate specific auditory processing deficits.

Environmental accommodations provide the individual with greater access to acoustic information. This may be accomplished by acoustically treating a room to reduce noise and reverberation, seating the individual closer to the sound source, fitting the individual with a personal FM or sound field system, or providing written notes to supplement verbal information. Accommodations may also include a variety of instructional techniques such as speaking clearly at a moderate rate, providing clear and concise directions, using familiar vocabulary and simple sentence structure, breaking utterances into smaller segments, and asking the individual to repeat critical information to ensure comprehension.

Compensatory strategies are introduced to strengthen higher-order resources including attention, language and cognition. This may include the use of memory and organizational techniques such as chunking, reauditorization, mnemonics, visualization, and written reminders. It may also focus on making use of linguistic and contextual cues to anticipate what is likely to be said and facilitate auditory closure.

Finally, direct therapy consists of intensive auditory training designed to remediate those specific auditory deficits identified during the assessment process. Activities may include formal exercises involving auditory discrimination, localization, temporal sequencing, sound blending, and understanding speech in noise, to name a few. Direct therapy usually takes place through individual sessions with an audiologist or speech-language pathologist, although various curricula and computer-based programs are available for individualized training outside the clinic environment, including the home.

Communication Methodology

Communication options for people with hearing loss can be generally divided into two major categories: those that are auditory based, emphasizing spoken language or speaking and listening, and those that are visually based, emphasizing manual communication or sign language. A third category, referred to as total communication, combines features common to both. Proponents of auditory-based approaches advocate for the use of speech and audition to facilitate adjustment and integration into the hearing world. It is their belief that learning to communicate orally provides hearing-impaired children with a greater number of social, educational, and vocational options during the course of their lifetime. In contrast, proponents of manual communication argue that children who learn to sign are able to communicate more quickly without frustration and therefore are able to learn at a faster pace. Advocates of manual communication also believe that signing serves to facilitate socialization with, and acceptance by, a child's hearing-impaired peers and other members of the Deaf Community, which ultimately has a positive impact on their self-identity and self-esteem.

The decision regarding which method to embrace can be extremely difficult, especially for parents of an infant who has just been identified with a hearing loss because they rarely have any experience in this area. It is helpful to ask parents what they desire for their child in terms of communication outcomes. Many factors need to be considered, including the amount of residual hearing, potential benefits from amplification, quality and availability of intervention and support services for the child and family, level of commitment to the selected approach by the child's family, presence of other disabilities, and personal preference. The preference of the child's parents is especially important because there are numerous complex personal and philosophical issues that must be considered. It is imperative that families receive accurate, unbiased information regarding the full range of options available. Professionals, in turn, must be sensitive to all aspects surrounding the communication issue and be prepared, if necessary, to advocate in the best interests of the child. It is beyond the scope of this chapter to discuss these issues with the depth required to do them justice. Rather, a brief overview of the nature of auditory and visually based communication approaches is provided.

AUDITORY-BASED APPROACHES

With the proliferation of early hearing detection and intervention programs and advancements in amplification technology, most children born today with hearing loss have the opportunity to make sufficient use of auditory information to develop spoken language and communication skills. Even in cases of profound hearing loss there is usually sufficient residual hearing to develop the auditory channel effectively. The best candidates for auditory-based approaches are those who are consistent users of amplification. Speech-reading skills may also be taken into consideration. There are differing opinions on this issue, however. Some professionals believe that speech-reading ability is an inherent skill and therefore should not be a determining factor in choosing a communication mode. Others believe that speech reading can be taught through formal instruction, and therefore speech-reading training is incorporated into the overall goals of the aural rehabilitation plan.

In terms of communication methods designed to promote the development of spoken language skills, currently two approaches have received considerable attention. The primary goal of each is to develop speech and communication skills necessary for full integration into the hearing world.

The first is the **auditory-verbal** approach whose overall goal is the development of spoken language through audition by focusing on the use of residual hearing through amplification. Because this approach strives to maximize an individual's listening skills, no forms of manual communication are used and the individual is discouraged from relying on speech reading. During training activities, this is accomplished by having parents and therapists eliminate the use of visual cues to promote reliance on listening alone. Limited visual cues are introduced only when the individual cannot understand through audition alone. This approach has been used extensively with children by way of one-on-one therapy and family-centered teaching activities designed to facilitate the early, consistent, and successful use of amplification.

The second method is the **auditory-oral** approach. Similar to the auditory-verbal approach, the auditory-oral approach teaches the individual to make maximum use of his of her residual hearing through amplification. Where it differs, however, is that it also emphasizes the use of visual cues such as speech reading to facilitate receptive communication. The use of any forms of manual communication, other than natural gestures, is strongly discouraged.

With both of these approaches, there is a strong emphasis on the development of verbal as well as auditory skills. Both approaches require extensive training and practice. The individual must be immersed in a speech-intensive, language-enriched environment both at home and at school, with the consistent use of amplification strictly enforced.

Speech-language pathologists and audiologists involved in early intervention model appropriate techniques and strategies for parents, who then incorporate them into the child's daily routine. A strong commitment on behalf of the family is vital to the success of either approach.

VISUALLY BASED APPROACHES

For those who cannot effectively utilize the acoustic speech signal, even through well-fitted amplification, some form of visually based manual communication is usually necessary. Manual communication, or sign language, allows information to be conveyed visually by way of the hands and has long been used by large numbers of deaf individuals to communicate with each other.

Depending on the specific type of manual communication system, signs can occur in isolation or in combination with speech, a process referred to as **simultaneous communication.** Individual signs are formed through the combination of four distinct parameters: hand shape, location of the hands relative to the body and to each other, palm orientation, and movement. Simply by altering any one of these parameters can significantly change the meaning of a sign. In addition, the meaning can be altered by varying the size, intensity, speed, and duration of the sign. Also of importance in conveying meaning are nonmanual cues such as facial expression, body position, head tilt, and eye gaze. These cues are particularly important for expressing feelings and emotions, for conveying spatial relationships between people and objects, and for differentiating statements, questions, and commands.

When attempting to distinguish the array of manual communication systems available, it is helpful to view them along a continuum bounded by forms of Manually Coded English (e.g., Signing Exact English) at one end and American Sign Language (ASL) at the opposite end (see Figure 14.14). As previously discussed, ASL is a language unto itself rather than a visual

Manually Coded English Signing Systems	⟶	American Sign Language (ASL)
Signed Exact English (SEE)	Pidgin Signed English (PSE)	
Word meaning is NOT considered (e.g., the word "right" will have the same sign regardless of context)	Signs used are more conceptual. One word may have many signs depending upon meaning.	Has its own vocabulary, grammar, and sentence structure. One sign may represent an entire thought.
All grammatical markers (articles, auxiliary verbs, plurals, etc.) are signed.	Grammatical markers may or may not be signed.	Does not have specific signs for grammatical markers.
	Facial expression and gestures are incorporated.	Facial expression, body position, space, and repetition are used extensively.

FIGURE 14.14

Sign-language continuum.

representation of an existing language such as English. The origin of ASL has been traced to France and was subsequently introduced to the United States in 1815 by Thomas Hopkins Gallaudet. It is very much a conceptual language with a single sign having the capability of conveying an entire thought, and because ASL and English are distinct languages with different grammatical structures, one cannot simultaneously speak syntactically correct English sentences while using ASL.

Pidgin signed english (PSE), sometimes referred to as **contact signing,** is an intermediate variety of the languages of ASL and English. In general, PSE is characterized by the use of ASL signs with English word order, thus preserving the conceptual integrity of ASL while integrating English syntax. As with ASL, facial expression, body position, gestures, and the use of space are important features, and function words such as "a," "an," and "the" are typically omitted. PSE is usually the type of manual communication taught in basic sign curricula for hearing people interested in learning to sign. New users of PSE tend to communicate using a structure that is more English-like, whereas experienced users tend to incorporate more features that are common to ASL.

Other forms of manual communication, referred to as **manually coded English,** have been developed for use with deaf children in educational settings to replicate spoken English more accurately. Unlike natural languages, these sign systems are contrived and operate under the premise that competency in spoken and written English is critical for academic achievement. Manually coded English uses two types of gestures: sign vocabulary, most of which comes from ASL to represent English words visually, and invented sign markers that visually represent English grammatical principles including common affixes (e.g., "-ly" and "-ing"). Signs are produced in the exact order in which they are spoken, which allows English to be modeled using

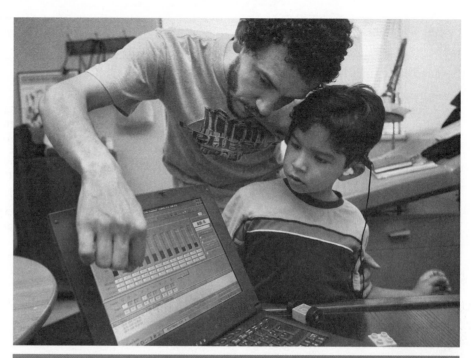

Preschool children may pose a special challenge for the audiologist.

visual and auditory modalities simultaneously. Several systems have been developed, and although there are subtle differences among each, their main purpose is to represent spoken English accurately in a visual form.

Two additional forms of manual communication are **fingerspelling** and **Cued Speech.** Fingerspelling consists of distinct handshapes used to visually represent each of the 26 letters of the English alphabet. Although not very efficient because each letter of a word must be manually produced, fingerspelling is routinely incorporated into ASL, PSE, and manually coded English systems to reference proper names, technical vocabulary, English words that have no corresponding sign, and words and concepts where the signer does not know the formal sign.

Cued Speech is a manual communication system designed to overcome the ambiguity associated with speech reading. One's dependence on visual cues provided through speech reading tends to increase as the degree of hearing loss becomes more severe. Unfortunately, by itself, speech reading is not an efficient means of receptive communication because approximately 50% of speech sounds are visually indistinguishable. For example, consider the phonemes /p/, /b/, and /m/. If you look in the mirror and produce all three without voice, you will notice that visually there are no differences. These sounds are referred to as **homophonous** because they look alike on the lips. Likewise, the words "palm," "bomb," and "mom" are visually indistinguishable and would be difficult to differentiate without the use of audition. This is the type of problem people encounter when their hearing loss prevents them from making fine distinctions between sounds that look alike.

Cued Speech was developed by Dr. Richard Orin Cornet in 1966 as a means of helping hearing-impaired persons identify speech sounds that are visually similar, as well as those that are not readily visible such as /g/ and /k/. Cued Speech combines the natural movements of the mouth produced while speaking with "cues" formed using eight unique hand shapes and four hand positions relative to the face. This system is designed to facilitate speech reading and the development of language and literacy skills. Users must have a good grasp of phonetics to use Cued Speech effectively, which may be why it is not as widely embraced as other approaches. Web links to sites providing information on Cued Speech and American Sign Language are available at the end of this chapter.

SUMMARY

The profession of audiology is a richly diverse field that offers the opportunity to work with many diverse populations in a wide variety of settings. The audiologist has the responsibility to assess auditory and vestibular function and to provide aural (audiological) habilitation/rehabilitation services. A hearing loss is caused by an interruption at one or more points along the auditory pathway spanning from the outer ear to the brain. The three types of hearing loss that affect the peripheral auditory system are conductive, sensorineural, and mixed. Audiologists are also concerned with problems affecting the central auditory system, including the brainstem, the subcortical auditory pathways, and the auditory cortex of the brain. Problems along these pathways generally result in an inability to use and interpret auditory information efficiently and effectively, referred to as an auditory processing disorder.

When describing hearing loss, audiologists use terminology such as *conductive, sensorineural, mixed,* and *central* to identify the portion of the auditory system that is affected. Another important set of terms describe the degree of hearing loss measured in decibels. Each degree of hearing loss corresponds to a specific decibel range. Individuals with hearing loss in the slight/mild to moderately severe range are often referred to as hard of hearing and depend as much as possible on the use of residual hearing for communication. For people with a severe to profound hearing loss, often referred to as "deaf," the auditory system provides little or no access to sound without proper amplification.

When evaluating the auditory system, audiologists rely on electroacoustic, electrophysiological, and behavioral measures. A battery of tests is administered to identify the presence of a hearing loss, determine its type, quantify its degree, and assess its impact on communication. Informational and personal adjustment counseling are critical to the entire process.

Aural (audiological) habilitation/rehabilitation refers to the services and procedures that are designed to minimize and alleviate communication difficulties presented by a hearing loss. *Aural habilitation* alludes to therapies that are used primarily with children to teach missing communication skills; *aural rehabilitation* refers to services provided to those who have lost their hearing later in life, after spoken communication skills have been established. The focus of aural rehabilitation is to help the person recover lost skills and to use compensatory strategies effectively. Areas typically considered in creating an individual aural rehabilitation program are the evaluation and fitting of amplification and hearing assistive technology, auditory training, communication strategy training, and determination of an appropriate mode of communication.

THOUGHT QUESTIONS

- In what settings are audiologists employed?
- What are the main functions of the outer, middle, and inner ear?
- Explain the differences between conductive, sensorineural, and mixed hearing loss.
- Explain how disorders of the peripheral auditory system differ from those of the central auditory system.
- What are some causes of different types of hearing loss?
- What effects may hearing loss have on communication and psychosocial well-being?
- Identify the methods used in evaluating hearing in children. How do they compare with methods used with adults?
- What are the goals of aural (audiological) habilitation and rehabilitation?
- Explain the types of intervention considered when developing an individualized aural (audiological) habilitation/rehabilitation plan.

SUGGESTED READINGS

Bellis, T. J. (2003). *Assessment and management of central auditory processing disorders in the educational setting: From science to practice.* San Diego, CA: Singular.

Clark, J. G., & English, K. (2004). *Audiologic counseling in clinical practice: Helping clients and families adjust to hearing loss.* Boston: Allyn and Bacon.

Martin, F. N., & Clark, J. G. (2009). Introduction to audiology (10th ed.). Boston: Pearson.

Tye-Murray, N. (2009). *Foundations of aural rehabilitation: Children, adults, and their family members* (3rd ed.). Clifton Park, NY: Delmar Cengage Learning.

ONLINE RESOURCES

American Academy of Audiology
www.audiology.org
General information about audiology.

www.audiologyonline.com
General information about audiology.

American Speech-Language-Hearing Association
www.asha.org
General information about audiology.

Better Hearing Institute
www.betterhearing.org
General information about hearing loss.

Cochlear Corporation
www.cochlear.com
Information about cochlear implants.

Dogs for the Deaf
www.dogsforthedeaf.org
Information about hearing dogs.

Healthy Hearing
www.healthyhearing.com
Information about hearing aids.

Hearing Education and Awareness for Rockers
www.hearnet.com
Information about noise/music-induced hearing loss for musicians and music lovers.

National Center for Hearing Assessment and Management
www.infanthearing.org
Information about early hearing detection and intervention.

National Coalition on Auditory Processing Disorders, Inc
www.ncapd.org
Information about auditory processing disorders.

National Cued Speech Association
www.cuedspeech.org
Resources and information on the use of Cued Speech.

National Institute on Deafness and Other Communication Disorders
www.nidcd.nih.gov
General information about hearing loss.

Roy Sullivan
www.rcsullivan.com/www/ears.htm
Roy Sullivan developed this Web site, which provides video-otoscopic images of various outer and middle ear disorders.

Scott Bradley's Web site
http://facstaff.uww.edu/bradleys/radio/hlsimulation/
Audio simulations of different types of hearing loss.

Signing Online
www.signingonline.com
Interactive Web-based instruction in American Sign Language.

Technology Access Program, Gallaudet University
tap.gallaudet.edu
Information about assistive technologies for the deaf.

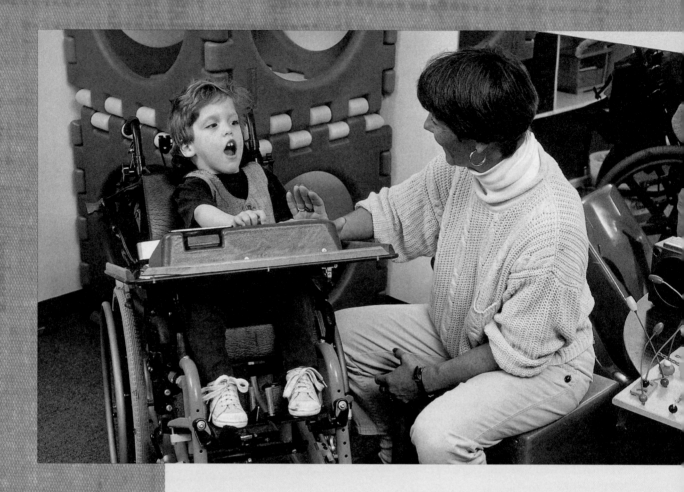

CHAPTER LEARNING GOALS

When you have finished this chapter, you should be able to:

- Describe the major types of unaided and aided AAC systems

- Explain how AAC needs change thoroughout the lifespan

- List the major concerns in client assessment for AAC

- Explain the major elements of intervention with AAC and what we know from EBP

15

Augmentative and Alternative Communication

Throughout this text, individuals have been mentioned who have severe speech and language impairments and might need either some additional support or an alternative method of communication. These forms of communication, referred to as **augmentative and alternative communication (AAC),** include gestures, signing, pictures, photographs, print, computerized communication, and voice production (Glennen & DeCoste, 1997). The American Speech-Language-Hearing Association (ASHA) defined AAC by saying,

> AAC is, foremost, a set of procedures and processes by which an individual's communication skills (i.e., production as well as comprehension) can be maximized for functional and effective communication. It involves supplementing or replacing natural speech and/or writing with aided (e.g., picture communication symbols, line drawings, Blissymbols, and tangible objects) and/or unaided symbols (e.g., manual signs, gestures, and finger spelling). (ASHA, 2002b, p. 98)

Use of the term AAC can be further clarified by understanding the difference between the words augmentative and alternative. *Augmentative* communication can be thought of as the process of supplementing existing speech abilities, whereas *alternative* refers to a substitute or replacement for speech (Glennen, 1997).

The importance of AAC can easily be seen when one considers that "approximately 12 of every 1000 people are unable to meet their daily communication needs through speech. . . . Unless these individuals receive effective AAC interventions and supports they will not have a 'voice' and will remain silenced" (Light et al., 2003, p. ix).

Individuals who might benefit from AAC include, but are not limited to, those with deafness, mental retardation (MR), autism spectrum disorder (ASD), aphasia, traumatic brain injury (TBI), motor-speech problems, cerebral

All typical communicators augment speech with other means of communication, such as gestures and facial expression.

palsy (CP), glossectomy, laryngectomy, dysarthria, and apraxia of speech, to name a few. More than at any time in human history, people with disabilities are meeting new challenges, participating in life to the fullest, and demanding that their voices be heard. As mentioned in Chapter 2, legislation, adaptations, and technology are helping to ensure this participation. Individuals are overcoming what were considered only a few years ago to be insurmountable barriers to independence. Case Study 15.1 presents the story of a child who uses AAC.

In this chapter, we explore AAC, describing what it is and how it works, and then focusing on assessment and intervention considerations. Most chapters in this book discuss specific types of communication disorders, whereas this chapter discusses an intervention approach that benefits people with many different types of communication disorders.

The goals for AAC intervention vary with each individual user; however, general treatment aims typically include one, or more, of the following:

1. Assist individuals with their daily communication needs.
2. Help facilitate the development of speech and language.
3. Help facilitate the return of speech and language. (Blackstone, 1989)

CASE STUDY 15.1
Case Study of a Child Requiring an Augmentative and Alternative Communication (AAC) System: Nicky

Nicky is an 8-year-old girl who is nonverbal, is diagnosed as having a developmental disability, and has difficulty with fine motor skills. She attends second grade in a blended classroom. When Nicky was a preschooler, she received early intervention services in her home where she was seen by a speech-language pathologist and an occupational therapist. Nicky is able to make some sounds, and she approximates the words *mom* and *dog;* in addition, she nods her head for yes and no. Although the speech-language pathologist working with Nicky has not ruled out the possibility that she could someday talk, at this stage, Nicky needs an alternative method of communication to supplement her few words, sounds, and gestures.

Last year, Nicky's speech-language pathologist tried teaching her sign language; however, given Nicky's fine motor issues, signing was difficult for her. In addition, none of the students in Nicky's class knew sign. Given the motor requirements of signing, Nicky's team elected to begin using a symbol-based system. Nicky learned to use several symbols to communicate a variety of messages including such things as "Hi," "My name is Nicky," "My favorite color is purple," "I love to swim," "Let's play a game," "I want a cookie," and "That's yucky!"

The speech-language pathologist worked with Nicky's classroom teacher, other school personnel, and Nicky's parents to ensure that new symbols added to Nicky's repertoire reflected priority needs across her environments. In addition, her team is now exploring the use of a voice output communication aid (VOCA) so that when Nicky touches a symbol, a girl's voice would speak the messages out loud—giving Nicky a voice.

As you read the chapter, think about:

- Why sign language was not the best choice for a communication system for Nicky.
- How you would begin to decide which symbols/ messages should be added to Nicky's device.
- What type of VOCA would be most appropriate for Nicky at this point in time.

Only careful and ongoing evaluation of a client's abilities, his or her needs, and the environment can ensure that these goals will be met effectively and efficiently.

TYPES OF AAC

AAC systems can be separated into two primary categories: unaided and aided. Unaided systems do not involve any external equipment and rely only on the individual's body (Lloyd et al., 1997). Aided systems involve the use of some type of equipment or device and range from very simple to extremely sophisticated options.

Unaided AAC

All of us use gestures to communicate. We shake our head, shrug our shoulders, point, and reach. Gesturing is a form of unaided AAC, as are signing, fingerspelling, Cued Speech, and writing.

Signing is a highly developed form of communication, as is speech. The sign system is the code or the language. As noted in Chapter 14, "Audiology and Hearing Loss," American Sign Language or ASL, the language of the Deaf Culture in the United States, is a language with its own vocabulary and syntax. Other sign systems in use in the United States are translations of English into sign and include Signed English, the most frequently taught sign system in the United States.

American Indian gestural or hand communication, called AmerInd, is a gestural system used with some nonspeaking individuals. It is a relatively grammar-free, nonsign system of 250 concept signals. Almost all gestures in AmerInd can be made with one hand, making it easier for those with hemiplegia, paralysis on one side of the body, or hemiparesis, weakness on one side.

Individual signs can be classified based on their ease of production or comprehension. In general, it is easier to produce signs that touch the body and that use both hands, and, when both hands are used, it is easier to produce signs that are symmetrical (both hands produce the same movement).

Some signs are easy to comprehend because they look like what they represent. These signs are called *iconic*. For example, the sign for "drink" in most systems is made by miming drinking from a cup. Unfortunately, few signs are of this type. Signs that are easily guessable, explainable, and memorable are called *transparent*. AmerInd has a high proportion of transparent signs. Signs, such as "apple," which are difficult to interpret, are called *opaque*. Examples of iconic, transparent, and opaque signs are presented in Figure 15.1.

Gestural communication systems can be differentiated based on their grammatical structure. As we have discussed, sign language, like ASL, have their own syntax or grammar, whereas sign systems like Signed English are based on, and follow, the rules of American English grammar; thus they are not separate languages.

> American Sign Language is a language, just as Spanish is a language.

ICONIC

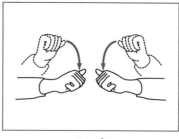

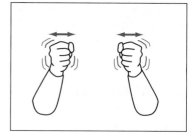

coat

Make an "A" shape with both hands. With thumbs, trace shape of jacket lapels.

cold *(adj.)*

Make an "S" shape with both hands. Draw hands close to body and shiver.

TRANSPARENT

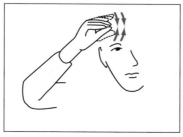

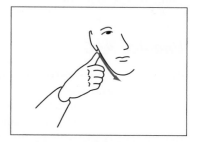

boy

With hand by forehead, snap a flat "O" shape twice, indicating the brim of a baseball cap.

girl

Make an "A" shape with right hand. Place thumb by right earlobe and move down jaw line.

OPAQUE

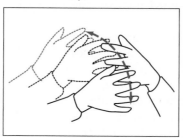

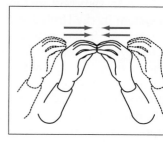

gray

Make a "5" shape with both hands, thumbs up, palms facing body. Move hands back and forth with Ⓡ fingers passing between Ⓛ ones.

more

Make a flat "O" shape with both hands, fingertips facing each other. Tap fingertips together twice.

FIGURE 15.1
. . . .

Examples of Iconic, transparent, and opaque signed English signs.

For most Deaf signers, fingerspelling is mixed with signs and used for new words or names. Fingerspelling, or the manual alphabet, may be a good alternative for older clients with both good cognitive and fine motor abilities. The client has ultimate flexibility because any word in the language can be spelled for transmission.

Unaided systems are not appropriate for every individual who needs either to enhance or replace his or her current method of communicating.

For example, an individual with severe motor involvement in the limbs as in some forms of CP may be unable to make the fine motor adjustments necessary for many signs. Another problem with gestural communication systems has to do with the number of possible communication partners available. Unfortunately, many individuals in the community (e.g., outside of a signer's home or school environments) are not familiar with sign and may not be able to understand what the signer is trying to communicate.

Aided AAC

Communication boards and electronic modes of communication are collectively called **assistive technologies,** a broad term that includes aids for daily living, communication aids, environmental controls, prosthetic and orthotic devices, sensory aids, seating and positioning systems, and mobility/transportation aids.

> AAC is part of a group of assistive technologies that support the needs of people with disabilities.

Aided systems differ in the type of system, the graphic means of representation, and the input and output modes. Selection of each is determined by ongoing careful assessment.

AIDED AAC SYSTEMS

Aided AAC systems vary from "no-tech" through "low-tech" to "high-tech" and can be represented by a continuum of technology (see Figure 15.2). No-tech systems are those that do not involve the use of any technology and use readily available materials (e.g., paper and pencil, writing the letters of the alphabet on a piece of paper so the user can spell out a message). Low-tech systems are those that are fairly simple and contain few moving parts (Mann & Lane, 1991). Examples of low-tech AAC systems include such devices as BIGmack, Step-by-Step, and VoicePal Max, to name a few. High-tech AAC systems are those electronic devices that are considerably more sophisticated, many of which are based on computer technology. Examples would include such devices as a DynaVox, a Lightwriter, or a Pathfinder.

GRAPHIC MEANS OF REPRESENTATION

Whether on a communication board or an electronic device, graphic symbols are just as important to aided AAC as words are to speech or signs to signing. Symbols may include pictures, various representational systems, and/or printed words. Some symbol systems have been specifically designed for AAC use.

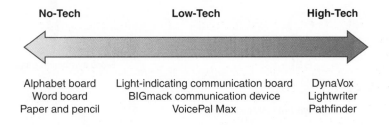

No-Tech	Low-Tech	High-Tech
Alphabet board	Light-indicating communication board	DynaVox
Word board	BIGmack communication device	Lightwriter
Paper and pencil	VoicePal Max	Pathfinder

FIGURE 15.2

Continuum of aided AAC technology with examples of each.

Graphic symbol systems include iconic representations, such as Picture Communication Symbols (PCS) and some Rebus Symbols, less iconic representations, such as Pictogram Ideogram Communication (PIC), and opaque symbol systems, such as Blissymbolics or spelling. These are presented in Figure 15.3. Symbolic systems are more rule-governed and generative, allowing for symbol combination and the creation of new symbols.

Graphic symbol systems may use a variety of means to express different concepts. Rebus symbols are line drawings of both concrete and abstract concepts and of sound sequences, originally developed as an aid for teaching reading. PIC contains ideograms used to represent an idea rather than the way a referent or concept appears in the real world. Ideograms and symbols, such as those used in Blissymbolics, can be used for abstract concepts just as words can. Blissymbols consist of 100 pictographic representations and arbitrary symbols that can be combined to create words.

> Graphic symbols may be selected directly by the AAC user or scanned, when each symbol is highlighted in turn until the desired one is reached.

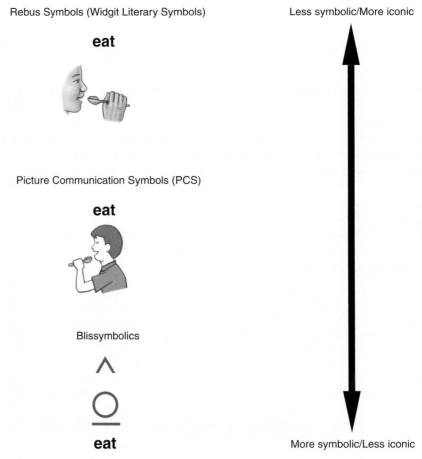

FIGURE 15.3

Iconography of aided symbol systems.

With very young children or more severely cognitively impaired individuals, SLPs may choose to use actual objects, product packaging, photographs, or drawings. These are very concrete and may not represent anything beyond the referent displayed. A system called Tangible Symbols (Rowland & Schweigert, 1989) attempts to bridge the gap between actual objects and graphic representations by using objects or pictures with a clear relationship to the referent. For example, a key or a shoelace might represent *car* or *shoe,* respectively.

AIDED SYSTEM INPUT

Input, or access method, is especially important, and great care must be exercised in choosing the appropriate interface between the client and the device. The two primary means of symbol selection are direct selection and scanning. The client may select the symbol directly by pointing with a finger, hand, head pointer, optical head pointer, or by operating a joystick. In cases of severe neuromuscular involvement, eye gaze, sometimes referred to as eye pointing, may be used to select symbols. Most users of communication boards indicate their message by direct selection.

Pointing may be aided by the use of either hand splints or pointing sticks that strengthen, or enable, the client's response. Optical head pointers may be used with both electronic and nonelectronic systems. For example, something as simple as a small flashlight or penlight attached by a headband to an individual's head communicates when the individual shines the light onto the desired symbol or message. Some electronic communication devices have sensors built into the device itself. The optical head pointers used with these devices typically utilize infrared (IR) technology. As the optical head pointer moves across the symbol display, the device's sensors light up, indicating to the user what symbol it is on. When the individual gets to the desired symbol, he or she stops for a predetermined period of time (called dwell time). Once the user has rested on that location for that period of time, the device "knows" that the user is selecting that symbol. The dwell time on most devices can be set depending on the needs and abilities of each individual.

Individuals using eye gaze may look at symbols on a clear acrylic board located between the user and the communication partner. The user gazes at desired symbols, which appear on both sides of the board.

Direct selection methods are difficult, especially for those with severe motor problems. The main difficulties are speed and accuracy. Although word prediction programs, including context specific prediction, have been proposed to increase efficient use, there do not seem to be statistically significant process and performance differences in actual performance using keystroke-based measures (Higginbotham et al., 2009).

Another access method for individuals with limited motor abilities is scanning. In scanning, the choices are presented sequentially to the user, who then signals when the desired symbol has been presented (Piché & Reichle, 1991; Quist & Lloyd, 1997). This can be done by another person's pointing to symbols on a communication board and the user's signaling when the symbol/message he or she wants to communicate has been presented. Although this form of manual scanning can be and is used, a more common form of scanning is electronic. In this case, the device presents choices to the user, and the user responds or signals by using some type of switch when the desired symbol occurs.

People with motor limitations can use many different types of input—simple pressure switches, pneumatic "sip and puff" switches, and eye blink switches. The type of switch an individual uses depends on his or her particular needs and abilities. Often, an SLP, along with an occupational therapist (OT), is involved in selecting the most appropriate type of switch for an individual to use to access his or her AAC system.

When scanning, an individual activates a switch to start the scanning process. The device then presents the choices. When the symbols are presented visually, either by a light in a corner of the symbol lighting up or by the appearance of an illuminated frame around the symbol, it is referred to as visual scanning. Auditory scanning works in a similar way, but in addition to the symbols being presented visually, there is also an auditory cue present. For example, imagine a lunch page on which the device has the symbols hamburger, hotdog, and pizza present. For visual scanning, when those symbols were presented, an illuminated frame would appear first around the hamburger. If no selection was made, the frame would move to the hotdog, and then if this selection was not made, it would move to pizza. To select pizza, when the pizza symbol was highlighted, the individual would activate his or her switch, and a message that said "I'd like pizza for lunch today" would be spoken by the device. If the individual was an auditory scanner, the device would work as just described, but with the addition of an auditory cue. So when the hamburger symbol was highlighted, the device would say "hamburger." If no selection was made, the illuminated frame would move to hotdog, and the device would say "hotdog." If no selection was made again, the illuminated frame would move to pizza and the device would say "pizza." If the individual activated his or her switch to select pizza, the device would speak the message that had been programmed into that location: "I'd like pizza for lunch today."

Scanning is a very effective option for individuals with significant motor limitations. However, it is an extremely slow and laborious process. The majority of an individual's time is spent waiting while extraneous things are presented. Scanning requires extended concentration and has the potential to be very frustrating, especially when symbols are missed and the process must be repeated.

Efficiency can be enhanced by placing symbols so that the most frequently used symbols are scanned most frequently. For example, if the cursor or indicator begins at the top of the display and returns there after each symbol selection, then the most frequently used symbols would be placed at the top. Obviously, such an arrangement requires constant monitoring by those in the user's environment to ensure peak efficiency. School-age children are more accurate in direct selection than in scanning, indicating the memory retrieval abilities required in scanning (Wagner & Jackson, 2006).

Anticipatory monitoring and the number of pulses required to reach the desired picture are important factors.

Various scanning methods can also increase efficiency (Venkatagiri, 2000). For example, in linear scanning each possible selection is presented in sequence. In contrast, both row-column and block scanning enable the user to scan larger areas, then refine the scan once the desired area has been highlighted. As an example, the user might press the switch to begin the scan. Rows are lighted in sequence until the desired one is found. The user presses the switch again and individual symbols within that row are highlighted one at a time.

Another option is to scan groups of related symbols (group-item display), such as food items, from which the AAC user then selects the desired symbol. Typically developing preschool children are more accurate using direct selection than group-item scanning. Although they required a greater number of cursor movements to select symbols with group-item scanning, there doesn't appear to be a difference in accuracy or the time required (Dropik & Reichle, 2008).

Obviously, the type of access method is as important as the symbol system used. In general, the SLP and client determine the most efficient and accurate access method given the client's cognitive and physical abilities and the environmental demands. Several individuals are presented using AAC devices on the accompanying CD-ROM.

AIDED SYSTEM OUTPUT

As in unaided AAC, with communication boards the partner interprets the message directly. With electronic AAC devices, a wide range of outputs are possible. Electronic output or transmission may be as simple as a light over or behind a symbol or as elaborate as a voice and printed message. SLPs help the client to find the most appropriate output for his or her needs. Several types of output options exist. In some situations, an individual may need written or printed output. For example, at school a device user may need to submit a hard copy of a speech he or she delivered in class, necessitating written output. In many other situations, spoken output or voice output would be the most natural and appropriate.

Voice output communication (VOC) can be either recorded or digitized, synthesized, or a combination of both. Because digitized output is actually prerecorded by a person, it is much more natural sounding, and it is relatively easy to age- and gender-match the voice on the device with the individual using it. However, a disadvantage to digitized VOC is that the only output an individual can produce on his or her device is messages that have already been anticipated and programmed, or stored, in the system's memory. In contrast, synthesized speech has more flexibility but often sounds mechanical or robotic. Instead of recording actual words or phrases, the speech synthesizer contains sounds and rules for combining them. Generally, messages are programmed into a device with synthesized speech by simply typing in the words and phrases/messages. The speech synthesizer then converts that text string into spoken output using the sounds and rules for combining them contained in its program.

Compared to natural speech, comprehension of synthesized speech, found on devices such as DECtalk1 and VeriVox2, requires increased focused attention by the partner. When attention is divided, partners comprehend significantly less synthesized speech (Drager & Reichle, 2001). In addition, partners tend to respond more slowly to synthesized speech (Reynolds & Jefferson, 2000). Although more research is needed on intelligibility, listeners to synthesized speech can improve their speech-sound perceptions through word recognition training (Francis et al., 2007). Even individuals with severe intellectual disabilities can become more proficient at recognizing synthetic speech as a result of repeated exposure to it (Koul & Hester, 2006). For preschool children, intelligibility of synthesized speech is increased if single words are placed within longer language units, such as sentences (Drager et al., 2006).

Decisions on the appropriate type of AAC are made only after careful evaluation. As the user's abilities or needs change, that decision may need to be revisited. Users may also employ multiple types of AAC communication. Training of both the user and others in the user's environment is essential for maximum efficacy.

SPEECH AND AAC

AAC use can change the communication process in ways that are not always predictable.

Obviously, AAC is not the same as speech. There are some important distinctions that may not be readily apparent. First, with the exception of expert signers, the typical AAC user is much slower than the typical speaker. This has implications for users as well as their communication partners. Communication partners may feel compelled to complete the message for the users or take more responsibility for the communication than during speech. The untrained communication partner may take control away from the AAC speaker unintentionally.

Second, some AAC communication is less face-to-face than speech. Both participants may be attending to the device in aided systems. In unaided systems, such as signing, it is easier to glance from hands to face and back, but eye contact will still be less than in speaking situations. With less face-to-face communication, shades of meaning expressed nonlinguistically may be missed.

Finally, although more research is needed, it seems that in actual practice aided AAC is not just speech translated into another form, especially when syntax is involved, as in forming complicated sentences (Trudeau et al., 2007). If, as some researchers believe, graphic symbols are selected prior to sentence formulation, then utterances are constructed directly in the graphic symbol modality. Although AAC users have demonstrated sophisticated linguistic skills, much research is still needed on the impact of AAC on language learning by young children (Blockberger & Johnston, 2001; Blockberger & Sutton, 2003; Fried-Oken & Bersani, 2000; Redmond & Johnston, 2001; Soto, 1999; Williams & Krezman, 2000).

Caregivers sometimes worry that learning a different means of communication will adversely affect an individual's natural speech. People often mistakenly believe that if a person uses AAC, "his or her natural speech will diminish or fail to develop" (Blischak et al., 2003, p. 29). In reality, the opposite is true. As you will see in the following section, learning to use an AAC system often enhances other aspects of communication and can facilitate production of natural speech (Schlosser & Wendt, 2008).

THEORY AND REALITY

Use of AAC has been documented to increase conversational participation, speech intelligibility, and conversational initiations (Dattilo & Camarata, 1991; Glennen & Calculator, 1985; Hunter et al., 1991; Spiegel et al., 1993). Training conversational partners as well as the client results in increased reciprocity in turn taking and initiations (Light et al., 1992).

In short, AAC facilitates the development of both communication and language. None of these positive statements about AAC suggests that it is the great panacea for "curing" all communication ills, but, as with any good intervention method, AAC works very well with certain clients.

Several factors can explain the effects of AAC. These are presented in Figure 15.4. For the user, production may be easier than speech because of reduced physical demands, removal of the pressure to speak, hand-over-hand shaping and modeling, and increased involvement of the right hemisphere. When others in the user's environment also use AAC, they increase the user's comprehension by producing the symbols at a slower rate than speech, by reducing the number of symbols and grammatical structures used, and by eliminating many irrelevant or wordy comments that often accompany speech.

Even the best of methods must be monitored by the SLP for progress and use within the everyday environment of the client. Sometimes AAC methods fail, especially when they are not a good match for the client's abilities and needs and the needs of the environment. For example, if no one in the client's home or school is willing to learn sign, sign usage will not generalize to these situations. Several other factors may account for lack of progress or failure to generalize. These include the lack of useful client-centered content, nonuse in the everyday environment, and inflexibility in the use of the means of communication. Inflexibility is an insistence by either the SLP or the client on the exclusive use of only one means of communication. The need for flexibility was summed up nicely by a young man who is an AAC user: "No one communication mode . . . could possibly meet all my communication needs all of the time. . . . I suggest that everyone needs more than one way to communicate" (Williams, 2004).

Generally, communication is best when multiple means can be used. For example, the client may have some usable speech, a few easily recognizable signs, and a communication board. If the client can easily produce a verbal "no," it seems inflexible to ignore that word and insist on the sign or symbol equivalent.

FIGURE 15.4

Why AAC facilitates communication as compared to speech.

Source: Based on information from "Augmentative and Alternative Communication," by L. L. Lloyd and K. A. Kangas (1994). In G. H. Shames, E. H. Wiig, and W. A. Secord (Eds.), *Human Communication Disorders* (4th ed.). Boston: Allyn and Bacon.

Simplification of input

    Irrelevant and parenthetical comments eliminated.

    Slower rate permits more processing time.

Response production advantages

    Pressure to speak removed.

    Physical demands decreased compared to speech.

    Physical manipulation of client's hands or other parts of body by trainer is possible.

    Client observation of physical manipulation facilitated.

Advantages for individuals with severe cognitive impairment

    Limited and functional vocabulary.

    Individual's attention easier to maintain.

Receptive language/auditory processing advantages

    Structure of language is simplified.

    Auditory short-term memory and/or auditory processing problems minimized.

Simultaneous processing/stimulus association advantages

    Visual nature of the symbol makes it more obvious.

    Visual symbols have more consistency.

    Duration of symbol is greater than spoken word.

    Visual symbols more easily associated with visual referents.

Symbolic representation advantages

    Supplement speech symbols.

    Symbols visually represent referents.

LIFESPAN ISSUES

AAC users may have other needs that call for the use of additional assistive technologies.

Severe communication impairments, whether developmental or acquired, often affect many aspects of an individual's life. In addition, those with severe communication deficits also may have a wide array of other disabling conditions.

Children with evident syndromes or impairments, those at risk, or those failing infant measures, such as hearing screenings, are candidates for early intervention (EI). For some of these children, especially those with CP or deafness, exposure to augmentative communication may begin within the first few months. Caregivers talk to the infant but supplement this input with sign or other visual input. AAC may or may not become the primary means of communication and the SLP will continue to work on oral

CASE STUDY 15.2
Jean's Story

Her parents eagerly anticipated Jean's birth. She was their first child. Although her motor behavior seemed rigid at birth, the pediatrician assured them that her behavior was typical reflexive behavior for an infant. They were saddened and confused when Jean was later diagnosed with spastic cerebral palsy.

Although her parents tried to give Jean a typical childhood, their task was complicated by her motor impairment. Jean was enrolled in a preschool, but her lack of speech and language inhibited her interactions with other children. She was later enrolled in a special preschool where she received speech and language services, daily living skills training, and academic preparation.

Unfortunately, Jean's SLP chose to emphasize speech intervention and AAC was not attempted. When she began first grade, Jean had only a few words that were understood by her immediate family, teacher, and the SLP. Her new SLP decided to use AAC with Jean but opted for signing primarily because other children in the school signed. Signing was not a good match for Jean because of the motor involvement of her hands.

Finally, after several frustrating years of less than adequate communication, Jean's new SLP suggested combined use of an electronic communication board, plus some of Jean's easily recognizable signs and words. Using creative funding and a state grant, the SLP was able to purchase an electronic device. The manual board was used when Jean was between these two sites or when she traveled in the car with her family. Although she used direct selection on her manual board, it was a slow, frustrating process. Her electronic board was accessed through the use of a joystick that enabled Jean to go to the desired symbol.

Now a young adult, Jean lives at home with her parents and attends vocational training at the local United Cerebral Palsy Association workshop. She continues to receive speech-language pathology services and has a large repertoire of graphic symbols at her disposal. She is able to request, to ask and answer questions, and to make conversational comments. Her life has become more fulfilling thanks to the many means she can use to communicate. It is hoped that soon she will be able to attempt an assisted living arrangement.

motor skills and sound production. Case Study 15.2 presents the story of one young woman whose life was changed by AAC.

Just as a developmental continuum exists for speech, so it does for AAC (Cress, 2001). Communication begins with an infant prior to development of speech, language, and AAC use. Experiencing AAC signs and symbols prior to using them directly facilitates a child's understanding of their nature and function (Romski & Sevcik, 1996; Rowland & Schweigert, 2000).

Later, the child may begin to use AAC to produce language. If exposed to signs, children with deafness begin to sign their first words at about 8 months of age. Unfortunately, some infants and toddlers with deafness live in nonsign environments and do not begin to learn sign until they attend a special preschool. Similarly, a child with CP or other disorders can benefit from early exposure to AAC systems.

Some children may not be identified as having a communication impairment until later. As you will recall, children with autism spectrum disorder (ASD) are often not identified until age 2 or older. AAC can provide initial communication and a motivation for learning language. For example, using behavior chain interruption, a technique in which the SLP stops a pleasurable activity and prompts the child to signal beginning again, the SLP can

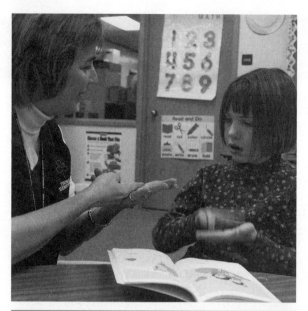

For children with good manual motor control, signing may offer a good means of communication.

establish initial meaningful communication with the child. Communication can then be expanded as new desires by the child are identified.

Inevitably, some children and adolescents experience acquired communication impairments because of accidents or illness. Many children and adolescents with TBI benefit from short-term or long-term use of AAC. In one case, a young man who had lost speech and language as the result of a gun-related suicide attempt was able to retrieve language and some speech by learning signs. His new communication system consists of vocalizations, verbalizations, gestures, and signs.

As AAC users mature, communication needs change. Approximately 20% enjoy full- or part-time employment and may benefit from AAC use on the job (Balandin & Morgan, 2001). Sadly for adults with severe acquired communication disorders, nursing home staffs rarely are knowledgeable in AAC use. Changes in hearing and vision with age may affect AAC use and necessitate system changes. Good communication skills can positively affect health, well-being, and safety (Straus et al., 1999).

For both children and adults with degenerative disorders, aided AAC may provide continued communication when speech is no longer possible. For one young man, it was extremely important to his family that he be able to express his needs and thoughts for as long as possible. Although he became less able to control his body's movements, he continued to communicate. His computer was modified and modified again as his ability to interface changed. Typing letters gave way to touching pictures, which in turn changed to scanning the same pictures. When he could no longer use his computer, a yes/no signal system and eye gaze were used. Throughout this process, the SLP worked closely with the family and the visiting caretakers.

In the early stages of intervention with individuals with degenerative neuromuscular conditions, intervention focuses on maintaining natural communication (Doyle & Phillips, 2001). During the middle stages, as motor function deteriorates, the individual may begin to use AAC in specific situations. As motor control and speech become severely impaired, the individual may rely on AAC. The SLP continually monitors the progress of the disease and modifies the AAC system and/or the interface between the client and the AAC device. As devices have become more sophisticated, many now offer the option of utilizing both digitized (recorded) and synthesized speech, and a process known as "voice banking" has begun to emerge. Before an individual loses his or her ability to speak and before speech is too compromised, he or she records and stores voice samples in an AAC system. This person may not need the AAC system yet but has preserved his or her own voice for the day when it will no longer be usable. There are many benefits of voice banking, not the least of which is that "it enables communication in his or her own voice, tone, and intonation pattern, which helps to preserve a part of his or her personality" (Costello, 2000, p. 141).

Typically functioning adults may also experience accidents and illness that affect communication. As with children, they may benefit from AAC use. Those with apraxia of speech may have very good hand coordination and may be primary candidates for AAC use. Likewise, individuals with aphasia or TBI may benefit from the use of graphic symbols or signs. Much visual information is interpreted in the right hemisphere. By tapping into this area of the brain, it is possible with some clients with aphasia or TBI to build a "bridge" to the damaged areas of the left hemisphere and to improve access to language.

It may be more difficult for an adult who once spoke typically to accept AAC. Embarrassment and shame may accompany the loss of speech or language. The SLP must counsel the client and family on the positive benefits of AAC use.

ASSESSMENT CONSIDERATIONS

It is not always clear whether a client will benefit from AAC use. If the SLP believes that AAC support may be beneficial in the future, the topic should be introduced early in the assessment and intervention process. Need becomes apparent if the client's communication abilities are being constrained by slowly recovering or developing speech. The following recommendations can help families accept AAC use (Zangari, 2001):

- Provide honest information
- Honor their concerns and provide information that addresses those concerns
- Recognize the emotional impact in realizing that a loved one may use AAC and try to address concerns that are stated and those that are not
- Address the client's strengths and the way in which AAC enhances them
- Provide specific rationales for your recommendations

As in other areas of speech-language pathology, careful thorough assessment of a client's abilities and needs is essential for determining the appropriate AAC system and the course of intervention services. Assessment should include not only the client's speech, language, and communication abilities and needs but also motor and perceptual skills, communication preferences, and the willingness of the environment to support AAC use. This data will be collected through the help of a team of professionals who will be identified as we discuss each element of the evaluation.

As noted in other assessments of communication impairment, assessment for AAC use is a team effort.

Speech considerations include the types of sounds and sound combinations produced, intelligibility, and connected speech. Spontaneous speech and imitative speech samples should be collected and analyzed. In addition, an oral peripheral examination with attention to different motor behaviors, swallowing, and oral movement imitation is essential.

Hearing is extremely important for speech production and feedback and should be assessed thoroughly by an audiologist. Seniors may have hearing loss that is unrelated or related to the acquired speech and/or language impairment. Individuals with developmental speech and/or language impairments may have hearing, perceptual, or central auditory processing impairments related to various syndromes or disorders.

Language and prelanguage skills, both receptive and expressive, will be important for programming content and selection of symbol systems, especially graphic. Although certain cognitive abilities seem to be needed for some types of symbol use, such as use of printed words, clients should not be excluded from AAC consideration because these abilities are still developing. Prelinguistic skills can be taught at the same time the client is learning to communicate with the AAC system.

The client's current communication skills are very important. The desire to communicate or to improve communication is the basis for AAC intervention and the motivation for learning. Although individuals with severe disabilities have great difficulty making clear and intentional signals, they often create their own individualistic gestures (Iacono et al., 1998; Yoder & Munson, 1995). The multimodal nature of AAC necessitates a systematic exploration of the role these gestures and other forms play in communication (Hunt-Berg, 2001; Reichle et al., 1998).

It is very difficult not to communicate. Consequently, one of the SLP's roles is to determine the communication method, or methods, currently used by the client. This is often more difficult than it sounds because sometimes the manner in which an individual is communicating is not always recognized as communication. For example, a young girl with severe disabilities was frequently observed to tap her cheek after coming in from the playground. It was not until the SLP began to look at that behavior more closely that people realized she was using that cheek tapping to indicate that she wanted a drink. Communication is often demonstrated when an individual engages in a consistent behavior (e.g., cheek tapping) in the same situations over time (e.g., after coming in from the playground). The SLP should also attempt to determine the current and future communication needs of the client.

An occupational (OT) and/or physical therapist (PT) can aid in motor assessment. Of interest is ambulation or the ability to move about, fine motor dexterity for signing or pointing, range of movement especially of the upper limbs, motor imitation skills, and the consistency and accuracy of motor responses. This data will be extremely important in deciding the appropriate aided or unaided system and the placement and size of graphic symbols.

Caregivers are part of the AAC intervention team.

Visual and auditory acuity and perception will be important for system selection and intervention. Vision, along with motor skills, will be used to decide the size of graphic symbols. A vision specialist will be an invaluable member of the team in assessing these abilities.

Occasionally, the environment will not support the use of AAC. Caregivers may be uncomfortable, feel inadequate, or just not want to be involved. The SLP may need to educate caregivers about the benefits of AAC to the client and to the home or school. Explaining the likely course of intervention may increase caregiver comfort levels.

Last, the SLP is interested in collecting a list of client preferences and of possible symbols to train. Likes and desires of the client will be important for intervention. This information can be gathered from client responses or choices, from caregiver suggestions, or through observation of the client. This portion of the assessment can be very positive with the focus on communication potential rather than on impairment. It is especially important for those with acquired communication disabilities, such as dysarthria, in which the focus tends to be on loss rather than potential (Klasner & Yorkston, 2001). A positive shift is welcome.

The actual assessment is only a first step. The SLP, in coordination with the family and other professionals, such as the OT, PT, audiologist, vision specialist, psychologist, rehabilitation engineer, and/or classroom teacher, uses the data from the assessment to make decisions on the appropriate AAC method, AAC symbol system, and potential vocabulary. These decisions will be adjusted and modified as the client progresses. A good fit increases the likelihood of success.

AAC System Selection

In deciding on the appropriate AAC system or method, the SLP considers the client's motor and cognitive abilities, the potential size of the client's vocabulary, the ease in learning and using the system, the acceptability of the system to the user and potential communication partners, and the flexibility and intelligibility of the system. For example, unaided systems are very portable and can be expanded easily without concern for limited storage or display space but allow for no permanent record, thus necessitating use of some graphic system for purposes such as homework. Many graphic symbols appear with the printed word, making them easy for communication partners to use, but these same symbols require the partner to concentrate on the graphic message to the exclusion of the user's face.

The potential user's motor abilities are very important in determining the best system to use. Individuals with severe motor impairments in their upper extremities may be poor candidates for unaided systems. However, poor pointing skills need not deter the individual from using a communication board or a device and accessing it via head pointing, eye gaze, or with an assistive device like a T-stick that allows the individual to hold the pointer in both hands while the bottom leg of the "T" serves to point to the desired symbol or location. In addition, poor motor abilities may dictate the use of certain selection methods (e.g., scanning) to access an electronic communication device.

Those in the potential user's communication environment also must find the AAC system acceptable. Lack of portability or embarrassment concerning use may lead to nonuse in certain situations or by some potential partners.

The selection of the AAC system can lead to further questions. For example, if the SLP decides to use a communication board, several considerations influence its final design. These include, but are not limited to, the construction material, overall size, arrangement and size of the symbols, placement and organization of the symbols, and the mounting of the board if necessary.

AAC Symbol Selection

Decisions on the appropriate symbol system will flow naturally from the method of communication chosen. If signing is deemed to be the appropriate method, the SLP must make decisions on the best gestural or sign system to use. In addition to the cognitive and motor abilities of the potential user, the SLP might consider the gestural or signing system used most frequently in the client's school or workplace and in the local community, the availability of teaching materials, and the ease in using these materials.

AAC system selection is much more than merely matching the client and the system.

Selection of aided symbol systems may be guided by the potential user's cognitive abilities, the ease of learning different graphic AAC systems, and the willingness of potential communication partners. Aided symbols form a continuum from actual objects, which may represent only themselves, to letters that can be used to spell words. As we move from concrete objects to abstract symbols and letters, the client gains increased communication flexibility. Although not all clients can spell or use an encryption code, potential partners may be uneasy with interpretation of pictures, photographs, or other symbols. If we expect the client to use the system at home or in school, then these partner concerns must be treated seriously.

AAC Vocabulary Selection

Vocabulary should reflect the client's current needs and communication potential.

The vocabulary chosen will have a great impact on future communication. Decisions about potential vocabulary will continue to be made as long as the client uses AAC. The best guideline is to select vocabulary that reflects the user's needs, desires, likes, and preferences and is functional or useful based on observation of the client and the communication environment. The resultant vocabulary should be highly individualized.

Several lists of potential vocabulary are available and may serve as a guide when matched with the client's communication needs. These lists may also suggest various communication intentions and semantic categories of language that are important for early language development with presymbolic clients. Individuals with acquired speech and language impairments may have very different needs and rarely must relearn language.

The order of teaching signs or symbols must also be guided by the client's immediate needs. In addition, the iconicity and transparency of different signs/symbols must be considered. Selecting appropriate and useful vocabulary can make or break how successful an AAC system will be for an individual. "Poorly selected or inappropriate vocabulary may be one of the primary deterrents to successful communication" (Yorkston et al., 1989, p. 101). The impact of vocabulary selection on AAC use cannot be underestimated.

INTERVENTION CONSIDERATIONS

Although intervention will be a team effort, it is important for services not to become fragmented (Beukelman & Mirenda, 1992). Rather, a coherent, holistic approach is needed—one that includes the user's natural environment and communication partners. Family members, whether parents of a child with a developmental communication impairment or spouses and children of an adult with an acquired communication impairment, must be integral members of the intervention team.

The SLP must be concerned with linguistic and communicative competence as well as operational competence for the AAC system being trained. It's not enough, however, for a child simply to have assistive technology and the skills to operate it. A child needs to be able to communicate spontaneously in family interactions and in everyday settings (Granlund et al., 2008).

Some important considerations for an SLP are as seemingly simple as the location of symbols on a communication board, whereas others involve the teaching of complex syntactic constructions. For example, both typically developing children and those with Down syndrome like drawings that share a color and are clustered together to create a subgroup, such as clothing or food, to facilitate both the speed and accuracy of locating the target symbol (Wilkinson et al., 2008).

Children with ID do not seem to induce English word order rules from the language spoken around them and apply these rules to their sign output (Grove & Dockrell, 2000; Smith & Grove, 1999). Occasionally, they change the form of the signs creatively, such as performing the sign "hit" in the location where the blow occurred, to indicate changes in meaning. In this way, signs are used more as gestures (Grove & Dockrell, 2000; Rudd et al., 2007; Woll et al., 1997).

In any case, production of longer grammatical utterances is slow if users are forming them from single symbols. One option for increasing the rate of production is to prestore potential utterances in the device. The disadvantage is that the utterance may not fit a communication situation exactly. This said, partners seem to prefer these less than precise but more quickly produced messages (McCoy et al., 2007).

Modeling is one method for teaching production of multisymbol messages (Binger & Light, 2007). The SLP points to two symbols on the child's AAC device, such as *mommy* and *eat,* while providing a grammatically complete spoken model, such as "Mommy is eating." This teaching can be enhanced by the use of matrix strategies in which all actions needed are combinable with all objects and by milieu language teaching strategies

FIGURE 15.5
....

Possible matrix format.

	Pencil	Book	Wagon	Car	Cocoa	Tea
Drop	Drop pencil	Drop book				
Pick up	Pick up pencil	Pick up book				
Push			Push wagon	Push car		
Pull			Pull wagon	Pull car		
Drink					Drink cocoa	Drink tea
Make					Make cocoa	Make tea

(Nigam et al., 2006). In milieu teaching, an SLP might perform an action while asking, "What am I doing?" If a child fails to respond or responds incorrectly, the SLP models the correct response and then asks again. A sample matrix is presented in Figure 15.5.

Intervention must include both the short-range and long-range needs of the client (Beukelman & Mirenda, 1997). As users move beyond the school years, there is a need for easily accessible vocabulary that reflects socially valued adult roles, such as being a college student or engaging in intimate relationships (Nelson Bryen, 2008).

Although many of the good intervention practices described in Chapter 4 are equally important when working with individuals using AAC, other intervention considerations apply more specifically to AAC (Zangari & Kangas, 1997). These include but are not limited to the following:

- Establish an environment of AAC
- Use everyday experiences as the training context
- Individualize the content as discussed earlier
- Train others to modify their interactional style
- Consider positioning for those with severe motor impairments
- Make communication real

Each of these are discussed in some detail.

Although individual client factors are important, two external factors that contribute to positive outcomes are community support and parent and family support (Lund & Light, 2007b). Such environmental support is very important. Abandonment of AAC technology usually is related to loss of facilitator/partner support rather than rejection of the technology (Fager et al., 2006).

An environment of augmentative communication is very important and highlights the need to have others, such as caregivers and teachers, involved. The AAC system should be used by others and aided systems should always be available for the user. We are reminded of one teacher who constructed a huge communication board on one wall of her classroom so that she could use it when addressing the entire class. Naturally, integration into the classroom requires a collaborative strategy involving both the classroom teacher and the SLP. AAC training for the entire educational team—teachers, instructional aides, SLPs, and parents—is a key element in success with children (Soto et al., 2001).

Intervention will be maximally effective if caregivers also use AAC along with speech. Caregivers can be taught a few simple signs, or they can learn to use an individual's communication board and point to a symbol while speaking their message. For individuals using an electronic device, caregivers can and should learn to use the device, and again, pair what they are saying with using the voice output of the device. This is referred to as augmented input, and it serves as a model for use of the communication device (Romski & Sevcik, 1996).

Caregivers are sometimes fearful that they will be expected to sign as if interpreting for a deaf audience. Nothing could be further from reality with most clients. Signs or graphic symbols can be used as gestures for important words in an utterance as the caregiver continues to speak.

One unintended consequence of AAC use by nonsymbolic children with profound multiple disabilities is that over time, a child becomes more and more dependent on one or two skilled interaction partners within the family. As a result, the child is less likely to interact with a range of partners within the family (Wilder & Granlund, 2006). This is especially true if a child learns to use an AAC mode, but family members do not develop sufficient skills in that mode (Thunstam, 2004). As much as possible we want to program so that the client has multiple partners in multiple situations to increase social integration, especially among peers. In one classroom, we trained partners to interact with AAC users and reinforced them when they did. Educators can also organize clubs and experiences, such as an integrated dramatic arts program, to promote AAC use (McCarthy & Light, 2001).

In short, the SLP must identify opportunities for communication, create a need for communication, and maximize the instructional benefit of these opportunities (Sigafoos, 2000). Partners will need instructional support if they are to function as effective communication partners for AAC users.

> All members of the intervention team should use the AAC system to provide multiple partners and multiple situations.

One method that holds some promise for children with ASD is *aided language modeling* (ALM), consisting of engaging children in interactive play activities and providing models of AAC symbol use during play (Drager, Postal et al., 2006). ALM is implemented in a natural play context in which the child is provided models of use of the AAC symbols on a communication board.

Clients with acquired communication impairments may elect, if possible, to continue to work. Self-reports indicate that access to appropriate AAC systems is an important factor in facilitating continued employment (McNaughton et al., 2001). In addition, job-related social networks can be maintained by e-mail and the Internet (Nelson Bryen, 2006).

Everyday events and routines provide *scripts* or personalized event sequences that enable each of us to participate. When circumstances are

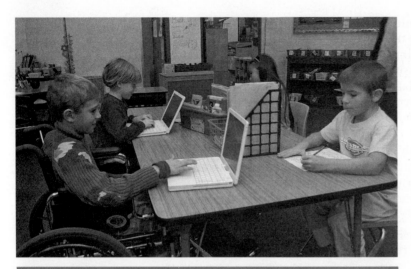

In order for AAD training to generalize to everyday use, important people in a user's life should be included in the intervention.

modified as in the use of AAC, we rely heavily on the script to help us. Use of the script frees "cognitive energy" to be applied to other aspects of the situation. In addition, the use of everyday events teaches the client to use AAC as the need arises. The SLP must use instructional strategies that integrate AAC into the different communication environments of the user (Ball et al., 2000; Rainforth et al., 1992). Even children using low-tech communication boards can have ample opportunities to use their AAC systems to communicate during the school day in greetings, academics, snack, sharing, and recess (Downey et al., 2004).

Acceptance of AAC is the degree to which the system is integrated into the life of the user (Lasker & Bedrosian, 2000). Optimal use occurs when AAC is used willingly and at every opportunity. Community-based training approaches in which the client becomes more comfortable and efficient using AAC in public may lead to optimal use (Lasker & Bedrosian, 2001). In these approaches, venues, such as the post office, grocery store, and fast-food outlets, are identified. Training begins with scripted interactions that are modified gradually to more spontaneous communication.

Unless trained, well-meaning communication partners may assume too active a role in their interaction with the AAC user. Partners need to offer real choices to AAC users, to acknowledge the user's communication attempts, and to allow time for the user to express the message.

Often because of the device, communication takes place at a very close distance, enabling the partner to be inside the user's space. To encourage social interaction by the AAC user, SLPs may want to do something as simple as increasing the communication distance (Sigafoos et al., 2009).

Because communication partners may be unfamiliar with AAC, it is important that systems and their purpose be explained carefully and demonstrated (Cress, 2001). Partners should also be trained to use AAC expressively, not because they need AAC to be understood, but because they can help the user acclimate to this new method of communication.

Partners should be consulted for their observations, suggestions, and ideas for intervention. As members of the intervention team, they become invested in the outcomes for the client.

For clients with severe motor impairments, such as CP, positioning is very important and can often be the determining factor in successful motor movement. Control of the head, shoulders, spine, and hips and alignment along the midline is essential.

Finally, the user of AAC must be involved in real communication and versatile with meaningful outcomes. Otherwise, for individuals with progressive disorders, such as ALS, communication becomes solely a means of regulating the behavior of others for basic needs and wants (Fried-Oken et al., 2006). It is all too easy for intervention to evolve into drill in which the client touches objects or pictures with no real outcome except a reinforcing word by the SLP or other partner. Training must include real communication choices, not just performance of a sign or locating a symbol. With meaningful communication, the grief and sense of loss that accompanies acquired communication impairments and laryngectomy and glossectomy can be replaced by a sense of empowerment (Fox & Rau, 2001).

Evidence-Based Practice

Although each client seen by an SLP is unique, those with AAC needs are especially so. This, plus the relatively low number of users seen by any one SLP, makes conducting clinical research especially difficult. As a result, many studies include only a single subject or a very small number of subjects, resulting in conclusions that cannot be generalized to most users. In addition, few studies of AAC intervention have evaluated the effects of intervention on the family and on broader social contacts (see Box 15.1)

BOX 15.1
Evidence-Based Practice with AAC

Overall

- Little long-term research exists. Longitudinal research is needed that focuses on everyday functioning of children and adults who use AAC.
- Improved speech intelligibility doesn't necessarily lead to enhanced participation in social interactions. Generalization to social situations must be included in intervention.
- With continued use, turn-taking becomes more equitable between the AAC user and speaking partner.

Symbol selection

- Scanning is especially difficult for young children. Direct selection is easier to teach.

Effect on speech production

- For children with autism spectrum disorder or mental retardation, AAC intervention does not impede speech production. Most studies report an increase in speech production, albeit rather modest in most cases. These results require that SLPs help families

and clients to have realistic expectations about speech gains.
- For children with autism spectrum disorder, the gains in overall communication from the use of sign are modest.

Syntax and morphology

- Although many individuals who use AAC can comprehend and express a wide range of grammatical structures, they tend to produce shorter utterances when they use graphic symbol-based AAC systems.

Family participation

- Few studies have investigated the effectiveness of AAC-specific aspects of intervention in a family context, making it difficult to draw any empirically based conclusions about the effectiveness of these interventions in family environments.

Source: Based on Binger & Light (2008); Granlund et al. (2008); Lund & Light (2006, 2007a); Millar et al. (2006); Schlosser & Wendt (2008); Schwartz & Nye (2006); Snell et al. (2006).

SUMMARY

Augmentative and alternative communication (AAC) includes many forms and the strategies and methods to assist individuals in using them to meet their communication needs. AAC may enhance or augment an individual's speech or may become the primary means of communication.

Although the specific goals of AAC intervention vary with each individual user, treatment aims include the following:

1. Assist individuals with their daily communication needs.
2. Help facilitate the development of speech and language.
3. Help facilitate the return of speech and language.

Decisions on the appropriate type of AAC may need to be revised as the user's abilities or needs change. Users may also employ multiple types of AAC communication. Training of both the user and others in the user's environment is essential for maximum efficacy.

A careful, thorough assessment of a client's abilities and needs is essential for determining the appropriate AAC system and the course of intervention services.

The SLP, in coordination with the family and other professionals, uses the data from the assessment to make decisions on the appropriate AAC method, AAC symbol system, and potential vocabulary.

The SLP must be concerned with linguistic and communicative competence as well as operational competence for the AAC system being trained. Intervention must include both the short-range and long-range communication needs of the client.

THOUGHT QUESTIONS

- What are the major types of unaided and aided AAC systems?
- How do AAC needs change throughout the lifespan?
- What are the major concerns in client assessment for AAC?
- What are the major elements of intervention with AAC?

SUGGESTED READINGS

Lloyd, L. L., Fuller, D. R., & Arvidson, H. H. (1997). *Augmentative and alternative communication: A handbook of principles and practices.* Boston: Allyn and Bacon.

Reichle, J., Halle, J. W., & Drasgow, E. (1998). Implementing augmentative communication systems. In A. Wetherby, S. Warren, & J. Reichle (Eds.), *Transitions in prelinguistic communication* (pp. 417–436). Baltimore: Brookes.

ONLINE RESOURCES

About.com
http://specialed.about.com/od/augmentativecommunication/Augmentative_
or_Alternative_Communication_Vendor_Sites_AAC.htm
About.com New York Times site has links to several manufacturers of assistive
devices.

American Speech-Language-Hearing Association
www.asha.org/public/speech/disorders/AAC.htm
ASHA Web site has detailed discussion of AAC.

**International Association for Augmentative and Alternative
Communication**
www.isaac-online.org/en/interactive/index.html
International Association for Augmentative and Alternative Communication
Web site is the professional site for those interested in AAC, containing discus-
sions and links.

University of California Northridge
www.aacintervention.com/boardmaker.html
University of California Northridge Web site with usable Boardmaker information and lots more.

Requirements for Becoming an Audiologist

After January 1, 2012, applicants for certification in audiology will need a **doctoral degree** from a graduate program accredited by the ASHA Council on Academic Accreditation in Audiology and Speech-Language Pathology (CAA).

The program of study includes the following:

- A minimum of **75 semester credit hours of academic course work and at least 12 months of full-time equivalent of supervised and verified clinical practicum**.
- Practicum should be of sufficient depth and breadth to achieve the knowledge and skills outcomes required.
- A variety of clinical practicum experiences in different work settings and with different populations so student can demonstrate skills across the scope of practice in audiology.
- The total of clinical experiences should equal 52 work weeks of at least 35 hours per week in direct patient/client contact, consultation, record keeping, and administrative duties.

KNOWLEDGE AND SKILLS OUTCOMES

Prerequisite knowledge and skills in the foundations of practice, prevention and identification, evaluation, and treatment, including:

- Oral and written or other communication
- Life sciences, physical sciences, behavioral sciences, and mathematics
- Professional codes of ethics and credentialing
- Patient characteristics and their relationship to clinical services

- Educational, vocational, and social and psychological effects of hearing impairment and their impact on treatment program development
- Anatomy and physiology, pathophysiology and embryology, and development of the auditory and vestibular systems
- Normal development of speech and language
- Phonologic, morphologic, syntactic, and pragmatic aspects of communication associated with hearing impairment
- Normal processes of speech and language production and perception through the lifespan
- Normal aspects of auditory physiology and behavior through the lifespan
- Psychoacoustic principles, methods, and applications
- Effects of chemical agents on the auditory and vestibular systems
- Instrumentation and bioelectrical hazards
- Infectious/contagious diseases and universal precautions
- Physical characteristics and measurement of acoustic stimuli and of electric and other nonacoustic stimuli
- Research principles and practices, including experimental design, statistical methods, and application to clinical populations
- Medical/surgical procedures for treatment of auditory and vestibular system disorders
- Health care and educational delivery systems
- Effects of cultural diversity on professional practice
- Supervisory processes and procedures
- Laws, regulations, policies, and management practices relative to audiology
- Use of manual communication, interpreters, and assistive technology

Competence in the prevention and identification of auditory and vestibular disorders, including the following:

- Interacting effectively with patients, families, other appropriate individuals, and professionals
- Preventing the onset and minimizing the development of communication disorders
- Identifying individuals at risk
- Screening individuals for
  - Hearing impairment and disability/handicap using clinically appropriate and culturally sensitive screening measures
  - Speech and language impairments and other factors affecting communication function using clinically appropriate and culturally sensitive screening measures
- Administering hearing conservation programs

Competence in the evaluation of individuals with suspected disorders of auditory, balance, communication, and related systems, including the following:

- Interacting effectively with patients, families, other appropriate individuals, and professionals
- Evaluating information from appropriate sources
- Obtaining a case history
- Performing an otoscopic examination
- Determining the need for removal of cerumen
- Administering clinically appropriate and culturally sensitive assessment
- Performing
  - Audiologic assessment using physiologic, psychophysical, and self-assessment measures
  - Electrodiagnostic test procedures
  - Balance system assessment and determination of the need for balance rehabilitation
  - Aural rehabilitation assessment
- Documenting evaluation procedures and results
- Interpreting results to establish type and severity of disorder
- Generating recommendations and referrals
- Providing counseling to facilitate understanding
- Maintaining records consistent with legal and professional standards
- Communicating results and recommendations orally and in writing
- Using instrumentation according to specifications and recommendations
- Determining instrumentation calibration

Competence in the treatment of individuals with auditory, balance, and related communication disorders, including:

- Interacting effectively with patients, families, other appropriate individuals, and professionals
- Developing and implementing treatment plan
- Discussing prognosis and treatment options
- Counseling patients, families, and other appropriate individuals
- Developing culturally sensitive and age-appropriate management strategies
- Collaborating with other service providers
- Performing hearing aid, assistive listening device, and sensory aid assessment
- Recommending, dispensing, and servicing prosthetic and assistive devices

- Providing hearing aid, assistive listening device, and sensory aid orientation
- Conducting aural rehabilitation
- Monitoring and summarizing treatment progress and outcomes
- Assessing efficacy of interventions
- Establishing criteria for treatment admission and discharge
- Serving as an advocate
- Documenting treatment procedures and results
- Maintaining records consistent with legal and professional standards
- Communicating results, recommendations, and progress
- Using instrumentation according to specifications and recommendations
- Determining instrumentation calibration

Demonstrate successful and verifiable achievement of the knowledge and skills: evidence of a **passing score on the ASHA-approved national examination in audiology** within 5 years prior to the certification application submission.

Continued professional development to maintain the Audiology Certificate of Clinical Competence, renewed every 3 years.

Adherence to the ASHA Code of Ethics.

Source: Based on information from ASHA (2009b).

Requirements for Becoming a Speech-Language Pathologist

Graduate degree from a regionally accredited institution of higher education.

Completion of a program of study (a minimum of 75 semester credit hours overall, including at least 36 at the graduate level) that includes:

- At least one course in each of the following areas: biological sciences, physical sciences, social/behavioral sciences, and mathematics.
- Demonstrated knowledge of
  - Basic human communication and swallowing processes, including their biological, neurological, acoustic, psychological, developmental, and linguistic and cultural bases; and the ability to integrate information pertaining to normal and abnormal human development across the life span, including basic communication processes and the impact of cultural and linguistic diversity on communication.
  - The nature of speech, language, hearing, and communication disorders and differences and swallowing disorders, including the etiologies, characteristics, anatomical/physiological, acoustic, psychological, developmental, linguistic, and cultural correlates. Specific knowledge must be demonstrated in articulation, fluency, voice and resonance including respiration and phonation, receptive and expressive language, hearing including the impact on speech and language, swallowing, cognitive and social aspects of communication, and communication modalities including augmentative and alternative communication techniques and assistive technologies.

- The principles and methods of prevention, assessment, and intervention for people with communication and swallowing disorders, including consideration of anatomical/physiological, psychological, developmental, and linguistic and cultural correlates of the disorders.

- Standards of ethical conduct.

- Processes used in research and the integration of research principles into evidence-based clinical practice.

- Contemporary professional issues.

- Certification, specialty recognition, licensure, and other relevant professional credentials.

Completion of a curriculum of academic and clinical education that follows an appropriate sequence of learning including:

- Supervised clinical experiences sufficient in breadth and depth to achieve the following skills outcomes:
  - Evaluation:
    - Conduct screening and prevention procedures (including prevention activities)
    - Collect case history information and integrate information
    - Select and administer appropriate evaluation procedures
    - Adapt evaluation procedures to meet client/patient needs
    - Interpret, integrate, and synthesize all information to develop diagnoses and make appropriate recommendations for intervention
    - Complete administrative and reporting functions
    - Refer clients/patients for appropriate services
  - Intervention:
    - Develop setting-appropriate intervention plans with measurable and achievable goals that meet clients'/patients' needs
    - Implement intervention plans
    - Select or develop and use appropriate materials and instrumentation for prevention and intervention
    - Measure and evaluate clients'/patients' performance and progress
    - Modify intervention plans, strategies, materials, or instrumentation as appropriate to meet the needs of clients/patients
    - Complete administrative and reporting functions necessary to support intervention
    - Identify and refer clients/patients for services as appropriate

- Interaction and personal qualities:
  - Communicate effectively, recognizing the needs, values, preferred mode of communication, and cultural/linguistic background of the client/patient, family, caregivers, and relevant others
  - Collaborate with other professionals in case management
  - Provide counseling regarding communication and swallowing disorders
  - Adhere to the ASHA Code of Ethics and behave professionally
  - Demonstrate skill in oral and written or other forms of communication sufficient for entry into professional practice.

- A minimum of **400 clock hours of supervised clinical experience** in the practice of speech-language pathology. Twenty-five hours must be spent in clinical observation, and 375 hours must be spent in direct client/patient contact. At least 325 of the 400 clock hours must be completed while the applicant is engaged in graduate study.

- Supervision must be provided by individuals who hold the Certificate of Clinical Competence in the appropriate area of practice. No less than 25 percent of the student's total contact should be with each client/patient and must take place periodically throughout the practicum.

- Supervised practicum must include experience with client/patient populations through the lifespan and from culturally/linguistically diverse backgrounds and with various types and severities of communication and/or related disorders, differences, and disabilities.

Demonstrate successful and verifiable achievement of the knowledge and skills: evidence of a **passing score on the ASHA-approved national examination** in speech-language pathology within 5 years prior to the certification application submission.

Continued professional development to maintain SLP Certificate of Clinical Competence, renewed every 3 years.

Adherence to the ASHA Code of Ethics.

Source: Based on information from ASHA (2009a).

Glossary

Abdominal aponeurosis   Broad sheet of connective tissue covering the front of the abdominal wall.

Acoustic immittance   The term used to refer to either the flow or opposition to the flow of energy through the middle.

Acoustic neuroma   A tumor of the vestibulocochlear (VIIIth) nerve.

Acquired   Occurring after birth.

Acquired immunodeficiency syndrome (AIDS)   A viral disease in which a person becomes susceptible to an assortment of other illnesses.

Acute laryngitis   Temporary swelling of the vocal folds, resulting in a hoarse voice quality.

Acute otitis media   Inflammation of the middle ear characterized by rapid onset, with resolution within approximately 3 weeks.

Addition   In articulation, the insertion of a phoneme that is not part of the word.

Adventitious   Occurring sometime after birth.

Affricate   A combination of a stop and fricative phoneme.

Agnosia   Sensory deficit accompanying some aphasias that make it difficult to understand incoming sensory information.

Agrammatism   Omission of spoken and written grammatical elements found in some aphasias in which individuals omit short unstressed words and morphological endings.

Agraphia   Writing difficulty accompanying some aphasias and characterized by mistakes and poorly formed letters.

AIDS   See *Acquired immunodeficiency syndrome.*

Air conduction   A method of evaluating hearing by transmitting sound to the inner ear via the outer and middle ear.

Alexia   Reading difficulties found in some aphasias in which the client may be unable to recognize even common words that he or she says.

Allophone   A phonemic variation.

Alport's syndrome   A hereditary disorder characterized by kidney disease and bilateral progressive sensorineural hearing loss.

Alveolar   Refers to the alveolar or gum ridge of the mouth. In speech, alveolar consonants are those produced with the tongue on the alveolar ridge.

Alveolar pressure   The pressure inside the lungs.

Alveolus   Area of the mandible and maxilla that houses the teeth.

Alzheimer's disease   A cortical pathology that affects primarily memory, language, or visuospatial skills as a result of diffuse brain atrophy; presenile dementia.

American Sign Language (ASL)   A complex non-vocal language containing elaborate syntax and semantics. Proficiency in its use is one of the primary methods by which a deaf individual becomes part of the Deaf Community.

Amplification   Technology such as hearing aids, cochlear implants, and assistive listening devices that improve access to sounds by electronically increasing their intensity.

Amyotrophic lateral sclerosis (ALS)   Commonly called Lou Gehrig's disease, ALS is a rapidly progressive degenerative disease in which the individuals gradually loses control of their musculature. It is characterized by fatigue, muscle atrophy or loss of bulk, involuntary contractions, and reduced muscle tone. Speech in the later stages is labored and slow with short phrasing, long pauses, hypernasality, and severely impaired articulation.

Anatomy   The study of the structures of the body and the relationship of these structures to one another.

Aneurysm   A type of hemorrhagic stroke resulting from the rupture of a sac-like bulging in a weakened artery wall.

Ankyloglossia   Tongue-tie; a relatively short lingual frenum.

Anomia   Difficulty naming entities.

Anomic aphasia   A fluent aphasia characterized by naming difficulties and mild to moderate auditory comprehension problems.

Anoxia   Deprivation of oxygen.

Aphasia   An impairment due to localized brain injury and affecting understanding, retrieving, and formulating meaningful and sequential elements of language.

Aplasia   Hearing loss due to the absence of the inner ear structures during embryonic development.

Approximant   Sometimes called a semivowel; an oral consonant that is produced with less constriction than the obstruents, includes glides and liquids.

Apraxia of speech   A neurological impairment of the ability to program—organize and plan—and execute movement of the speech muscles, unrelated to muscle weakness, slowness, or paralysis.

Arteriovenous malformation   A poorly formed tangle of arteries and veins that may result in a rare type of stroke in which arterial walls are weak and give way under pressure.

Articulation   Rapid and coordinated movement of the tongue, teeth, lips, and palate to produce speech sounds.

Articulatory/resonating system   Structures used during sound production including the oral cavity, nasal cavity, tongue, and soft palate.

Aryepiglottic folds   The membrane and muscle that connect the sides of the epiglottis to the arytenoid cartilages in the larynx.

Asperger syndrome (AS)   Mild form of pervasive developmental disorder (PDD) characterized by normal intelligence and typical language development with deficits in social and communication skills.

Aspiration   Inhaling; used to mean the inhalation of fluid or food into the lungs; in phonology, a puff of air that is released in the production of various allophones.

Assessment of communication disorders   The systematic process of obtaining information from many source, through various means, and in different settings to verify and specify communication strengths and weaknesses, identify possible causes, and make plans to address them.

Assistive listening devices (ALD)   The general term applied to electronic devices designed to enhance the reception of sound by those who are hearing-impaired.

Assistive technologies   Aids for daily living, communication, environmental controls; prosthetic or orthotic devices; sensory aids; seating and positioning systems; and mobility/transportation aids.

Ataxia   Disorder of muscle coordination.

Ataxic cerebral palsy   A congenital disorder characterized by uncoordinated movement and disturbed balance. Movements lack direction, and hypotonic muscles lack adequate force and rate and have poor directional control.

Ataxic dysarthria   A motor-speech disorder involving a combination of muscle weakness or reduced tone or hypotonia and problems with muscle coordination. Little or no paralysis exists, and the problem is one involving the accuracy, timing, and direction of movement. Speech is characterized by excessive and equal stress and imprecise articulation, especially in repetitive movements.

Atresia   Congenital disorder resulting in complete closure of the external auditory meatus.

Attention deficit hyperactivity disorder (ADHD)   Hyperactivity and attentional difficulties in children who do not manifest other characteristics of learning disabilities.

Audibility   The ability to detect the presence of sound.

Audiogram   A graph on which results of pure tone audiometry are recorded.

Audiologist   A professional whose distinguishing role is to identify, assess, manage, and prevent disorders of hearing and balance.

Audiometer   A device used to regulate and deliver pure tone and speech stimuli during audiometric testing.

Auditory Brainstem Response (ABR)   A type of electrophysiological test that records neural responses along the ascending auditory pathways occurring within the first 5 to 6 ms following stimulus presentation.

Auditory closure   The process of filling in the missing pieces when the listener hears only part of a spoken message.

Auditory evoked potentials (AEP)   Refers to small neuroelectic responses to auditory stimulation by the ascending auditory pathways leading from the cochlea to the cortex of the brain.

Auditory neuropathy/auditory Dys-synchrony (AN/AD)   A disorder of the inner ear whereby auditory nerve fibers fail to fire in unison in response to acoustic stimulation.

Auditory training   Listening activities designed to maximize a hearing-impaired person's ability to detect, discriminate, identify, and comprehend auditory information.

Auditory-oral   A training method for hearing-impaired persons that emphasizes the use of residual hearing and speech reading (lipreading).

Auditory-verbal   A training method for hearing-impaired persons that emphasizes the use of residual hearing rather than vision.

Augmentative and alternative communication (AAC)   Gestures, signing, picture systems, print, computerized communication, and voice production used to complement or supplement speech for persons with severe communication impairments.

Aural (audiological) habilitation/rehabilitation   Services and procedures designed to improve communication deficits that result from hearing loss.

Authentic data   Information about an individual that is based on real life.

Autism spectrum disorder (ASD)   Term used to characterize individuals at the severe end of the pervasive developmental disorder (PDD) continuum. ASD is an impairment in reciprocal social interaction with a severely limited behavior, interest, and activity repertoire that has its onset before 30 months of age.

Automaticity   The ease with which a person uses a particular skill without apparent thought.

Babbling   Single-syllable nonpurposeful consonant-vowel (CV) or vowel-consonant (VC) vocalizations that begin at about 4 months of age.

Basal ganglia   Large subcortical nuclei that regulate motor functioning and maintain posture and muscle tone.

Baseline data   Information about client performance before intervention begins.

Basilar membrane   The membrane that forms the floor of the organ of Corti. It is nonuniform in width, thickness, and stiffness, allowing it to respond differently to different frequencies of sound (tonotopically). The basilar membrane contains thousands of hair cells, the receptor cells for the auditory system.

Behavior modification   A systematic method of changing behavior through careful target selection, stimulation, client response, and reinforcement.

Behavioral observation audiometry (BOA)   A method of assessing infant hearing by presentation of different stimuli and watching for any changes in activity that signals a response.

Bifid uvula   A uvula that is split in half.

Bilabial   Pertaining to two lips, as phonemes produced with both lips.

Bilateral   Both sides.

Binaural integration   The process of assimilating different information presented to each ear into a single unit.

Blend   Creating a word from individual sounds and syllables.

Bolus   A chewed lump of food ready for swallowing.

Bone-anchored hearing aid   A type of amplification in which some of the components are surgically implanted into the temporal bone of the skull, stimulating the cochlea via bone conduction.

Bone conduction   A method of evaluating hearing by transmitting sound to the inner ear by mechanically vibrating the bones of the skull.

Booster treatment   Additional therapy, based on retesting, offered after treatment has been terminated.

Bound morpheme   A morpheme that must be attached to a free morpheme to communicate meaning; grammatical morpheme.

Brainstem   Comprises the midbrain, pons, and medulla. Important for regulating respiration, chewing, swallowing, and automatic functions of the body.

Breathiness   Perception of audible air escaping through the glottis during phonation.

Broca's aphasia   A nonfluent aphasia that is characterized by short sentences with agrammatism; anomia; problems with imitation of speech because of overall speech problems; slow, labored speech and writing; and articulation and phonological errors.

Bulbar palsy   A progressive neurological condition resulting in flaccid dysarthria characterized by muscle atrophy and by rapid, random, irregular, and minute contractions (vasiculation) of nerve bundles.

Carryover   Transference or generalization; the use of the corrected form outside of the clinical setting.

Case history   Background information on a client.

(Central) Auditory processing disorder (C)APD   A disorder resulting from impairment to the auditory structures leading from the brainstem to the cortex of the brain.

Central nervous system   Comprises the brain and spinal cord.

Cerebellopontine angle   The angle formed by the cerebellum and the pons located at the level of the brainstem.

Cerebellum   A lower brain structure consisting of two hemispheres that smoothly regulates and coordinates the control of purposeful movement, including very complex and fine motor activities. The cerebellum revises the transmission from the cortex's motor strip to produce accurate, precise movements. It is also important for motor skill learning.

Cerebral arteriosclerosis   A type of ischemic stroke resulting from a thickening of the walls of cerebral arteries in which elasticity is lost or reduced, the walls become weakened, and blood flow is restricted.

Cerebral palsy (CP)   A heterogeneous group of neurogenic disorders that result in difficulty with motor movement; were acquired before, during, or shortly after birth; and affect one or more limbs.

Cerebrovascular accident (CVA)   Stroke, the most common cause of aphasia, results when the blood supply to the brain is blocked or when the brain is flooded with blood.

Cerumen (earwax)   A substance produced by glands in the ear canal that provides lubrication and protects the ear from the invasion of insects and other foreign objects.

Chin tuck   A posture with the chin down that is helpful with some patients who have a swallowing disability.

Cholesteatoma   A tumor-like mass of epithelial (skin) cells, keratin, and fats such as cholesterol that migrates into the middle ear cavity.

Chorea   A form of hyperkinetic dysarthria characterized by rapid or continual, random, irregular, and or abrupt hyperkinesia. Speech, when affected, may be characterized by inappropriate silences caused by voice stoppage; intermittent breathiness, strained harsh voice, and hypernasality; imprecise articulation with prolonged pauses; and forced inspiration and expiration resulting in excessive loudness variations.

Chronemics   The study of the effect of time on communication.

Chronic laryngitis   Vocal abuse during acute laryngitis that leads to vocal fold tissue damage.

Chronic otitis media   Inflammation of the middle ear lasting longer than 8 weeks.

Cleft   An abnormal opening in an anatomical structure.

Cleft palate team   A team of professionals including a surgeon, orthodontist, a speech-language pathologist, and one additional specialist according to the requirements of the American Cleft Palate-Craniofacial Association.

Closed syllable   A syllable, or basic acoustic unit of speech, that ends in one or more consonants.

Cluttering   Disfluent speech that is characterized by overuse of fillers and circumlocutions associated with word-finding difficulties, rapid speech, and word and phrase repetitions. Cluttering does not seem to contain the fear of words or situations found in stuttering.

Cochlea   The portion of the inner ear that contains the sensory cells of the auditory system. It is composed of two concentric labyrinths. The outer one is composed of bone and the inner one of membrane.

Cochlear implant   An electronic amplification device that is surgically placed in the cochlea and provides electrical stimulation to the surviving auditory nerve fibers.

Code switching   Process in which bilingual speakers transfer between two languages based on the listener, context, or topic.

Cognitive rehabilitation   A treatment regimen for individuals with TBI that is designed to increase functional abilities for everyday life by improving the capacity to process incoming information.

Columella   A strip of tissue connecting the tip of the nose to the base.

Communication   An exchange of ideas between sender(s) and receivers(s).

Communication disorder   An impairment in the ability to receive, send, process, or comprehend concepts of verbal, nonverbal, or graphic symbol systems.

Compensatory articulation error   Gross sound substitution errors that are an attempt to make up for the physical inability to produce a given sound correctly.

Complete cleft   A total separation of a normally fused structure.

Concha   The deep bowllike depression on the pinna.

Conditioned play audiometry (CPA)   A method of assessing the hearing of children ages $2\frac{1}{2}$ to 3 years and older by instructing them to put a block in a bucket, a ring on a peg, or other action whenever they hear the test signal.

Conduction aphasia   A fluent aphasia in which the individual's conversation is abundant and quick. Characterized by anomia, mildly impaired auditory comprehension if at all, extremely poor repetitive or imitative speech, and paraphasia.

Conductive hearing loss   A loss of auditory sensitivity due to malformation or obstruction of the outer and/or middle ear.

Congenital   Present at birth.

Congenital laryngeal webbing   Extraneous tissue on the anterior aspects of the vocal folds that can interfere with breathing; present at birth.

Consistent aphonia   Persistent absence of voice.

Consonant   A phoneme that is produced with some vocal tract constriction or occlusion.

Contact signing   See *pidgin signed English (PSE)*.

Contact ulcer   A benign lesion that may develop on the posterior surface of the vocal folds.

Conversion aphonia   Psychologically based loss of voice.

Conversion disorder   Condition in which emotion is suppressed and transformed into a sensory or motor disability.

Correlate   Something that tends to exist in the presence of something else or be associated with it, but without a demonstrated causal relationship.

Craniofacial anomalies   Congenital malformations involving the head (*cranio:* above the upper eyelid) and face (*facial:* below the upper eyelid).

Craniosynostosis   Premature closing of the sutures of the skull, which greatly disfigures the forehead.

Critical literacy   Reader's ability to actively interpret between the lines, to analyze, and synthesize information and to be able to explain content.

Criterion referenced   An evaluation of an individual's strengths and weaknesses with regard to specific skills.

Cued Speech   A visual communication system that combines the mouth movements of speech with manual cues designed to facilitate the identification of speech sounds that are visually similar, as well as those that are not readily visible.

Deaf Community   A group of persons who share a common means of communication (American Sign Language) that facilitates group cohesion and identity.

Deaf Culture   A view of life manifested by the mores, beliefs, artistic expression, understandings, and language (ASL) that is particular to Deaf people.

Decibel (dB)   A mathematically derived unit based on the pressure exerted by a particular sound vibration.

Decoding   Breaking or segmenting a written word into its component sounds and then blending them together to form a recognizable word.

Decontextualized   Outside of a conversational context. When we write, we construct the context with our writing rather than having it constructed by our conversational partner(s).

Dementia   An acquired pathological condition or syndrome that is characterized by intellectual decline, especially memory, due to neurogenic causes. Additional deficits include poor reasoning or judgment, impaired abstract thinking, inability to attend to relevant information, impaired communication, and personality changes.

Dentition   The number, type, and arrangement of teeth.

Developmental apraxia of speech (DAS)   An impairment in programming the musculature for speech without apparent muscle weakness or paralysis. Apraxia of speech in children is characterized by multiple articulation errors including addition of speech sounds, sound and syllable repetitions, and sound prolongations.

Developmental disfluency or developmental stuttering   Whole-word repetitions and other self-conscious nonfluency that is apparent in many young children.

Developmental verbal dyspraxia (DVD)   See *Developmental apraxia of speech.*

Diagnosis   A statement distinguishing an individual's difficulties from the broad range of possibilities.

Diagnostic therapy   Ongoing assessment and evaluation as intervention takes place.

Dialect   A linguistic variation that is attributable primarily to geographic region or foreign language background. It includes features of form, content, and use.

Dialogic reading   Picture book interactive sharing between a caregiver and a young child, in which parents try to get children involved in the reading process by asking them questions about the story or allowing the child to tell the story.

Dichotic   The simultaneous presentation of different stimuli to each ear.

Diphthong   Two vowels said in such close proximity that they are treated as a single phoneme.

Diplophonia   The perception of two vocal frequencies.

Disability   The functional consequence of an impairment.

Distinctive features   The attributes of phonemes that differentiate one from another on the basis of a binary principle.

Distortion   In articulation, a deviant production of a phoneme.

Double swallow   A technique in which the patient swallows more than once per bolus.

Down syndrome   A congenital condition that is characterized by multiple defects and varying degrees of intellectual deficit.

Dynamic   Characterized by energy or effective energy, changing over time.

Dynamic assessment Nonstandardized assessment approach that can take the form of test-teach-test to determine a child's ability to learn.

Dynamic literacy Reader's ability to interrelate content to other knowledge through both deductive and inductive reasoning.

Dysarthria One of several motor-speech disorders that involve impaired articulation, respiration, phonation, or prosody as a result of paralysis, muscle weakness, or poor coordination. Motor function may be excessively slow or rapid, decreased in range or strength, and have poor directionality and timing.

Dyskinesia Impairment in the ability to control voluntary movement; sometimes due to prolonged use of certain medications.

Dyslexia A disability that is characterized by difficulty comprehending printed symbols and recognizing words. Children with dyslexia often exhibit delayed language development, listening comprehension problems, and poor phonological awareness.

Dysphagia A disorder of swallowing.

Dysplasia Hearing loss due to malformation or incomplete development of the inner ear structures during embryonic development.

Dystonia A form of hyperkinetic dysarthria that is characterized by a slow, sustained increase and decrease of hyperkinesia involving either the entire body or localized sets of muscles. As a result, there are excessive pitch and loudness variations, irregular articulation breakdowns, and vowel distortions.

Eardrum See *Tympanic membrane*.

Echolalia An immediate imitation of another speaker. Among children with ASD, it may represent the storage and production of unanalyzed whole units of language.

Edema Swelling due to an accumulation of fluid.

Effectiveness The probability of benefit to individuals in a defined population from a specific intervention applied to a given communication problem under *average everyday* clinical conditions.

Efficacy The probability of benefit to individuals in a defined population from a specific intervention applied for a given communication problem under *ideal* conditions.

Efficiency Application of the quickest intervention method involving the least effort and the greatest positive benefit, including unintended effects.

Electrocochleography (ECochG) A type of electrophysiological testing that records neural responses occurring within 1.5 to 2 ms following stimulus presentation.

Electropalatography (EPG) A technique used to teach correct placement of the articulators for speech production. It uses an artificial palatal plate fitted in the client's mouth that contains electrodes. The electrodes are connected to a computer. When the tongue contacts the electrodes during speech production, the articulatory patterns can be viewed on the computer screen.

Electrolarynx Battery-powered device that sets air in the vocal tract into vibration.

Embolism A blood clot, fatty materials, or an air bubble that may travel through the circulatory system until it blocks the flow of blood in a small artery. If it travels to the brain, it may cause a stroke.

Endolymph The fluid that fills the membranous labyrinth of the cochlea and vestibular system.

Endoscope A lens coupled with a light source used for viewing internal bodily structures, including the vocal folds.

Episodic aphonia Uncontrolled and unpredictable occasional loss of voice.

Esophageal atresia The absence of a normal open passageway from the esophagus to the stomach.

Esophageal speech Speech that is produced by using burping as a substitute for the laryngeal voice.

Esophagostomy A surgical hole in the esophagus through which a feeding tube may be inserted.

Etiology Cause or origin of a problem; also the study of cause.

Eustachian tube The tube that connects the middle ear cavity with the nasopharynx.

Evidence-based practice The process of making decisions regarding individual client care and specific courses of treatment based on current well-designed research.

Examination of the peripheral speech mechanism Sometimes called *oral peripheral exam;* assessment of the structure and function of the visible speech system.

Executive function An aspect of metacognition used in self-regulation and including the ability to attend; to set reasonable goals; to plan and organize to achieve each goal; to initiate, monitor, and evaluate your performance in relation to that goal; and to revise plans and strategies based on feedback.

Explicit Clearly defined.

External auditory meatus or canal The tubular structure that extends from the concha of the pinna to the tympanic membrane.

External error sound discrimination   Perceiving differences in the production of the target phoneme in another person's speech.

Failure to thrive   The absence of healthy growth and development.

Fast mapping   Process in which a child infers the meaning of a word form context and uses it in a similar context at a later time. A fuller definition evolves over time. Fast mapping enables preschool children to expand their vocabularies quickly by being able to use a word without fully understanding the meaning.

Fetal alcohol syndrome (FAS)   Overuse of alcohol during pregnancy, which severely impairs the neurological and physical development of the fetus, resulting in growth deficiencies, craniofacial disorders, central nervous system dysfunction, limited cognitive development, and, in some cases, sensorineural hearing loss.

Fiberoptic endoscopic evaluation of swallowing (FEES)   A laryngoscopic technique for viewing swallowing.

Figurative language   Nonliteral phrases consisting of idioms, metaphors, similes, and proverbs.

Filler   Utterances such as "er," "um," and "you know" that are used within productions. Sometimes characteristic of dysfluent speech and/or stuttering.

Fingerspelling   A form of manual communication system consisting of 26 distinct handshapes that visually represent each letter of the English alphabet.

Flaccid dysarthria   Speech disorder caused by weak, soft, flabby muscle tone, called hypotonia. May result in hypernasality, breathiness, and imprecise articulation.

Fluency   Smoothness of rhythm and rate.

Fluent   Speech that is relatively smooth and free of disruptions.

Fluent aphasia   Speech characterized by word substitutions, neologisms, and often verbose verbal output. Also called Wernicke's aphasia.

FM system   A type of hearing assistive technology that transmits sound to a hearing-impaired person via FM radio waves. The system consists of a microphone, transmitter, and a wireless receiver.

Follow-up testing   Assessment after dismissal from therapy to ensure that skills have been maintained.

Free morpheme   The portion of a word that can stand alone and designate meaning; root morpheme.

Frequency   An acoustical term that refers to the number of sound wave cycles that are completed within a specific time period. Subjectively, it is perceived as the pitch of the sound.

Fricative   A consonant phoneme that is produced by exhaling air through a narrow passageway.

Frontonasal process   Embryonic structure that develops into the nasomedial processes and the lateral nasal processes during the fifth week of gestation.

Functional   Having no known organic cause; perhaps psychogenic or learned.

Fundamental frequency   The lowest frequency component of a complex vibration.

Gastroesophageal reflux (GER)   Movement of food or acid from the stomach back into the esophagus.

Genderlect   Variations in language associated with males or females; gender-based dialect.

Generalization   The extending of a skill learned in a clinical setting to other "natural" environments or skills; carryover or transference.

Generative   Capable of being freshly created; refers to the infinite number of sentences that can be created through the application of grammatical rules.

Glide   Phoneme in which the articulatory posture changes from consonant to vowel.

Global or mixed aphasia   A profound language impairment in all modalities as a result of brain damage.

Glossectomy   The surgical removal of the tongue.

Glottal   Relating to, or produced in or by the glottis, the space between the vocal cords.

Glottal stop   A compensatory behavior where a stoppage of air occurs at the level of the glottis rather than in the oral cavity.

Grammar   The rules of a language.

Granuloma   A nodular lesion due to injury or infection. May occur on the vocal folds and be caused by a breathing tube placed through the glottis.

Habitual pitch   The basic frequency level that an individual uses most of the time.

Hair cells   Auditory receptor cells located in the organ of Corti that are responsible for encoding auditory information.

Handicap   The psychosocial consequence of a disability.

Hard glottal attacks   Abrupt initiation of voicing using hypertensive vocal fold adduction.

Hard of hearing   Slight/mild to moderately severe hearing loss. Hard-of-hearing individuals usually depend as much as possible on their hearing for communication and learning of new concepts.

Harmonics Frequencies in a complex sound that are integer multiples of the fundamental frequency.

Head-back position A posture with the head held back that is useful for some clients with a swallowing disability.

Head rotation A posture with the head turned toward the impairment, used for some clients with a swallowing disability.

Head tilt position A posture with the head away from the impairment, used for some individuals with a swallowing disability.

Hearing assistive technology (HAT) The general term applied to electronic devices designed to enhance the reception of sound by those who are hearing impaired.

Hematoma Blood trapped in an organ or skin tissue owing to injury or surgery.

Hemianopsia Blindness in the left or right visual field of both eyes caused by lesions on the temporal or lower parietal lobe.

Hemiparesis Muscle weakness on one side of the body, resulting in reduced strength and control.

Hemiplegia Paralysis on one side of the body.

Hemisensory impairment Loss of the ability to perceive sensory information on one side of the body.

Hemorrhagic stroke A type of stroke resulting from the weakening of arterial walls that burst under pressure.

Hertz (Hz) Number of complete vibrations or cycles per second.

Hesitation A pause before or between parts of utterances. If used excessively, it may be considered a sign of dysfluency or stuttering.

HIV/AIDS See *Human immunodeficiency virus* and *Acquired immunodeficiency syndrome*.

Hoarseness A voice quality that is characterized by a rough, usually low-pitched quality.

Holistic Pertaining to the whole; multidimensional.

Homophonous Phonemes that are visually indistinguishable when spoken, such as /p/ and /b/.

Human immunodeficiency virus (HIV) The organism responsible for AIDS.

Huntington's chorea An inherited progressive disease also known as Huntington's disease, resulting from a genetic defect on chromosome 4.

Hyperadduction Excessive movement toward the midline, often resulting in a tense voice quality.

Hyperfluent speech Very rapid speech found in people with fluent aphasia and characterized by few pauses, incoherence, inefficiency, and pragmatic inappropriateness.

Hyperkinetic dysarthria A speech disorder characterized by increased movement, such as tremors and tics, and by inaccurate articulation.

Hyperlexia A mild form of pervasive developmental disorder (PDD) characterized by an inordinate interest in letters and words and by early ability to read but with little comprehension.

Hypertonia A condition in which there is too much muscle tone, especially in those muscles that oppose the bending of joints and help us to stand erect. Also called spasticity.

Hypoadduction Reduced movement toward the midline of the vocal folds, often resulting in a breathy voice quality.

Hypokinesia Abnormally decreased motor function or activity.

Hypokinetic dysarthria A speech disorder that is characterized by a decrease or lack of appropriate movement as muscles become rigid and stiff, resulting in monopitch and monoloudness and imprecise articulation.

Hyponasality A lack of nasal resonance.

Hypotonia Poor muscle tone and weakness.

Idiolect An individual's unique way of speaking, a personal dialect.

Impairment A loss of structure or function.

Implicit Assumed but not directly expressed.

Inappropriate pitch Pitch judged to be outside the normal range for age and/or sex.

Incidental teaching Using a natural activity to train targets.

Incomplete cleft A separation of a normally fused structure that involves only a portion of the structure.

Incus The middle bone of the ossicular chain in the middle ear. It articulates with the malleus at the top and has a projection that is joined to the stapes at the bottom.

Infarction Death of bodily tissue due to deprivation of the blood supply.

Inferior longitudinal muscle (tongue) Intrinsic muscle of the tongue that shortens the tongue.

Informational counseling The process of imparting information to clients and their families.

Inner ear The interior section of the ear containing the cochlea and vestibular system. It supplies information to the brain regarding balance, spatial orientation, and hearing.

Intellectual disability See *mental retardation*.

Intelligibility The ability to understand what has been detected auditorily.

Intensity A measure of the magnitude of a sound, generally expressed in decibels.

Intentionality Goal directedness in interactions. It is first demonstrated at about 8 months of age primarily through gestures.

Interdental Between the teeth; see *Linguadental*.

Internal auditory meatus The bony canal housing the vestibulocochlear (VIIIth) nerve that runs from the cochlea to the brainstem.

Internal error sound discrimination Judging the accuracy of one's own phoneme production; intrapersonal error sound discrimination.

Interpersonal error sound discrimination See *External error sound discrimination*.

Intonation Pitch movement within an utterance.

Intrapersonal error sound discrimination See *Internal error sound discrimination*.

Ischemic stroke A cerebrovascular accident resulting from a complete or partial blockage or occlusion of the arteries transporting blood to the brain.

Jargon In infancy, long strings of unintelligible sounds with adultlike intonation that develop at about 8 months of age and exhibit the pitch and intonational pattern of the language to which the child is exposed. Jargon may sound like questions, commands, and statements. In some aphasias, jargon refers to meaningless or irrelevant speech, characterized by typical intonational patterns and frequently correct syntax.

Kernahan's Striped Y A visual classification system for cleft lip and palate.

Kinesics The study of bodily movement and gesture. Also known as body language.

Labiodental Pertaining to lips and teeth; phonemes produced with lip and tooth contact.

Language A socially shared code for representing concepts through the use of arbitrary symbols and rule-governed combinations of those symbols.

Language impairment A heterogeneous group of deficits and/or immaturities in the comprehension and/or production of spoken or written language.

Language-learning disability Term used to describe the approximately 75% of children with learning disability (LD) who have difficulty primarily with learning and using symbols.

Language sample A systematic collection and analysis of a person's speech or writing. Sometimes called a corpus; used as a part of language assessment.

Laryngeal cancer Carcinoma of supraglottal, glottal, or subglottal structures.

Laryngeal papilloma Wartlike growth on the vocal folds.

Laryngeal system Structures of the larynx used for sound production.

Larynx The superior termination of the trachea that protects the lower airways and is the primary sound source for speech production.

Lateral nasal processes Primitive embryological tissue that gives rise to the nasal alae.

Lexicon An individual's personal dictionary of words and meanings.

Linguadental Pertaining to tongue and teeth; phonemes produced with tongue and tooth contact.

Linguistic intuition A language user's underlying knowledge about the system of rules pertaining to his or her native language; linguistic competence.

Liquid Refers to the oral resonant consonants /r/ and /l/.

Literacy Use of visual modes of communication, specifically reading and writing.

Localization The process of determining where sound originates in space.

Loudness variation Speaking too loudly or too softly for a particular vocal situation.

Lungs Pair of air-filled elastic sacs that change in size and shape and allow us to breathe.

Maintaining cause The perpetuating cause that keeps a problem from self-correcting; for example, parents of an 8-year-old considering a lisp "cute."

Malar hypoplasia Underdevelopment of the cheek bones.

Malleus The largest of the ossicles. It is fastened to the eardrum and articulates with the incus, the next bone in the chain.

Malocclusion Improper alignment of the maxillary (upper) and mandibular (lower) dental arches.

Mandibular processes Primitive embryological tissue that gives rise to the mandible.

Manually coded English Sign communication systems designed to duplicate spoken English manually for teaching children who are deaf.

Maternal rubella German measles contracted during pregnancy that may result in various disorders in the developing fetus.

Maxillary processes Primitive embryological tissue that gives rise to the lateral aspects of the maxilla and palatal shelves.

Maximal contrast A minimal pair in which the differing phonemes differ in more than one distinctive feature, for example, "say" (/se/) and "bay" (/be/).

Maximal opposition See *Maximal contrast.*

Mean length of utterance (MLU) The average length of utterances measured in morphemes. In English, this is an important measure of preschool development because language becomes more complex as it becomes longer.

Meniere's disease A condition resulting from excessive endolymph in the inner ear, resulting in vertigo, tinnitus, aural fullness, and sensorineural hearing loss.

Meningitis An inflammation of the meninges, or layers of tissue covering the brain and spinal cord.

Mental retardation/intellectual disabilities A disorder characterized by substantial limitations in intellectual functioning, concurrent related limitations in adaptive skill areas, and manifestation before age 18.

Metacognition Knowledge about knowledge and cognitive processes, including self-appraisal.

Metalinguistic skills Abilities that enable a child to consider language in the abstract, to make judgments about its correctness, and to create verbal contexts, such as in writing.

Metaphon An approach to phonological therapy that is based on the premise that phonological disorders in children are developmental language learning disorders.

Metaphonological skills The ability to analyze, think about, and manipulate speech sounds.

Micrognathia Underdeveloped mandible.

Microtia Congenital disorder resulting in a small malformed pinna or ear canal.

Middle ear The section of the ear containing the ossicles. It is bounded laterally by the tympanic membrane and medially by the cochlea.

Middle ear space or tympanic cavity The cube-shaped area between the outer and middle ear containing the ossicles.

Minimal pair Two words that differ in a single phoneme, for example, "say" (/se/) and "bay" (/be/).

Mixed dysarthrias Symptoms or areas of brain injury that cross several dysarthrias as a result of degenerative disorders, toxins, metabolic disorders, stroke, trauma, tumors, or infectious diseases.

Mixed hearing loss The simultaneous presence of conductive and sensorineural hearing loss.

Modified barium swallow study An X-ray procedure that is used to visualize the swallowing process. Also known as *videofluoroscopy.*

Monoloudness Voice lacking normal variations of intensity that occur during speech.

Monopitch Voice that lacks normal inflection in tone.

Monotone Voice that is produced without varying the fundamental frequency.

Morpheme The smallest meaningful unit of language.

Morphology Aspect of language concerned with rules governing change in meaning at the intra-word level.

Morphophonemic contrast Change in pronunciation as a result of morphological changes.

Mucosal tissue Pinkish tissue lining the inside of the mouth.

Multiple oppositions approach A phonologically based therapy approach that targets multiple sound errors at one time using phoneme word pairs that are maximally contrasted (i.e., differ according to place, manner, and voicing).

Multiple sclerosis (MS) A progressive disease characterized by demyelinization of nerve fibers of the brain and spinal cord.

Multiview videofluoroscopy Motion picture X-rays recorded from various angles.

Muscular dystrophy A group of genetic diseases characterized by progressive weakness and degeneration of the muscles that control movement. Forms differ in the pattern of inheritance, age of onset, rate of progression, and distribution of muscle weakness.

Myasthenia gravis A disorder characterized by fatigability and rapid weakening of muscles, a cause of flaccid dysarthria.

Myelination Development of a protective myelin sheath or sleeve around the cranial nerves.

Myofunctional disorder See *Tongue thrust.*

Myringotomy A small surgical incision made in the surface of the tympanic membrane.

Nasal Phoneme that is produced with nasal resonance.

Nasal alae Lateral flaring of the nostrils.

Nasalance score A numerical score that reflects the magnitude of hypernasality when measured by a nasometer.

Nasal emission Air escaping through the nose during speech production.

Nasogastric tube (NG tube) A tube placed into the nose and then through the pharynx and esophagus by which liquefied food may be fed.

Nasomedian processes Primitive embryological tissue that gives rise to the anterior portion of the upper lip and premaxilla.

Nasometer A commercially available device that is used to measure nasality.

Nasopharynx The space within the skull that is behind the nose and above the roof of the mouth.

Neologism A novel word that does not exist in the language. Neologisms are created and used quite confidently by some individuals with aphasia.

Neural plasticity Physiological and functional changes within the central nervous system in response to auditory stimulation.

Neurogenic stuttering Disorder of fluency associated with some form of brain damage.

Neuron The basic unit of the central nervous system consisting of the cell body, axon, and dendrites.

Noise-induced hearing loss Hearing impairment resulting from exposure to high levels of occupational or recreational noise.

Nonorganic hearing loss A condition in which a patient portrays having a hearing loss when one does not truly exist or exaggerates the degree of a true auditory deficit.

Nonvocal Without voice.

Norm referenced A comparison that is usually based on others of the same gender and similar age.

Obstruent In articulation refers to speech sounds that are produced with a significant amount of constriction in the vocal tract (stops, fricatives, affricates); also called nonresonant phonemes.

Odynophagia Painful swallowing.

Olfactory pits Depressions between the nasomedian and lateral nasal processes that will ultimately become the right and left nasal cavities.

Omission In articulation, the absence of a phoneme that has not been produced or replaced.

Open syllable A syllable, or basic acoustic unit of speech, that ends in a vowel.

Optimal pitch level A particularly suitable pitch level for an individual largely determined by vocal fold structure.

Oral apraxia A neurological impairment in programming and executing speech and nonspeech movements of the mouth.

Organ of Corti The intricate structure that runs along the center of the membranous labyrinth of the cochlea and contains the auditory sensory receptor cells.

Organic Physiological.

Orthodontist A dental specialist who is concerned primarily with alignment of the teeth.

Ossicles or ossicular chain The small bones housed within the middle ear. They include the malleus, the incus, and the stapes.

Otitis media Inflammation of the middle ear.

Otitis media with effusion (OME) Inflammation of the middle ear with fluid.

Otoacoustic emissions (OAEs) Measurable low-level sounds or echoes, occurring either spontaneously or in response to acoustic stimulation, due to outer hair cell motility within the cochlea.

Otolith system The portion of the vestibular system responsible for sensing linear acceleration.

Otosclerosis A disorder characterized by the formation of spongy bone in the region of the stapes footplate, resulting in a progressive conductive hearing loss.

Otoscope A small handheld device used to visually inspect the external auditory canal and tympanic membrane.

Ototoxic Refers to drugs and chemical agents that are potentially damaging to the inner ear.

Outer ear The section of the ear comprised of the pinna and the external auditory meatus or ear canal.

Oval window A small oval membrane located on the lateral wall of the cochlea, behind the stapes footplate.

Palatal Refers to the front area of the roof of the mouth. In speech, palatal consonants are produced with the tongue touching or approximating the hard palate.

Palatal obturator A plate that covers a portion of the soft palate. It is useful for individuals who have had palatal surgery.

Palatal shelves Wedge-shaped tissue masses that will become the bony hard palate.

Palatoplasty Surgical correction of a cleft palate.

Paraphasia Word substitutions that are found in some individuals with aphasia who may talk fluently and grammatically.

Parkinson disease A progressive neurogenic disorder that is characterized by resting tremors, slowness of movement, and difficulty initiating voluntary movements. Speech may be rapid, breathy, and reduced in loudness, pitch range, and stress.

Pedunculated polyp Polyp that appears to be attached to the vocal fold by a stalk.

Perilymph The fluid that fills the bony labyrinth of the cochlea and vestibular system.

Peripheral nervous system Comprises the cranial and spinal nerves that receive and transmit information from the brain to the body.

Perpetuating cause See *Maintaining cause.*

Permanent threshold shift (PTS) A permanent change in hearing acuity associated with exposure to high-intensity noise.

Personal adjustment counseling The process of assisting clients and their families in dealing with the emotional consequences of hearing loss.

Personal hearing aid Personal amplification device ranging from tiny completely-in-the-canal models to those worn behind the ear.

Pervasive developmental disability (PDD) Any of several disorders of childhood that are characterized by markedly atypical behaviors and severe impairment in the ability to relate to others, including infantile autism and childhood schizophrenia.

Pharyngeal flap A secondary surgical procedure to correct velopharyngeal incompetence.

Pharyngostomy A surgical hole in the pharynx through which a feeding tube may be placed.

Pharynx The anatomical passageway connecting the nasal and oral cavities.

Phonation Production of sound by vocal fold vibration.

Phonemic awareness Ability to manipulate sounds, such as blending sounds to create new words or segmenting words into sounds.

Phonemic regression Difficulty understanding speech that is far greater than expected based on the degree of hearing loss.

Phonetically balanced (PB) Refers to words used in auditory word recognition testing where each phoneme is represented in the same proportion in which it occurs in everyday English.

Phonetically consistent forms (PCFs) Consistent vocal patterns that function as meaningful "words" for the infant. These are a transition to words.

Phonics Sound-letter or phoneme-grapheme correspondence.

Phonological awareness Knowledge of sounds and syllables and of the sound structure of words.

Phonology The study of the sound systems of language.

Phonotactic The study of the way in which phonemes are combined and arranged in syllables and words of a particular language or dialect.

Physiology The branch of biology that is concerned with the process and function of parts of the body.

Pidgin signed English (PSE) A sign system that incorporates ASL signs while maintaining English word order.

Pierre Robin syndrome A congenital condition resulting in a small mandible, cleft lip, cleft palate, and other facial abnormalities.

Pinna The funnel-shaped outermost part of the ear that serves to collect sound waves and channel them into the ear canal.

Pitch The perceptual counterpart to fundamental frequency associated with the speed of vocal fold vibration.

Pitch breaks Sudden uncontrolled upward or downward changes in pitch.

Postlingually After the development of speech and language.

Posttherapy testing Assessment following intervention.

Prader-Willi syndrome A congenital condition characterized by obesity and intellectual deficit.

Pragmatics The use, function, or purpose of communication; the study of communicative acts and contexts.

Precipitating cause Factors that trigger a disorder (e.g., a stroke).

Predisposing cause Underlying factors that contribute to a problem (e.g., a genetic basis).

Prelingually Prior to the development of speech and language.

Premaxilla The anterior portion of the hard palate to the incisive foramen.

Presbycusis Hearing loss incurred as a result of the aging process.

Pressure equalization (PE) tube A small-diameter tube that is surgically placed in the eardrum to provide ventilation of the middle ear space via the external auditory meatus.

Prevalence The total number of cases of a disorder at a particular point in time in a designated population.

Primary auditory cortex Heschl's gyrus located in the temporal lobe that is concerned with the analysis and elaboration of speech.

Primary motor cortex A 2-cm-wide gyrus immediately in front of the central sulcus of the brain that controls voluntary motor movements.

Primary progressive aphasia A degenerative disorder of language in which other mental functions and activities of daily living are preserved. There is no marked dementia or loss of cognitive functioning.

Print awareness Knowledge of the meaning and function of print, including recognition of words and letters and terminology, such as letter, word, or sentence.

Prognosis An informed prediction of the outcome of a disorder.

Prolabium Central prominence of the lip; also isolated soft tissue mass in unrepaired bilateral clefts.

Prolongation In fluency analysis, the process of holding a phoneme longer than is typical; for example, "sssssso."

Prolonged speech A group of speech rate reduction techniques (e.g., prolonged, continuous phonation;

gentle voicing onsets; light articulatory contacts) used to treat stuttering and establish stutter-free speech.

Prosthodontist   A dental specialist who is concerned with the replacement of missing teeth and other oral structures with various appliances.

Proxemics   The study of physical distance between people.

Pseudobulbar palsy   A condition that resembles progressive bulbar palsy, characterized by spastic dysarthria and dysphagia.

Psychogenic   Caused by psychological factors.

Pure tone audiometry   A procedure that is used to assess hearing sensitivity at discrete frequencies.

Pure tones   Sounds that contain energy at only a single frequency, such as 250 Hz, 500 Hz, 1000 Hz, 2000 Hz, 4000 Hz, and 8000 Hz, and are used in pure tone audiometry.

Purulent   Pus formation and discharge by the tissue of the middle ear cavity.

Pyloric stenosis   A narrowing of the sphincter connecting the stomach to the small intestine, resulting in a blockage to the intestines.

Range of motion   The extent of movement of a joint from maximum extension to maximum flexion.

Rate   The speed at which something occurs. In speech this may be the number of words or syllables in a given period of time.

Recurrent branch   Branch of the tenth cranial nerve that innervates muscles of the larynx.

Reduplicated babbling   Long strings of consonant-vowel syllable repetitions, such as "ma-ma-ma-ma-ma."

Reformulation   An adult response to a child's utterance in which the adult adds to the child's utterance to provide a more complex example of what the child has said.

Reinforcement   A procedure that follows a response with the intent of perpetuating or extinguishing it; used in conditioning.

Repetition   In fluency analysis, the process of repeating a word or a part of a word, as in "the-the-the" or "b-b-ball."

Representation   Process of having one thing stand for another, such as a piece of paper used as a blanket for a doll.

Residual hearing   Any hearing that remains following the onset of hearing loss.

Resonant   A consonant phoneme that is produced with resonance occurring throughout the vocal tract; refers to nasals, liquids, and glides.

Respiratory system   Stuctures, including the lungs, bronchi, trachea, larynx, mouth, and nose, that are used in breathing for life and speech.

Resting tidal breathing   Breathing to sustain life.

Reverberation   The short echo effect caused by the reflection of sound waves off solid surfaces within a confined space.

Right hemisphere damage (RHD)   A group of neuromuscular, perceptual, and/or linguistic deficits that result from damage to the right hemisphere of the brain and may include epilepsy, hemisensory impairment, and hemiparesis or hemiplegia.

Scintigraphy   A computerized technique for measuring aspiration during or after a swallow.

Segmentation   Creating a word when a phoneme or syllable is deleted.

Self-monitoring   The ability to recognize one's own errors and correct them.

Semantic features   The pieces of meaning that come together to define a particular word.

Semantic-pragmatic disorder   A mild form of pervasive developmental disorder characterized by limited vocabulary, concrete definitions, and poor conversational skills.

Semantics   The study of word and language meaning.

Semicircular canals   Series of three canals located in the inner ear that senses angular acceleration.

Sensorimotor training   Articulatory training that emphasizes tactile and proprioceptive sensations and sound, syllable, and word production.

Sensorineural hearing loss   Permanent hearing loss as the result of absence, malformation, or damage to the structures of the inner ear.

Sensory-motor approach   Articulatory training that emphasizes tactile and proprioceptive sensations and sound, syllable, and word production.

Serous otitis media   Inflammation of the middle ear with sterile fluid.

Sessile polyp   Polyp with a broad-based attachment to the vocal fold.

Silent aspiration   Lack of coughing when food or liquid enters the airway.

Simultaneous communication   The use of sign language in combination with speech.

SLP   See *Speech language pathologist*.

Sociolinguistics   The study of influences such as cultural identity, setting, and participants on communicative variables.

Soft-voice syndrome   Compensatory behavior in which a child with velopharyngeal incompetence purposely reduces vocal intensity to prevent air escape through the nose and reduce hypernasality.

Somatogenic   Coming from the body; organic or physiological.

Sound field amplification   A type of assistive listening device whereby sound is transmitted via a microphone to loudspeakers that are strategically placed within a room.

Spasmodic dysphonia (SD)   A voice disorder characterized by hyperadduction of the vocal folds resulting in strained/strangled voice production with intermittent stoppages.

Spastic cerebral palsy   A congenital disorder that is characterized by increased muscle tone, such that when a muscle contracts, the opposing muscle may react abnormally to stretch by increasing muscle tone too much. Muscle movements are described as jerky, labored, and slow.

Spastic dysarthria   Speech that is characterized as slow with jerky, imprecise articulation and reduction of the rapidly alternating movements of speech because of stiff and rigid muscles.

Specific Language Impairment (SLI)   Language impairment in the absence of hearing, oral structural or functioning, cognitive, or perceptual deficits.

Speech bulb   An obturator that fills the velopharyngeal space, closing the velopharyngeal portal.

Speech community   A group of people who share a common understanding of the rules and restrictions that govern communicative situations.

Speech-language pathologist (SLP)   A professional whose distinguishing role is to identify, assess, treat, and prevent speech, language, communication, and swallowing disorders.

Speech Recognition Threshold (SRT) test   A test procedure used in speech audiometry that measures the lowest (quietest) level at which a person can recognize approximately 50% of the spondee words presented for a given number of trials.

Speech sample   A systematic collection and analysis of a person's speech, a corpus; used in language assessment.

Spina bifida   A congenital malformation of the spinal column.

Spondees   Two-syllable compound words that are spoken with equal emphasis on both syllables and used in Speech Recognition Threshold testing.

Spontaneous recovery   A natural recovery process that proceeds without professional intervention.

Stacked ABR   A procedure used to sum the neural activity across the entire frequency region of the cochlea to assist in identifying small acoustic nerve tumors.

Stapedius muscle   The small muscle that attaches to the neck of the stapes and contracts in response to high-intensity sound.

Stapes   The third and smallest of the ossicles in the middle ear.

Stenosis   Narrowing of the external auditory meatus.

Stereocilia   Small hairlike projections situated on the top of the hair cells in the organ of Corti.

Stimulability   The ability to imitate a target phoneme when given focused auditory and visual cues.

Stimulus   Anything that is capable of eliciting a response.

Stoma   A small opening: for example, a surgical hole in the external neck region extending into the pharynx to permit breathing following laryngectomy.

Stop   Consonant phoneme produced by building air pressure behind the point of constriction.

Story grammar   Common elements and event sequences in narratives.

Strain and struggle   Difficulty initiating and maintaining voice.

Stridor   Noisy breathing or involuntary sound that accompanies inspiration and expiration.

Stroke   Cerebrovascular accident (CVA), the most common cause of aphasia, resulting when the blood supply to the brain is blocked or when the brain is flooded with blood.

Stuttering   A disorder of speech fluency characterized by hesitations, repetitions, prolongations, tension, and avoidance behaviors.

Subacute otitis media   Inflammation of the middle ear lasting between 3 and 8 weeks.

Subcortical aphasia   Fluent aphasia as the result of lesions in the thalamus and basal ganglia below the level of the cortex.

Subglottal pressure   Pressure beneath the vocal folds that sets them into vibration.

Substitution   In articulation, the production of one phoneme in place of another.

Support group   Individuals with similar problems who meet together to share feelings, information, and ideas.

Suppurative otitis media   Pus formation and discharge by the tissue of the middle ear cavity.

Synapse   The minuscule space between the axon of one neuron and the dendrites of the next, where "communication" between neurons occurs.

Syndactyly   Webbing of the fingers and toes.

Syndrome   A combination of symptoms that occur together in predictable and consistent combinations of traits.

Syntax   How words are arranged in sentences.

Symbolization   Using an arbitrary symbol, such as a word or sign, to stand for something.

Tactiles   Touching behaviors.

Tardive dyskinesia   Involuntary, repetitive facial, tongue, or limb movements that sometimes occur as a side effect of certain medications.

TBI   See *Traumatic brain injury.*

Tectorial membrane   The gelatinous tongue-shaped structure that forms the roof of the organ of Corti.

Teletypewriter (TTY)   A portable keyboard used for remote text conversations over regular phone lines by those who are deaf.

Temporary threshold shift (TTS)   A temporary change in hearing acuity followed by spontaneous recovery that is associated with short-term exposure to high-intensity noise.

Tensor veli palatine   Muscle of the soft palate that opens the auditory tube.

Teratogens   Chemical or environmental agents that produce congenital abnormalities.

Thalamus   Paired egg-shaped structure in the brain that serves as a relay station for incoming and outgoing information. The thalamus may set the tone for the brain, alerting it to prepare to receive or to transmit information.

Threshold   The lowest (quietest) presentation level (measured in decibels) at which a person can barely detect a stimulus 50% of the time it is presented.

Thrombosis   A blood clot within a blood vessel of the body. It may result in an ischemic stroke.

Tics   Involuntary, rapid and repetitive, stereotypic movements.

Tinnitus   The perception of sound (ringing, buzzing) in the ears or head when there is no external source present.

Tongue thrust   Swallowing with a forward movement of the tongue, resulting in misarticulation of various phonemes. Also known as *myofunctional disorder.*

Tonotopic organization   Refers to the coding of frequency information by the auditory system whereby certain areas within a structure are spatially arranged to respond to different frequencies.

Trachea   Cartilaginous membraneous tube by which air moves to and from the lungs.

Tracheo-esophageal shunt (TEP)   A device that directs air from the trachea to the esophagus for esophageal speech.

Tracheostomy tube   A tube that is inserted into the trachea to relieve a breathing obstruction.

Traditional motor approach   An articulation treatment approach that emphasizes discrete skill learning, beginning first with auditory discrimination of the error sound, followed by production training of the sound in isolation, in nonsense syllables, and then in words, phrases, sentences, and conversation.

Transcortical motor aphasia   A nonfluent aphasia that is characterized by impaired conversational speech, good verbal imitative abilities, and mildly impaired auditory comprehension.

Transcortical sensory aphasia   A rare fluent aphasia that is characterized by word substitutions, lack of nouns and severe anomia, and poor auditory comprehension, but the ability to repeat or imitate words, phrases, and sentences.

Traumatic brain injury (TBI)   Damage to the brain resulting from bruising and laceration caused by forceful contact with the relatively rough inner surfaces of the skull or from secondary edema or swelling, infarction or death of tissue, and hematoma or focal bleeding.

Treacher Collins syndrome   An inherited disorder that is characterized by excessive muscle tone in the face and jaw.

Tympanic cavity   See *middle ear space.*

Tympanic membrane or eardrum   The thin cone-shaped structure composed of three layers of tissue located at the end of the external auditory meatus. It is set into vibration as acoustic energy strikes its surface.

Tympanogram   The graph generated during acoustic immittance testing that depicts compliance of the eardrum relative to changes in air pressure.

Tympanostomy tube   See *pressure equalization (PE) tube.*

Ultrasonography   Ultrasound.

Ultrasound   A technique that uses high-frequency sound waves to visualize internal bodily organs.

Unilateral hearing loss   Loss of hearing on one side.

Usher's syndrome   A hereditary disorder characterized by sensorineural hearing impairment and progressive blindness.

Uvula   Small, pendulous structure suspended from the soft palate.

Variegated babbling   Long strings of consonant-vowel syllables, in which adjacent and successive syllables in the string are not identical.

Vasiculation   Rapid, random, irregular, and minute contractions of nerve bundles.

Veau system Roman numeral classification system for describing clefts of the lip and/or palate.

Velar Refers to the posterior area of the roof of the mouth. In speech, velar consonants are produced with the tongue touching or approximating the velum or soft palate.

Velopharyngeal closure Contact of the velum with the lateral and posterior pharyngeal walls, thus separating the oral and nasal cavities.

Velopharyngeal inadequacy (VPI) Inability of the velopharyngeal mechanism to separate the oral and nasal cavities during swallowing and speech.

Verbal stereotype An expression that is repeated over and over; characteristic of some individuals with aphasia.

Vermilion Pinkish to brown coloration of the lips.

Vertigo The sensation of spinning relative to one's surroundings.

Vestibular system Structures of the inner ear responsible for supplying information to the brain regarding balance and spatial orientation.

Vestibulocochlear nerve or VIIIth nerve The cranial nerve that runs from the base of the cochlea to the cochlear nucleus of the brainstem. It is comprised of the vestibular and cochlear branches.

Video fluoroscopy See *Modified barium swallow study*.

Visual Reinforcement Audiometry (VRA) A method of hearing assessment in which a child is rewarded for localizing to a test signal through the use of moving toys and/or flashing lights.

Vocal abuse Any of several behaviors, including smoking and yelling, that can result in damage to the laryngeal mechanism.

Vocal fold paralysis Immobilized vocal fold usually due to nerve damage.

Vocal hygiene Proper care of the voice.

Vocal nodules Localized growths on the vocal folds that are associated with vocal abuse.

Vocal polyp A fluid-filled lesion of the vocal fold that results from mechanical stress.

Vocal tremor Variations in the pitch and loudness of the voice that are involuntary.

Voice Vocal tone and resonance.

Vowel Any of several voiced phonemes that are produced with a relatively open vocal tract.

Waardenburg's syndrome A hereditary disorder characterized by pigmentary discoloration, particularly in the irises and hair; craniofacial malformation of the nasal area; and severe to profound hearing impairment.

Wernicke's aphasia A fluent aphasia that is characterized by rapid-fire strings of sentences with little pause for acknowledgment or turn taking. Content may seem to be a jumble and may be incoherent or incomprehensible, although fluent and well articulated.

Word recognition test (WRT) A test procedure used in speech audiometry to measure an individual's ability to recognize single-syllable words presented at a predetermined level above their auditory threshold.

References

Agency for Health Care Policy and Research. (1999). *Diagnosis and treatment of swallowing disorders (dysphagia) in acute-care stroke patients.* Rockville, MD: Author.

Air, D. H., Wood, A. S., & Neils, J. R. (1989). Considerations for organic disorders. In N. A. Creaghead, P. W. Newman, & W. A. Secord (Eds.), *Assessment and remediation of articulatory and phonological disorders* (2nd ed.). Columbus, OH: Merrill.

Ali, W., & O'Connell, R. (2007). The effectiveness of early cochlear implantation for infants and young children with hearing loss. *NZHTA Technical Brief, 6*(5).

Alzheimer's Association (2005). http://www.alz.org/AboutAD/Statistics.asp. Retrieved October 22, 2005.

Alzheimer's Association. (2009, May 11). *2009 Alzheimer's disease facts and figures.* Retrieved May 27, 2009, from www.alz.org/national/ documents/report_alzfactsfigures2009.pdf

Ambrose, N., Yairi, E., & Cox, N. (1993). Genetic aspects of early childhood stuttering. *Journal of Speech and Hearing Research, 36,* 701–706.

American Association on Intellectual and Developmental Disabilities. (2009). *Definition of intellectual disability.* Retrieved June 2, 2009, at www.aaidd.org/content_100.cfm?navID=21

American Psychiatric Association. (1987). *Diagnostic and statistical manual of mental disorders* (3rd ed. rev.). Washington, DC: Author.

American Psychiatric Association. (1994). *Diagnostic and statistical manual of mental disorders* (4th ed.). Washington, DC: Author.

American Psychiatric Association. (2000). *Diagnostic and statistical manual of mental disorders* (4th ed.). Washington, DC: American Psychiatric Association.

American Speech-Language-Hearing Association (ASHA). (1992, March). Instrumental diagnostic procedures for swallowing. *Asha, 34* (Suppl. 7), 25–33.

American Speech-Language-Hearing Association (ASHA). (1993). Definitions of communication disorders and variations. *Asha, 35* (Suppl. 10), pp. 40–41.

American Speech-Language-Hearing Association (ASHA). (1995). *Guidelines for the training, credentialing, use, and supervision of speech-language pathology assistants.* Rockville, MD: Author.

American Speech-Language-Hearing Association (ASHA). (1997). *Preferred practice patterns for the profession of speech-language pathology.* Rockville, MD: Author.

American Speech-Language-Hearing Association (ASHA). (2000a). Council on Professional Standards. Background information for the standards and implementation for the certificate of clinical competence in speech-language pathology. (Effective date: January 1, 2005). Available from http://professional.asha.org/library/slp_standards.htm

American Speech-Language-Hearing Association (ASHA). (2000b). Council on Professional Standards. Background information for the standards and implementation for the certificate of clinical competence in audiology. (Effective date: January 1, 2007). Available from http:// professional.asha.org/library/audiology_standards.htm

American Speech-Language-Hearing Association (ASHA). (2000c). Fact Sheet: Speech-Language Pathology. Available at http://professional.asha.org/students/careers/slp.htm

American Speech-Language-Hearing Association (ASHA). (2001a, December 26). Code of ethics (revised). *ASHA Leader, 6*(23), 2.

American Speech-Language-Hearing Association (ASHA). (2001b). Council on Academic Accreditation. Standards for accreditation of graduate education programs in audiology and speech-language pathology. Available at http://professional.asha.org/students/caa_programs/standards.htm

American Speech-Language-Hearing Association (ASHA). (2001c). Fact Sheet: Audiology. Available at http://professional.asha.org/students/careers/audiology.htm

American Speech-Language-Hearing Association (ASHA). (2001d). *Roles and responsibilities of speech-language pathologists with respect to reading and writing in children and adolescents* (Position paper, technical report, and guidelines). Rockville, MD: Author.

American Speech-Language-Hearing Association (ASHA). (2001e). Roles of Speech-Language Pathologists in Swallowing and Feeding Disorders: Technical Report [Technical Report]. Available from www.asha.org/policy

American Speech-Language-Hearing Association (ASHA). (2002a). About ASHA: Mission statement. Available at http://professional.asha.org/services/about_asha.com

American Speech-Language-Hearing Association (ASHA). (2002b). Augmentative and alternative communication: Knowledge and skills for service delivery. *ASHA Supplement 22*, 97–106.

American Speech-Language-Hearing Association (ASHA). (2003). *2003 Omnibus survey: Practice trends in audiology*. Rockville, MD: Author.

American Speech-Language-Hearing Association (ASHA). (2004). Scope of practice in audiology. *ASHA Supplement, 24*.

American Speech-Language-Hearing Association (ASHA). (2005). *(Central) auditory processing disorders*. Available at http://www.asha.org/members/deskref-journals/deskref/default

American Speech-Language-Hearing Association. (2007). Childhood Apraxia of Speech [Position statement]. Available from www.asha.org/policy

American Speech-Language-Hearing Association (ASHA). (2008). Incidence and Prevalence of Speech, Voice, and Language Disorders in Adults in the United States: 2008 Edition. Available at www.nsslha.org/research/reports/speech_voice_language.htm

American Speech-Language-Hearing Association. (2009a, March 24). *2005 Standards and implementation procedures for the certificate of clinical competence in speech-language pathology* (revised March 2009). Retrieved May 29, 2009, at www.asha.org/certification/handbooks/slp/slp_standards.htm

American Speech-Language-Hearing Association. (2009b, May 19). *2007 standards and implementation procedures for the certificate of clinical competence in audiology* (revised March 2009). Retrieved May 29, 2009, at www.asha.org/certification/aud_standards_new.htm

American Speech-Language-Hearing Association. (2009c) *About the American Speech-Language-Hearing Association (ASHA)*. Retrieved May 30, 2009, at www.asha.org/about_asha.htm

American Speech-Language-Hearing Association. (2005c). SLP health care survey 2005: Caseload characteristics. Available from www.asha.org/about/membership-certification/member-data/healthcare_survey.htm

Anderson, K. L. (2002). Early Listening Function: Discovery tool for parents and caregivers of infants and toddlers. Available from http://www.phonak.com

Anderson, R. C., Hiebert, E., Scott, J. A., & Wilkenson, J. A. (1985). *Becoming a nation of readers*. Washington, DC: National Institute of Education.

Andrews, G., Craig, A., Feyer, A. M., Hoddinott, S., Howie, P., & Neilson, M. (1983). Stuttering: A review of research findings and theories circa 1982. *Journal of Speech and Hearing Disorders, 48*, 226–246.

Angelo, J. (1992). Comparison of three computer scanning modes as an interface method for persons with cerebral palsy. *American Journal of Occupational Therapy, 46*, 217–222.

Apel, K., & Masterson, J. (2001). Theory-guided spelling assessment and intervention: A case study. *Language, Speech, and Hearing Services in Schools, 32*, 182–194.

Apel, K., & Self, T. (2003). Evidence-based practice: The marriage of research and clinical practice. *The ASHA Leader, 8*(16), 6–7.

Aram, D. M. (1997). Hyperlexia: Reading without meaning in young children. *Topics in Language Disorders, 17*(3), 1–13.

Archibald, L. M. D., & Gathercole, S. E. (2006). Visuospatial immediate memory in specific language impairment. *Journal of Speech, Language, and Hearing Research, 49*, 265–277.

Aronson, A. E. (1990). *Clinical voice disorders*. New York: Thieme.

Arvedson, J. (2000). Evaluation of children with feeding and swallowing problems. *Language, Speech, and Hearing Services in Schools, 31*, 28–41.

Arvedson, J. (2009, June 19). Pediatric feeding and swallowing disorders. Treatment Efficacy Summary. Retrieved June 24, 2009, at www.asha.org/NR/

rdonlyres/EEE3706F-215C-428B-A461-3ABFA8 C0787A/0/TESPediatricFeedingandSwallowing.pdf

Arvedson, J., & Brodsky, L. (2002). *Pediatric swallowing and feeding: Assessment and management* (2nd ed.). Albany, NY: Singular.

Ashford, J. R., Logemann, J. A., & McCullough, G. (2009a, June 19). Swallowing disorders (dysphagia) in adults. *Treatment efficacy summary.* Retrieved June 23, 2009, at www.asha.org/NR/rdonlyres/ 1EC1FFDC-CDD2-4569-AB57-319987BFB858 /0/TESDysphagiainAdults.pdf

Ashford, J. R., McCabe, D., Wheeler-Hegland, K., Frymark, T., et al. (2009b). Evidence-based systematic review: Oropharyngeal dysphagia behavioral treatments: Part III. Impact of dysphagia treatments on populations with neurological disorders. *Journal of Rehabilitation Research & Development, 46,* 195–204.

Aviv, J. E., Sataloff, R. T., Cohen, M., et al. (2001). Cost effectiveness of two types of dysphagia care in head and neck cancer: A preliminary report. *Ear, Nose, and Throat Journal, 80,* 553–558.

Azuma, T., & Bayles, L. A. (1997). Memory impairments underlying language difficulties in dementia. *Topics in Language Disorders, 18*(1), 58–71.

Balandin, S., & Morgan, J. (2001). Preparing for the future: Aging and alternative and augmentative communication. *Augmentative and Alternative Communication, 17,* 99–108.

Ball, L. J., Marvin, C. A., Beukelman, D. R., Lasker, J., & Rupp, D. (2000). Generic talk use by preschool children. *Augmentative and Alternative Communication, 16,* 145–155.

Balsamo, L., Xu, B., Grandin, C., Petrella, J., et al. (2002). A functional magnetic resonance imaging study of left hemisphere language dominance in children. *Archives of Neurology, 59,* 1168–1174.

Bankson, N. W., & Bernthal, J. E. (1998a). Factors related to phonologic disorders. In J. E. Bernthal & N. W. Bankson (Eds.), *Articulation and phonological disorders* (4th ed.). Boston: Allyn and Bacon.

Bassotti, G., Germani, U., Pagliaricci, S., Plesa, A., Giulietti, O., Mannarino, E., & Morelli, A. (1998). Esophageal manometric abnormalities in Parkinson's disease. *Dysphagia, 13*(1), 28–31.

Bates, E. (1997). On the nature and nurture of language. In E. Bizzi, P. Catissano, & V. Volterra (Eds.), *Frontiere della Biologia:* The brain of Homo sapiens Rome: Giovanni Trecani.

Bayles, K. A., & Kazniak, A. W. (1987). *Communication and cognition in normal aging and dementia.* Boston: Little, Brown.

Bayles, K., & Tomoeda, C. K. (1994). *Functional Linguistic Communication Inventory.* East Aurora, NY: Slosson.

Bear, D. R., Invernizzi, M., Templeton, S., & Johnston, F. (2000). *Words their way: Word study for phonics, vocabulary, and spelling instruction* (2nd ed.). Upper Saddle River, NJ: Prentice Hall.

Bear, D. R., Invernizzi, M., Templeton, S., & Johnston, F. (2004). *Words their way: Word study with phonics, vocabulary, and spelling instruction* (3rd ed.). Upper Saddle River, NJ: Merrill/Prentice Hall.

Bedore, L. M., & Leonard, L. B. (2001). Grammatical morphological deficits in Spanish-speaking children with specific language impairment. *Journal of Speech, Language, and Hearing Research, 44,* 905–924.

Beebe, S. A., Beebe, S. J., & Redmond, M. V. (1996). *Interpersonal communication: Relating to others.* Boston: Allyn and Bacon.

Behrman, A., & Orlikoff, R. F. (1997). Instrumentation in voice assessment and treatment: What's the use? *American Journal of Speech-Language Pathology, 6,* 9–16.

Bellis, T. J. (2003a). *Assessment and management of central auditory processing disorders in the educational setting: From science to practice.* San Diego, CA: Singular.

Bellis, T. J. (2003b). Auditory processing disorders: It's not just kids who have them. *The Hearing Journal, 56,* 10–19.

Bello, J. (1994). Prevalence of speech, voice, and language disorders in the United States. *Communication facts, 1994 ed.* Rockville, MD: American Speech-Language-Hearing Association.

Belmonte, M. K., & Bourgerone, T. (2006). Fragile X syndrome and autism at the intersection of genetic and neural networks. *Nature, 9*(10), 1221–1225.

Benelli, B., Belacchi, C., Gini, G., & Lucanggeli, D. (2006). 'To define means to say what you know about things': The development of definitional skills as metalinguistic acquisition. *Journal of Child Language, 33,* 71–97.

Ben-Yishay, Y., & Diller, L. (1993). Cognitive remediation in traumatic brain injury: Update and issues. *Archives of Physical Medicine and Rehabilitation, 74,* 204–213.

Bergman, R. L., Piacentini, J., & McCracken, J. (2002). Prevalence and description of selective mutism in a school-based sample. *Journal of the American Academy of Child and Adolescent Psychiatry, 41,* 938–946.

Bernhardt, B. H., & Holdgrafer, G. (2001). Beyond the basics I: The need for strategic sampling from indepth phonological analysis. *Language, Speech, and Hearing Services in Schools, 32*, 18–27.

Berninger, V. W. (2000). Development of language by hand and its connections with language by ear, mouth, and eye. *Topics in Language Disorders, 20*(4), 65–84.

Berninger, V. W., Abbott, R. D., Billingsley, F., & Nagy, W. (2001). Processes underlying timing and fluency of reading: Efficiency, automaticity, coordination, and morphological awareness. In M. Worf (Ed.), *Dyslexia, fluency, and the brain* (pp. 383–413). Timonium, MD: York.

Berninger, V. W., Cartwright, A., Yates, C., Swanson, H. L., & Abbott, R. (1994). Developmental skills related to writing and reading acquisition in the intermediate grades: Shared and unique variance. *Reading and Writing: An Interdisciplinary Journal, 6*, 161–196.

Berninger, V. W. Vaughan, K., Abbott, R., Brooks, A., Abbott, S., Reed, E., Rogan, L., & Graham, S. (1998). Early intervention for spelling problems: Teaching spelling units of varying size within a multiple connections framework. *Journal of Educational Psychology, 90*, 587–605.

Bernstein Ratner, N. (2006). Evidence-based practice: An examination of its ramifications for the practice of speech-language pathology. *Language, Speech, and Hearing Services in Schools, 37*, 257–267.

Bernthal, J., Bankson, N., & Flipson, P. (2009). *Articulation and phonological disorders: Speech Sound Disorders in Children*. Boston: Pearson.

Bess, F. H., Dodd-Murphy, J., & Parker, R. A. (1998). Children with minimal sensorineural hearing loss: Prevalence, educational performance, and functional status. *Ear and Hearing, 19*, 339–354.

Beukelman, D., & Mirenda, P. (1997). *Augmentative and alternative communication: Management of severe communication disorders in children and adults* (2nd ed.). Baltimore, MD: Brookes.

Beukelman, D. R., & Mirenda, P. (1992). *Augmentative and alternative communication: Management of severe communication disorders in children and adults*. Baltimore: Brookes.

Binger, C., & Light, J. (2007). The effect of aided AAC modeling on the expression of multisymbol messages by preschoolers who use AAC. *Augmentative and Alternative Communication, 23*, 30–43.

Blackstone, S. (1989). Augmentative communication services in the schools. *Asha, 31*(1), 61–64.

Blalock, J., & Johnson, D. (1987). *Adults with learning disabilities: Clinical studies*. New York: Grune & Stratton.

Blischak, D., Lombardino, L., & Dyson, A. (2003). Use of speech-generating devices: In support of natural speech. *Augmentative and Alternative Communication, 19*(1), 29–35.

Blockberger, S., & Johnston, J. R. (2001). Grammatical morphology acquisition by children with extremely limited speech. *Augmentative and Alternative Communication, 19*, 207–221.

Blockberger, S., & Sutton, A. (2003). Toward linguistic competence: Language experience and knowledge of children with extremely limited speech. In J. Light, D. Beukelman, & J. Reichle (Eds.), *Communicative competence for people who use AAC: From research to effective practice* (pp. 63–106). Baltimore: Brookes.

Blood, G. W., & Blood, I. M. (2004). Bullying in adolescents who stutter: Communicative competence and self-esteem. *Contemporary Issues in Communication Science and Disorders, 31*, 69–79.

Bloodstein, O. (1995). *A handbook on stuttering*. San Diego, CA: Singular.

Bloom, L. (1970). *Language development: Form and function of emerging grammars*. Cambridge, MA: MIT Press.

Bloom, R. L., & Ferrand, C. T. (1997). Neuromotor speech disorders. In C. T. Ferrand & R. L. Bloom (Eds.), *Introduction to organic and neurogenic disorders of communication: Current scope of practice*. Boston: Allyn and Bacon.

Boburg, E., & Kully, D. (1995). The comprehensive stuttering program. In C. W. Starkweather & H. F. M. Peters (Eds.), *Stuttering: Proceedings of the First World Congress on Fluency Disorder* (pp. 305–308). Munich: International Fluency Association.

Bonita, R. (1992). Epidemiology of stroke. *Lancet*, 339–320.

Boone, D., & McFarlane, S. (1993). A critical view of the yawn-sigh as a voice therapy technique. *Journal of Voice, 7*, 75–80.

Boone, D. R., & McFarlane, S. C. (2000). *The voice and voice therapy* (4th ed.). Boston: Allyn and Bacon.

Bosman, A., & van Orden, G. (1997). Why spelling is more difficult than reading. In C. Perfetti, L. Riebert, & M. Fayol (Eds.), *Learning to spell: Research, theory, and practice across languages* (pp. 173–194). Mahwah, NJ: Erlbaum.

Boswell, S. (2004). International agreement brings mutual recognition of certification. *The ASHA Leader, 9*(19), 1, 22.

Bothe, A., Davidow, J., Bramlett, R., & Ingham, R. (2006). Stuttering treatment research 1970–2005: I. Systematic review incorporating trial quality assessment of behavioral, cognitive, and related approaches. *American Journal of Speech-Language Pathology, 15*, 321–341.

Bottenberg, D. E., & Hanks, J. M. (1986). Language and speech of physically handicapped children. In V. A. Reed (Ed.), *An introduction to children with language disorders* (pp. 201–219). New York: Macmillan.

Boudreau, D. (2005). Use of a parent questionnaire in emergent and early literacy assessment of preschool children. *Language, Speech, and Hearing Services in Schools, 36*, 33–47.

Boudreau, D. M., & Chapman, R. (2000). The relationship between event representation and linguistic skills in narratives of children and adolescents with Down syndrome. *Journal of Speech, Language, and Hearing Research, 43*, 1146–1159.

Boudreau, D. M., & Hedberg, N. L. (1999). A comparison of early literacy skills in children with specific language impairment and their typically developing peers. *American Journal of Speech-Language Pathology, 8*, 249–260.

Boudreau, D. M., & Larson, J. (2004). *Strategies for teaching narrative abilities to school-aged children.* Paper presented at the annual convention of the American Speech-Language-Hearing Association, Philadelphia.

Brackenbury, T., Burroughs, E., & Hewitt, L. E. (2008). A qualitative examination of current guidelines for evidence-based practice in child language intervention. *Language, Speech, and Hearing Services in Schools, 39*, 78–88.

Brackenbury, T., & Pye, C. (2005). Semantic deficits in children with language impairments: Issues for clinical assessment. *Language, Speech, and Hearing Services in Schools, 36*, 5–16.

Bradley, D. P. (1997). Congenital and acquired velopharyngeal inadequacy. In K. R. Bzoch (Ed.), *Communicative disorders related to cleft lip and palate* (4th ed., pp. 223–243). Austin, TX: PRO-ED.

Bradshaw, M. L., Hoffman, P. R., & Norris, J. A. (1998). Efficacy of expansions and cloze procedures in the development of interpretations by preschool children exhibiting delayed language development. *Language, Speech and Hearing Services in Schools, 29*, 85–95.

Brand Robertson, S., & Ellis Weismer, S. (1999). Effects of treatment on linguistic and social skills in toddlers with delayed language development. *Journal of Speech, Language, and Hearing Research, 42*, 1234–1248.

Brault, M. W. (2005). Americans with Disabilities, 2005. *Current Population Reports*, pp. 70–117. Washington, DC: U.S. Census Bureau.

Brinton, B., & Fujiki, M. (2004). Social and affective factors in children with language impairment: Implications for literacy learning. In C. A. Stone, E. R. Silliman, B. J. Ehren, & K. Apel (Eds.), *Handbook of language and literacy: Development and disorders* (pp. 130–153). New York: Guilford.

Brinton, B., Fujiki, M., & Powell, J. M. (1997). The ability of children with language impairment to manipulate topic in a structured task. *Language, Speech, and Hearing Services in Schools, 28*, 3–11.

Brinton, B., Spackman, M. P., Fujiki, M., & Ricks, J. (2007). What should Chris say? The ability of children with specific language impairment to recognize the need to dissemble emotions in social situations. *Journal of Speech, Language, and Hearing Research, 50*, 798–811.

Broen, P., Devers, M., Doyle, S., Prouty, J., & Moller, K. (1998). Acquisition of linguistic and cognitive skills by children with cleft palate. *Journal of Speech, Language, and Hearing Research, 41*, 676–687.

Brown, S., Ingham, R., Ingham, J., Laird, A., & Fox, P. (2005). Stuttered and fluent speech production: An ALE meta-analysis of normal neuroimaging studies. *Human Brain Mapping, 25*, 105–117.

Bryan, K. L. (1989). *The right hemisphere language battery.* Leicester, UK: Far Communications.

Bulow, M., Olsson, R., & Ekberg, O. (2001). Videomanometric analysis of supraglottic swallow, effortful swallow, and chin tuck in patients with pharyngeal dysfunction. *Dysphagia, 16*, 190–195.

Burgess, S., & Turkstra, L. S. (2006). Social skills intervention for adolescents with autism spectrum disorders: A review of the experimental evidence. *EBP Briefs, 1*(4).

Burns, M. M., Halper, A. S., & Mogil, S. I. (1985). *Clinical management of right hemisphere dysfunction.* Rockville, MD: Aspen.

Butkowsky, I. S., & Willows, D. M. (1980). Cognitive-motivational characteristics of children varying in reading ability: Evidence of learned helplessness in poor readers: *Journal of Educational Psychology, 72*, 408–422.

Byl, F. M. J. (1984). Sudden hearing loss: Eight years experience and suggested prognostic table. *Laryngoscope, 94*, 647–651.

Bzoch, K. R. (1997). Introduction to the study of communicative disorders in cleft palate and related craniofacial anomalies. In K. R. Bzoch (Ed.), *Communicative disorders related to cleft lip and palate* (4th ed., pp. 3–44). Austin, TX: Pro-Ed.

Caccamise, D., & Snyder, L. (2005). Theory and pedagogical practices of text comprehension. *Topics in Language Disorders, 25*(1), 1–20.

Cain, K. Patson, N., & Andrews, L. (2005). Age- and ability-related differences in young readers' use of conjunctions. *Journal of Child Language, 32*, 877–892.

Calculator, S. (1997). Fostering early language acquisition and AAC use: Exploring reciprocal influences between children and their environments. *Augmentative and Alternative Communication, 13*, 149–157.

Calvert, D. (1982) Articulation and hearing impairments. In Lass, L., Northern, J., Yoder, D., & McReynolds, L. (Eds.), *Speech, language, and hearing* (Vol. 2). Philadelphia: Saunders.

Camicioli, R., Oken, B. S., Sexton, G., Kaye, J. A., & Nutt, J. G. (1998). Verbal fluency task affects gait in Parkinson's disease with motor freezing. *Journal of Geriatric Psychiatry and Neurology, 11*, 181–185.

Carr, S. C., & Thompson, B. (1996). The effects of prior knowledge and schema activation strategies on the inferential reading comprehension of children with and without learning disabilities. *Learning Disability Quarterly, 19*, 48–61.

Casby, M. W. (1997). Symbolic play of children with language impairment: A critical review. *Journal of Speech, Language, and Hearing Research, 40*, 468–479.

Castrogiovanni, A. (1999a). Incidence and prevalence of hearing impairment in the United States. *Communication facts, 1999 ed.* Rockville, MD: American Speech-Language-Hearing Association.

Castrogiovanni, A. (1999b). Incidence and prevalence of speech, voice, and language disorders in the United States. *Communication facts, 1999 ed.* Rockville, MD: American Speech-Language-Hearing Association.

Castrogiovanni, A. (1999c). Special populations: Dysphagia. *Communication facts, 1999 ed.* Rockville, MD: American Speech-Language-Hearing Association.

Catten, M., Gray, S., Hammond, T., Zhou, R., & Hammond, E. (1998). Analysis of cellular location and concentration in vocal fold lamina propria. *Archives of Otolaryngology—Head & Neck Surgery, 118*, 663–666.

Catts, H. W. (1997). The early identification of language-based reading disabilities. *Language, Speech, and Hearing Services in Schools, 28*, 86–89.

Catts, H. W., Adlof, S. M., & Ellis Weismer, S. (2006). Language deficits in poor comprehenders: A case for the simple view of reading. *Journal of Speech, Language, and Hearing Research, 49*, 278–293.

Catts, H. W., Fey, M. E., Zhang, X., & Tomblin, J. B. (1999). Language basis of reading and reading disabilities: Evidence from a longitudinal investigation. *Scientific Studies in Reading, 3*, 331–361.

Catts, H. W., Fey, M. E., Zhang, X., & Tomblin, J. B. (2001). Estimating the risk of future reading difficulties in kindergarten children: A research-based model and its clinical implementation. *Language, Speech, and Hearing Services in Schools, 32*, 38–50.

Catts, H. W., & Kamhi, A. (2005). Causes of reading disabilities. In H. W. Catts & A. G. Kamhi (Eds.), *Language and reading disabilities* (2nd ed., pp. 94–126). Boston: Allyn and Bacon.

Causino Lamar, M. A., Obler, L. K., Knoeful, J. E., & Albert, M. L. (1994). Communication patterns in end-stage Alzheimer's disease: Pragmatic analysis. In R. L. Bloom, L. K. Obler, S. DeSanti, & J. L. Ehrlich (Eds.), *Discourse analysis and application: Studies in adult clinical populations* (pp. 217–235). Hillsdale, NJ: Erlbaum.

Centers for Disease Control and Prevention (2003). http://www.cdc.gov/doc.do/id/0900f3ec800101e8. Retrieved October 22, 2005.

Chang, S., Ohde, R., & Conture, E. (2002). Coarticulation and formant transition rate in young children who stutter. *Journal of Speech, Language, and Hearing Research, 45*, 676–688.

Chapman, S. B. (1997). Cognitive-communication abilities in children with closed head injury. *American Journal of Speech-Language Pathology, 6*(2), 50–58.

Chapman, S. B., Watkins, R., Gustafson, C., Moore, S., Levin, H., & Kufera, J. A. (1997). Narrative discourse in children with closed head injury, children with language impairment, and typically developing children. *American Journal of Speech-Language Pathology, 6*(2), 66–76.

Charman, T., Drew, A., Baird, C., & Baird, G. (2003). Measuring early language development in preschool children with autism spectrum disorder using the

MacArthur Communicative Development Inventory (Infant Form). *Journal of Child Language, 30,* 213–236.

Chermak, G. D., & Musiek, F. E. (1997). *Central auditory processing disorders: New perspectives.* San Diego: Singular.

Cherney, L. R. (1994). Dysphagia in adults with neurologic disorders: An overview. In L. R. Cherney (Ed.), *Clinical management of dysphagia in adults and children.* Gaithersburg, MD: Aspen.

Cherney, L. R., Patterson, J. P., Raymer, A., Frymark, T., & Schooling, T. (2008). Evidence-based systematic review: Effects of intensity of treatment and constraint-induced language therapy for individuals with stroke-induced aphasia. *Journal of Speech, Language, and Hearing Research, 51,* 1282–1299.

Chisolm, T. H., Johnson, C. E., Danhauer, J. L., Portz, L. J., Abrams, H. B., Lesner, S., McCarthy, P. A., & Newman, C. W. (2007). A systematic review of health-related quality of life and hearing aids: Final report of the American Academy of Audiology Task Force on the Health-Related Quality of Life Benefits of Amplification in Adults. *Journal of the American Academy of Audiology, 18,* 151–83.

Chomsky, N. (1965). *Aspects of the theory of syntax.* Cambridge, MA: MIT Press.

Chomsky, N., & Halle, M. (1968). *The sound patterns of English.* New York: Harper & Row.

Choudhury, N., & Benasich, A. A. (2003). A family aggregation study: The influence of family history and other risk factors on language development. *Journal of Speech, Language, and Hearing Research, 46,* 261–272.

Chouinard, M. M., & Clark, E. V. (2003). Adult reformulations of child errors as negative evidence. *Journal of Child Language, 30,* 637–669.

Church, C., Alisanski, S., & Amanullah, S. (2000). The social, behavioral, and academic experiences of children with Asperger syndrome. *Focus on Autism and Other Developmental Disabilities, 15*(1), 12–20.

Cirrin, F. M., & Gillam, R. B. (2008). Language intervention practices for school-age children with spoken language disorders: A systematic review. *Language, Speech, and Hearing Services in Schools, 39,* 110–137.

Clark, H., Lazarus, C., Arvedson, J., Schooling, T., & Frymark, T. (2009). Evidence-based systematic review: Effects of neuromuscular electrical stimulation on swallowing and neural activation. *American Journal of Speech-Language Pathology, 18,* 361–375.

Clark, H. M. (2004). Neuromuscular treatment for speech and swallowing: A tutorial. *American Journal of Speech-Language Pathology, 12,* 400–415.

Clarke, C. E., Gullaksen, E., Macdonald, S., et al. (1998). Referral criteria for speech and language therapy assessment of dysphagia caused by idiopathic Parkinson's disease. *Acta Neurologica Scandinavica, 97*(1), 27–35.

Cleave, P. L., & Fey, M. E. (1997). Two approaches to the facilitation of grammar in children with language impairments: Rationale and description. *American Journal of Speech-Language Pathology, 6*(1), 22–32.

Coelho, C. A. (1997). Cognitive-communicative disorders following traumatic brain injury. In C. T. Ferrand & R. L. Bloom (Eds.), *Introduction to organic and neurogenic disorders of communication: Current scope of practice* (pp. 110–137). Boston: Allyn and Bacon.

Coelho, C. A., DeRuyter, F., Kennedy, M. R. T., & Stein, M. (2008). Cognitive-communication disorders resulting from traumatic brain injury. *Treatment Efficacy Summary.* Retrieved June 28, 2009, at www.asha.org/NR/rdonlyres/4BAF3969-9ADC-4C01-B5ED-1334CC20DD3D/0/TreatmentEfficacySummaries2008.pdf

Coelho, C. A., Liles, B. Z., & Duffy, R. J. (1995). Impairments of discourse abilities and executive functions in traumatically brain injured adults. *Brain Injury, 9,* 471–477.

Coffin, J. M., Baroody, S., Schneider, K., & O'Neill, J. (2005). Impaired cerebellar learning in children with prenatal alcohol exposure: A comparative study of eyeblink conditioning in children with ADHD and dyslexia. *Cortex, 41,* 389–398.

Colasent, R., & Griffith, P. (1998). Autism and literacy: Looking into the classroom with rabbit stories. *The Reading Teacher, 51*(5), 414–420.

Colton, R. H., & Casper, J. K. (1990). *Understanding voice problems: A physiological perspective for diagnosis and treatment.* Baltimore, MD: Williams & Wilkins.

Colton, R. H., & Casper, J. K. (1996). *Understanding voice problems: A physiological perspective for diagnosis and treatment* (2nd ed.). Baltimore: Williams & Wilkins.

Condouris, K., Meyer, E., & Tager-Flusberg, H. (2003). The relationship between standardized measures of language and measures of spontaneous speech in children with autism. *American Journal of Speech-Language Pathology, 12,* 349–358.

Connell, P. J., & Stone, C. (1992). Morpheme learning of children with specific language impairments under controlled conditions. *Journal of Speech and Hearing Research, 35,* 844–852.

Conti-Ramsden, G., & Botting, N. (2004). Social difficulties and victimization in children with SLI at

11 years of age. *Journal of Speech, Language, and Hearing Research, 47*, 145–161.

Conti-Ramsden, G., & Durkin, K. (2008). Language and independence in adolescents with and without a history of specific language impairment (SLI). *Journal of Speech, Language, and Hearing Research, 51*, 70–83.

Conti-Ramsden, G., Simkin, Z., & Pickles, A. (2006). Estimating familial loading in SLI: A comparison of direct assessment versus personal interview. *Journal of Speech, Language, and Hearing Research, 49*, 88–101.

Conture, E. G. (1990a). Childhood stuttering: What is it and who does it? In J. Cooper (Ed.), *Research needs in stuttering: Roadblocks and future directions* (ASHA Reports 18, pp. 2–14). Rockville, MD: American Speech-Language-Hearing Association.

Conture, E. G. (1990b). *Stuttering* (2nd ed.). Englewood Cliffs, NJ: Prentice Hall.

Conture, E. G. (1996). Treatment efficacy: Stuttering. *Journal of Speech and Hearing Research, 39*, S18–S26.

Conture, E. G., & Guitar, B. (1993). Evaluating efficacy of treatment of stuttering: School-age children. *Journal of Fluency Disorders, 18*, 253–287.

Conture, E. G., & Yaruss, J. S. (2009, June 19). Stuttering. *Treatment Efficacy Summary*. Retrieved June 23, 2009, at www.asha.org/NR/rdonlyres/85BCEC0C-FBF5-43C7-880D-EF2D3219F807/0/TESStuttering.pdf

Convit, A., deLeon, J. J., Tarshish, C., DeSanti, S., Tsui, W., Rusinek, H., & George, A. (1995). *Hippocampal volume in pre-clinical and early Alzheimer's dementia: Relationship to cognitive function.* Austin, TX: Pro-Ed.

Cooper, E. B. (1984). Personalized fluency control therapy: A status report. In M. Peins (Ed.), *Contemporary approaches to stuttering therapy* (pp. 1–38). Boston: Little, Brown.

Cooper, P. V. (1990). Discourse production and normal aging: Performance on oral picture description tasks. *Journal of Gerontology: Psychological Sciences, 45*, 210–214.

Corriveau, K., Posquine, E., & Goswami, U. (2007). Basic auditory processing skills and specific language impairment: A new look at an old hypothesis. *Journal of Speech, Language, and Hearing Research, 50*, 647–666.

Costello, J. (2000). AAC intervention in the intensive care unit: The Children's Hospital Boston model. *Augmentative and Alternative Communication, 16*, 137–153.

Coyle, J., Davis, L., Easterling, C., Graner, D., et al. (2009). Oropharyngeal dysphagia assessment and treatment efficacy: Setting the record straight (Response to Campbell-Taylor). *Journal of the American Medical Directors Association*, pp. 62–66.

Crago, M. B., Eriks-Brophy, A., Pesco, D., & McAlpine, L. (1997). Culturally based miscommunication in classroom interaction. *Language, Speech, and Hearing Services in Schools, 28*, 245–254.

Craig, A., & Calvert, P. (1991). Following up on treated stutterers: Studies of perception of fluency and job status. *Journal of Speech and Hearing Research, 34*, 279–284.

Craig, A., Hancock, H., Chang, E., McCready, C., et al. (1996). A controlled clinical trial for stuttering in persons aged 9 to 14 years. *Journal of Speech and Hearing Research, 39*, 808–826.

Cress, C. J. (2001). Language and AAC intervention in young children: Never too early or too late to start. *American Speech-Language Hearing Association Special Interest Division 1, Language Learning and Education Newsletter, 8* (1), 3–4.

Crites, L. S., Fischer, K. L., McNeish-Stengel, M., & Siegel, C. J. (1992). Working with families of drug-exposed children: Three model programs. *Infant-Toddler Intervention: The Transdisciplinary Journal, 2*,(1), 13–23.

Crowe, L. K. (2003). Comparison of two reading feedback strategies in improving the oral and written language performance of children with language-learning disabilities. *American Journal of Speech-Language Pathology, 12*, 16–27.

Cruickshanks, K. J., Wiley, T. L., Tweed, T. S., Klein, B. E. K., Klein, R., Mares-Perlman, J. A., et al. (1998). Prevalence of hearing loss in older adults in Beaver Dam, Wisconsin: The epidemiology of hearing loss study. *American Journal of Epidemiology, 148*(9), 879–885.

Cummings, J. L., & Benson, D. F. (1992). *Dementia: A clinical approach* (2nd ed.). Boston: Butterworth-Heinemann.

Cummings, L. (2008). *Clinical linguistics*. Edinburgh: Edinburgh University Press.

Cupples, L., & Iacono, T. (2000). Phonological awareness and oral reading skill in children with Down syndrome. *Journal of Speech, Language, and Hearing Research, 43*, 595–608.

Dale, P. S., Price, T. S., Bishop, D. V. M., & Plomin, R. (2003). Outcomes of early language delay: I. Predicting persistent and transient language difficulties at 3 and 4 years. *Journal of Speech, Language, and Hearing Research, 46*, 544–560.

Dalston, R. M. (1995). The use of nasometry in the assessment and remediation of velopharyngeal inadequacy. In K. R. Bzoch (Ed.), *Communicative disorders related to cleft lip and palate* (4th ed., pp. 331–346). Austin, TX: Pro-Ed.

Dalston, R. (2004). The use of nasometry in the assessment and remediation of velopharyngeal inadequacy. In K. Bzoch (Ed.), *Communicative disorders related to cleft lip and palate* (5th ed.). Austin, TX: Pro-Ed.

Dalston, R. M., & Seaver, E. J. (1990). Nasometric and phototransductive measurements of reaction times in normal adult speakers. *Cleft Palate Journal, 27*, 61–67.

Daly, D., Simon, C., & Burnett-Stolnack, M. (1995). Helping adolescents who stutter focus on fluency. *Language, Speech, and Hearing Services in Schools, 26*, 162–168.

Damico, J. S. (1997, April). *Authentic classroom assessment for the speech-language pathologist.* Workshop presented at annual convention of the New York State Speech-Language-Hearing Association, Buffalo.

Darley, F., Aronson, A., & Brown, J. (1975). *Motor speech disorders.* Philadelphia: Saunders.

Dattilo, J., & Camarata, S. (1991). Facilitating conversation through self-initiated augmentative communication treatment. *Journal of Applied Behavior Analysis, 24*, 369–378.

Davis, A. (1993). *A survey of adult aphasia and related language disorders.* Englewood Cliffs, NJ: Prentice Hall.

Davis, B., Jakielski, K., & Marquardt, T. (1998). Developmental apraxia of speech: Determiners of differential diagnosis. *Clinical Linguistics and Phonetics, 12*, 25–45.

Dawson, G., Carver, L., Meltzoff, A. N., Panagiotides, H., McPartland, J., & Webb, S. J. (2002). Neural correlates of face and object recognition in young children with autism spectrum disorder, developmental delay, and typical development. *Child Development, 73*, 700–712.

Dawson, J., & Tattersall, P. (2001). *Structured Photographic Articulation Test II—Featuring Dudsberry.* DeKalb, IL: Janelle.

Dean Qualls, C., O'Brien, R. M., Blood, G. W., & Scheffner Hammer, C. (2003). Contextual variation, familiarity, academic literacy, and rural adolescents' idiom knowledge. *Language, Speech, and Hearing Services in Schools, 34*, 69–79.

DeBonis, D., & Moncrieff, D. (2008). Auditory processing disorders: An update for speech-language pathologists. *American Journal of Speech-Language Pathology, 17*, 4–18.

Deevy, P., & Leonard, L. B. (2004). The comprehension of wh-questions in children with specific language impairment. *Journal of Speech, Language, and Hearing Research, 47*, 802–815.

DeKosky, S. T. (2008, May 13). *Alzheimer's disease: Current and future research.* Public Policy Forum, Alzheimer's Association, Washington, DC.

Denk, D. M., Swoboda, H., Schima, W., & Eibenberger, K. (1997). Prognostic factors for swallowing rehabilitation following head and neck cancer surgery. *Acta Otolaryngolica, 117*(5), 769–774.

Dennis, M. (1992). Word finding in children and adolescents with a history of brain injury. *Topics in Language Disorders, 13*(1), 66–82.

DePippo, K. L., Holas, M. A., & Reding, M. J. (1992). validation of the 3-oz water swallow test for aspiration following stroke. *Archives of Neurology, 49*(12), 1259–1261.

DeRuyter, F., Fromm, D., Holland, A., & Stein, M. (2008). Aphasia resulting from left hemisphere stroke. *Treatment Efficacy Summary.* Retrieved June 28, 2009, at www.asha.org/NR/rdonlyres/4BAF3969-9ADC-4C01-B5ED-1334CC20DD3D/0/TreatmentEfficacySummaries2008.pdf

DeSanti, S. (1997). Differentiating the dementias. In C. T. Ferrand & R. L. Bloom (Eds.), *Introduction to organic and neurogenic disorders of communication: Current scope of practice* (pp. 84–109). Boston: Allyn and Bacon.

Deutsch, G. K., Dougherty, R. F., Bammer, R., Siok, W. T., Gabrieli, J. D., & Wandell, B. (2005). Children's reading performance is correlated with white matter structure measured by diffusion tensor imaging. *Cortex, 41*, 354–363.

Diefendorf, A. (1988). Pediatric audiology. In J. Lass, L. McReynolds, J. Northern, & D. Yoder (Eds.), *Handbook of speech language pathology and audiology* (pp. 1315–1338). Toronto, Ontario, Canada: B. C. Decker.

Diehl, S. F., Ford, C., & Federico, J. (2005). The communication journey of a fully included child with an autism spectrum disorder. *Topics in Language Disorders, 25*(4), 375–387.

Dole, J. A., Brown, K. J., & Trathen, W. (1996). The effects of strategy instruction on the comprehension performance of at-risk students. *Reading Research Quarterly, 31*, 62–88.

Dollaghan, C. A. (2004). Evidence-based practice in communication disorders: What do we know, and when do we know it? *Journal of Communication Disorders, 37*, 391–400.

Donahue, M. L., & Foster, S. K. (2004). Social cognition, conversation, and reading comprehension: How to read a comedy of manners. In C. A. Stone, E. R. Silliman, B. J. Ehren, & K. Apel (Eds.), *Handbook of language and literacy: Development and disorders* (pp. 363–379). New York: Guilford.

Dore, J., Franklin, M., Miller, R., & Ramer, A. (1976). Transitional phenomena in early language acquisition. *Journal of Child Language, 3,* 13–28.

Downey, D., Daugherty, P., Helt, S., & Daugherty, D. (2004). Integrating AAC into the classroom. *The ASHA Leader, 9*(17), 6–7, 36.

Downey, D. M., & Snyder, L. E. (2000). College students with LLD: The phonological core as risk for failure in foreign language classes. *Topics in Language Disorder, 21*(1), 82–92.

Doyle, M., & Phillips, B. (2001). Trends in augmentative and alternative communication use by individuals with amyotrophic lateral sclerosis. *Augmentative and Alternative Communication, 17,* 167–178.

Drager, K. D. R., & Reichle, J. E. (2001). Effects of age and divided attention on listeners' comprehension of synthesized speech. *Augmentative and Alternative Communication, 17,* 109–119.

Drager, K. D. R., Clark-Serpentine, E. A., Johnson, K. E., & Roeser, J. L. (2006). Accuracy of repetition of digitized and synthesized speech for young children in background noise. *American Journal of Speech-Language Pathology, 15,* 155–164.

Drager, K. D. R., Postal, V. J., Carrolus, L., Castellano, M., Gagliano, C., & Glynn, J. (2006). The effect of aided language modeling on symbol comprehension and production in 2 preschoolers with autism. *American Journal of Speech-Language Pathology, 15,* 112–125.

Dromi, E., Leonard., L. B., Adam, G., & Zadunaisky-Ehrlich, S. (1999). Verb agreement morphology in Hebrew-speaking children with specific language impairment. *Journal of Speech, Language, and Hearing Research, 42,* 1414–1431.

Dropik, P. L., & Reichle, J. (2008). Comparison of accuracy and efficiency of directed scanning and group-item scanning for augmentative communication selection techniques with typically developing preschoolers. *American Journal of Speech-Language Pathology, 17,* 35–47.

Duchan, J. F. (2002). What do you know about the history of speech-language pathology? And why is it important? *The ASHA Leader, 7*(23), 4–5, 29.

Duffy, J. R. (1995). *Motor speech disorders; Substrates, differential diagnosis, and management.* St. Louis, Mo: Mosby Year Book.

Duffy, J. (2005). *Motor speech disorders: Substrates, differential diagnosis, and management* (2nd ed.). St. Louis, MO: Elsevier, Mosby.

Duffy, J. R., Peach, R. K., & Strand, E. A. (2006). Progressive apraxia of speech as a sign of motor neuron disease. *American Journal of Speech-Language Pathology, 16,* 198–208.

Eadie, T. L., Yorkston, K. M., Klasner, E. R., Dudgeon, B. J., Deitz, J. C., Baylor, C. R., Miller, R. M., & Amtmann, D. (2006). Measuring communicative participation: A review of self-report instruments in speech-language pathology. *American Journal of Speech-Language Pathology, 15,* 307–320.

EBP Compendium. (2009, February). Review of Nasser et al. (2008), Interventions for the Management of Submucous Cleft Palate, *Cochrane Database of Systematic Reviews* (1). Retrieved June 23, 2009, at www.asha.org/members/ebp/compendium/reviews/review188

Eckert, M. A., Leonard, C. M., Wilke, M., Eckert, M., Richards, T., Richards, A., & Berninger, V. (2004). Anatomical signatures of dyslexia in children: Unique information from manual and voxel based morphometry brain measures. *Cortex, 41,* 304–315.

Ehren, B. J. (2005). Looking for evidence-based practice in reading comprehension instruction. *Topics in Language Disorders, 25,* 310–321.

Ehren, B. J. (2006). Partnerships to support reading comprehension for students with language impairment. *Topics in Language Disorders, 26,* 42–54.

Ehri, L. C. (2000). Learning to read and learning to spell: Two sides of a coin. *TLD, Topics in Language Disorders, 20*(3), 19–36.

Eigsti, L., & Cicchetti, D. (2004). The impact of child maltreatment on the expressive syntax at 60 months. *Developmental Science, 7,* 88–102.

Eisenberg, S. L., Ukrainetz, T. A., Hsu, J. R., Kaderavek, J. N., Justice, L. M., & Gillam, R. B. (2008). Noun phrase elaboration in children's spoken stories. *Language, Speech, and Hearing Services in Schools, 39,* 145–157.

Elliott, N., Sundberg, J., & Gramming, P. (1997). Physiological aspects of a vocal exercise. *Journal of Voice, 11,* 171–177.

Ellis Weismer, S., Plante, E., Jones, M., & Tomblin, J. B. (2005): A functional magnetic resonance imaging investigation of verbal working memory in adolescents with specific language impairment. *Journal of Speech, Language, and Hearing Research, 48,* 405–425.

Englert, C. S., Raphael, T. E., Anderson, L. M., Anthony, H. M., Fear, K. L., & Gregg, S. L. (1988). A case for writing intervention: Strategies for writing informational text. *Learning Disabilities Focus, 3*(2), 98–113.

English, K. (2002). Psychosocial aspects of hearing impairment and counseling basics. In R. L. Schow & M. A. Nerbonne (Eds.), *Introduction to audiologic rehabilitation.* (4th ed., pp. 225–246). Boston: Allyn and Bacon.

English, K. (2007). Psychosocial aspects of hearing impairment and counseling basics. In R. L. Schow & M. A. Nerbonne (Eds.), *Introduction to audiologic rehabilitation.* (5th ed., pp. 245–268). Boston: Pearson.

Erber, N. (1982). *Auditory training.* Washington, DC: Alexander Graham Bell Association for the Deaf.

Ertmer, D. J., Strong, L. M., & Sadagopan, N. (2003). Beginning to communicate after cochlear implantation: Oral language development in a young child. *Journal of Speech, Language, and Hearing Research, 46,* 328–340.

Ervalahti N., Korkman M., Fagerlund Å., Autti-Rämö I., Loimu L., & Hoyme H. E. (2007). Relationship between dysmorphic features and general cognitive function in children with fetal alcohol spectrum disorders. *American Journal of Medical Genetics, Part A, 143A,* 2916–2923.

Fager, S., Hux, K., Beukelman, D., & Karantounis, R. (2006). Augmentative and alternative communication use and acceptance by adults with traumatic brain injury. *Augmentative and Alternative Communication, 22,* 37–47.

Fagundes, D. D., Haynes, W. O., Haak, N. J., & Moran, M. J. (1998). Task variability effects on the language test performance of southern lower socioeconomic class African American and Caucasian 5-year-olds. *Language, Speech, and Hearing Services in Schools, 29,* 148–157.

Farber, J. G., & Klein, E. R. (1999). Classroom-based assessment of a collaborative intervention program for kindergarten and first-grade students. *Language, Speech, and Hearing Services in Schools, 30,* 83–91.

Farley, B., Fox, C., Ramig, L., & McFarland, D. (2008). Intensive amplitude-specific thereputic approaches for Parkinson disease: Toward a neuroplasticity-principled rehabilitation model. *Topics in Geriatric Rehabilitation, 24*(2), 99–114.

Feinberg, M. (1997). The effects of medications on swallowing. In B. C. Sonies (Ed.), *Dysphagia: A continuum of care.* Gaithersburg, MD: Aspen.

Feldman, H. M., Dollaghan, C. A., Campbell, T. F., Colborn, D. K., Janosky, J., Kurs-Lasky, M., Rockette, H. E., Dale, P. S., & Paradise, J. L. (2003). Parent-reported language skills in relation to otitis media during the first 3 years of life. *Journal of Speech, Language, and Hearing Research, 46,* 273–287.

Felsenfeld, S. (1997). Epidemiology and genetics of stuttering. In R. F. Curlee & G. M. Siegel (Eds.), *Nature and treatment of stuttering: New directions* (2nd ed., pp. 3–23). Boston: Allyn and Bacon.

Felsenfeld, S., Kirk, K. M., Zhu, G., Statham, D. J., Neale, M. C., & Martin, N. G. (2000). A study of genetic and environmental etiology of stuttering in a selected twin sample. *Behavior Genetics, 30*(5), 359–366.

Fey, M. E., Long, S. H., & Finestack, L. H. (2003). Ten principles of grammar facilitation for children with specific language impairment. *American Journal of Speech-Language Pathology, 12,* 3–15.

Filipek, P., Accordo, P., Baranek, G., Cook, E., Dawson, G., Gordon, B., et al. (1999). The screening and diagnosis of autism spectrum disorders. *Journal of Autism and Developmental Disorders, 29,* 49–58.

Flax, J. F., Realpe-Bonilla, T., Hirsch, L. S., Brzustowicz, L. M., Bartlett, C. W., & Tallal, P. (2003). Specific language impairment in families: Evidence for co-occurrence with reading impairments. *Journal of Speech, Language, and Hearing Research, 46,* 530–543.

Fleming, J., & Forester, B. (1997). Infusing language enhancement into reading curriculum for disadvantaged adolescents. *Language, Speech, and Hearing Services in Schools, 28,* 177–180.

Flipsen, P. (2003). Articulation rate and speech-sound normalization failure. *Journal of Speech, Language, and Hearing Research, 46,* 724–737.

Fluharty, N. B. (2000). *Fluharty Preschool Speech and Language Screening Test,* 2nd edition. Austin, TX: Pro-Ed.

Foster, W. A., & Miller, M. (2007). Development of the literacy achievement gap: A longitudinal study of kindergarten through third grade. *Language, Speech, and Hearing Services in Schools, 38,* 173–181.

Fowler, G. (1982). Developing comprehension skills in primary students through the use of story frames. *Reading Teacher, 36,* 176–179.

Fox, C., Boliek, C., & Ramig, L., (2006, March). The impact of intensive voice treatment (LSVT®) on speech intelligibility in children with spastic cerebral palsy. Poster presented at the Conference on Motor Speech, Austin, TX.

Fox, C., Morrison, C., Ramig, L., & Sapir, S. (2002). Current perspectives on the Lee Silverman Voice Treatment (LSVT) for individuals with idiopathic Parkinson disease. *American Journal of Speech-Language Pathology, 11,* 111–123.

Fox, L. E., & Rau, M. T. (2001). Augmentative and alternative communication for adults following glossectomy and laryngectomy surgery. *Augmentative and Alternative Communication, 17*, 161–166.

Foy, J. G., & Mann, V. (2003). Home literacy environment and phonological awareness in preschool children: Differential effects for rhyme and phoneme awareness. *Applied Psycholinguistics, 24*, 59–88.

Francis, A. L., Nusbaum, H. C., & Fenn, K. (2007). Effects of training on the acoustic-phonetic representation of synthetic speech. *Journal of Speech, Language, and Hearing Research, 50*, 1445–1465.

Fridriksson, J., Moser, D., Ryalls, J., Bonilha, L., Rorden, C., & Baylis, G. (2009). Modulation of frontal lobe speech areas associated with the production and perception of speech movements. *Journal of Speech and Hearing Research, 52*, 812–819.

Fried-Oken, M., & Bersani, H. A., Jr. (2000). *Speaking up and spelling it out: Personal essays on augmentative and alternative communication.* Baltimore: Brookes.

Fried-Oken, M., Fox, L., Rau, M. T., Tullman, J., Baker, G., Hindal, M., et al. (2006). Purposes of AAC device use for persons with ALS as reported by caregivers. *Augmentative and Alternative Communication, 22*, 209–221.

Frome Loeb, D., & Leonard, L. B. (1991). Subject case marking and verb morphology in normally developing and specifically language-impaired children. *Journal of Speech and Hearing Research, 34*, 340–346.

Fuchs, D., Fuchs, L. S., Thompson, A., Otaiba, S. A., Yen, L., Yang, N. J., Braun, N., & O'Connor, N. E. (2001). Is reading important in reading-readiness programs? A randomized field trial with teachers as program implementers. *Journal of Educational Psychology, 93*, 251–267.

Gaeth, J. H. (1948). *A study of phonemic regression in relation to hearing loss.* Unpublished doctoral dissertation, Northwestern University, Evanston, IL.

Galaburda, A. L. (2005). Neurology of learning disabilities: What will the future bring? The answer comes from the successes of the recent past. *Journal of Learning Disabilities, 28*, 107–109.

Garcia, J. M., Cannito, M. P., & Dagenais, P. A. (2000). Hand gestures: Perspectives and preliminary implications for adults with acquired dysarthria. *American Journal of Speech-Language Pathology, 9*, 107–115.

Gelb, A. B., Medeiros, L. J., Chen, Y. Y., Weiss, L. M., & Weidner, N. (1997). Hodgkin's disease of the esophagus. *American Journal of Clinical Pathology, 108*(5), 593–598.

Gelfer, M. P. (1996). *Survey of communication disorders: A social and behavioral perspective.* New York: McGraw-Hill.

Gerber, A., & Klein, E. R. (2004). *Teacher/tutor assisted literacy learning in the primary grades, a speech-language approach to early reading: T. A. L. L. while small.* Paper presented at the annual convention of the American Speech-Language-Hearing Association, Philadelphia.

German, D. J., & Simon, E. (1991). Analysis of children's word-finding skills in discourse. *Journal of Speech and Hearing Research, 34*, 309–316.

Gibbon, F. E., & Wood, S. E. (2003). Using electropalatography (EPG) to diagnose and treat articulation disorders associated with mild cerebral palsy: A case study. *Clinical Linguistics and Phonetics, 17*, 365–374.

Gibbs, D. P., & Cooper, E. B. (1989). Prevalence of communication disorders in students with learning disabilities. *Journal of Learning Disabilities, 22*, 60–63.

Gierut, J. A. (1998). Treatment efficacy: Functional phonological disorders in children. *Journal of Speech, Language, and Hearing Research, 41*(1), S85–S100.

Gierut, J. A. (2001). Complexity in phonological treatment: Clinical factors. *Language, Speech, and Hearing Services in Schools, 32*, 229–241.

Gierut, J. A. (2005). Phonological intervention: The how or the what? In A. Kamhi & K. Pollock (Eds.), *Phonological disorders in children: Clinical decision making in assessment and intervention* (pp. 201–210). Baltimore, MD: Brookes.

Gierut, J. A. (2009, June 19). Phonological disorders in children. *Treatment Efficacy Summary.* Retrieved June 23, 2009, from www.asha.org/NR/rdonlyres/F251004F-005C-47D9-8A2C-B85C818F3D33/0/TESPhonologicalDisordersinChildren.pdf

Gierut, J. A., Morrisette, M. L., Hughes, M. T., & Rowland, S. (1996). Phonological treatment efficacy and developmental norms. *Language, Speech, Hearing Services in Schools, 27*, 215–230.

Gillam, R. B. (1999). Computer-assisted language intervention using Fast For Word: Theoretical and empirical considerations for clinical decision making. *Language, Speech, and Hearing Services in Schools, 30*, 363–370.

Gillam, R. B., & Gorman, B. K. (2004). Language and discourse contributions to word recognition and text interpretation. In E. R. Silliman & L. C. Wilkinson (Eds.), *Language and literacy learning in schools* (pp. 63–97). New York: Guilford.

Gillon, G. T. (2000). The efficacy of phonological awareness intervention for children with spoken language impairment. *Language, Speech, and Hearing Services in Schools, 31*, 126–141.

Girolametto, L., Hoaken, L., Weitzman, E., & van Lieshout, R. (2000). Patterns of adult-child linguistic interaction in integrated day care groups. *Language, Speech, and Hearing Services in Schools, 31*, 155–168.

Girolametto, L., Weitzman, E., & Greenberg, J. (2003). Training day care staff to facilitate children's language. *American Journal of Speech-Language Pathology, 12*, 299–311.

Girolametto, L., Weitzman, E., Wiigs, M., & Steig Pearce, P. (1999). The relationship between maternal language measures and language development in toddlers with expressive vocabulary delays. *American Journal of Speech-Language Pathology, 8*, 364–374.

Glattke, T. J., & Robinette, M. S. (2007). Otoacoustic emissions. In R. J. Roeser, M. Valente, & H. H. Dunn (Eds.), *Audiology: Diagnosis* (2nd ed., pp. 478–496). New York: Thieme.

Glennen, S. (1997). Introduction to augmentative and alternative communication. In S. Glennen & D. DeCoste (Eds.), *Handbook of augmentative and alternative Communication* (p. 3–19). San Diego, CA: Singular.

Glennen, S., & Calculator, S. (1985). Training functional communication board use: A pragmatic approach. *Augmentative and Alternative Communication, 1*, 134–145.

Glennen, S. L., & DeCoste, C. (1997). *Handbook of augmentative communication*. San Diego, CA: Singular.

Golder, C., & Coirier, P. (1994). Argumentative text writing: Developmental trends. *Discourse Processes, 18*, 187–210.

Golding-Kushner, K. (1995). Treatment of articulation and resonance disorders associated with cleft palate and VPI. In R. J. Shprintzen & J. Bardach (Eds.), *Cleft palate speech management: A multidisciplinary approach*. St. Louis, MO: Mosby.

Goldman, R., & Fristoe, M. (2000). *Goldman-Fristoe test of articulation-Second edition (GFTA-2)*. Circle Pines, MN: American Guidance Service.

Goldstein, H., & Prelock, P. (2008). Child language disorders. *Treatment efficacy summary*. Retrieved June 28, 2009, from www.asha.org/NR/rdonlyres/4BAF3969-9ADC-4C01-B5ED-1334CC20DD3D/0/TreatmentEfficacySummaries2008.pdf

Goodglass, H., & Kaplan, E. (1983a). *The Boston diagnostic aphasia examination*. Philadelphia: Lea & Febiger.

Goodglass, H., & Kaplan, E. (1983b). *Boston naming test*. Philadelphia: Lea & Febiger.

Goswarni, U. C. (1988) Children's use of analogy in learning to spell. *British Journal of Developmental Psychology, 6*, 1–22.

Gottwald, S., & Starkweather, W. C. (1995). Fluency intervention for preschoolers and their families in the public schools. *Language, Speech, and Hearing Services in Schools, 26*, 117–126.

Grabb, W. C., Rosenstein, S. W., & Bzoch, K. R. (1971). *Cleft lip and palate: Surgical, dental, and speech aspects*. Boston: Little, Brown.

Graham, S. (1999). Handwriting and spelling instruction for students with learning disabilities: A review. *Learning Disability Quarterly, 22*, 78–98.

Graham, S., & Freeman, S. (1986). Strategy training and teacher- vs. student-controlled study conditions: Effects on LD students' performance. *Learning Disability Quarterly, 9*, 15–22.

Graham, S., & Harris, K. R. (1996). Addressing problems in attention, memory, and executive functioning: An example from self-regulated strategy development. In G. Reid Lyon & N. A. Krasnegor (Eds.), *Attention, memory and executive function* (pp. 349–365). Baltimore: Brookes.

Graham, S., & Harris, K. R. (1997). Self-regulation and writing: Where do we go from here? *Contemporary Educational Psychology, 22*, 102–114.

Graham, S., & Harris, K. R. (1999). Assessment and intervention in overcoming writing difficulties: An illustration from the self-regulation strategy development model. *Language, Speech, and Hearing Services in Schools, 30*(3), 255–264.

Graham, S., Harris, K., & Loynachan, C. (1994). The spelling for writing list. *Journal of Learning Disability, 27*, 210–217.

Graham, S., Harris, K., MacArthur, C. A., & Schwartz, S. S. (1991). Writing and writing instruction for students with learning disabilities: A review of a program of research. *Learning Disability Quarterly, 14*, 89–114.

Granlund, M., Björck-ÄKesson, E., Wilder, J., & Ylvén, R. (2008). AAC Interventions for children in a family environment: Implementing evidence in practice. *Augmentative and Alternative Communication, 24*, 207–219.

Gravel, J. S., & Wallace, I. F. (1999). Language, speech, and educational outcomes of otitis media. *Journal of Otolaryngology, 27*(Suppl. 2), 17–25.

Graves, A., Montague, M., & Wong, Y. (1990). The effects of procedural facilitation on the composition of learning disabled students. *Learning Disabilities Research, 5,* 88–93.

Gray, S. (2004). Word learning by preschoolers with specific language impairment: Predictors and poor learners. *Journal of Speech, Language, and Hearing Research, 47,* 1117–1132.

Gray, S., Plante, E., Vance, R., & Henrichsen, M. (1999). The diagnostic accuracy of four vocabulary tests administered to preschool-age children. *Language, Speech, and Hearing Services in Schools, 30,* 196–206.

Gray, S. D., Titze, I. R., & Lusk, R. P. (1987). Electron microscopy of hyperphonated canine vocal cords. *Journal of Voice, 1,* 109–115.

Greenamyre, J. T., & Shoulson, I. (1994). Huntington's disease. In D. Calne (Ed.), *Neurodegenerative diseases* (pp. 685–704). Philadelphia: Saunders.

Greenberg, D., Ehri, L., & Perin, D. (1997). Are word reading processes the same or different in adult literacy students and 3rd–5th graders matched for reading level? *Journal of Educational Psychology, 89,* 262–275.

Greene, J. F. (1996). Psycholinguistic assessment: The clinical base for identity of dyslexia. *Topics in Language Disorders 16*(2), 45–72.

Greenhalgh, K. S., & Strong, C. J. (2001). Literate language features in spoken narratives of children with typical language and children with language impairments. *Language, Speech, and Hearing Services in Schools, 32,* 114–126.

Greenough, W. T. (1975). Experimental modification of the developing brain. *American Science, 63,* 37–46.

Gregory, R. L. (1981). *Mind in science.* New York: Cambridge University Press.

Grice, H. (1975). Logic and conversation. In D. Davidson & G. Harmon (Eds.), *The logic of grammar.* Encino, CA: Dickenson Press.

Grice, S. J., Halit, H., Farroni, T., Baron-Cohen, S., Bolton, P., & Johnson, M. H. (2005). Neural correlates of eye-gaze detection in young children with autism. *Cortex, 41,* 327–341.

Griffith, P. (1991). Phonemic awareness helps first graders invent spellings and third graders remember correct spelling. *Journal of Reading Behavior, 23,* 215–233.

Grigorenko, E. L. (2005). A conservative meta-analysis of linkage and linkage-association studies of developmental dyslexia. *Scientific Studies of Reading, 9,* 285–316.

Grove, N., & Dockrell, J. (2000) Multisign combinations by children with intellectual impairments: An analysis of language skills. *Journal of Speech, Language and Hearing Research, 43,* 309–323.

Grunwell, P. (1987). *Clinical phonology* (2nd ed.). London: Chapman & Hall.

Guitar, G. (2006). *Stuttering: An integrated approach to its nature and treatment.* Philadelphia: Lippincott Williams & Wilkins.

Gummersall, D. M., & Strong, C. J. (1999). Assessment of complex sentence production in a narrative context. *Language, Speech, and Hearing Services in Schools, 30,* 152–164.

Gumperz, J. J., & Hymes, D. (1972). *Directions in sociolinguistics: The ethnography of communication.* New York: Holt, Rinehart and Winston.

Guo, L.-Y., Tomblin, J. B., & Samelson, V. (2008). Speech disruptions in the narratives of English-speaking children with specific language impairment. *Journal of Speech, Language, and Hearing Research, 51,* 722–738.

Gurd, J. M., Bessell, N., Watson, I., & Coleman, J. (1998). Motor speech vs. digit control in Parkinson's disease: A cognitive neuropsychology investigation. *Clinical Linguistics and Phonetics, 12,* 357–378.

Gutierrez-Clellen, V. F. (2000). Dynamic assessment: An approach to assessing children's language-learning potential. *Seminars in Speech and Language, 21,* 215–222.

Guyatt, G., & Rennie, D. (Eds.). (2002). *User's guides to the medical literature: A manual for evidence-based clinical practice.* Chicago: American Medical Association Press.

Hadley, P. A. (1998). Language sampling protocols for eliciting text-level discourse. *Language, Speech, and Hearing Services in Schools, 29,* 132–147.

Hadley, P. A., Simmerman, A., Long, M., & Luna, M. (2000). Facilitating language development in inner-city children: Experimental evaluation of a collaborative classroom-based intervention. *Language, Speech, and Hearing Services in Schools, 31,* 280–295.

Hagan, C., & Malkamus, D. (1979, November). *Interaction strategies for language disorders secondary to head trauma.* Paper presented at the annual convention of the American Speech-Language-Hearing Association, Atlanta, GA.

Hall, J. W. (2007). *New handbook of auditory evoked potentials.* Boston: Pearson.

Hall, J. W., & Grose, J. H. (1993). The effect of otitis media with effusion on the masking-level difference and the auditory brainstem response. *Journal of Speech and Hearing Research, 36*, 210–217.

Hall, K. (2001). *Pediatric dysphagia resource guide.* San Diego, CA: Singular.

Hall, P. K., Jordan, L. S., & Robin, D. A. (1993). *Developmental apraxia of speech: Theory and clinical practice.* Austin, TX: Pro-Ed.

Hambly, C., & Riddle, L. (2002, April). *Phonological awareness training for school-age children.* Paper presented at the annual convention of the New York State Speech-Language-Hearing Association, Rochester, NY.

Hane, A. A., Feldstein, S., & Dernetz, V. H. (2003). The relation between coordinated interpersonal timing and maternal sensitivity in four-month-olds. *Journal of Psycholinguistic Research, 32*, 525–539.

Hardin-Jones, M., Chapman, K., & Scherer, N. J. (2006, June 13). Early intervention in children with cleft palate. *The ASHA Leader, 11*(8), 8–9, 32.

Hardy, E., & Robinson, N. M. (1993). *Swallowing disorders treatment manual.* Bisbee, AZ: Imaginart.

Harlaar, N., Hayiou-Thomas, M. E., Dale, P. S., & Plomin, R. (2008). Why do preschool language abilities correlate with later reading? A twin study. *Journal of Speech, Language, and Hearing Research, 51*, 688–705.

Hart, K. I., Fujiki, M., Brinton, B., & Hart, C. H. (2004). The relationship between social behavior and severity of language impairment. *Journal of Speech, Language, and Hearing Research, 47*, 647–662.

Hayden, D., & Square, P. (1999). *Verbal motor production assessment for children.* San Antonio, TX: Psychological Corporation.

Haynes, W. O., & Pindzola, R. H. (1998). *Diagnosis and evaluation in speech pathology* (5th ed.). Boston: Allyn and Bacon.

Hegde, M. N. (1998). *Treatment procedures in communicative disorders* (3rd ed.). Austin, TX: Pro-Ed.

Heiss, W. D., Kessler, J., Thiel, A., Ghaemi, M., & Karbe, H. (1999). Differential capacity of left and right hemisphere areas for compensation of part-stroke aphasia. *Annals of Neurology, 45*, 430–438.

Helm-Estabrooks, N., & Albert, M. C. (1991). *Manual of aphasia therapy.* Austin, TX: Pro-Ed.

Henderson, E. H. (1990). *Teaching spelling* (2nd ed.). Boston: Houghton Mifflin.

Hewat, S., Onslow, M., Packman, A., & O'Brain, S. (2006). A phase II clinical trial of self-imposed time-out treatment for stuttering in adults and adolescents. *Disability and Rehabilitation, 28*, 33–42.

Hewlett, N. (1990). The processes of speech production and speech development. In P. Grunwell (Ed.), *Developmental speech disorders: Clinical issues and practical implications.* Edinburgh, UK: Churchill Livingstone.

Hicks, C. B., Tharpe, A. M., & Ashmead, D. H. (2000). Behavioral auditory assessment of young infants: Methodologic limitations or natural lack of auditory responsiveness? *American Journal of Audiology, 9*, 124–130.

Higginbotham, D. J., Bisantz, A. M., Sunm, M., Adams, K., & Yik, F. (2009). The effect of context priming and task type on augmentative communication performance. *Augmentative and Alternative Communication, 25*(1), 19–31.

Hill, A. J., Theodoros, D. G., Russell, T. G., Cahill, L. M., Ward, E. C., & Clark, K. M. (2006). An internet-based telerehabilitation system for the assessment of motor speech disorders: A pilot study. *American Journal of Speech-Language Pathology, 15*, 45–56.

Hirano, M., Vennard, W., & Ohala, J. (1970). Regulation of register, pitch, and intensity of voice. *Folia Phoniatrica et Logopaedica, 22*, 1–20.

Hixon, T., & Hoit, J. (2005). *Evaluation and management of speech breathing disorders: Principles and methods.* Tucson, AZ: Redington Brown.

Hixon, T., Weismer, G., & Hoit, J. (2008). *Preclinical speech science: Anatomy, physiology, acoustics, and perception.* San Diego, CA: Plural.

Ho, A., Iansek, R., Marigliani, C., Bradshaw, J., & Gates, S. (1998). Speech impairment in a large sample of patients with Parkinson's disease. *Behavioral Neurology, 11*, 131–137.

Hodson, B. (2004). *Hodson assessment of phonological patterns* (3rd ed.). Austin, TX: Pro-Ed.

Hodson, B., & Paden, E. (1991). *Targeting intelligible speech: A phonological approach to remediation* (2nd ed.). Austin, TX: Pro-Ed.

Hoffman, R., Norris, J. & Monjure, J. (1990). Comparison of process targeting and whole language treatment for phonologically delayed preschool children. *Language, Speech, and Hearing Services in Schools, 21*, 102–109.

Hogan, T., & Catts, H. W. (2004). *Phonological awareness test items: Lexical and phonological characteristics affect performance.* Paper presented at the annual convention of the American Speech-Language-Hearing Association, Philadelphia.

Hoit, J., & Hixon, T. (1987). Age and speech breathing. *Journal of Speech and Hearing Research, 30*, 351–366.

Holland, A. L. (1980). *Communication abilities in daily living: A test of functional communication for adults*. Baltimore: University Park Press.

Holland, A., & Fridriksson, J. (2001). Aphasia management during the early phases of recovery following stroke. *American Journal of Speech-Language Pathology, 10*, 19–28.

Hollien, H. (2002). *Forensic voice identification*. San Diego, CA: Academic Press.

Hopper, T. (2005, November 8). Assessment and treatment of cognitive-communication disorders in individuals with dementia. *The ASHA Leader, 10*(15), 10–11.

Horn, E. (1954). *Teaching spelling*. Washington, DC: American Education Research Association.

Houston-Price, C., Plunkett, K., & Haris, P. (2005). Word-learning wizardry at 1;6. *Journal of Child Language, 32*, 175–189.

Howell, J., & Dean, E. (1994). *Treating phonological disorders in children: Metaphon—theory to practice* (2nd ed.). London: Whurr.

Howell, P. (2004). Assessment of some contemporary theories of stuttering that apply to spontaneous speech. *Contemporary Issues in Communication Science and Disorders, 31*, 69–79. 123–140.

Huaqing Qi, C., & Kaiser, A. P. (2004). Problem behaviors of low income children with language delays: An observation study. *Journal of Speech, Language, and Hearing Research, 47*, 595–609.

Hugdahl, K., Gundersen, H., Brekke, C., Thomsen, T., Rimol, L. M., Ersland, L., et al. (2004). fMRI brain activation in a Finnish family with specific language impairment compared with a normal control group. *Journal of Speech, Language, and Hearing Research, 47*, 162–172.

Hughes, M., & Searle, D. (1997). *The violet E and other tricky sounds: Learning to spell from kindergarten to grade 6*. York, ME: Stenhouse.

Hunt-Berg, M. (2001). Gestures in development: Implications for early intervention in AAC. *American Speech-Language Hearing Association Special Interest Division 1, Language Learning and Education Newsletter, 8*(1), 5–8.

Hunter, L., Pring, T., & Martin, S. (1991). The use of strategies to increase speech intelligibility in cerebral palsy: An experimental evaluation. *British Journal of Disorders of Communication, 26*, 163–174.

Hurst, M., & Cooper, G. (1983). Employer attitudes towards stuttering. *Journal of Fluency Disorders, 8*, 1–12.

Hustad, K. C. (2007). Contribution of two sources of listener knowledge to intelligibility of speakers with cerebral palsy. *Journal of Speech, Language, and Hearing Research, 50*, 1228–1240.

Hustad, K. C., & Beukelman, D. R. (2001). Effects of linguistic cues and stimulus cohesion on intelligibility of severely dysarthric speech. *Journal of Speech, Language, and Hearing Research, 44*, 497–510.

Hustad, K. C., & Cahill, M. A. (2003). Effects of presentation mode and repeated familiarization on intelligibility of dysarthric speech. *American Journal of Speech-Language Pathology, 12*, 198–208.

Hutchinson, J., & Marquardt, T. P. (1997). Functional treatment approaches to memory impairment following brain injury. *Topics in Language Disorders, 18*(1), 45–57.

Iacono, T., Carter, M., & Hook, J. (1998). Identification of international communication in students with severe and multiple disabilities. *Augmentative and Alternative Communication, 14*, 102–114.

Iglesias, A., & Goldstein, B. (1998). Language and dialectical variations. In J. E. Bernthal, & N. W. Bankson (Eds.), *Articulation and phonological disorders* (4th ed.). Boston: Allyn and Bacon.

Ingham, R. J., & Cordes, A. K. (1997). Self-measurement and evaluating stuttering treatment efficacy. In R. F. Curlee & G. M. Siegel (Eds.), *Nature and treatment of stuttering: New directions* (2nd ed., pp. 413–437). Boston: Allyn and Bacon.

Ingram, K., Bunta, F., & Ingram, D. (2004). Digital data collection and analysis: Application for clinical practice. *Language, Speech, and Hearing Services in Schools, 35*, 112–121.

Ingham, R. J., Ingham, J. C., Finn, P., & Fox, P. T. (2003). Towards a functional neural systems model of developmental stuttering. *Journal of Fluency Disorders, 28*, 297–318.

The Internet Stroke Center (2005). http:// www.stroke-center.org/path/stats.htm. Retrieved October 22.

Isshiki, N. (1964). Regulatory mechanism of voice intensity of voice variation. *Journal of Speech and Hearing Research, 7*, 17–29.

Izumikawa, M., Minoda, R., Kawamoto, K., Abrashkin, K. A., Swiderski, D. L., Dolan, D. F., et al. (2005). Auditory hair cell replacement and hearing improvement by *Atohl* gene therapy in deaf mammals. *Nature Medicine, 11*, 271–276.

Jacobs, B. J., & Thompson, C. K. (2000). Cross-modality generalization effects of training non-canonical sentence comprehension and production in agrammatic aphasia. *Journal of Speech, Language, and Hearing Research, 43*, 5–20.

James, J. (1981a). Self-monitoring of stuttering: Reactivity and accuracy. *Behaviour Research and Therapy, 19*, 291–296.

James, J. (1981b). Behavioral self-control of stuttering using time-out from speaking. *Journal of Applied Behavioral Analysis, 14,* 25–37.

Jarvis, J. (1989). Taking a Metaphon approach to phonological development: A case study. *Child Language Teaching and Therapy, 5,* 16–32.

Jelm, J. M. (1994). Treatment of feeding and swallowing disorders in children: An overview. In L. R. Cherney (Ed.), *Clinical management of dysphagia in adults and children.* Gaithersburg, MD: Aspen.

Jerome, A. C., Fujiki, M., Brinton, B., & James, S. L. (2002). Self-esteem in children with specific language impairment. *Journal of Speech, Language, and Hearing Research, 45,* 700–714.

Jewett, D. L., Romano, M. N., & Williston, J. S. (1970). Human auditory evoked potentials: Possible brain stem components detected on the scalp. *Science, 167,* 1517–1518.

Johns Hopkins. (2000). Help when it's hard to swallow. *Johns Hopkins Medical Letter, Health after 50, 11* (12), 6–7.

Johnson, C. J. (2006). Getting started in evidence-based practice for childhood speech-language disorders. *American Journal of Speech-Language Pathology, 15,* 20–35.

Johnson, C. J., & Yeates, E. (2006). Evidence-based vocabulary instruction for elementary students via storybook reading. *EBP Briefs, 1* (3).

Johnston, B. T., Colcher, A., Li, Q., et al. (2001). Repetitive proximal esophageal contractions: A new manometric finding and a possible link between Parkinson's disease and achalasia. *Dysphagia, 16,* 186–189.

Johnston, J. R. (2001). An alternative MLU calculation: Magnitude and variability of effects. *Journal of Speech, Language, and Hearing Research, 44,* 156–164.

Johnston, P. H., & Winograd, P. N. (1985). Passive failure in reading. *Journal of Reading Behavior, 4,* 156–164.

Jung, T. T. K., & Hanson, J. B. (1999). Otitis media: Surgical principles based on pathogenesis. *Otolaryngologic Clinics of North America, 32,* 369–383.

Justice, L. M., & Ezell, H. K. (1999). Vygotskian theory and its application to assessment: An overview for speech-language pathologists. *Contemporary Issues and Science and Disorders, 26,* 111–118.

Justice, L. M., & Ezell, H. K. (2002). Use of storybook reading to increase print awareness in at-risk children. *American Journal of Speech-Language Pathology, 11,* 17–29.

Justice, L. M., & Kaderavek, J. N. (2004). Embedded-explicit emergent literacy intervention I: Background and description of approach. *Language, Speech, and Hearing Services in Schools, 35,* 201–211.

Justice, L. M., & Pence, K. (2007). Parent-implemented interactive language intervention: Can it be used effectively? *EBP Briefs, 2*(1).

Kaderavek, J. N., & Justice, L. M. (2004). Embedded-explicit emergent literacy intervention II: Goal selection and implementation in the early childhood classroom. *Language, Speech, and Hearing Services in Schools, 35,* 212–228.

Kaderavek, J. N., & Sulzby, E. (1998). Parent-child joint book reading: An observational protocol for young children. *American Journal of Speech-Language Pathology, 7* (1), 33–47.

Kamhi, A. (1998). Trying to make sense of developmental language disorders. *Language, Speech, and Hearing Services in Schools, 29,* 35–44.

Kamhi, A. G. (2003). The role of the SLP in improving reading fluency. *The ASHA Leader, 8* (7), 6–8.

Kamhi, A. G. (2006a). Prologue: Combining research and reason to make treatment decisions. *Language, Speech, and Hearing Services in Schools, 37,* 225–256.

Kamhi, A. G. (2006b). Treatment decisions for children with speech-sound disorders. *Language, Speech, and Hearing Services in Schools, 37,* 271–279.

Kamhi, A. G., & Catts, H. W. (2005). Language and reading: Convergences and divergences. In H. W. Catts & A. G. Kamhi (Eds.), *Language and reading disabilities* (2nd ed., pp. 1–25). Boston: Allyn and Bacon.

Kamhi, A. G., Gentry, B., Mauer, D., & Gholson, B. (1990). Analogical learning and transfer in language-impaired children. *Journal of Speech and Hearing Disorders, 55,* 140–148.

Kamhi, A. G., & Hinton, L. N. (2000). Explaining individual differences in spelling ability. *Topics in Language Disorders, 20*(3), 37.

Karagiannis, A., Stainback, W., & Stainback, S. (1996). Historical overview of inclusion. In S. Stainback & W. Stainback (Eds.), *Inclusion: A guide for educators.* Baltimore: Brookes.

Katz, R. C., & Wertz, R. T. (1997). The efficacy of computer-provided reading treatment for chronic aphasic adults. *Journal of Speech, Language, and Hearing Research, 40,* 493–507.

Katz, W. F. (2003). From basic research in speech science to answers in speech-language pathology. *The ASHA Leader, 8* (1), 6–7, 20.

Katz, W. F., Bharadwaj, S. V., & Carstens, B. (1999). Electromagnetic articulography treatment for an adult with Broca's aphasia and apraxia of speech.

Journal of Speech, Language, and Hearing Research, 42, 1355–1366.

Kaufman, N. (1995). *Kaufman Speech Praxis Test for Children*. Detroit, MI: Wayne State University Press.

Kavé, G., & Levy, Y. (2003). Morphology in picture descriptions provided by persons with Alzheimer's disease. *Journal of Speech, Language, and Hearing Research, 46*, 341–352.

Kavrie, S., & Neils-Strunjas, J. (2002). Dysgraphia in Alzheimer's disease with mild cognitive impairment. *Journal of Medical Speech-Language Pathology, 10*(1), 73–85.

Kay-Raining Bird, E., & Chapman, R. S. (1994). Sequential recall in individuals with Down syndrome. *Journal of Speech, Language, and Learning Research, 37*, 1369–1380.

Kay-Raining Bird, E., Cleave, P. L., White, D., Pike, H., & Helmkay, A. (2008). Written and oral narratives of children and adolescents with Down syndrome. *Journal of speech, Language, and Hearing Research, 51*, 436–450.

Kearns, K. P., & Simmons, N. N. (1988). Motor speech disorders: The dysarthrias and apraxia of speech. In N. J. Lass, L. V. McReynolds, & D. E. Yoder (Eds.), *Handbook of speech-language pathology and audiology* (pp. 592–621). Burlington, Ontario, Canada: B. D. Decker.

Keele, S. W. (1968). Movement control in skilled motor performance. *Psychological Bulletin, 70*, 387–403.

Kemker, F. J. (1995). Audiologic management of patients with cleft palate and related disorders. In K. R. Bzoch (Ed.), *Communicative disorders related to cleft lip and palate* (4th ed., pp. 245–260). Austin, TX: Pro-Ed.

Kemp, D. T. (1978). Stimulated acoustic emissions from within the human auditory system. *Journal of the Acoustical Society of American, 64*, 1386–1391.

Kemper, S., Thompson, M., & Marquis, J. (2001). Longitudinal change in language production: Effects of aging and dementia on grammatical complexity and prepositional content. *Psychology and Aging, 16*, 600–614.

Kemper, T. (1984). Neuroanatomical and neuropathological changes in normal aging and in dementia. In M. L. Albert (Ed.), *Clinical neurology of aging*. New York: Oxford University Press.

Kent, R. D. (1997). *The speech sciences*. San Diego, CA: Singular.

Kent, R. D., Duffy, J. R., Slama, A., Kent, J. F., & Clift, A. (2001). Clinicoanatomic studies in dysarthria: Review, critique, and directions for research. *Journal*

of Speech, Language, and Hearing Research, 44, 535–551.

Kent, R. D., Finley Kent, J., Duffy, J. R., Thomas, J. E., Weismer, G., & Stuntebeck, S. (2000). Ataxic dysarthria. *Journal of Speech, Language, and Hearing Research, 43*, 1275–1289.

Kertesz, A., & McCabe, P. (1982). *Western Aphasia Battery*. New York: Grune & Stratton.

Kertesz, A., & McCabe, P. (1997). Recovery patterns and prognosis in aphasia. *Brain, 100*, 100–118.

Kessels, R. P. C., (2003). Patients' memory for medical information. *Journal of Royal Society of Medicine 96*, 219–222.

Kidd, K. (1984). Stuttering as a genetic disorder. In R. F. Curlee & W. H. Perkins (Eds.), *Nature and treatment of stuttering: New directions* (pp. 149–169). Boston: Allyn and Bacon.

Kiernan, B., Snow, D., Swisher, L., & Vance, R. (1997). Another look at nonverbal rule induction in children with specific language impairment: Testing a flexible reconceptualization hypothesis. *Journal of Speech and Hearing Research, 40*, 75–82.

Kintsch, W. (1998). *Comprehension: A paradigm for cognition*. New York: Cambridge University Press.

Kirk, C., & Gillon, G. T. (2008, October 24). Integrated morphological awareness intervention as a tool for improving literacy. *Language, Speech, and Hearing Services in Schools*. Retrieved June 6, 2008, from http://lshss.asha.org/cgi/rapidpdf/0161-1461_2008_08-0009v1?maxtoshow=&HITS=10&hits=10&RESULTFORMAT=&author1=kirk&andorexactfulltext=and&searchid=1&FIRSTINDEX=0&sortspec=relevance&resourcetype=HWCIT

Kirshner, H. S. (1995). *Handbook of neurological speech and language disorders*. New York: Marcel Dekker.

Klasner, E. R., & Yorkston, K. M. (2001). Linguistic and cognitive supplementation strategies as augmentative and alternative communication techniques in Huntington's disease: Case study. *Augmentative and Alternative Communication, 17*, 154–160.

Kleim, J. A., & Jones, T. A. (2008). Principles of experience-dependent neural plasticity: Implications for rehabilitation after brain damage. *Journal of Speech, Language, and Hearing Research, 51*, S225–S239.

Kochkin, S. (2005). MarkeTrak VII: Hearing loss population tops 31 million. *The Hearing Review, 12*(7): 16–29.

Koo, E., & Price, D. (1993). The neurobiology of dementia. In P. Whitehouse (Ed.), *Dementia* (pp. 55–91). Philadelphia: F. A. Davis.

Koppenhaver, D., & Erickson, K. (2003). Natural emergent literacy supports for preschoolers with autism and severe communication impairments. *Topics in Language Disorders, 23*(4), 283–292.

Koul, R., & Hester, K. (2006). Effects of repeated listening experiences on the recognition of synthetic speech by individuals with severe intellectual disabilities. *Journal of Speech, Language, and Hearing Research, 49*, 47–57.

Kouri, T. A., Selle, C. A., & Riley, S. A. (2006). Comparison of meaning and graphophonemic feedback strategies for guided reading instruction of children with language delays. *American Journal of Speech-Language Pathology, 15*, 236–246.

Koutsoftas, A. D., Harmon, M., & Gray, S. (2008, October 24). The Effect of Tier 2 Intervention for Phonemic Awareness in a Response-to-Intervention Model in Low-Income Preschool Classrooms. *Language, Speech, and Hearing Services in Schools.* Retrieved June 6, 2009, from http://lshss.asha.org/cgi/rapidpdf/0161-1461_2008_07-0101v1?maxtoshow=&HITS=10&hits=10&RESULTFORMAT=&authorl=Koutsoftas&andorexactfulltext=and&searchid=1&FIRSTINDEX=0&sortspec=relevance&resourcetype

Kristensen, H. (2000). Selective mutism and comorbidity with developmental disorder/delay, anxiety disorder, and elimination disorder. *Journal of the American Academy of Child and Adolescent Psychiatry, 39*, 249–256.

Kuehn, D. (1991). New therapy for treating hypernasal speech using continuous positive airway pressure (CPAP). *Plastic and Reconstructive Surgery, 88*, 959–966.

Kuehn, D., & Henne, L. (2003). Speech evaluation and treatment for patients with cleft palate. *American Journal of Speech-Language Pathology, 12*, 103–109.

Kuehn, D., Imrey, P., Tomes, L., et al. (2002). Efficacy of continuous positive airway pressure (CPAP) treatment of hypernasality. *Cleft Palate-Craniofacial Journal, 39*, 267–276.

Kummer, A. W. (2001). *Cleft palate and craniofacial anomalies: The effects on speech and resonance.* San Diego, CA: Singular Thomson Learning.

Laguaite, J. K. (1972). Adult voice screening. *Journal of Speech and Hearing Disorders, 37*, 147–151.

Langford, S., & Cooper, E. (1974). Recovery from stuttering as viewed by parents of self-diagnosed recovered stutterers. *Journal of Communication Disorders, 7*, 171–181.

Langmore, S. E., Terpenning, M. S., Schork, A., Chen, Y., Murray, J. T., Lopatin, D., & Loesche, W. J. (1998). Predictors of aspiration pneumonia: How important is dysphagia? *Dysphagia, 13*(2), 69–81.

Lanter, E., & Watson, L. R. (2008). Promoting literacy in students with ASD: The basics for the SLP. *Language, Speech, and Hearing Services in Schools, 39*, 33–43.

La Paro, K. M., Justice, L., Skibbe, L. E., & Pianta, R. C. (2004). Relations among maternal, child, and demographic factors and the persistence of preschool language impairment. *American Journal of Speech-Language Pathology, 13*, 291–303.

Lapko, L., & Bankson, N. (1975). Relationship between auditory discrimination, articulation stimulability and consistency of misarticulation. *Perceptual and Motor Skills, 40*, 171–177.

Larrivee, L., & Catts, H. (1999). Early reading achievement in children with expressive phonological disorders. *American Journal of Speech-Language Pathology, 8*, 118, 128.

Larson, V. L., & McKinley, N. L. (1998). Characteristics of adolescents' conversation: A longitudinal study. *Clinical Linguistics and Phonetics, 12*, 183–203.

Lasker, J. P., & Bedrosian, J. L. (2000). Acceptance of AAC by adults with acquired disorders. In D. Beukelman, K. Yorkston, & J. Reichle (Eds.), *Augmentative communication for adults with neurogenic and neuromuscular disabilities* (pp. 107–136). Baltimore: Brookes.

Lasker, J. P., & Bedrosian, J. L. (2001). Promoting acceptance of augmentative and alternative communication by adults with acquired communication disorders. *Augmentative and Alternative Communication, 17*, 141–153.

Lass, N. J., & Pannbacker, M. (2008). The application of evidence-based practice to nonspeech oral motor treatments. *Language, Speech, and Hearing Services in Schools, 39*, 408–421.

Lau, C., & Kusnierczyk, I. (2001). Quantitative evaluation of infant's nonnutritive and nutritive sucking. *Dysphagia, 16*, 58–67.

Law, J., Garrett, Z., & Nye, C. (2004). The efficacy of treatment for children with developmental speech and language delay/disorder: A meta-analysis. *Journal of Speech, Language, and Hearing Research, 47*, 924–943.

Le Blanc, E. M., & Cisneros, G. J. (1995). The dynamics of speech and orthodontic management in cleft lip and palate. In R. J. Shprintzen & J. Bardach (Eds.), *Cleft palate speech management: A multidisciplinary approach.* St. Louis, MO: Mosby.

Leblanc, R. (1996). Familial cerebral aneurysms. *Stroke, 27*, 1050–1054.

Leder, S. B., Sasaki, C. T., & Burrell, M. I. (1998). Fiberoptic endoscopic evaluation of dysphagia to identify silent aspiration. *Dysphagia, 13* (1), 19–21.

Lee, J., Croen, L. A., Lindan, C., Nash, K. B., Yoshida, C. K., Ferriero, D. M., et al. (2005). Predictors of outcome in perinatal arterial stroke: A population-based study. *Annals of Neurology, 58*(2), 303–308.

Lehman Blake, M. (2006). Clinical relevance of discourse characteristics after right hemisphere brain damage. *American Journal of Speech-Language Pathology, 15,* 255–267.

Lehman Blake, M. (2007). Perspectives on treatment for communication deficits associated with right hemisphere brain damage. *American Journal of Speech-Language Pathology, 16,* 331–342.

Lehman Blake, M., & Tompkins, C. A. (2008). Cognitive-communication disorders resulting from right hemisphere damage. *Treatment Efficacy Summary.* Retrieved June 28, 2009, from www.asha.org/NR/rdonlyres/4BAF3969-9ADC-4C01-B5ED-1334CC20DD3D/0/TreatmentEfficacySummaries2008.pdf

Lennox, C., & Siegel, L. S. (1996). The development of phonological rules and visual strategies in average and poor spellers. *Journal of Experimental Child Psychology, 62,* 60–83.

Lesar, S. (1992). Prenatal cocaine exposure: The challenge to education. *Infant-Toddler Intervention: The Transdisciplinary Journal, 2*(1), 37–52.

Lewis, B. A., O'Donnell, B., Freebairn, L. A., & Taylor, H. G. (1998). Spoken language and written expression—interplay of delays. *American Journal of Speech-Language Pathology, 7*(3), 77–84.

Lieven, E., Behrens, H., Speares, J., & Tomasello, M. (2003). Early syntactic creativity: A usage-based approach. *Journal of Child Language, 30,* 333–370.

Light, J. (1989). Toward a definition of communication competence for individuals using augmentative and alternative communication systems. *Augmentative and Alternative Communication, 5,* 137–144.

Light, J. (1997). "Let's go star fishing": Reflections on the contexts of language learning for children who use aided AAC. *Augmentative and Alternative Communication, 13,* 158–171.

Light, J., Beukelman, D., & Reichle, J. (2003). *Communicative competence for individuals who use AAC: From research to effective practice.* Baltimore: Brookes.

Light, J., & Lindsay, P. (1991). Cognitive science and augmentative and alternative communication. *Augmentative and Alternative Communication, 7,* 186–203.

Liiva, C. A., & Cleave, P. L. (2005). Roles of initiation and responsiveness in access and participation for children with specific language impairment. *Journal of Speech, Language, and Hearing Research, 48,* 868–883.

Lincoln, M., & Onslow, M. (1997). Long-term outcome of early intervention for stuttering. *American Journal of Speech-Language Pathology, 6,* 51–58.

Liss, J. M., Krein-Jones, K., Wszolek, Z. K., & Caviness, J. N. (2006). Speech characteristics of patients with pallido-ponto-nigral degeneration and their application to presymptomatic detection in at-risk relatives. *American Journal of Speech-Language Pathology, 15,* 226–235.

Lloyd, L. L. Fuller, D., & Arvidson, H. (1997). *Augmentative and alternative communication: A handbook of principles and practices.* Boston: Allyn and Bacon.

Logemann, J. A. (1996). Screening, diagnosis, and management of neurogenic dysphasia. *Seminars in Neurology, 16*(4), 319–327.

Logemann, J. A. (1997). Structural and functional aspects of normal and disordered swallowing. In C. T. Ferrand & R. L. Bloom (Eds.), *Introduction to organic and neurogenic disorders of communication: Current scope of practice.* Boston: Allyn and Bacon.

Logemann, J. A. (1998). *Evaluation and treatment of swallowing disorders* (2nd ed.). Austin, TX: Pro-Ed.

Logemann, J., Gensler, G., Robbins, J., Lindblad, J., et al. (2008). A randomized study of three interventions for aspiration of thin liquids in patients with dementia or Parkinson's disease. *Journal of Speech, Language, and Hearing Research, 51,* 173–183.

Logemann, J., Kahrilas, P., Kobara, M., & Vakil, N. (1989). The benefit of head rotation on pharyngeoesophageal dysphagia. *Archives of Physical Medicine Rehabilitation, 70,* 767–771.

Long, S. (1994). Language and other special populations of children. In V. Reed (Ed.), *An introduction to children with language disorders* (2nd ed.). Upper Saddle River, NJ: Merrill/Prentice Hall.

Lonsbury-Martin, B. L. (2005). Otoacoustic emissions: Where are we today? *ASHA Leader, 10,* 6–7, 19.

Lord, C. (1988). Enhancing communication in adolescents with autism. *Topics in Language Disorders, 9*(1), 72–81.

Losh, M., & Capps, L. (2003). Narrative ability in high-functioning children with autism or Asperger's syndrome. *Journal of Autism and Developmental Disorders, 33,* 239–251.

Lotze, M. (1995). Nursing assessment and management. In S. R. Rosenthal, J. J. Sheppard, & M. Lotze (Eds.), *Dysphagia and the child with developmental disabilities: Medical, clinical, and family interventions.* San Diego, CA: Singular.

Love, R. J. (1992). *Childhood motor speech disability.* New York: Macmillan.

Love, R., & Webb, W. (2001). *Neurology for the speech-language pathologist* (4th ed.). Boston: Butterworth–Heinemann.

Lubinski, R., & Masters, M. G. (2001). Special populations, special settings: New and expanding frontiers. In R. Lubinski & C. Frattali (Eds.), *Professional issues in speech-language pathology and audiology* (2nd ed.). San Diego, CA: Singular.

Lubker, B. B. (1997). Language learning disorders in children with chronic health conditions: Epidemiologic perspectives. *American Speech-Language-Hearing Association, Special Interest Divisions, Language Learning and Education, 4*(1), 2–5.

Lukens, C., & Linscheid, T. (2008). Development and validation of an inventory to assess mealtime behavior problems in children with autism. *Journal of Autism Developmental Disorders, 38,* 342–352.

Lund, N., & Duchan, J. (1993). *Assessing children's language in naturalistic contexts* (3rd ed.). Englewood Cliffs, NJ: Prentice Hall.

Lund, S., & Light, J. (2006). Long-term outcomes for individuals who use augmentative and alternative communication: Part I—What is a good outcome? *Augmentative and Alternative Communication, 22,* 284–299.

Lund, S., & Light, J. (2007a). Long-term outcomes for individuals who use augmentative and alternative communication: Part II—What is a good outcome? *Augmentative and Alternative Communication, 23,* 1–15.

Lund, S., & Light, J. (2007b). Long-term outcomes for individuals who use augmentative and alternative communication: Part III—Contributing factors. *Augmentative and Alternative Communication, 23,* 323–335.

Lyon, G. R., Shaywitz, S. E., & Shaywitz, B. A. (2003). Defining dyslexia, comorbidity, teachers' knowledge of language and reading: A definition of dyslexia. *Annals of Dyslexia, 53,* 1.

Maas, E., Robin, D. A., Austermann Hula, S. N., Freedman, S. E., Wulf, G., & Ballard, K. J. (2008). Principles of motor learning in treatment of motor speech disorders. *American Journal of Speech-Language Pathology, 17,* 277–298.

MacArthur, C. A. (1999). Word processing with speech synthesis and word prediction: Effects on the dialogue journal writing of students with learning disabilities. *Learning Disability Quarterly, 21,* 1–16.

MacArthur, C. A., & Graham, S. (1987). Learning disabled students composing under three methods of text production: Handwriting, word processing, and dictation. *Journal of Special Education, 21,* 22–42.

MacArthur, C. A., Graham, S., Haynes, J. A., & DeLaPaz, S. (1996). Spelling checkers and students with learning disabilities: Performance comparisons and impact on spelling. *Journal of Special Education, 30,* 35–57.

MacArthur, C. A., Graham, S., Schwartz, S. S., & Schafer, W. (1995). Evaluation of a writing instruction model that integrated a process approach, strategy instruction, and word processing. *Learning Disability Quarterly, 18,* 278–291.

MacDonald, C. C. (1992). Perinatal cocaine exposure: Predictor of an endangered generation. *Infant-Toddler Intervention: The Transdisciplinary Journal, 2*(1), 1–12.

Mackay, L. E., Bernstein, B. A., Chapman, P. E., Morgan, A. S., & Milazzo, L. S. (1992). Early intervention in severe head injury: Long-term benefits of a formalized program. *Archives of Physical Medicine and Rehabilitation, 73,* 635–641.

Madell, J. R. (2008). Using behavioral observation audiometry to evaluate hearing in infants. In J. R. Madell & C. Flexer (Eds.), *Pediatric audiology* (pp. 54–64). New York: Thieme.

Magaziner, J., German, P., Itkin Zimmerman, S., Mainela-Arnold, E., Evans, J. J., & Alibali, M. W. (2006). Understanding conservation delays in children with specific language impairment: Task representations revealed in speech and gesture. *Journal of Speech, Language, and Hearing Research, 49,* 1267–1279.

Mann, G., & Hankey, G. J. (2001). Initial clinical and demographic predictors of swallowing impairment following acute stroke. *Dysphagia, 16,* 205–216.

Mann, W., & Lane, J. (1991). *Assistive technology for persons with disabilities: The role of occupational therapy.* Rockville, MD: American Occupational Therapy Association.

Margolis, R. H. (2004). What do your patients remember? *Hearing Journal, 57,* 10–17.

Marini, A., Boewe, A., Caltagirone, C., & Carlomagno, S. (2005). Age-related differences in the production of textual descriptions. *Journal of Psycholinguistic Research, 34,* 439–464.

Markel, N., Meisels, M., & Houck, J. (1964). Judging personality from voice quality. *Journal of Abnormal Social Psychology, 69*, 458–463.

Marshall, R. C. (1997). Aphasia treatment in the early postonset period: Managing our resources effectively. *American Journal of Speech-Language Pathology, 6*(1), 5–11.

Martin, B. J. (1994). Treatment of dysphagia in adults. In L. R. Cherney (Ed.), *Clinical management of dysphagia in adults and children.* Gaithersburg, MD: Aspen.

Martin, F. N., & Clark, J. G. (2003). *Introduction to audiology* (8th ed.). Boston: Allyn and Bacon.

Martin, R., & Haroldson, S. (1981). Stuttering identification: Standard definition and moment of stuttering. *Journal of Speech and Hearing Research, 46*, 59–63.

Martin, R., & Lindamood, L. (1986). Stuttering and spontaneous recovery: Implications for the speech-language pathologist. *Language, Speech, and Hearing Services in Schools, 17*, 207–218.

Martin, R. E., Neary, M. A., & Diamant, N. E. (1997). Dysphagia following anterior cervical spine surgery. *Dysphagia, 12*(1), 2–10.

Marton, K., & Schwartz, R. G. (2003). Working memory capacity and language processes in children with specific language impairment. *Journal of Speech, Language, and Hearing Research, 46*, 1138–1153.

Marvin, C. A., & Wright, D. (1997). Literacy socialization in the homes of preschool children. *Language, Speech, and Hearing Services in Schools, 28*, 154–163.

Masterson, J. J., & Apel, K. (2000). Spelling assessment: Charting a path to optimal intervention. *Topics in Language Disorders, 20*(3), 50–65.

Masterson, J. J., & Bernhardt, B. (2001). *Computerized articulation and phonology evaluation.* Austin, TX: Pro-Ed.

Masterson, J. J., & Crede, L. A. (1999). Learning to spell: Implications for assessment and intervention. *Language, Speech, and Hearing Services in Schools, 30*, 243–354.

Masterson, J. J., & Pagan, F. (1993). *Interactive system for phonological analysis: Version 1.0* (Macintosh Computer Program). San Antonio, TX: The Psychological Corporation.

Max, L., & Caruso, A. J. (1997). Contemporary techniques for establishing fluency in the treatment of adults who stutter. *Contemporary Issues in Communication Science and Disorders, 24*, 45–52.

Max, L., Guenther, F., Gracco, V., Ghosh, S., & Wallace, M. (2004). Unstable or insufficiently activated internal models and feedback-biased motor control as sources of dysfluency: A theoretical model of stuttering. *Contemporary Issues in Communication Science and Disorders, 31*, 105–122.

McCarthy, J., & Light, J. (2001). Instructional effectiveness of an integrated theatre arts program for children using augmentative and alternative communication and their nondisabled peers: Preliminary study. *Augmentative and Alternative Communication, 17*, 88–98.

McCauley, R., & Strand, E. (2008). A review of standardized tests of nonverbal oral and speech motor performance in children. *American Journal of Speech-Language Pathology, 17*, 81–91.

McCoy, K. F., Bedrosian, J. L., Hoag, L. A., & Johnson, D. E. (2007). Brevity and speed of message delivery trade-offs in augmentative and alternative communication. *Augmentative and Alternative Communication, 23*, 76–88.

McDonald, E. T. (1964). *Articulation testing and treatment: A sensory-motor approach.* Pittsburgh, PA: Stanwix House.

McFadden, T. U. (1998). Sounds and stories: Teaching phonemic awareness in interactions around text. *American Journal of Speech-Language Pathology, 7*(2), 5–13.

McFarland, C., & Cacase, T. (2006). Current controversies in CAPD: From Procrustes bed to Pandora's box. In T. K. Parthasarathy (Ed.), *An introduction to auditory processing disorders in children* (pp. 247–263). Mahwah, NJ: Erlbaum.

McGinty, A. S., & Justice, L. M. (2006). Classroom-based versus pull-out interventions: A review of the experimental evidence. *EBP Briefs, 1*(1).

McGregor, K. K. (2000). The development and enhancement of narrative skills in a preschool classroom: Toward a solution to clinician-client mismatch. *American Journal of Speech-Language Pathology, 9*, 55–71.

McGregor, K. K., Sheng, L., & Smith, B. (2005). The precocious two-year-old: Status of the lexicon and links to the grammar. *Journal of Child Language, 32*, 563–585.

McKinlay, W. W., Brooks, D. N., Bond, M. R., Martinage, D. P., & Marshall, M. M. (1981). The shortterm outcome of severe blunt head injury as reported by the relatives of the injured person. *Journal of Neurology, Neurosurgery, and Psychiatry, 44*, 527–533.

McLeod, S., & Searl, J. (2006). Adaptation to an electropalatograph palate: Acoustic, impressionistic, and perceptual data. *American Journal of Speech-Language Pathology, 15*, 192–206.

McNaughton, D., Hughes, C., & Ofiesh, N. (1997). Proofreading for students with learning disabilities:

Integrating computer use and strategic use. *Learning Disabilities Research and Practice, 12,* 16–28.

McNaughton, D., Light, J., & Groszyk, L. (2001). "Don't give up": Employment experiences of individuals with amyotrophic lateral sclerosis who use augmentative and alternative communication. *Augmentative and Alternative Communication, 17,* 179–195.

McNeilly, L. (2005). HIV and communication. *Journal of Communication Disorders, 38,* 303–310.

McWilliams, B. J., Morris, H. L., & Shelton, R. L. (1990). *Cleft palate speech* (2nd ed.). Philadelphia: B. C. Decker.

Mecham, M. (1996). *Cerebral palsy* (2nd ed.). Austin, TX: Pro-Ed.

Mental Health Research Association. (2007). *Childhood schizophrenia.* Retrieved July 20, 2007, from www.narsad.org/dc/childhood_disorders/schizophrenia.html

Meilijson, S. R., Kasher, A., & Elizur, A. (2004). Language performance in chronic schizophrenia: A pragmatic approach. *Journal of Speech, Language, and Hearing Research, 47,* 695–713.

Mentis, M., & Lundgren, K. (1995). Effects of prenatal exposure to cocaine and associated risk factors on language development. *Journal of Speech and Hearing Research, 38,* 1303–1318.

Merrell, A. W., & Plante, E. (1997). Norm-referenced test interpretation in the diagnostic process. *Language, Speech, and Hearing Services in Schools, 28,* 50–58.

Metsala, J. L., & Walley, A. C. (1998). Spoken vocabulary growth and the segmental restructuring of lexical representations: Precursors to phonemic awareness and early reading ability. In J. L. Metsala & L. C. Ehri (Eds.), *Word recognition in beginning literacy* (pp. 89–120). Mahway, NJ: Erlbaum.

Meyers, P. S. (1999). *Right hemisphere damage.* San Diego, CA: Singular.

Miccio, A. W., Elbert, M., & Forrest, K. (1999). The relationship between stimulability and phonological acquisition in children with normally developing and disordered phonologies. *American Journal of Speech-Language Pathology, 8,* 347–363.

Miccio, A. W., & Ingrisano, D. (2000). The acquisition of fricatives and affricates: Evidence from a disordered phonological system. *American Journal of Speech-Language Pathology, 9,* 214–229.

The Michael J. Fox Foundation for Parkinson's Research. (2006). Available from www.michaeljfox.org/living_aboutParkinsons_parkinsons101.cfm#q1

Michi, K., Yamashita, Y., Imai, S., Suzuki, N., & Yoshida, H. (1993). Role of visual feedback treatment for defective /s/ sounds in patients with cleft palate. *Journal of Speech and Hearing Research, 36,* 277–285.

Millar, D. C., Light, J. C., & Schlosser, R. W. (2006). The impact of augmentative and alternative communication intervention on the speech production of individuals with developmental disabilities: A research review. *Journal of Speech, Language, and Hearing Research, 49,* 248–264.

Miller, C. A., Kail, R., Leonard, L. B., & Tomblin, J. B. (2001). Speed of processing in children with specific language impairment. *Journal of Speech, Language, and Hearing Research, 44,* 416–433.

Miller, C. A., Leonard, L. B., Kail, R. V., Zhang, X., Tomblin, J. B., & Francis, D. J. (2006). Response time in 14-year-olds with language impairment. *Journal of Speech, Language, and Hearing Research, 49,* 712–728.

Miller, L. (1993, January). Testing and the creation of disorder. *American Journal of Speech Language Pathology, 2,* 13–16.

Miniutti, A. (1991). Language deficiencies in inner-city children with learning and behavioral problems. *Language, Speech, and Hearing Services in Schools, 22,* 31–38.

Mitchell, R. E., & Karchmer, M. A. (2004). Chasing the mythical ten percent: Parental hearing status of deaf and hard of hearing students in the United States. *Sign Language Studies, 4,* 138–163.

Moats, L. (1995). *Spelling development, disability, and instruction.* Baltimore: York Press.

Montague, M., Graves, A., & Leavell, A. (1991). Planning procedural facilitation, and narrative composition of junior high students with learning disabilities. *Learning Disabilities Research and Practice, 6,* 219–224.

Montgomery, J. W., & Leonard, L. B. (2006). Effects of acoustic manipulation on the real-time inflectional processing of children with specific language impairment. *Journal of Speech, Language, and Hearing Research, 49,* 1238–1256.

Morgan, D. L., & Guilford, A. M. (1984). *Adolescent Language Screening Test.* Austin, TX: Pro-Ed.

Mullins, T. (2004). Depression in older adults with hearing loss. *ASHA Leader, 21,* 12–13, 27.

Murray, L. L. (2000). Spoken language production in Huntington's and Parkinson's diseases. *Journal of Speech, Language, and Hearing Research, 43,* 1350–1366.

Murray, L. L., Holland, A. L., & Beson, P. M. (1997). Auditory processing in individuals with mild aphasia: A study of resource allocation. *Journal of Speech, Language, and Hearing Research, 40,* 792–808.

Murray, L. L., Holland, A. L., & Beson, P. M. (1998). Spoken language of individuals with mild fluent aphasia under focused and divided-attention conditions. *Journal of Speech, Language, and Hearing Research, 41,* 213–225.

Nagaya, M., Kachi, T., Yamada, T., & Sumi, Y. (2004). Videofluorographic observations on swallowing in patients with dysphagia due to neurodegenerative diseases. *Nagoya Journal of Medical Sciences, 67,* 17–23.

Naremore, R. C. (2001). *Narrative frameworks and early literacy.* Seminar presented for Rochester Hearing and Speech Center and Nazareth College, Rochester, NY.

Nathan, L., Stackhouse, J., Goulandris, N., & Snowling, M. J. (2004). The development of early literacy skills among children with speech difficulties: A test of the "critical age hypothesis." *Journal of Speech, Language, and Hearing Research, 47,* 377–391.

Nation, K., & Frazier Norbury, C. (2005). Why reading comprehension fails. *Topics in Language Disorders, 25,* 21–32.

Nation, K., & Hulme, C. (1997). Phonemic segmentation, not onset-rime segmentation, predicts early reading and spelling skills. *Reading Research Quarterly, 32,* 154–167.

Nation, K., & Norbury, C. F. (2005). Why reading comprehension fails: Insights into developmental disorders. *Topics in Language Disorders, 25*(1), 21–32.

National Center for Hearing Assessment and Management. (2009). State summary statistics: Universal newborn hearing screening. Retrieved May 27, 2009, from www. infanthearing.org/status/unhsstate.html

National Center for Injury Prevention and Control. (2009, March 18). What Is traumatic brain injury? Centers for Disease Control and Prevention. Retrieved May 27, 2009, from www.cdc.gov/ncipc/tbi/TBI.htm

National Institute of Neurological Disorders and Stroke, National Institute of Health. (2005). http://www.minds.nih.gov/disorders/aphasia/aphasia.htm. Retrieved October 22, 2005.

National Joint Committee on Learning Disabilities. (1991). Learning disabilities: Issues on definition (A position paper). *Asha, 33* (Suppl. 5), 18–20.

National Reading Panel. (2000). *National Reading Panel Progress Report.* Bethesda, MD: Author.

National Institute of Neurological Disorders and Stroke, National Institutes of Health. (2009). Parkinson's disease: Challenges, progress, and promise. Available from www.ninds.nih.gov/disorders/parkinsons_disease/parkinsons_research.htm

Neils-Strunjas, J., Groves-Wright, K., Mashima, P., & Harnish, S. (2006). Dysgraphia in Alzheimer's disease: A review for clinical and research purposes. *Journal of Speech, Language, and Hearing Research, 49,* 1313–1330.

Nelson H. D., Bougatsos C., & Nygren P. (2008). Universal newborn hearing screening: Systematic review to update the 2001 U.S. Preventive Services Task Force recommendation. *Pediatrics, 122,* 266–276.

Nelson, N. W. (1994). Curriculum-based language assessment and intervention across grades. In G. P. Wallach & K. G. Butler (Eds.), *Language learning disabilities in school-age children and adolescents* (pp. 104–131). Boston: Allyn and Bacon.

Nelson, N. W. (1998). *Childhood language disorders in context: Infancy through adolescence,* (2nd ed.). Boston: Allyn and Bacon.

Nelson, N. W., & Van Meter, A. M. (2002). Assessing curriculum-based reading and writing samples. *Topics in Language Disorders, 22*(2), 35–59.

Nelson Bryen, D. (2006). Job-related social networks and communication technology. *Augmentative and Alternative Communication, 22,* 1–9.

Nelson Bryen, D. (2008). Vocabulary to support socially-valued adult roles. *Augmentative and Alternative Communication, 24,* 294–301.

Newell, A. F., Booth, L., Arnott, J., & Beattie, W. (1992). Increasing literacy levels by the use of linguistic prediction. *Child Language Teaching and Therapy, 8,* 138–187.

Nicholas, M., Barth, C., Obler, L. K., Au, R., & Albert, M. J. (1997). Naming in normal aging and dementia of the Alzheimer's type. In H. Goodglass & A. Wingfield (Eds.), *Anomia: Neuroanatomical and cognitive correlates* (pp. 166–188). San Diego, CA: Academic Press.

Nicholas, M., Connor, L. T., Obler, L. K., & Albert, M. L. (1998). Aging, language, and language disorders. In M. T. Sarno (Ed.), Acquired aphasia (3rd ed., pp. 413–449). San Diego, CA: Academic Press.

Nicholas, M. L., Helm-Estabrooks, N., Ward-Lonergan, J., & Morgan, A. R. (1993). Evolution of severe aphasia in the first two years post onset.

Archives of Physical Medicine and Rehabilitation, 74, 830–836.

Nicolson, R., Lenane, M., Singaracharlu, S., Malaspina, D., Giedd, J. N., Hamburger, S. D., et al. (2000). Premorbid speech and language impairments in childhood-onset schizophrenia: Association with risk factors. *American Journal of Psychiatry, 157,* 794–800.

Nigam, R., Schlosser, R. W., & Lloyd, L. L. (2006). Concomitant use of the matrix strategy and the mand-model procedure in teaching graphic symbol combinations. *Augmentative and Alternative Communication, 22,* 160–177.

Nilsson, H., Ekberg, O., Olsson, R., & Hindfelt, B. (1998). Dysphagia in stroke: A prospective study of quantitative aspects of swallowing in dysphagic patients. *Dysphagia, 13*(1), 32–38.

Nippold, M. A., Hesketh, L. J., Duthie, J. K., & Mansfield, T. C. (2005). Conversational vs. expository discourse: A study of syntactic development in children, adolescents, and adults. *Journal of Speech, Language, and Hearing Research, 48,* 1048–1064.

Nippold, M. A., Mansfield, T. C., & Billow, J. L. (2007). Peer conflict explanations in children, adolescents, and adults: Examining the development of complex syntax. *American Journal of Speech-Language Pathology, 16,* 179–186.

Nippold, M. A., Ward-Lonergan, J. M., & Fanning, J. L. (2005). Persuasive writing in children, adolescents, and adults: A study of syntactic, semantic, and pragmatic development. *Language, Speech, and Hearing Service in Schools, 36,* 125–138.

Odderson, M. D., Keaton, J. C., & McKenna, B. S. (1995). Swallow management in patients on an acute stroke pathway: Quality is cost effective. *Archives of Physical Medicine and Rehabilitation, 76*(12), 1130–1133.

Oetting, J. B., & Morohov, J. E. (1997). Past-tense marking by children with and without specific language impairment. *Journal of Speech, Language, and Hearing Research, 40,* 62–74.

Office of Technology Assessment. (1978). *Assessing the efficacy and safety of medical technologies.* OTA-H-75. Washington, DC: U.S. Government Printing Office.

Olivier, C., Hecker, L., Klucken, J., & Westby, C. (2000). Language: The embedded curriculum in postsecondary education. *Topics in Language Disorders, 21*(1) 15–29.

Oller, J. W., Kim, K., & Choe, Y. (2001). Can instructions to nonverbal tests be given in pantomime? Additional applications of a general theory of signs. *Semiotica, 133,* 15–44.

Olmsted, D. (1971). *Out of the mouth of babes.* The Hague, Netherlands: Mouton.

Olswang, L., Bain, B., & Johnson, G. (1990). Using dynamic assessment with children with language disorders. In S. Warren & J. Reichle (Eds.), *Causes and effects of communication and language intervention.* Baltimore: Paul H. Brookes.

Olswang, L. B., Rodriguez, B., & Timler, G. (1998). Recommending intervention for toddlers with specific language learning difficulties: We may not have all the answers, but we know a lot. *American Journal of Speech-Language Pathology, 7*(1), 23–32.

Olswang, L. B., Svennson, L., Coggins, T. E., Beilinson, J. S., & Donaldson, A. L. (2006). Reliability issues and solutions for coding social communication performance in classroom settings. *Journal of Speech, Language, and Hearing Research, 49,* 1058–1071.

O'Neil-Pirozzi, T. M. (2003). Language functioning of residents in family homeless shelters. *American Journal of Speech-Language Pathology, 12,* 229–242.

Onslow, M., Packman, A., & Harrison, E. (2003). *The Lidcombe program of early stuttering intervention: A clinician's guide.* Austin, TX: Pro-Ed.

Oram, J., Fine, J., Okamoto, C., & Tannock, R. (1999). Assessing the language of children with attention deficit hyperactivity disorder. *American Journal of Speech-Language Pathology, 8,* 72–80.

Orange, J. B., Lubinsky, R. B., & Higginbotham, D. J. (1996). Conversational repair by individuals with dementia of the Alzheimer's type. *Journal of Speech, Language, and Hearing Research, 39,* 881–895.

Ors, M., Ryding, E., Lindgren, M., Gustafsson, P., Blennow, G., & Rosén, I. (2005). SPECT findings in children with specific language impairment. *Cortex, 41,* 316–326.

Orsolini, M., Sechi, E., et al. (2001). Nature of phonological delay in children with specific language impairment. *International Journal of Language and Communication Disorders, 36,* 63–90.

Owen, A. J., Dromi, E., & Leonard, L. B. (2001). The phonology-morphology interface in the speech of Hebrew-speaking children with specific language impairment. *Journal of Communication Disorders, 34,* 323–337.

Owens, R. E. (2008). *Language development: An introduction* (7th ed.). Boston, Allyn and Bacon.

Owens, R. E. (2010). *Language disorders, a functional approach to assessment and intervention* (5th ed.). Boston: Allyn and Bacon.

Owens, R. E., & Kim, K. (2007, November). *Holistic reading and semantic investigation intervention with struggling readers.* Paper presented at the annual convention of the American Speech-Language-Hearing Association, Boston.

Pannabacker, M. (2004). Velopharyngeal incompetence: The need for speech standards. *American Journal of Speech-Language Pathology, 13*, 195–201.

Papsin, B. K., Gysin, C., Picton, N., Nedzelski, J., & Harrison, R. V. (2000). Speech perception outcome measures in prelingually deaf children up to four years after cochlear implantation. *Annals of Otology, Rhinology & Laryngology Supplement, 185*, 38–42.

Paradis, J. (2005). Grammatical morphology in children learning English as a second language: Implications of similarities with specific language impairment. *Language, Speech, and Hearing Services in Schools, 36*, 172–187.

Paratore, J. R. (1995). Assessing literacy: Establishing common standards in portfolio assessment. *Topics in Language Disorders, 16*(1), 67–82.

Pataraia, E., Simos, P. G., Castillo, E. M., Billingsley-Marshall, R. L., McGregor, A. L., Breier, J. I., et al. (2004). Reorganization of language-specific cortex in patients with lesions or mesial temporal epilepsy. *Neurology, 63*, 1825–1832.

Patel, R., & Salata, A. (2006). Using computer games to mediate caregiver-child communication for children with severe dysarthria. *Journal of Medical Speech-Language Pathology, 14*, 279–284.

Patterson, J. L. (2000). Observed and reported expressive vocabulary and word combinations in bilingual toddlers. *Journal of Speech, Language, and Hearing Research, 43*, 121–128.

Paul, R. (1991). Outcomes of early expressive language delay. *Journal of Childhood Communication Disorders, 15*, 7–14.

Paul, R. (1995). *Language disorders from infancy through adolescence: Assessment and intervention*. St. Louis, MO: Mosby.

Paul-Brown, D., & Goldberg, L. R. (2001). Current policies and new directions for speech-language pathology assistants. *Language, Speech, and Hearing Services in Schools, 32*, 4–17.

Peach, R. K. (2001). Further thoughts regarding management of acute aphasia following stroke. *American Journal of Speech-Language Pathology, 10*, 29–36.

Peña, E. D., Gillam, R. B., Malek, M., Ruiz-Felter, R., Resendiz, M., Fiestas, C., & Sabel, T. (2006). Dynamic assessment of school-age children's narrative ability: An experimental investigation of classification accuracy. *Journal of Speech, Language, and Hearing Research, 49*, 1037–1057.

Peña, E., Iglesias, A., & Lidz, C. S. (2001). Reducing test bias through dynamic assessment of children's word learning ability. *American Journal of Speech-Language Pathology, 10*, 138–154.

Peña, E. D., & Quinn, R. (1997). Task familiarity: Effects on the test performance of Puerto Rican and African American children. *Language, Speech and Hearing Services in Schools, 28*, 323–332.

Pena-Brooks, A., & Hedge, M. (2007). *Assessment and treatment of articulation and phonological disorders in children* (2nd ed.). Austin, TX: Pro-Ed.

Pence, K. L., Justice, L. M., & Wiggins, A. K. (2008). Preschool teachers' fidelity in implementing a comprehensive language-rich curriculum. *Language, Speech, and Hearing Services in Schools, 39*, 329–341.

Perez, K., Ramig, L., Smith, M., & Dromey, C. (1996). The Parkinson larynx: Tremor and videostroboscopic findings. *Journal of Voice, 10*, 354–361.

Perez, I., Smithard, D. G., Davies, H., & Kaira, L. (1998). Pharmacological treatment of dysphagia in stroke. *Dysphagia, 13*(1), 12–16.

Peterson, R., Pennington, B., Shriberg, L., & Boada, R. (2009). What influences literacy outcome in children with speech sound disorder? *Journal of Speech. Language. and Hearing Research, 52*, 1175–1188.

Peterson-Falzone, S., Hardin-Jones, M., & Karnell, M. (2010). *Cleft palate speech* (4th ed.). St. Louis, MO: Mosby.

Peterson-Falzone, S. J., & Imagire, R. (1997). Basic genetic concepts in cranialfacial anomalies. In K. R. Bzoch (Ed.), *Communicative disorders related to cleftlip and palate* (4th ed.). Austin, TX: Pro-Ed.

Peterson-Falzone, S. J., Trost-Cardamone, J., Karnell, M., & Hardin-Jones, M. (2006). *The clinician's guide to treating cleft palate speech*. St. Louis, MO: Mosby.

Piché, L., & Reichle, J. (1991). Teaching scanning selection techniques. In J. Reichle, J. York, & J. Sigafoos (Eds.), *Implementing augmentative and alternative communication: Strategies for learners with severe disabilities* (p. 257–274). Baltimore B, rookes.

Pimental, P. A., & Kingsbury, N. A. (1989). *Mini inventory of right brain injury*. Austin, TX: Pro-Ed.

Pindzola, R. (1993). Materials for use in vocal hygiene programs for children. *Language, Speech, and Hearing Services in the Schools, 24*, 174–176.

Pinker, S. (1995). *The language instinct: How the mind creates language*. New York: Harper Perennial.

Plaut, D. C., & Kello, C. T. (1999). The emergence of phonology from the interplay of speech comprehension and production: A distributed connectionist approach. In B. MacWhinney (Ed.), *The emergence of language*. Mahwah, NJ: Erlbaum.

Poeppel, D. (1996). A critical review of PET studies of phonological processing. *Brain and Language, 55*(3), 352–379.

Porch, B. E. (1981). *Porch index of communicative ability* (3rd ed.). Palo Alto, CA: Consulting Psychologists Press.

Postma. A., & Kolk, H. H. J. (1993). The covert repair hypothesis: Prearticulatory repair processes in normal and stuttered disfluencies. *Journal of Speech and Hearing Research, 36,* 472–487.

Poyatos, F. (1983). *New perspectives in nonverbal communication: Studies in cultural anthropology, social psychology, linguistics, literature and semiotics.* Oxford, UK: Pergamon Press.

Prather, E., Hedrick, D., & Kern, C. (1975). Articulation development in children aged two to four years. *Journal of Speech and Hearing Disorders, 40,* 179–191.

Prelock, P. A. (2000). Prologue: Multiple perspectives for determining the roles of speech-language pathologists in inclusionary classrooms. *Language, Speech, and Hearing Services in Schools, 31,* 213–218.

Prelock, P. A. (2008). Autism spectrum disorders. *Treatment efficacy summary.* Retrieved June 28, 2009, from www.asha.org/NR/rdonlyres/4BAF3969-9ADC-4C01-B5ED-1334CC20DD3D/0/TreatmentEfficacySummaries2008.pdf

Prelock, P. A., Beatson, J., Bitner, B., Broder, C., & Ducker, A. (2003). Interdisciplinary assessment of young children with autism spectrum disorder. *Language, Speech, and Hearing Services in Schools, 34,* 194–202.

Prins, D., & Ingham, R. (2009). Evidence-based treatment and stuttering—historical perspective. *Journal of Speech, Language, and Hearing Research, 52,* 254–263.

Prizant, B. M., Schuler, A. L., Wetherby, A. M., & Rydell, P. (1997). Enhancing language and communication: Language approaches. In D. Cohen & F. Volkmar (Eds.), *Handbook of autism and pervasive developmental disorders* (2nd ed., pp. 572–605). New York: Wiley.

Prontnicki, J. (1995). Presentation: Symptomatology and etiology of dysphasia. In S. R. Rosenthal, J. J. Sheppard, & M. Lotze (Eds.), *Dysphagia and the child with developmental disabilities: Medical, clinical, and family interventions.* San Diego, CA: Singular.

Pry, R., Petersen, A., & Baghdadli, A. (2005). The relationship between expressive language level and psychological development in children with autism 5 years of age. *International Journal of Research and Practice, 9,* 179–189.

Pugh, S., & Klecan-Aker, J. S. (2004). *Effects of phonological awareness training on students with learning disabilities.* Paper presented at the annual convention of the American Speech-Language-Hearing Association, Philadelphia.

Pulvermuller, F. B., Neininger, B., Elbert, T., Mohr, B., Rockstroh, B., Koebbel, P., et al. & (2001). Constraint-induced therapy of chronic aphasia after stroke. *Stroke, 32,* 1621–1626.

Qi, C. H., Kaiser, A. P., Milan, S. E., Yzquierdo, Z., & Hancock, T. B. (2003). The performance of low-income African American children on the Preschool Language Scale-3. *Journal of Speech, Language, and Hearing Research, 46,* 576–590.

Queensland Health. (2008). A systematic review of the literature on early intervention for children with a permanent hearing loss. Technical report produced for Queensland Health, Brisbane, Australia. Retrieved June 16, 2009, from www.health.qld.gov.au/healthyhearing/pages/publications.asp

Quist, R., & Lloyd, L. (1997). Principles and uses of technology. In L. Lloyd, D. Fuller, & H. Arvidson (Eds.), *Augmentative and alternative communication: A handbook of principles and practices* (pp. 107–126). Boston: Allyn and Bacon.

Rainforth, B., York, J., & MacDonald, C. (1992). *Collaborative teams for students with severe disabilities: Integrating therapy and educational services.* Baltimore: Brookes.

Ramig, L. (1994). Voice disorders. In F. Minifie (Ed.), *Introduction to communication sciences and disorders* (pp. 481–520). San Diego, CA: Singular.

Ramig, L. (2002). The joy of research. *The ASHA Leader, 7*(8), 6–7, 19.

Ramig, L., & Verdolini, K. (1998). Treatment efficacy: Voice disorders. *Journal of Speech-Language-Hearing Research, 41,* S101–S116.

Ramig, L. O., Fox, C., & Sapir, S. (2004). Parkinson's disease: Speech and voice disorders and their treatment with the Lee Silverman Voice Treatment. *Seminars in Speech and Language, 25,* 169–180.

Ramig, L. O., Sapir, S., Countryman, S., Pawlas, A., et al. (2001). Intensive voice treatment (LSVT®) for individuals with Parkinson's disease: A 2-year follow-up. *Journal of Neurology, Neurosurgery, and Psychiatry, 71,* 493–498.

Ramig, L. O., & Verdolini, K. (2009, June 19). Laryngeal-based voice disorders. *Treatment Efficacy Summary.*

Retrieved June 23, 2009, from www.asha.org/NR/rdonlyres/5B211B91-9D44-42D2-82C7-55A1315D8CD6/0/TESLaryngealBasedVoiceDisorders.pdf

Raymer, A. M., Beeson, P., Holland, A., Kendall, D., Mahe, L. M., Martin, N., et al. (2008). Translational research in aphasia: From neuroscience to neurorehabilitation. *Journal of Speech, Language, and Hearing Research (Neuroplasticity Supplement), 51,* S259–S275.

Redmond, S. M. (2003). Children's production of the affix-ed in past tense and past participle contexts. *Journal of Speech, Language, and Hearing Research, 46,* 1095–1109.

Redmond, S. M., & Johnston, S. S. (2001). Evaluating the morphological competence of children with severe speech and physical impairments. *Journal of Speech, Language, and Hearing Research, 44,* 1362–1375.

Redmond, S. M., & Rice, M. L. (2001). Detection of irregular verb violations by children with and without SLI. *Journal of Speech, Language, and Hearing Research, 44,* 655–669.

Reichle, J., Halle, J. W., & Drasgow, E. (1998). Implementing augmentative communication systems. In A. Wetherby, S. Warren, & J. Reichle (Eds.), *Transitions in prelinguistic communication* (pp. 417–436). Baltimore: Brookes.

Rescorla, L. (2005). Age 13 language and reading outcomes in late talking toddlers. *Journal of Speech, Language, and Hearing Research, 48,* 459–473.

Rescorla, L., & Alley, A. (2001). Validation of the Language Development Survey (LDS): A parent report tool for identifying language delay in toddlers. *Journal of Speech, Language, and Hearing Research, 44,* 434–445.

Reynolds, M. E., & Jefferson, L. (2000). Natural and synthetic speech comprehension: Comparison of children from two age groups. *Augmentative and Alternative Communication, 16,* 174–182.

Rhea, P. (1997). Facilitating transitions in language development in children who use AAC. *Augmentative and Alternative Communication, 13,* 141–148.

Rice, M. L., Cleave, P. L., & Oetting, J. B. (2000). The use of syntactic cues in lexical acquisition by children with SLI. *Journal of Speech, Language, and Hearing Research, 34,* 582–594.

Rice, M. L., Redmont, S. M., & Hoffman, L. (2006). Mean length of utterance in children with specific language impairment and in younger control children shows concurrent validity and stable and parallel growth trajectories. *Journal of Speech, Language, and Hearing Research, 49,* 793–808.

Rice, M. L., Tomblin, J. B., Hoffman, L., Richman, W. A., & Marquis, J. (2004). Grammatical tense deficits in children with SLI and nonspecific language impairment: Relationships with nonverbal IQ over time. *Journal of Speech, Language, and Hearing Research, 47,* 816–834.

Rieber, R. W., & Wollock, J. (1977). The historical roots of the theory and therapy of stuttering. *Journal of Communication Disorders, 10,* 3–24.

Riley, G., & Riley, J. (1981). *Stuttering prediction instrument for young children.* Tigard, OR: C. C. Publications.

Ringo, C. C., & Dietrich, S. (1995). Neurogenic stuttering: An analysis and critique. *Journal of Medical Speech-Language Pathology, 2,* 111–122.

Riski, J. E. (1995). Secondary surgical procedures to correct postoperative velopharyngeal incompetencies found after primary palatoplasties. In K. R. Bzoch (Ed.), *Communicative disorders related to cleft lip and palate,* (4th ed., pp. 121–152). Austin, TX: Pro-Ed.

Rittle-Johnson, B., & Siegler, R. S. (1999). Learning to spell: Variability, choice, and change in children's strategy use. *Child Development, 70,* 332–348.

Ritvo, E. R., & Freeman, B. J. (1978). National Society for Autistic Children definition of the syndrome of autism. *Journal of Autism and Childhood Schizophrenia, 8,* 162–167.

Roberts, J. E., Long, S.H., Malkin, C., Barnes, E., Skinner, M., Hennon, E. A., et al. (2005). A comparison of phonological skills with fragile X syndrome and Down syndrome. *Journal of Speech, Language, and Hearing Research, 48,* 980–995.

Roberts, J. E., Mirrett, P., & Burchinal, M. (2001). Receptive and expressive communication development in young meales with fragile X syndrome. *American Journal of Mental Retardation, 106,* 216–231.

Robey, R. R. (1994). The efficacy of treatment for aphasic persons: A meta-analysis. *Brain and Language, 47,* 585–608.

Robey, R. R. (1998). A meta-analysis of clinical outcomes in the treatment of aphasia. *Journal of Speech, Language, and Hearing Research, 41,* 172–187.

Robey, R. R., & Schultz, M. C. (1998). A model for conducting clinical-outcome research: An adaptation of the standard protocol for use in aphasiology. *Aphasiology, 12*(9), 787–810.

Rogers, B., Arvedson, J., Buck, G., et al. (1994). Characteristics of dysphagia in children with cerebral palsy. *Dysphagia, 9*(1), 69–73.

Romski, M. A., & Sevcik, R. A. (1996). *Breaking the speech barrier: Language development through augmented means.* Baltimore: Brookes.

Rosen, K. M., Kent, R. D., Delaney, A. L., & Duffy, J. R. (2006). Parametric quantitative acoustic analysis of conversation produced by speakers with dysarthria and healthy speakers. *Journal of Speech, Language, and Hearing Research, 49,* 395–411.

Rosenbek, J. C., LaPointe, L. L., & Wertz, R. T. (1989). *Aphasia: A clinical approach.* Austin, TX: Pro-Ed.

Rosenbek, J. C., Lemme, M., Ahern, M., Harris, E., & Wertz, R. (1973). A treatment for apraxia of speech in adults. *Journal of Speech and Hearing Disorders, 43,* 462–472.

Rosenfeld, R. M., Vertrees, J. E., Carr, J., Cipolle, R. J., Uden, D. L., Giebink, G. S., et al. (1994). Clinical efficacy of antimicrobial drugs for acute otitis media: Meta-analysis of 5400 children from thirty-three randomized trials. *Journal of Pediatrics, 124,* 355–367.

Rosenthal, S. R., Sheppard, J. J., & Lotze, M. (1995). *Dysphagia and the child with developmental disabilities: Medical, clinical, and family interventions.* San Diego, CA: Singular.

Ross, K. B., & Wertz, R. T. (2003). Discriminative validity of selected measures of differentiating normal from aphasic performance. *American Journal of Speech-Language Pathology, 12,* 312–319.

Roth, F. P. (2000). Narrative writing: Development and teaching with children with writing difficulties. *Topics in Language Disorders, 20*(4), 15–28.

Roth, F. P. (2004). Word recognition assessment framework. In C. A. Stone, E. R. Silliman, B. J. Ehren, & K. Apel (Eds.), *Handbook of language and literacy: Development and disorders* (pp. 461–480). New York: Guilford.

Roth, F. P., Spekman, N. J., & Fye, E. C. (1991, November). *Written syntactic patterns of stories produced by learning disabled students.* Paper presented at the annual convention of the American Speech-Language-Hearing Association, Atlanta, GA.

Rowland, C., & Schweigert, P. (1989). Tangible symbols: Symbolic communication for individuals with multisensory impairments. *Augmentative and Alternative Communication, 5,* 226–234.

Rowland, C., & Schweigert, P. (2000). Tangible symbols, tangible outcomes. *Augmentative and Alternative Communication, 16,* 61–78.

Rowland, C. F., Pine, J. M., Lieven, E. V. M., & Theakston, A. L. (2005). The incidence of error in young children's wh-questions. *Journal of Speech, Language, and Hearing Research, 48,* 384–404.

Roy, N. (2005). Teachers with voice disorders: Recent clinical trials research. *The ASHA Leader, 10,* 8–9, 11.

Roy, N., Gray, S., Simon, M., Dove, M., Dove, H., Corbin-Lewis, K., et al. (2001). An evaluation of the effects of two treatment approaches for teachers with voice disorders: A prospective randomized clinical trial. *Journal of Speech, Language, and Hearing Research, 44,* 286–296.

Roy, N., Merrill, R. M., Thibeault, S., Parsa, R. A., Gray, S. D., & Smith, E. M. (2004). Prevalence of voice disorders in teachers and the general population. *Journal of Speech, Language, and Hearing Research, 47,* 281–293.

Rubin, K. H., Burgess, K. B., & Coplan, R. J. (2002). Social withdrawal and shyness. In P. K. Smith & C. H. Hart (Eds.), *Blackwell handbook of childhood social development* (pp. 329–352). Malden, MA: Blackwell.

Rudd, H., Grove, N., & Pring, T. (2007). Teaching productive sign modifications to children with intellectual disabilities. *Augmentative and Alternative Communication, 23,* 154–163.

Russell, N. (1993). Educational considerations in traumatic brain injury: The role of the speech-language pathologist. *Language, Speech, and Hearing Services in Schools, 24,* 67–75.

Rvachew, S. (2006). Longitudinal predictors of implicit phonological awareness skills. *American Journal of Speech-Language Pathology, 15,* 165–176.

Rvachew, S. R., & Grawburg, M. (2006). Correlates of phonological awareness in preschoolers with speech sound disorders. *Journal of Speech, Language, and Hearing Research, 49,* 74–87.

Ryan, B. P. (1974). *Programmed therapy for stuttering children and adults.* Springfield, IL: Charles C. Thomas.

Ryan, B. P., & Van Kirk Ryan, B. (1983). Programmed stuttering therapy for children: Comparisons of four established programs. *Journal of Fluency Disorders, 8,* 291–321.

Ryan, B. P., & Van Kirk Ryan, B. (1995). Programmed stuttering treatment for children: Comparisons of two established programs through transfer, maintenance, and follow-up. *Journal of Speech and Hearing Research, 38,* 61–75.

Sabol, J., Lee, L., & Stemple, J. (1995). The value of vocal function exercises in the practice regimen of singers. *Journal of Voice, 9,* 27–36.

Saint-Exupéry, A. de (1968). *The little prince.* New York: Harcourt Brace.

Sameroff, A., & Fiese, B. (1990). Transactional regulation and early intervention. In S. Meisels & J. Shonkoff (Eds.), *Early intervention: A handbook of theory, practice, and analysis.* New York: Cambridge University Press.

Sanders, E. (1972). When are speech sounds learned? *Journal of Speech and Hearing Disorders, 37,* 55–63.

Sanders, L. D., & Neville, H. J. (2000). Lexical, syntactic, and stress-pattern cues for speech segmentation. *Journal of Speech, Language, and Hearing Research, 43,* 1301–1321.

Sanford, A. J., & Garrod, S. M. (1998). The role of scenario mapping in text comprehension. *Discourse Processes, 26,* 159–190.

Sapir, S., Ramig, L., & Fox, C. (2006). Lee Silverman Voice Treatment [LSVT®] for voice, speech, and other orofacial disorders in people with Parkinson's Disease. *Future Neurology, 1,* 563–570.

Sapir, S., Spielman, J. L., Ramig, L. O., Story, B. H., & Fox, C. (2007). Effects of intensive voice treatment (the Lee Silverman Voice Treatment [LSVT]) on vowel articulation in dysarthric individuals with idiopathic Parkinson disease: Acoustic and perceptual findings. *Journal of Speech, Language, and Hearing Research, 50,* 899–912.

Sarno, M. T. (1969). *Functional Communication Profile.* Rehabilitation Monographs 42. New York: New York University Medical Center.

Sarno, M. T., Buonaguro, A., & Levita, E. (1986). Characteristics of verbal impairment in closed head injury. *Archives of Physical Medicine and Rehabilitation, 67,* 400.

Sawyer, D. J. (2006). Dyslexia: A generation of inquiry. *Topics in Language Disorders, 26,* 95–109.

Schlosser, R. W. (2004). Evidence-based practice in ACC: 10 points to consider. *The ASHA Leader, 9*(12), 6–7, 10.

Schlosser, R. W., & Wendt, O. (2008). Effects of augmentative and alternative communication intervention on speech production in children with autism: A systematic review. *American Journal of Speech-Language Pathology, 17,* 212–230.

Schow, R. L., & Nerbonne, M. A. (2007). *Introduction to audiologic rehabilitation.* Boston: Pearson.

Schraeder, T., Quinn, M., Stockman, I. J., & Miller, J. (1999). Authentic assessment as an approach to preschool speech-language screening. *American Journal of Speech-Language Pathology, 8,* 195–200.

Schuell, H. (1972). *The Minnesota test for the differential diagnosis of aphasia.* Minneapolis: University of Minnesota Press.

Schwartz, H. (1993). Adolescents who stutter. *Journal of Fluency Disorders, 18,* 291–321.

Schwartz, J. B., & Nye, C. (2006). Improving communication for children with autism: Does sign language work? *EBP Briefs, 1*(2).

Schwarz, S. M., Corredor, J., Fisher-Medina, J., et al. (2001). Diagnosis and treatment of feeding disorders in children with developmental disabilities. *Pediatrics, 108,* 671–676.

Scott, A. (1998). NICE and easy. *Advance for Speech-Language Pathologists and Audiologists, 8*(24), 16–17.

Scott, C. M. (1999). Learning to write. In H. W. Catts & A. G. Kamhi (Eds.), *Language and reading disabilities* (pp. 224–258). Boston: Allyn and Bacon.

Scott, C. M. (2000). Principles and methods of spelling instruction: Applications for poor spellers. *Topics in Language Disorder, 20*(3), 66–82.

Scott, C. M., & Windsor, J. (2000). General language performance measures in spoken and written narrative and expository discourse of school-age children with language learning disabilities. *Journal of Speech, Language, and Hearing Research, 43,* 324–339.

Seagle, M. B. (1997). Primary surgical correction of cleft palate. In K. R. Bzoch (Ed.), *Communicative disorders related to cleft lip and palate* (4th ed., pp. 115–120). Austin, TX: Pro-Ed.

Sebat, J., Lakshmi, B., et al. (2007, April 20). Strong association of de novo copy number mutations with autism. *Science, 20,* 445–449.

Segebart DeThorne, L., Hart, S. A., Petrill, S. A., Deater-Deckard, K., Thompson, L. A., Schatschneider, C., et al. (2006). Children's history of speech-language difficulties: Genetic influences and association with reading-related measures. *Journal of Speech, Language, and Hearing Research, 49,* 1280–1293.

Segebart DeThorne, L., & Watkins, R. V. (2001). Listeners' perceptions of language use in children. *Language, Speech, and Hearing Services in Schools, 32,* 142–148.

Seung, H., & Chapman, R. (2000). Digit span in individuals with Down syndrome and in typically developing children: Temporal aspects. *Journal of Speech, Language, and Hearing Research, 43,* 609–620.

Shadden, B. B., & Toner, M. A. (Eds.). (1997). *Aging and communication: For clinicians by clinicians.* Austin, TX: Pro-Ed.

Shaker, R., Easterling, C., Kern, M., Nitschke, T., et al. (2002). Rehabilitation of swallowing by exercise in tube-fed patients with pharyngeal dysphagia secondary to abnormal UES opening. *Gastroenterology, 122,* 1314–1321.

Sharkawi, A., Ramig, L., Logemann, J., Pauloski, B., Rademaker, A., Smith, C., et al. (2002). Swallowing and voice effects of Lee Silverman Voice Treatment (LSVT): A pilot study. *Journal of Neurology, Neurosurgery, & Psychiatry, 2,* 31–36.

Shapiro, L., Swinney, D., & Borsky, S. (1998). Online examination of language performance in normal and neurologically impaired adults. *American Journal of Speech-Language Pathology, 7*(1), 49–60.

Shekim, L. (1990). Dementia. In L. L. LaPointe (Ed.), *Aphasia and related neurogenic language disorders* (pp. 210–220). New York: Thieme.

Shekim, L., & LaPointe, L. L. (1984, February). *Production of discourse in patients with Alzheimer's dementia.* Paper presented at the International Neuropsychology Society meeting, Houston, TX.

Sheppard, J. J. (1991). Managing dysphagia in mentally retarded adults. *Dysphagia, 6*(2), 83–87.

Sheppard, J. J. (1995). Clinical evaluation and treatment. In S. R. Rosenthal, J. J., Sheppard, & M. Lotze (Eds.), *Dysphagia and the child with developmental disabilities: Medical, clinical, and family interventions.* San Diego, CA: Singular.

Sheppard, J. (2008). Using motor learning approaches for treating swallowing and feeding disorders: A review. *Language, Speech, and Hearing Services in the Schools, 39,* 227–236.

Shipley, K. G., & McAfee, J. G. (1998). *Assessment in speech-language pathology: A resource manual* (2nd ed.). San Diego, CA: Singular.

Shprintzen, R. J. (1995). A new perspective on clefting. In R. J. Shprintzen & J. Bardach (Eds.), *Cleft palate speech management: A multidisciplinary approach.* St. Louis, MO: Mosby.

Shprintzen, R. J., & Goldberg, R. (1995). The genetics of clefting and associated syndromes. In R. J. Shprintzen & J. Bardach (Eds.), *Cleft palate speech management: A multidisciplinary approach.* St. Louis, MO: Mosby.

Shriberg, L. (1997). Developmental phonological disorders: One or many. In B. Hodson & M. Edwards (Eds.), *Perspectives in applied phonology* (pp. 105–127). Gaithersburg, MD: Aspen.

Shriberg, L. D., Austin, D., Lewis, B. A., McSweeney, J. L., & Wilson, D. L. (1997). The percentage of consonants correct (PCC) metric: Extensions and reliability data. *Journal of Speech, Language, and Hearing Research, 40*(4), 708–722.

Shriberg, L. D., & Kent, R. D. (1995). *Clinical phonetics* (2nd ed.). Boston: Allyn and Bacon.

Shriberg, L. D., & Kwiatkowski, J. (1994). Developmental phonological disorders. I: A clinical profile.

Journal of Speech and Hearing Research, 37, 1100–1126.

Shugart, Y. Y., Mundorff, J., Kilshaw, J., Doheny, K., Doan, B., Wanyee, J., Green, E. D., & Drayna, D. (2004). Results of a genome-wide linkage scan for stuttering. *American Journal of Medical Genetics Part A, 124*(2), 133–135.

Sigafoos, J. (2000). Creating opportunities for augmentative and alternative communication: Strategies for involving people with developmental disabilities. *Augmentative and Alternative Communication, 16,* 183–190.

Sigafoos, J., Green, V. A., Payne, D., Son, S-H., O'Reilly, M., & Lancioni, G. E. (2009). A comparison of picture exchange and speech-generating devices: Acquisition, preference, and effects on social interaction. *Augmentative and Alternative Communication, 25*(2), 99–109.

Silliman, E. R., & Wilkinson, L. C. (2004). Collaboration for language and literacy learning. In E. R. Silliman & L. C. Wilkinson (Eds.), *Language and literacy learning in schools* (pp. 3–38). New York: Guilford.

Silverman, F. H. (1995). *Communication for the speechless* (3rd. ed.). Boston: Allyn and Bacon.

Simmons-Mackie, N., Damico, J. S., & Damico, H. L. (1999). A qualitative study of feedback in aphasia treatment. *American Journal of Speech-Language Pathology, 8,* 218–230.

Singer, B. D., & Bashir, A. S. (2004). EmPOWER, A strategy of teaching students with language learning disabilities how to write expository text. In E. R. Silliman & L. C. Wilkinson (Eds.), *Language and literacy learning in schools* (pp. 239–272). New York: Guilford.

Singh, R., Cohen, S. N., & Krupp, R. (1996). Racial differences in cerebrovascular disease. *Neurology, 46* (Suppl. 2), A440–A441.

Skarakis-Doyle, E., Dempsey, L., & Lee, C. (2008). Identifying language comprehension impairment in preschool children. *Language, Speech, and Hearing Services in Schools, 39,* 54–65.

Skibbe, L. E., Grimm, K. J., Stanton-Chapman, T. L., Justice, L. M., Pence, K. L., & Bowles, R. P. (2008). Reading trajectories of children with language difficulties from preschool through fifth grade. *Language, Speech, and Hearing Services in Schools, 39,* 475–486.

Sloan, G. (2000). Posterior pharyngeal flap and sphincter pharyngoplasty: The state of the art. *Cleft Palate-Craniofacial Journal, 37,* 112–122.

Small, J. A., & Perry, J. (2005). Do you remember? How caregivers question their spouses who have

Alzheimer's disease and the impact on communication. *Journal of Speech, Language, and Hearing Research, 48*(1), 125–136.

Small, L. H. (1999). *Fundamentals of phonetics: A practical guide for students.* Boston: Allyn and Bacon.

Smith, M., & Grove, N. (1999). The bimodal situation of children learning language using manual and graphic signs. In F. T. Loncke, J. Clibbens, H. Arvidson, & L. L. Lloyd (Eds.), *Augmentative and alternative communication: New directions in research and practice* (pp. 8–30). London: Whurr.

Smith-Myles, B., Hilgenfeld, T., Barnhill, G., Griswold, D., Hagiwara, T., & Simpson, R. (2002). Analysis of reading skills in individuals with Asperger syndrome. *Focus on Autism and Other Developmental Disabilities, 17*(1), 44–47.

Snell, M., Chen, L. Y., & Hoover, K. (2006) Teaching augmentative and alternative communication to students with severe disabilities: A review of intervention research 1997–2003. *Research and Practices for Persons with Severe Disabilities, 31,* 203–214.

Snow, C. E., Scarborough, H. S., & Burns, M. S. (1999). What speech-language pathologists need to know about early reading. *Topics in Language Disorders, 20*(1), 48–58.

Snowling, M., & Frith, U. (1986). Comprehension in "hyperlexic" readers. *Journal of Experimental Child Psychology, 42,* 392–415.

Sohlberg, M., & Mateer, C. (1989). *Introduction to cognitive rehabilitation: Theory and practice.* New York: Guilford Press.

Sohlberg, M. M., Mateer, C. A., & Stuss, D. T. (1993). Contemporary approaches to the management of executive control dysfunction. *Journal of Head Trauma Rehabilitation, 8,* 45–58.

Solomon, N. P., McKee, A. S., Larson, K. J., Nawrocki, M. D., Tuite, P. J., Eriksen, S., Low, W. C., & Maxwell, R. E. (2000). Effects of pallidal stimulation on speech in three men with severe Parkinson's disease. *American Journal of Speech-Language Pathology, 9,* 241–256.

Sommers, R. K., & Caruso, A. J. (1995). Inservice training in speech-language pathology: Are we meeting the needs for fluency training? *American Journal of Speech-Language Pathology, 4*(3), 22–28.

Sonies, B. C. (1997). Evaluation and treatment of speech and swallowing disorders associated with myopathies. *Current Opinion in Rheumatology, 9*(6), 486–495.

Sonies, B. C., & Frattali, C. M. (1997). Critical decisions regarding service delivery across the health care continuum. In B. C. Sonies (Ed.), *Dysphagia: A continuum of care.* Gaithersburg, MD: Aspen.

Soto, G., Muller, E., Hunt, P., & Goetz, L. (2001). Critical issues in the inclusion of students who use augmentative and alternative communication: An educational team perspective. *Augmentative and Alternative Communication, 17,* 62–72.

Southwood, F., & Russell, A. F. (2004). Comparison of conversation, freeplay, and story generation as methods of language elicitation. *Journal of Speech, Language, and Hearing Research, 47,* 366–376.

Sparks, R. W., Helm, N., & Albert, M. (1974). Aphasia rehabilitation resulting from melodic intonation therapy. *Cortex, 10,* 303–316.

Sparks, R. W., & Holland, A. L. (1976). Method: Melodic intonation therapy for aphasia. *Journal of Speech and Hearing Disorders, 41,* 287–297.

Spaulding, T. J, Plante, E., & Farinella, K. A. (2006). Eligibility criteria for language impairment: Is the low end of normal always appropriate? *Language, Speech, and Hearing Services in Schools, 37,* 61–72.

Sperry, E., & Klich, R. (1992). Speech breathing in senescent and younger women during oral reading. *Journal of Speech and Hearing Research, 35,* 1246–1255.

Spiegel, B., Benjamin, B. J., & Spiegel, S. (1993). One method to increase spontaneous use of an assistive communication device: A case study. *Augmentative and Alternative Communication, 9,* 111–117.

Spielman, J., Borod, J., & Ramig, L. (2003). The effects of intensive voice treatment on facial expressiveness in Parkinson disease: Preliminary data. *Cognitive and Behavioral Neurology, 16,* 177–188.

Stach, B. A., Spretnjak, M. I., & Jerger, J. (1990). The prevalence of central presbycusis in a clinical population. *Journal of the American Academy of Audiology, 2,* 109–115.

Stanovich, K. (1986). "Matthew effects" in reading: Some consequences of individual differences in acquisition of literacy. *Reading Research Quarterly, 4,* 360–407.

Starch, S., & Falltrick, E. (1990). The importance of home evaluation for brain injured clients: A team approach. *Cognitive Rehabilitation, 8,* 28–32.

Starkweather, W. (1987). *Fluency and stuttering.* Englewood Cliffs, NJ: Prentice Hall.

Starkweather, W. (1997). Therapy for younger children. In R. F. Curlee & G. M. Siegel (Eds.), *Nature and treatment of stuttering: New directions* (2nd ed., pp. 143–166). Boston: Allyn and Bacon.

Stecker, N. A. (1998). Overview and update of central auditory processing disorders. In M. G. Masters,

N. A. Stecker, & J. Katz (Eds.), *Central auditory processing disorders: Mostly management.* Boston: Allyn and Bacon.

Steele, C. M., Greenwood, C., Ens, I., et al. (1997). Mealtime difficulties in a home for the aged: Not just dysphagia. *Dysphagia, 12*(1), 43–51.

Stoel-Gammon, C., & Dunn, C. (1985). *Normal and disordered phonology in children.* Austin, TX: Pro-Ed.

Stoicheff, M. (1981). Speaking fundamental frequency characteristics of nonsmoking female adults. *Journal of Speech and Hearing Research, 24,* 437–441.

Story, B. (2002). An overview of the physiology, physics, and modeling of the sound source for vowels. *Acoustical Science and Technology, 23,* 195–206.

Strand, E., & McCauley, R. (2008, August 12). Differential diagnosis of severe speech impairment in young children. *The ASHA Leader, 13*(10), 10–13.

Strand, E., & Skinder, A. (1999). Treatment of developmental apraxia of speech: Integral stimulation methods. In A. Caruso & E. Strand (Eds.), *Clinical management of motor speech disorders in children* (pp. 109–148). New York: Thieme.

Strand, E., Stoeckel, R., & Baas, B. (2006). Treatment of severe childhood apraxia of severe childhood apraxia of speech: A treatment efficacy study. *Journal of Medical Speech Pathology, 14,* 297–307.

Strand, E. A., & McCauley, R. (1997, November). *Differential diagnosis of phonological impairment and developmental apraxia of speech.* Paper presented at the American Speech-Language-Hearing Association annual convention, Boston.

Strange, W., & Broen, P. (1980). Perception and production of approximant consonants by 3-year-olds: A first study. In G. Yeni-Komshian, J. Kavanaugh, & C. A. Ferguson (Eds.), *Child phonology: Vol. 2. Perception.* New York: Academic Press.

Straus, D., Cable, W., & Shavelle, R. (1999). Causes of excess mortality in cerebral palsy. *Developmental Medicine and Child Neurology, 41,* 580–585.

Streb, J., Hemighausen, E., & Rösler, F. (2004). Different anaphoric expressions are investigated by event-related brain potentials. *Journal of Psycholinguistic Research, 33,* 175–201.

Stredler-Brown, A., & Johnson, D. C. (2003). Functional auditory performance indicators: An integrated approach to auditory development. Available at www.cde.state.co.us/cdesped/Specific DisabilityHearing.htm

Striano, T., Rochat, P., & Legerstee, M. (2003). The role of modeling and request type on symbolic comprehension of objects and gestures in young children. *Journal of Child Language, 30,* 27–45.

Suiter, D., & Leder, S. (2008). Clinical utility of the 3-ounce water swallow test. *Dysphagia, 23,* 244–250.

Sullivan, P. (2008). Gastrointestinal disorders in children with neurodevelopmental disabilities. *Developmental Disabilities Research Reviews, 14,* 128–136.

Sutcliffe, P. A., Bishop, D. V. M., Houghton, S., & Taylor, M. (2006). Effect of attentional state on frequency discrimination: A comparison of children with ADHD on and off medication. *Journal of Speech, Language, and Hearing Research, 49,* 1072–1084.

Tanner, D. C. (1980). Loss and grief: Implications for the speech-language pathologist and audiologist. *Asha, 22,* 916–928.

Tattershall, S. (2004). *SLPs contributing to and learning within the writing process.* Paper presented at the annual convention of the American Speech-Language-Hearing Association, Philadelphia.

Templeton, S. (2003). The spelling/meaning connection. *Voices from the Middle, 10*(3), 56–57.

Templeton, S. (2004). Instructional approaches to spelling: The window on students' word knowledge in reading and writing. In E. R. Silliman & L. C. Wilkinson (Eds.), *Language and literacy learning in schools* (pp. 273–291). New York: Guilford.

Thal, D., Jackson-Maldonado, D., & Acosta, D. (2000). Validity of a parent-report measure of vocabulary and grammar for Spanish-speaking toddlers. *Journal of Speech, Language, and Hearing Research, 43,* 1087–1100.

Thiemann, K. S., & Goldstein, H. (2004). Effects of peer training and written text cueing on social communication of school-age children with pervasive developmental disorder. *Journal of Speech, Language, and Hearing Research, 47,* 126–144.

Thomas, C., Englert, C. S., & Morsink, C. (1984). Modifying the classroom program in language. In C. V. Morsink (Ed.), *Teaching special needs students in regular classrooms* (pp. 239–276). Boston: Little, Brown.

Thomas, L. (1979). *The medusa and the snail: More notes of a biology watcher.* New York: Viking.

Thompson, C. K. (2004). Neuroimaging: Applications for studying aphasia. In L. L. LaPointe (Ed.), *Aphasia and related disorders* (pp. 19–38). New York: Thieme.

Thompson, C. K., Shapiro, L. P., Kiran, S., & Sobecks, J. (2003). The role of syntactic complexity in treatment of sentence deficits in agrammatic aphasia: The Complexity Account of Treatment Efficacy (CATE). *Journal of Speech, Language, and Hearing Research, 46,* 591–607.

Thunstam, L. (2004). *Social networks and communication for children with deafness and additional impairments.* Unpublished master's thesis, Mälardalens University, Sweden.

Tierney, L. M., Jr. (1993). *Current medical diagnosis and treatment, 1994.* Los Altos, CA: Appleton & Lange.

Tierney, L. M., Jr., McPhee, S. J., & Papadakis, M. A. (2000). *Current medical diagnosis and treatment* (39th ed.). New York: Lange Medical Books/McGraw-Hill.

Timler, G. R., Vogler-Elias, D., & McGill, K. F. (2007). Strategies for promoting generalization of social communication skills in preschoolers and school-aged children. *Topics in Language Disorders, 27,* 167–181.

Titze, I. R. (1994). *Principles of voice production.* Englewood Cliffs, NJ: Prentice Hall.

Tjaden, K., & Turner, G. (2000). Segmental timing in amyotropic lateral sclerosis. *Journal of Speech, Language, and Hearing Research, 43,* 683–696.

Tomblin, J. B., Zhang, X., Buckwalter, P., & O'Brien, M. (2003). The stability of primary language disorder: Four years after kindergarten diagnosis. *Journal of Speech, Language, and Hearing Research, 46,* 1283–1296.

Tomes, L. A., Kuehn, D. P., & Peterson-Falzone, S. J. (1997). Behavioral treatment of velopharyngeal impairment. In K. R. Bzoch (Ed.), *Communicative disorders related to cleft lip and palate* (4th ed.; pp. 529–562). Austin, TX: Pro-Ed.

Tompkins, C. A. (1995). *Right hemisphere communication disorders: Theory and management.* San Diego, CA: Singular.

Tompkins, C. A., Baumgaertner, A., Lehman, M. T., & Fassbinder, W. (2000). Mechanisms of discourse comprehension impairment after right hemisphere brain damage: Suppression of lexical ambiguity resolution. *Journal of Speech, Language, and Hearing Research, 43,* 62–78.

Toner, M. A. (1997). Targeting dysphagia in the elderly: Prevention, assessment, and intervention. In B. B. Shadden & M. A. Toner (Eds.), *Aging and communication: For clinicians by clinicians.* Austin, TX: Pro-Ed.

Torgesen, J. K. (1980). Conceptual and educational implications of the use of efficient task strategies by learning disabled children. *Journal of Learning Disabilities, 13,* 19–26.

Torgesen, J. K. (2000). Individual difference in response to early interventions in reading: The lingering problem of treatment resisters. *Learning Disabilities Research and Practice, 15,* 55–64.

Torgesen, J. K. (2005). Recent discoveries from research on remedial interventions for children with dyslexia. In M. Snowling & C. Hulme (Eds.), *The science of reading: A handbook* (pp. 521–537). Oxford, UK: Blackwell.

Torgesen, J. K., al Otaiba, S., & Grek, M. L. (2005). Assessment and instruction for phonemic awareness and word recognition skills. In H. W. Catts & A. G. Karnhi (Eds.), *Language and reading disabilities* (2nd ed., pp. 127–156). Boston: Allyn and Bacon.

Towey, M., Whitcomb, J., & Bray, C. (2004). *Printsound-story-talk, a successful early reading first program.* Paper presented at the annual convention of the American Speech-Language-Hearing Association, Philadelphia.

Trail, M., Fox, C., Ramig, L., Sapir, S., Howard, J., & Lai, E. (2005). Speech treatment for Parkinson's disease. *NeuroRehabilitation, 20,* 205–221.

Treffert, D. A. (2009). *Hyperlexia: Reading precociousness or savant skill?* Wisconsin Medical Society. Retrieved June 6, 2009, from www.wisconsinmedicalsociety.org/savant_syndrome/savant_articles/hyperlexia

Treiman, R. (1993). *Beginning to spell.* New York: Oxford University Press.

Treiman, R. (1997). Spelling in normal children and dyslexics. In B. Blachman (Ed.), *Foundations of reading acquisition and dyslexia: Implications for early intervention* (pp. 191–218). Mahwah, NJ: Erlbaum.

Treiman, R., & Cassar, M. (1997). Spelling acquisition in English. In C. A. Perfetti, L. Rieben, & M. Fayol (Eds.), *Learning to spell: Research, theory, and practice across languages* (pp. 61–80). Mahwah, NJ: Erlbaum.

Troia, G. A., Graham, S., & Harris, K. R. (1999) Teaching students with learning disabilities to mindfully plan when writing. *Exceptional Children, 65,* 235–252.

Trudeau, N., Sutton, A., Dagenais, E., de Broeck, S., & Morford, J. (2007). Construction of graphic symbol utterances by children, teenagers, and adults: The effect of structure and task demands. *Journal of Speech, Language, and Hearing Research, 50,* 1314–1329.

Tsao, F., Liu, H., & Kuhl, P. K. (2004). Speech perception in infancy predicts language development in the second year of life: A longitudinal study. *Child Development, 75*, 1067–1084.

Tyler, A., & Watterson, K. (1991). Effects of phonological versus language intervention in preschoolers with both phonological and language impairment. *Child Language Teaching and Therapy, 7*, 141–160.

Ukrainetz, T. A., Harpell, S., Walsh, C., & Coyle, C. (2000). A preliminary investigation of dynamic assessment with Native American kindergarteners. *Language, Speech, and Hearing Services in Schools, 31*, 142–154.

U.S. Department of Health and Human Services. (2007). *Child maltreatment, 2007*. Retrieved June 12, 2007, from www.acf.hhs.gov/programs/cb/pubs/cm07/summary.htm

Vace, N. N. (1987). Word processor versus handwriting: A comparative study of writing samples produced by mildly mentally handicapped students. *Exceptional Children, 54*, 156–165.

Valian, V., & Aubry, S. (2005). When opportunity knocks twice: two-year-olds' repetition of sentence subjects. *Journal of Child Language, 32*, 617–641.

Valian, V., & Casey, L. (2003). Young children's acquisition of *wh*-questions: The role of structured input. *Journal of Child Language, 30*, 117–143.

Vallecorsa, A. L., & Garriss, E. (1990). Story composition skills or middle-grade students with learning disabilities. *Exceptional Children, 57*, 48–54.

van der Merwe, A. (2004). The voice use reduction program. *American Journal of Speech-Language Pathology, 13*, 208–218.

Van Kleeck, A. (1995). Emphasizing form and meaning separately in prereading and early reading instruction. *Topics in Language Disorders, 16*(1), 27–49.

van Kleeck, A., Vander Woude, J., & Hammett, L. (2006). Fostering literal and inferential language skills in Head Start preschoolers with language impairment using scripted book-sharing discussions. *American Journal of Speech-Language Pathology, 15*, 85–95.

Van Meter, A. M., Nelson, N. W., & Ansell, P. (2004). *Developing spelling and vocabulary skills in curriculum writing activities*. Paper presented at the annual convention of the American Speech-Language Hearing Association, Philadelphia.

Van Riper, C. (1982). *The nature of stuttering*. Englewood Cliffs, NJ: Prentice-Hall.

Van Riper, C. (1992). *The nature of stuttering* (2nd ed.). Prospect Heights, IL: Waveland Press.

Van Riper, C., & Emerick, L. (1984). *Speech correction: An introduction to speech pathology and audiology* (7th ed.). Englewood Cliffs, NJ: Prentice Hall.

Varnhagen, C. K., McCallum, M., & Burstow, M. (1997). Is children's spelling naturally stage-like? *Reading and Writing: An Interdisciplinary Journal, 9*, 451–481.

Vaughn, S., & Klingner, J. (2004). Teaching reading comprehension to student with learning disabilities. In C. A. Stone, E. R. Silliman, B. J. Ehren, & K. Apel (Eds.), *Handbook of language and literacy: Development and disorders* (pp. 541–555). New York: Guilford.

Venkatagiri, H. S. (2000). Efficient keyboard layouts for sequential access in augmentative and alternative communication. *Augmentative and Alternative Communication, 16*, 126–134.

Wagner, B. T., & Jackson, H. M. (2006). Developmental memory capacity resources of typical children retrieving picture communication symbols using direct selection and visual linear scanning with fixed communication displays. *Journal of Speech, Language, and Hearing Research, 49*, 113–126.

Wagner, R. K., Torgesen, J. K., & Rashotte, C. A. (1999). *Comprehensive test of phonological processing (CTOPP)*. Austin, TX: Pro-Ed.

Wahlberg, T., & Magliano, J. P. (2004). The ability of high-functioning individuals with autism to comprehend written discourse. *Discourse Processes, 38*(1), 119–144.

Wallach, G. P., & Butler, K. G. (1995). Language learning disabilities: Moving in from the edge. *Topics in Language Disorders, 16*(1), 1–26.

Waltzman, S. B., & Roland, J. T. (2005). Cochlear implantation in children younger than 12 months. *Pediatrics, 116*, e487–e493.

Wambaugh, J., & Bain, B. (2002). Make research methods an integral part of your clinical practice. *The ASHA Leader, 7*(21), 1, 10–13.

Warburton, E., Price, C. J., Swinburn, K., & Wise, R. J. (1999). Mechanisms of recovery from aphasia: Evidence of positron emission tomography studies. *Journal of Neurology, Neurosurgery, and Psychiatry, 66*, 155–161.

Watzlawick, P., Beavin, J. H., & Jackson, D. D. (1967). *Pragmatics of human communication: A study of interactional patterns, pathologies, and paradoxes*. New York, NY: W. W. Norton & Company.

Weiller, C., Isensee, C., Rijntjes, R., Huber, W., Muller, S., Bier, D., et al. (1995). Recovery from Wernicke's aphasia: A positron emission tomographic study. *Annals of Neurology, 37*, 723–732.

Weismer, S. E., Evans, J., & Hesketh, L. J. (1999). An examination of verbal working memory capacity in children with specific language impairment. *Journal of Speech, Language, and Hearing Research, 23,* 1234–1248.

Weismer, S. E., & Hesketh, L. J. (1996). Lexical learning by children with specific language impairment: Effects of linguistic input presented at varying speaking rates. *Journal of Speech and Learning Research, 39,* 177–190.

Weismer, S. E., Tomblin, J. B., Zhang, X., Buckwalter, P., Gaura Chynoweth, J., & Jones, M. (2000). Non-word repetition performance in school-age childen with and without language impairment. *Journal of Speech, Language, and Hearing Research, 43,* 865–878.

Wertz, R. T., LaPointe, L. L., & Rosenbek, J. C. (1991). *Apraxia of speech in adults: The disorder and its management.* San Diego, CA: Singular.

Westby, C. E. (1997). There's more to passing than knowing the answers. *Language, Speech, and Hearing Services in Schools, 28,* 244–287.

Westby, C. E. (2004). A language perspective on executive functioning, metacognition, and self-regulation in reading. In C. A. Stone, E. R. Silliman, B. J. Ehren, & K. Apel (Eds.), *Handbook of language and literacy: Development and disorders* (pp. 398–427). New York: Guilford.

Westby, C. E. (2005). Assessing and remediating text comprehension problems. In H. W. Catts & A. G. Kamhi (Eds.), *Language and reading disabilities* (2nd ed., pp. 157–232). Boston: Allyn and Bacon.

Whitehurst, G. J., & Lonigan, C. J. (2001). Emergent readers: Development from prereaders to readers. In S. B. Neuman & D. K. Dickinson (Eds.), *Handbook of early literacy research* (pp. 11–29). New York: Guilford.

Whitmire, K. A. (2000). Adolescence as a developmental phase: A tutorial. *Topics in Language Disorders, 20*(2), 1–14.

Wiig, E. H., Zureich, P. Z., & Chan, H. H. (2000). A clinical rationale for assessing rapid automatized naming with language disorders. *Journal of Learning Disabilities, 33,* 359–374.

Wilcox, K., & Morris, S. (1999). *Children's speech intelligibility measure.* San Antonio, TX: Psychological Corporation.

Wilder, J., & Granlund, M. (2006). Presymbolic children in Sweden: Interaction, family accommodation and social networks. In *Proceedings from the 12th ISAAC Research Conference, Düsseldorf, August.*

Wilkinson, K., Carlin, M., & Thistle, J. (2008). The role of color cues in facilitating accurate and rapid location of aided symbols by children with and without Down syndrome. *American Journal of Speech-Language Pathology, 17,* 179–193.

Williams, A. (2000). Multiple oppositions: Case studies of variables in phonological intervention. *American Journal of Speech-Language Pathology, 9,* 282–288.

Williams, M., & Krezman, C. (2000). *Beneath the surface: Creative expressions of augmented communicators.* Toronto, Ontario, Canada: International Society for Augmentative and Alternative Communication.

Williams, M. B. (2004). *Reflections of a multimodal man [DVD].* Verona, WI: Attainment.

Wilson, D. (1987). *Voice problems in children* (3rd ed.). Baltimore: Williams and Wilkins.

Wilson, W. R. (1994). Sudden sensorineural hearing loss. In G. M. English (Ed.), *Otolaryngology.* Philadelphia: Lippincott.

Windsor, J., & Hwang, M. (1999). Testing the generalized slowing hypothesis in specific language impairment. *Journal of Speech, Language, and Hearing Research, 42,* 1205–1218.

Windsor, J., Scott, C. M., & Street, C. K. (2000). Verb and noun morphology in the spoken and written language of children with language learning disabilities. *Journal of Speech, Language, and Hearing Research, 43,* 1322–1336.

Winograd, P. N., & Niquette, G. (1988), Assessing learned helplessness in poor readers. *Topics in Language Disorders, 8*(3), 38–55.

Witzel, M. A. (1995). Communicative impairment associated with clefting. In R. J. Shprintzen & J. Bardach (Eds.), *Cleft palate speech management: A multidisciplinary approach.* St. Louis, MO: Mosby.

Wixson, K., Bosky, A., Yochum, M., & Alvermann, D. (1984). An interview for assessing students' perceptions of classroom reading tasks. *The Reading Teacher, 37,* 346–352.

Wolk, S., & Schildroth, A. N. (1986). Deaf children and speech intelligibility: A national study. In A. N. Schildroth & M. A. Karchmer (Eds.), *Deaf children in America* (pp. 139–159). San Diego, CA: College-Hill.

Woll, B., Grove, N., & Kenchington, D. (1997) Spoken language, sign language and gesture: Using a natural case study to understand their relationships and implications for language development in children with Down syndrome. In E. Bjorck-Akesson & P. Lindsay (Eds.), *Communication . . . naturally:*

Theoretical and methodological issues in AAC (pp. 76–91). Västerås, Sweden: Mälardalen University Press.

Wong, B. Y. (2000). Writing strategies instruction for expository essays for adolescents with and without learning disabilities. *Topics in Language Disorders, 20*(4), 244.

Wong, B. Y., Butler, D. L., Ficzere, S. A., & Kuperis, S. (1996). Teaching low achievers and students with learning disabilities to plan, write, and revise opinion essays. *Journal of Learning Disabilities, 29*(2), 197–212.

Wood, P., & Emick-Herring, B. (1997). Dysphagia: A Screening tool for stroke patients. *Journal of Neuroscientific Nursing, 29*(5), 325–329.

Woods, E. K. (1995). The influence of posture and positioning on oral motor development and dysphagia. In S. R. Rosenthal, J. J. Sheppard, & M. Lotze (Eds.), *Dysphagia and the child with developmental disabilities: Medical, clinical, and family interventions*. San Diego, CA: Singular.

Woods, J. J., & Wetherby, A. M. (2003). Early identification of and intervention for infants and toddlers who are at risk for autism spectrum disorder. *Language, Speech, and Hearing Services in Schools, 34*, 180–193.

Wooi, M., Scott, A., & Perry, A. (2001). Teaching speech pathology students the interpretation of videofluoroscopic swallowing studies. *Dysphagia, 16*, 32–39.

World Health Organization. (1980). *International classification of impairments, disabilities, and handicaps. A manual relating to the consequences of disease*. Geneva, Switzerland: Author.

Xue, S. A., & Hao, G. J. (2003). Changes in the human vocal tract due to aging and the acoustic correlates of speech production: A pilot study. *Journal of Speech, Language, and Hearing Research, 46*, 689–701.

Yairi, E. (1981). Disfluencies of normally speaking 2-year-old children. *Journal of Speech Language, and Hearing Research, 24*, 301–307.

Yairi, E. (1982). Longitudinal studies of disfluencies in 2-year-old children. *Journal of Speech and Hearing Research, 25*, 402–404.

Yairi, E. (1983). The onset of stuttering in 2- and 3-year-old children: A preliminary report. *Journal of Speech and Hearing Disorders, 48*, 171–177.

Yairi, E. (2004). The formative years of stuttering: A changing portrait. *Contemporary Issues in Communication Science and Disorders, 31*, 92–104.

Yairi, E., & Ambrose, N. (1992a). A longitudinal study of children: A preliminary report. *Journal of Speech and Hearing Research, 35*, 755–760.

Yairi, E., & Ambrose, N. (1992b). Onset of stuttering in preschool children: Selected factors. *Journal of Speech and Hearing Research, 35*, 782–788.

Yairi, E., & Ambrose, N. (2004). Stuttering: Recent developments and future directions. *The ASHA Leader, 18*, 4–5, 14–15.

Yairi, E., Ambrose, N., & Nierman, B. (1993). The early months of stuttering: A developmental study. *Journal of Speech and Hearing Research, 36*, 521–528.

Yairi, E., Watkins, R., Ambrose, N., et al. (2001). What is stuttering? [Letter to the editor]. *Journal of Speech, Language, and Hearing Research, 44*, 585–592.

Yang, M. T., Ko, F. T., Cheng, N. Y., et al. (1996). Clinical experience of esophageal ulcers and esophagitis in AIDS patients. *Kao Hsiung I Hsueh Ko Hsueh Tsa Chih, 12*(11), 624–629.

Yaruss, J. S. (1997). Clinical measurement of stuttering behaviors. *Contemporary Issues in Communication Science and Disorders, 24*, 33–44.

Yavas, M. (1998). *Phonolgy: Development and disorders*. San Diego, CA: Singular.

Yavas, M., & Goldstein, B. (1998). Phonological assessment and treatment of bilingual speakers. *American Journal of Speech-Language Pathology, 7*(2), 49–60.

Ylvisaker, M. (1994). Collaboration in assessment and intervention after TBI. *Topics in Language Disorders, 15*(1), 1–81.

Ylvisaker, M., & DeBonis, D. (2000). Executive function impairment in adolescence: TBI and ADHD. *Topics in Language Disorders, 20*(2), 29–57.

Ylvisaker, M., & Feeney, T. (1995). Traumatic brain injury in adolescence: Assessment and reintegration. *Seminars in Speech and Language, 16*, 32–44.

Ylvisaker, M., & Szekeres, S. F. (1989). Executive and metacognitive impairments in head injured children and adults. *Topics in Language Disorders, 9*(2), 34–49.

Ylvisaker, M., Szekeres, S. F., & Feeney, T. (1998). Cognitive rehabilitation: Executive functions. In M. Ylvisaker (Ed.), *Traumatic brain injury rehabilitation: Children and adolescents* (pp. 221–269). Boston: Butterworth-Heinemann.

Yoder, D., & Munson, L. (1995). The social correlates of co-ordinated attention to adults and objects in mother-infant interaction. *First Language, 15*, 219–230.

Yont, K. M., Hewitt, L. E., & Miccio, A. W. (2000). A coding system for describing conversational breakdowns in preschool children. *American Journal of Speech Language Pathology, 9*, 300–309.

Yorkston, K. M., Beukelman, D. R., & Bell, K. R. (1988). *Clinical management of dysarthric speakers.* Boston: College Hill Press.

Yorkston, K., & Beukelman, D. (2004). Dysarthria: Tools for clinical decision-making. *The ASHA Leader, 9*, 4–21.

Yorkston, K., Honsinger, M., Dowden, P., & Marriner, N. (1989). Vocabulary selection: A case report. *Augmentative and Alternative Communication, 5*(2), 101–108.

Yorkston, K. M., Miller, R. M., & Strand, E. A. (1995). *Management of speech and swallowing disorders in degenerative disease.* Tucson, AZ: Communication Skill Builders.

Yorkston, K. M., Smith, E., & Beukelman, D. R. (1990). Extended communication samples of augmentative communicators: I. A comparison of individualized versus standard single-word vocabularies. *Journal of Speech and Hearing Disorders, 55*, 217–224.

Yorkston, K. M., Strand, E. A., Miller, R. M., Hillel, A., & Smith, K. (1993). Speech deterioration in amyotrophic lateral sclerosis: Implications for the timing of intervention. *Journal of Medical Speech-Language Pathology, 1*, 35–46.

Yoshinaga-Itano, C., Sedley, A. L., Coulter, D. K., & Mehl, A. L. (1998). Language of early and later identified children with hearing loss. *Pediatrics, 102*, 1161–1171.

Yunusova, Y, Weismer, G., Westbury, J. R., & Lindstrom, M. J. (2008). Articulatory movements during vowels in speakers with dysarthria and healthy controls. *Journal of Speech, Language, and Hearing Research, 51*, 596–611.

Zangari, C. (2001). Helping families gain acceptance of AAC strategies. *American Speech-Language Hearing Association Special Interest Division 1, Language Learning and Education Newsletter, 8*(1), 14–17.

Zangari, C., & Kangas, K. A. (1997). Intervention principles and procedures. In L. L. Lloyd, D. R. Fuller, & H. H. Arvidson (Eds.), *Augmentative and alternative communication: A handbook of principles and practices.* Boston: Allyn and Bacon.

Zemlin, W. R. (1998). *Speech and hearing sciences: Anatomy and physiology* (4th ed.). Boston: Allyn and Bacon.

Zeuschner, R. (1997). *Communicating today* (2nd ed.). Boston: Allyn and Bacon.

Zhang, Y., Brooks, D. W., Fields, T., & Redelfs, M. (1995). Quality of writing by elementary students with learning disabilities. *Journal of Research on Computing in Education, 27*, 483–499.

Zhao X., et al. (2007, July 31). A unified genetic theory for sporadic and inherited autism. *Proceedings of the National Academy of Science, 31*, 12831–12836.

Name Index

Subject Index